PROGRAM PEACE

Self-Care Exercises to Reprogram Your Mind and Body

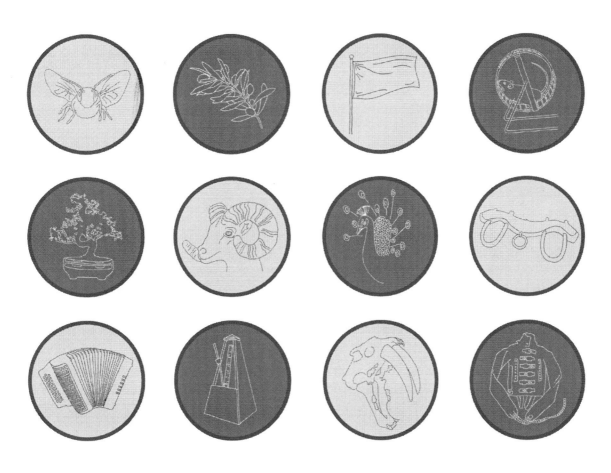

JARED EDWARD RESER, Ph.D.

ISBN: 979-8-9855151-0-7

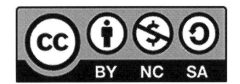

Table Of Contents

Preface

About Program Peace

Program Peace is a self-care system that will guide you through more than 200 activities and exercises designed to help your body function optimally. Organs throughout the human body learn to function suboptimally due to daily stress, strain, and negative emotions. Even a good night's sleep doesn't completely reverse these effects, and they accumulate over time. Stress, especially when chronic, dysregulates the nervous system and impairs the performance of the muscular, respiratory, and cardiovascular systems. The results of these changes are wide-ranging and harmful to our mental and physical health. Using the corrective exercises offered here will help you rehabilitate the damage, freeing you from pain and allowing you to feel comfortable in your own body. This system was designed to help you experience more energy, increased self-confidence, improved posture, and the ability to breathe freely.

Your goal will be to unlearn the submissive and aggressive nonverbal behaviors that cause us so much stress and to replace them with healthy ways of breathing, moving, and thinking. The text will explain how stress and physical trauma are rooted in defensive nonverbal behavior that we share with other mammals and lay out the Program Peace method of overcoming them. Throughout the book, I combine modern science with my personal experiences to explain key concepts related to optimal well-being. Each chapter addresses a different bodily system and explains why you should use the exercises, how they can help you, and what you can expect your progress to look and feel like.

A little more background on the book: I started developing it, along with its philosophy on life, morality, and healing in early childhood. I have been working weekly on the present text for more than 20 years. Much of the material in it has been available on my blog for more than ten years. I have been training clients to perform the exercises for more than five. I have read hundreds of related books and hundreds of scientific journal articles to inform and refine the content. The intended audience is everyone including people without a hint of anxiety or depression. However, it is also for physicians, psychiatrists, psychologists, social workers, life coaches, personal trainers, and other health and wellness professionals looking for safe, effective, and free ways to bring about growth and progress in their clients.

The Importance of Diaphragmatic Breathing

The Program Peace methodology is applied to organ systems all over the body but begins with the breath. After introducing the method in Chapters 1 and 2, Chapter 3 will teach you how to breathe in a way that activates the resting and healing division of your nervous system. The key is to breathe with maximal activation of the diaphragm. Mammals in a calm and peaceful state breathe diaphragmatically. When they are exposed to adversity, they instead breathe without the diaphragm, relying on the breathing muscles in their upper torsos. Known as distressed breathing, this is the body's way of preparing itself for a threatening and hostile environment. Distressed breathing is an integral part of how animals survive in the wild, but too much of it promotes chronic hyperventilation. An animal that experiences ongoing mental or emotional trauma will eventually turn distressed breathing into a deep-seated habit. Due to how this affects its brain, the animal ends up in constant fear for its life.

Our nervous system will always prioritize short-term survival over long-term well-being as long as it assumes our environment is dangerous. This strategy holds even though it is completely unnecessary in the modern world where we are rarely in immediate physical danger. Most 21st-century humans are stuck in a state of distress because non-diaphragmatic breathing has been ingrained in their nervous system. It convinces their bodies that death may be imminent, dramatically increases muscle tension, and results in constant fatigue. Non-diaphragmatic breathing may be the primary reason why so many people endure persistent pain, age rapidly, experience unceasing negative emotions, and can never fully catch their breath.

Like most adult mammals, you and I have learned to stifle and strain our diaphragm. Cumulatively, the non-peaceful moments in our lives have programmed us to breathe shallowly. Program Peace is designed to teach you how to reverse this by recruiting the diaphragm with every breath. This is the process of transitioning from short, shallow breaths to long, deep breaths. As your diaphragm strengthens from consistent use, its range of motion increases and your neurological control over it improves, allowing you to breathe more deeply and easily without even trying. It will take months, but the results are worth it. Adopting diaphragmatic breathing is one of the most significant changes you can make in your life because your body interprets it as indisputable proof that your environment is friendly and safe.

Shortcomings of This Book

I created the reprogramming exercises in this book to heal my anxiety. As I developed them, I thought they were original. After researching the details, I came to find that variations on some of them already existed in different clinical, spiritual, and self-improvement circles. It is difficult to look for precedent in self-help literature because it is not organized as well as academic literature. This book focuses on methods rather than recounting a history of past contributors. I apologize in advance if I have not given proper credit to similar work. However, I am quite confident that most of the exercises in these chapters cannot be found anywhere else.

Some readers may find the technical terms in this book to be overwhelming. I have tried my best to make sentences with jargon accessible so that you can get the gist even if you don't know the word. I wanted to keep the science in the text for the science-minded and other interested parties, but please don't get frustrated by it. If you encounter some unfamiliar terminology, just power through it and try to enjoy the read. There are only a few unfamiliar words that you will need to memorize because they pop up over and over. These include "parasympathetic nervous system," "developmental plasticity," and "partial muscular contraction."

The book is very long. Skim through it if you have to. You can get an overview by reading the bullet points at the end of each chapter. Please take your time reading and don't feel pressured to finish it or to read it linearly. Chapters 3 and 11 may be the most valuable to people trying to change their breathing. By all means, dog-ear the pages, highlight text you like, and write your notes in the margins. This will increase its usefulness to you and allow you to more easily reference the passages or exercises you found helpful. The book can seem repetitive at times. I intentionally structured it this way to get the therapeutic and big-picture messages across from different angles. I also often use imperative sentences, but I am not trying to be bossy—just a helpful coach.

These pages contain over 800 illustrations. I created most of them by tracing photographs that I took. Each of the illustrations on the cover of the book corresponds to an analogy in the text. I hoped that it would be fun for the reader to uncover the hidden meanings and have a way to reference some of the major principles of Program Peace at a glance.

Much of This Book Is Theoretical

I must be clear that much of what is written in this book is speculative. I have strong convictions about it coming from scientific knowledge and personal experience. However, as with much else in alternative health, there is no authority to confirm these hypotheses. The writing alternates between offering personal anecdotes and theories and reporting on clinical findings and research literature. To help readers discern between speculation and fact, I try to make it clear which statements are supported by scientific evidence. They are often accompanied by a bibliographical citation of which there are over 350. Many of the uncited claims are my opinions. I think of them as unproven but heavily informed by scientific knowledge and based on a new synthesis of diverse fields.

It would be difficult to reach a quick and firm conclusion about the efficacy of the techniques outlined here. Empirically validating clinical methods in psychology often takes decades. It can take just as long in medicine. The Program Peace activities and exercises have not been subjected to controlled, large-scale experimental studies. You can't just assign randomly selected people to the treatment conditions like you would with drugs and placebos. To benefit from the exercises takes time, dedication, and discipline that only comes from having a deep understanding of why and how the exercises are beneficial in the long run. Of course, that's exactly what this book attempts to provide.

I have spent the last ten years stringently testing the exercises. In this time, I have used myself as a guinea pig to evaluate and hone the techniques. Since doing this, I have trained dozens of clients in the Program Peace method. Working with individuals, listening to their feedback, and seeing their bodies and minds transform have given me conviction that the exercises here can help you. I hope that as you read about them and perform them yourself, you can see clearly how and why they lead to improvement. Even if you never perform any of the exercises but simply read the book, you will learn actionable rules of thumb for maintaining and improving the condition of your body.

This book's exercises are subject to validation through your experience. I am quite confident you will quickly see and feel results that place you on a path toward expressing your optimal genetic potential. If this book helps enough people, it will influence scientists and doctors in behavioral medicine to look at the proposed methods carefully and further test and refine them. The present copy is merely the first iteration of this book. Future revisions will reflect further user feedback and research-based findings. I welcome community criticism and collaboration. I also want anyone to feel free to create content based on what is written here. If the program works for you and you think it can help others, please share it. I sincerely hope that the Program Peace method will be successful in expanding your repertoire of self-regulatory healing practices.

Disclaimer

I cannot guarantee that the activities recommended here are completely safe for everyone. Some of them ask you to perturb traumatized areas of the body that could become injured or lead to any number of medical complications. Although most of the activities here are harmless, some have the potential to cause damage if performed incorrectly or by someone with a preexisting injury or condition. The exercises that have the highest potential to cause harm are noted.

The method and accompanying documentation are furnished "as is" and without warranty. You assume the entire risk as to the results you may obtain by use or misuse of the exercises. Please perform them with caution, restraint, and common sense. **Most importantly, none of these exercises should produce pain or discomfort after the exercise is completed. If it hurts afterward or even the next day, you are doing it wrong.** Discontinue participation in any exercise or activity that causes pain. In such an event, medical consultation should be obtained immediately.

The materials, information, and techniques in this book are general in nature, reflect the opinions of Jared Reser, and are not intended to be a substitute for medical counsel. The content provided is for informational purposes only and is not intended to diagnose, treat, cure, or prevent any disease. No specific claims are made regarding the treatment of medical diseases or disorders. Always consult your doctor or health care provider before making any medical decisions. Many of the psychological topics brought up here should be explored with a qualified mental health professional. Importantly, the Program Peace activities and exercises are to be used with traditional therapies and not in place of mainstream treatment.

How to Support

This entire book was never copyrighted and can be found for free at www.programpeace.com as a series of webpages and also as a single downloadable PDF. I chose to self-publish the printed version of this book to keep the price as low as possible. There is zero profit margin as the price only covers the printing and distribution costs. All illustrations are in the public domain. The dedicated app, available for iOS and Android, is also free. The tutorial videos are free on YouTube. However, if you would like to contribute to Program Peace, you can do so through the Patreon link here: patreon.com/programpeace. You can also make a donation via PayPal here: paypal.me/programpeace. Your help goes toward future content and updates. Thank you for your consideration. To support, you can also join or engage with our online community. Find us on Instagram (@program_peace), Twitter (@programpeace1), and Facebook and YouTube (just type in "Program Peace").

Acknowledgments

I express my gratitude to my brother, William Reser, and my parents, Daniel Reser and Paula Freund, for fruitful and encouraging discussions. I would especially like to thank my mother for providing incisive feedback on the manuscript. Special thanks to Tyran Grillo Ph.D., Matt Harvey Ph.D., and Beverly Gearreald, each of whom edited multiple chapters. Any remaining mistakes are my own. Thank you to Laura Duffy Design for help with the book cover. I want to thank my friends, clients, and all the people who have written emails, posted comments, and made other contributions to this work. I greatly appreciate the thoughtful insights and criticisms of everyone who has been involved, and I dedicate this book to these cherished friends.

About the Author

Jared Edward Reser has been developing the Program Peace exercises for over a decade. He holds a Ph.D. and Master's degree in brain and cognitive science from the University of Southern California. He also has a Master's in psychology from Pepperdine University. He has been certified as a personal trainer and health coach. He specializes in writing theoretical research articles and emphasizes an interdisciplinary approach to integrative biology, cognitive neuroscience, and artificial intelligence. You can find out more about his research at http://www.jared-research.com.

Welcome to Program Peace.

Jared Edward Reser, Ph.D.

Program Peace: *Testimonials and Praise*

The following are unsolicited message board comments about Program Peace:

Anonymous
"I found this site several months ago and it has been such a blessing. Your method sounded too good to be true, but it made perfect sense and it worked. Thank you so much for sharing this with us."

Andrew S.
"After looking through the techniques used in this article, I knew there was something to this…So I started doing it myself, 5 days a week, for about half an hour… and it works. "

Jinu G.
"I had immediate relief… I am going to try this every day. "

Jennifer L.
"Wow! So happy to finally find a resource about all of this! Seriously…this is a life changer. Thank you. "

Dalia M.
"Wow. Just wow… I just went through the whole routine and my splitting headache has been relieved. This is my new favorite thing to do. Thank you! "

Jill
"I bet I'm clearing away all sorts of garbage. I actually feel "clear headed" – like brain fog is just going away. I can't wait to keep going. This is profound. "

Anonymous
"Fantastic, instant relief. "

Jay M.
"This has caused me a great deal of depression and anxiety in the past years of my life. Now I feel that a huge weight has been lifted. I can't wait to continue with this for the rest of my life.

Brian S.
"Suffice to say that finding your website has been an absolute godsend. In the past I had never found a guide that actually taught me how to breathe diaphragmatically and not just faking it with stomach movement. Within a few months practice I have experienced a massive reduction in all negative emotions. I feel substantially happier, healthier, and more like myself.

Chapter 1: **Optimal Quality of Life Training**

My experience with chronic stress was an extreme version of the same issue that everyone on this planet contends with. Thus, recounting my story of recovery provides a vivid case study with which to compare your experience. It also allows me to describe how the Program Peace exercises relieved my symptoms so that you can see how they can relieve yours. My symptoms were pretty bad.

My breathing was shallow and rapid. My eyebrows were constantly raised. I was always squinting and had purple creases under my eyes. I couldn't maintain eye contact for long before my eyes would dart away of their own accord. I had an enduring lump in my throat and a hoarse and high voice. I had persistent kinks in my neck, tweaks in my lower back, and a clenched jaw. I mumbled and stammered when I spoke. I held my breath during conversations. I gasped between sentences and looked at the floor when speaking. I had almost no capacity to glare, frown, flare my nostrils, or straighten my neck in the company of others.

Throughout my twenties, I was deeply afflicted by anxiety, depression, and bodily discomfort. I was unaware that the symptoms described in the previous paragraph were causal factors in this discomfort. All I knew is that I felt perpetually distressed and couldn't figure out why. The feeling would not abate and was resulting in chronic, low-grade pain. This made me wonder: "Where in my body do I hold this pain, and how can I access and extinguish it?" I found the physical manifestations of my stress to be completely elusive. I tried many different clinical and alternative methods to improve my condition without success. Popular breathing exercises, medical recommendations, psychological therapy, and stress reduction programs did nothing for me. So, I began experimenting on myself using methods derived from my knowledge of social cognition, neuroplasticity, and mammalian biology. The result was a system designed to train the body to reflect an optimal environment.

The core idea is this: Had you been raised in a perfect world with zero negativity, the way you hold your body would be painless and symptom-free. But no one is raised in an ideal world. Our spines, facial muscles, breathing musculature, and brains have internalized trauma over our life course. Trillions of individual cells are altered on a molecular level. The alterations cause muscles and soft tissues throughout the body to become stiff and sore. These insidious changes rob us of our composure and put us in a metaphorical straitjacket. That straitjacket constricts more and more with the passage of time. Left unchecked, it fits a little tighter every day until death. The system presented here will teach you how to recompose yourself to escape this stranglehold.

This book presents activities and exercises for you to practice, each accompanied by relevant scientific background for perspective. The focus will be on *comparative physiology*, explaining how our bodies function by comparing us with other animals. Considering these parallels helps us make inferences about ideal functioning in humans. We saw an example of this in the Preface: When mammals are calm, they breathe with the respiratory diaphragm. When they are distressed, they tense the diaphragm and breathe with other respiratory muscles. The more traumatized a mammal becomes, the more tense and inactive its diaphragm becomes.

In fact, the diaphragm is one of your body's main repositories of trauma. The tightening stranglehold discussed above partially corresponds to cumulative changes to your breathing style that make you breathe more shallowly, unevenly, and rapidly. You can release this trauma by training your diaphragm, which we will start later in this chapter before focusing on it in depth in Chapter 3. You will learn a series of methods to make your breathing permanently deeper, smoother, and slower. This sends an "it's okay to relax" message to the entire body.

By training your diaphragm to preside over your breathing, you can convince your body to assume that it resides in a habitat free from danger. The remainder of the book will guide you through exercises that combine this form of peaceful breathing with various postures, expressions, and forms of body language. In performing them, you will reprogram yourself for confidence, health, and peace.

Stress Resides in the Way We Carry Ourselves

Most of us have, knowingly or not, experienced intense, long-term periods of stress. In my case, it happened throughout my twenties. In the morning, I would wake up feeling anxious. After just a few social encounters, my heart would be racing and my adrenaline overwhelming. Friends and acquaintances were often alarmed by the way I behaved, wondering what I could possibly be so stressed about. I would greet a friend, and the expression on my face would cause them to scan the immediate environment for threats because the fear on my face suggested to them we were in immediate danger. People would ask me: "What is it that you're so worried about?" To which I would reply: "I'm rarely worried about anything specific. It must be biological."

Under conditions of chronic stress, symptoms continually worsen over time. My default stress level had been elevated over many years. Upon going to bed, instead of allowing myself to return to a tranquil baseline, I fell asleep more frantic than the night before. When this happens, the body's systems become stuck in a state of overdrive. Thought processes become overclocked. It becomes hard to fall asleep, difficult to rest, and impossible to relax. Many of us reach a point at which our experience of life is like a "bad trip," infused with the sensations of both withdrawal and overdose. As tolerance to the sensations of stress builds, many people barely notice how deranged they have allowed themselves to become.

Pressing social concerns and professional responsibilities cause us to ignore the symptoms. As we habituate to the physical and mental anguish, our body continues making long-term adjustments that further entrench us in overexertion. This is compounded by the fact that it has historically been very difficult to successfully treat chronic stress. Modern medicine has no real solution aside from drugs and rest. This is why most people do little to nothing about it.

After a particularly bad day, while lying in bed trying to meditate, I had an epiphany. I recognized the way I was holding my body as the source of my mental suffering. For the first time, I could feel my anxiety not as diffuse and psychological, but as aching localized in my gut, stiffness in distinct spinal muscles, as agonizing contortions of my face, and as the misery of stiff, shaky breathing.

Recognizing that I did not hold my body in this way as a child, I immediately wanted to know how I had come to do it. From that point on, I have been working to discover how the body and mind compensate after being exposed to trauma. In creating this system, I spent countless hours analyzing my behavior and how I carried myself in minute detail. After comparing my mannerisms with the scientific literature on the manifestations of stress in mammalian biology, I came to realize I was a model of precisely what not to do. This process of self-deconstruction took me from being the most nervous person I knew to the calmest.

Why is stress so extensive in humans? It is because it had survival benefits. As a result of our prehistoric past, we react to minor threats as if they were matters of life and death. Most modern human stress derives from mundane frustrations that our body's evolved mechanisms misinterpret as life-threatening dangers. Although most people don't realize it, most of these minor "threats" are ultimately social in nature. I believe that the predominant source of stress is the apprehension of social conflict and the tension that it creates. Deep down, we are afraid that others will reject us if we are too calm. We make ourselves feel uneasy and excitable, so that our outward manifestations of stress communicate goodwill. I hope this book will convince you that you don't need to manufacture and advertise stress to avoid conflict and make friends.

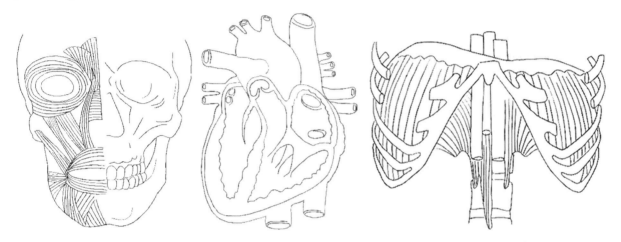

Illustration 1.1: A. Facial muscles; B. Cross-section of the heart; C. Diaphragm and bottom of the rib cage.

Submissive Nonverbal Behavior Is in Our Genes

Nonverbal social displays perpetuate the majority of our bodily tension. In biology, a "display" is an innate behavior that has evolved to serve a communicative purpose in members of the same species. Many such signals are observed in the animal kingdom. They are often used to negotiate conflict. For example, among wolves, the pack leader has a dominant posture: head and ears up, chest forward, tail stiff, and a confident swagger.[1] The other members of the pack (especially if unrelated to the leader) walk with heads lowered, ears back, and tails low and wagging. They remain behind the pack leader when traveling. If the alpha wolf challenges them, they will back away, bend down, or even lie on the ground exposing their vulnerable underbellies. It is clear to see that constant submissive signaling imprisons beta wolves in a suboptimal state of being.

Subordinate dogs use much of the same body language.[2] They lick or swallow nervously, display submissive grins, freeze, and tremble. Many dogs in the act of submission will dribble urine or pee on themselves without even lifting their leg. Canines are not unique in this. All mammals resort to their own set of subordination displays. They do it to avoid the escalation from contest to attack. To avoid outright fighting and bodily harm, lower-ranking individuals send a message: "You don't need to undermine me, because I am already undermining myself."

Due to how social primates are, submissive displays may be more important to them than to any other order of mammal. As primates, humans constantly send out signals about inferiority and resignation. Indeed, much of our nonverbal behavior exists to communicate deference to other humans. When we encounter a dominant member of our species, we restrict our breathing, subvert our posture, speak in a high voice, and tighten our faces.[3] Monkeys and apes routinely do the same.[4] It is essential to realize that these displays are controlled by innate, unconscious processes.[5] Although you may not think you are inferior, we were all born with neural pathways that cause us to adopt postures signifying inferiority. These pathways are encoded in our DNA and soldered into our nervous system before birth.

Samuel Johnson said, "No two people can be half an hour together, but one shall acquire an evident superiority over the other."[6] If this is true, the average person acts submissive at least 50% of the time. Even when we meet someone new, regardless of their status, we stoop our necks, stop flexing our buttocks, raise our shoulders, and stand shorter to make certain we do not offend them. This is the equivalent of the principal mammalian submissive display of rolling over to expose the belly.

We have all known since preschool that bullies don't want us to appear calmer than they are. If they think we are too relaxed, they are often willing to become violent. To address this, we learn to use anxiety as a form of social lubrication. I would go as far as to say that very little of my anxiety was due to the usual purported cause: physical trauma and rumination about it. I was not a victim of domestic abuse as a child and have never been molested. I believe that most of my anxiety and depression was due to the cumulative effects of submissive signaling.

These ritualized, self-destructive displays extend to our breathing. We unconsciously assume that to be respectful and friendly, we must make our breathing shallow. We are afraid that if our breaths are deep and long, other people will find it offensive. Again, shallow breathing is inherited from our mammalian ancestry. It shows other individuals that we are taking the present encounter seriously rather than being too relaxed.

The use of submissive "tells" communicates a history of victimization. They can also communicate that we are tired, distressed, possibly crippled, and are not poised for fighting. Instead, they show we are poised for flight. This would have kept humans safe during hunting and gathering times. It may also have kept us safe from larger kids on elementary school playgrounds. But it only holds us back in modern adulthood. Unless, of course, you are in prison.

For an inmate to avoid attracting negative attention in jail, criminologists recommend using submissive body language. Their advice? Never puff up your chest, minimize eye contact, don't whistle, don't sing, don't dance, and, above all, keep your head down (pointed toward the ground). Nonsubmissive body language is taken as disrespectful. Acting depressed keeps others from wanting to attack you. This was probably a major concern for our ancestors as many experts today believe the major predator of prehistoric humans was other humans.

People who have close encounters with 400-pound silverback gorillas in the wild must do the same. The more subdued they act, the less likely they are to be attacked. So, primatologists in the field slump over, act sheepish, move very slowly, and look straight at the ground, avoiding any eye contact. Even though they are perfect strangers amid adult gorillas and their young, as long as they continue to do these things, they are usually completely safe. But you don't live among wild gorillas, and you are likely not reading this book from a jail cell, so don't resort to conciliatory gestures. It is not your responsibility to placate anyone with postural concessions. Instead, we should make it our responsibility to overcome our genetic inclinations to do so and influence others to do the same, even if only by example.

Handicapping Signals Buy Mercy

Animal behaviorists point out that the costs of handicapping signals may enhance their perceived value. Because submissive behaviors hurt us, others recognize them as valid. Tensing our muscles and using inefficient postures usually results in an energy deficit, meaning that a subordinate individual is "spending" energy to "buy" mercy. The crouching and cringing that nondominant wolves exhibit require extra energy and come with personal costs (such as muscular strain) yet communicate that they are loyal, servile members of the pack. Thus, capitulation responses are authentic signals that we are operating with an impediment.

Blushing and crying have been conceptualized in a similar way.[7] Indeed, a blush can be unwanted, but often the costs to the blusher can be outweighed by the benefits. The involuntary aspect of a blush declares sensitivity to social norms and proves to others that you feel shame or guilt and value the group. Crying is an extreme form of self-handicapping. Some scientists believe that its evolved purpose is to self-sabotage normal vision. It also simulates respiratory distress. Sobbing thus signals acquiescence to a potential assailant. It convinces the aggressor that we are no longer a threat. There are many similar displays among animals, all of which are ways of saying, "Look, I'm going to all this extra trouble just to prove to you that I'm not an enemy."

Chimpanzees have obvious ways to signal that they have been defeated: walking in an apathetic way, covering their face, hitting themselves, and lying prostrate. Primates depend on these submissive displays because they constantly compete with members of their close-knit group for mating opportunities and food. Generally, hierarchies among males govern access to fertile females, whereas female hierarchies govern access to food resources, as these are a limiting factor for pregnancy and lactation. As modern humans, we usually don't fight physically over sex or meals, so why are our inclinations for submission so strong?

The answer is that humans don't just self-handicap to display deference. Unfortunately for us, we also do it to be likable. In humans, signaling a handicap can communicate modesty, conveying that one is not shameless or brazen. We demonstrate anxiety to build rapport with others, smooth over issues, and prove our friendliness. We do our best to act ingratiating, taking on bodily tension to do so. It is part of people-pleasing and the need to be accepted, but it is incredibly draining. This book will introduce a philosophy for dealing with these pressures, describing how to be a calm, confident, likable person without recourse to submissive signaling.

We use submissive displays around those we see as our superiors, our equals, and even our inferiors. Even very dominant people use subordination displays to be endearing and get people to open up and trust them. Therefore, it is not always clear whether submissive signaling is better characterized as weakness or as a form of social intelligence. It depends on the circumstances: primarily on the specific display in question and how long it is used. Before we discuss this let's look at comparable displays in other animals.

17

Submissive and Dominant Displays in Animals

Dominant and submissive displays occur in almost all animal species, from insects to fish to the great apes.[8] Threatening intimidation displays are meant to impress, making the animal bigger or emphasizing its physical dominance. They involve bristling hair, ruffling feathers, raising skin folds, baring teeth, displaying horns, emitting loud sounds, making quick and powerful movements, and adopting exaggerated postures.

When a western silverback gorilla wants to intimidate a rival, he will start throwing objects, pounding his chest, kicking his legs, and running sideways when approached. The fur of dominant chimps stands on end to make them appear larger, and they walk with exaggerated weight. They gallop, run in circles, hit things, perform somersaults, and produce a wide range of loud barking and hooting vocalizations.

Dominant lizards perform pushups, bobbing their heads up and down, displaying their muscles and athletic prowess for others to see. This display shows off the bright coloring on their throats and sides and indicates that they are in prime physical condition. Many male lizards raise themselves on their legs and arch their backs to signify territorial dominance. And remember, lizards are not utterly distinct from people. Three hundred million years ago, before mammals, our ancestors were reptiles crawling the earth. We have inherited many of our most primal instincts and social signals—as well as the structure of the oldest and most reflexive parts of our brains—from these miniature dragons. This inheritance is the reason that the dominance displays of modern reptiles seem so familiar.

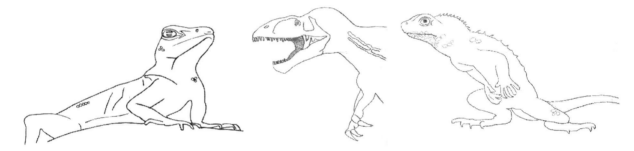

Illustration 1.2: A. Common lizard; B. Tyrannosaurus rex; C. Iguana.

Submissive displays, on the other hand, usually make the animal look smaller and weaker. They involve bowing, cowering, stooping, shaking, and exerting efforts to minimize the appearance of physical assets. Some animals have bizarre, ritualistic signals, as with some lizard species that display submission by raising a front leg and waving it in a slow, circular motion. Like a loyal subject genuflecting in the presence of royalty, chimpanzees with poor fighting records cower immediately during a confrontation. They shrink down and whimper. They may vomit, their legs shake, and their posture collapses.

For the most part, these displays are hardwired. For example, young male rhesus monkeys that have never been exposed to adult males will give subordination displays instinctively when they first encounter them. They involuntarily bow the head and adopt a bent-over posture. We don't realize it or think about it, but our subordination displays are similarly instinctive.

Submissive Displays in Apes	Dominant Displays in Apes
Withdrawal, flight, crouching, screaming, gaze aversion, ceasing activity, freezing, grimacing or grinning, peeking, trembling, pulling the limbs close to the body, moving out of the way of dominant members, and startling in response to their actions	Open-mouthed threat, nostril flare, direct stare, thumping the ground, lunging, tense mouth, strutting, mounting, chasing, yawning, genital display, chest-beating, sprawling, gnashing teeth, barking/roaring, destroying vegetation, breaking up fights, dragging branches, drumming on trees

Table 1.1: Common Hierarchical Displays Used by Chimps, Bonobos, Gorillas, Orangutans, and Gibbons

Too often, being fair, fun, and friendly toward others involves suboptimal displays. This is because the neural circuits responsible for submissive behavior were repurposed by natural selection to help us get along. Just as adult pair bonding in mammals evolved from the same brain machinery that was initially responsible for creating the mother/infant bond,[9] so many of our affiliative instincts evolved from submissive displays.

Involuntary Submissive Displays are the Source of Our Stress

Ordinarily, we don't use optimal postures because we are afraid they will be threatening to others. This is why, for instance, we rarely stand completely straight or lift our hands above our heads. This is unfortunate because when authentic and combined with positive affect, dominant displays can be calming and reassuring to people around us. Any good leader uses them to this effect. But because most of us never learn to use dominant displays in positive ways, we grow up associating them with bad experiences. For instance, classmates might have seen us walking with our heads up, taken offense, and tried to intimidate us into adopting a compliant, head-down posture. Experiences like these are the reason that performing optimal displays makes you breathe shallowly and become tense.

The table below lists submissive (suboptimal) displays and their dominant (optimal) counterparts. These are just a handful of those considered in this book, but they are a good start. While reading the table below, make a mental determination of which displays you use most and to what extent. Think about how you employ these displays in different scenarios, such as when you are by yourself at home, when you are with friends, and when you are in public.

Submissive Display	Dominant Display
Breathing short, quick, shallow, uneven, and through the mouth	Breathing long, slow, deep, smooth, and through the nose
Muscles tense and strained	Muscles calm and relaxed
Eyes looking down	Eyes looking up
Darting gaze	Eyes capable of holding a prolonged gaze
Minimized eye contact	Steady eye contact
Eyes blinking	Eyes unblinking
Eyes squinting	Eyes wide open
Raised eyebrows	Relaxed eyebrows
Face tense and wincing	Face completely relaxed
Jaw and chin tense	Jaw and chin completely relaxed
Trembling movement	Smooth, steady movement
Flinching and startling	Zero flinch or startle
Tense sneering, blushing, and crying facial muscles	Relaxed sneering, blushing, and crying facial muscles
Neck hunched	Neck straight
Head facing down	Head horizontal or up
Gluteus limp, hips tilted forward, genitals retracted	Gluteus flexed, hips neutral, genitals thrust forward
Middle back curved and tight	Middle back straight and relaxed
Shoulders raised	Shoulders down
Abdominals either flaccid or tense	Abdominals appropriately toned
Voice high, soft, and speaking quickly	Voice deep, loud, and commanding
Mumbling, stuttering, stammering	Articulating clearly and with conviction
Stilted, halting body language	Free, open body language
Body taking up as little space as possible	Body taking up as much space as possible

Table 1.2: Submissive Displays vs. Dominant Displays in Humans

We often refrain from using the dominant displays in Table 1.2 above because they might make people feel uncomfortable. The more we suppress them, the more our ability to use dominant nonverbals withers away due to disuse. This book will provide a thorough description of healthy, safe, well-functioning use of dominant nonverbal behavior.

How we carry ourselves has been molded by other people's reactions to our posture. Hundreds of elements of our body language have individual learning histories and have been either positively or negatively reinforced until they reached their current settings. This reinforcement is sometimes outright, as when our parents tell us not to stare, but is often subtle, as when peers ignore us until we take the bass out of our voice. The people who influence you to send them submissive signals may not be doing so because they dislike you. It may just be because they take it as flattery and don't want you to stop flattering them. Regardless, you did not choose your current postural settings; they were inadvertently chosen throughout the trial and error of your social learning. Most of them were selected during childhood and adolescence when you were surrounded by immature people and relatively immature yourself.

As you step out of your room, get out of your car, or walk into the grocery store, you are constantly trying to determine how you should hold your body. You are gauging how much impunity you can walk around with. You unconsciously scan each area to see whether there is anyone you will have to cower before. This behavior traces back to experiences you had in kindergarten. Even in adulthood, we relate to people as if they are about to physically attack us. We overcompensate by being chummy and compliant, totally out of proportion with any existing social threat. This keeps us from being our authentic selves. Prepare to leave all that in the past and hold your body like there is nothing and no one to be afraid of.

Use activities 1 and 2 below to get a sense of where you sit on this continuum, between the two extremes of submission and dominance, in your neighborhood.

Introductory Activity #1.1: *An Optimal Walk Around the Block*
Take a walk around your block. While doing so, observe your use of submissive displays. Remember that the docile you is not the real you. It is a fake character you have come to play to get along with people. As you read through this book, you are going to dismantle this role, and you can start now. Think about the behaviors in Table 1.2 above and try to determine how submissive your posture and body language are. As you walk, experiment with using dominant displays. How many of them can you use at the same time before you start to feel self-conscious?

Introductory Activity #1.2: *An Invisible Walk Around the Block*
Take another walk around the block, but this time either put on a coat, hat, and sunglasses or simply pretend that you are invisible. Think: "No one can judge me because no one can see me." If you were truly invisible, how would you comport yourself? How would your body language change? During this exercise, many people notice themselves using fewer suboptimal displays. What did you notice?

In the past, I thought that interpreting social interactions in terms of status wasn't productive or informative because the concepts of dominance and submission were passé. This proclamation of indifference toward the social hierarchy made me feel insightful and unique. It took time to realize that this stance was a play for status in itself.

Most people publicly pretend that the status hierarchy doesn't exist and that there is nothing submissive about them. However, many experts see dominance and submission as the fundamental concepts in social science, the same way mass and energy are the fundamental concepts in physics.[10] They are also key concepts of most relationships, including working relationships, in which individuals rely on one another to achieve their goals. As such, it is crucial to identify and efficiently navigate dominance games. This book is not trying to influence you to think about status more than you already do. It is meant to get you to think about it, and be negatively affected by it, less.

A Description of My Submissiveness

At this point it is helpful to use my history as an example. From my teens through my twenties, I hung out with a rough crowd. A number of my friends were convicted criminals and former gang members. Several were brawny athletes, while others were drug addicts. I enjoyed their companionship, but I was unaware of the extent to which I felt compelled to send them subordination signals. I didn't realize it at the time, but around them, I acted modestly at best and timid at worst.

Incarcerated people adopt exaggeratedly meek displays and carry these with them after being released from jail. Burly athletes commonly demand tribute from others in the form of deferential body language. Drug addicts exhibit some of the worst composure and breathing habits of anyone. Having these people as companions caused me to unknowingly amplify my existing submissive signaling to prove that I was an ally, not a competitor. I often felt courteous and gracious while sending these displays, but even minuscule nonoptimal displays become entrenched over the long term. Moreover, the more often you are submissive, the more others expect that behavior, and the more likely they are to be offended when you try to switch to more assertive behavior.

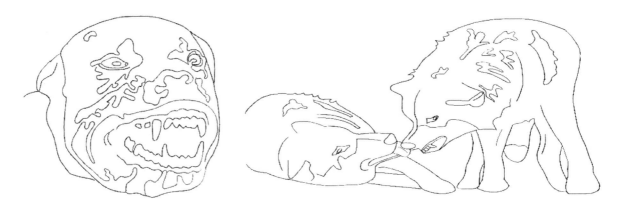

Illustration 1.3: A. Snarling dog; B. Subordinate wolf licking the dominant wolf.

You may have experienced trying to become more confident and assertive only to face social rejection. Here's how it happened to me. In my twenties, I tried to be more assertive at work. Away from my friends, I attempted to reduce my subordination signaling, doing my best to be calm and confident on the job. But my coworkers could tell from my breathing and facial tension that I was accustomed to using inferior mannerisms. They saw that I was attempting to withhold submissive signals from them. This made them angry, caused them to dislike me, and led to social rejection.

Submissive habits, social reinforcement, and accumulating tension continue to snowball once they start rolling. By my late twenties, I couldn't even pretend to be calm around anyone I knew. Each new acquaintance immediately assumed, from the way I presented myself, that I was their underling. I constantly felt that people were condescending and dismissive.

I couldn't see it, but it was my own fault. People couldn't respect me because I acted like I didn't respect myself. The condescension started to make me into a bitter, resentful person.

Crucially, the social dynamics at play are not about *what* you say but *how* you say it. It's the nonverbal behaviors that matter. If you saw a written transcript of my speech as a stressed-out 28-year-old, you might think I seemed chivalrous. But if you saw a video, you would immediately perceive me as fainthearted and jittery. At the time, I thought that people mistakenly perceived my kindness as weakness. Rather, they perceived my shortness of breath, my cowering posture, and cringing expressions as weakness.

Submissiveness is not just a social phenomenon. Once submissive actions become ingrained quirks, the stress and heartache they promote will negatively affect your mental and physical health. In my case, the symptoms were extreme. In addition to anxiety and depression, I showed other psychiatric symptoms of stress, such as a disrupted attention span, a working memory deficit, and panic attacks. I developed medical complications related to stress, including diagnoses such as esophageal achalasia, dyshidrotic eczema, male pattern balding, low testosterone, and outbreaks of cherry hemangiomas. I had back pain, frozen shoulder, tennis elbow, coccydynia, excessive cervical and lumbar lordosis, forward head posture, hip bursitis, unequal leg length, plantar fasciitis, Osgood-Schlatter disease, temporomandibular joint dysfunction, and numerous other structural misalignments and asymmetries. Medical professionals recognize each of these as linked to chronic stress.

Since I developed the exercises in this book, all those conditions, disorders, and symptoms have disappeared, and none have returned. Having had this experience and familiarizing myself with the vast body of scientific literature that relates stress to disease, I have concluded that submissive displays and the associated bodily tension are among the most pressing public health problems worldwide. However, it is not only preventable; it is also entirely reversible.

Even if all environmental sources of stress disappeared from your life, it would still be challenging to eliminate the lasting trauma already present in your body. Once your breathing has become hurried and your muscles have developed knots, it is very difficult to reverse this without employing the techniques in this book. Healing yourself with the Program Peace exercises can feel uncomfortable. To be free of trauma, you must work with and through its physical manifestations. Self-massaging achy muscles, overriding your shallow breathing style, flexing your way into better posture, and performing the various exercises within this book require resolve and determination. The good news? Even a little at a time adds up fast.

Chronic Use of Submissive Displays Leads to Deep Trauma

We often maintain a specific submissive display for long stretches of time. Many displays never abate. For example, some people spend their lives speaking in a voice that is much higher in pitch than is comfortable for them. Everyone overuses displays like this, allowing them to become fundamental components of their personality. These are rarely considered because we are usually utterly unconscious of them and lose perspective on how destructive they can be. Society has done little to recognize them, so there is scant relevant scientific research. Nevertheless, they constitute "bad form" that, when used habitually, comes at a steep price.

As we will discuss in Chapter 5, any muscle that is significantly contracted for more than a few minutes, and thus deprived of rest, will begin to take on damage. Most submissive displays, such as squinting or stooping the neck, last for several minutes or even hours. Even when it is unnoticeable, strain accumulates. At first, you might only slightly raise your shoulders and your eyebrows. Over time, however, knots develop in those muscles, keeping them permanently raised. The knots starve the muscle of blood and force it to atrophy. This eventually makes the muscle achy, weak, and dormant, leaving it perpetually fatigued and creating a source of chronic pain.[11] I will build on this concept of strain accumulation in almost every chapter of this book as we work through techniques for undoing its effects on different body parts.

I believe that I developed each of the medical symptoms listed in the last section as either a direct or indirect consequence of submissive muscular strain that went on too long. Muscles that are strained repetitively send continuous pain messages to the brain's emotional centers[12]. Sounds bad, right? Consider that the predominant form of social breathing in humans—shallow breathing in which the diaphragm is not utilized—increases muscle tension throughout the body. This dramatically compounds the strain and spreads it to the entire musculoskeletal system[13]. Below, Table 1.3 shows how prolonged use of the submissive displays listed in Figure 1.2 strains muscles, leading to unhealthy consequences.

Submissive Display	Unhealthy Consequences of Strain
Breathing short, quick, and shallow	Chronic nervousness, respiratory distress, whole-body tension
Eyes looking down	Atrophy of the muscles that help you look up
Minimized eye contact	Eye contact triggers startle
Eyes squinting	Eyes tired with bags and dark circles
Raised eyebrows	Brow strained and wrinkled
High voice	Voice permanently high and hoarse
Face tense and wincing	Facial muscle strain and atrophy, increased inflammation, and facial fat
Sneering muscles tense	Permanent sneer burned into the face
Jaw and chin tense	Jaw and chin knotted and painful
Head facing down	Difficulty facing up
Neck hunched	Neck humped and deformed
Gluteus limp, hips tilted forward	Weak core, stiff lower back and hips
Shoulders raised	Shoulders permanently raised
Abdominals either lax or tense	Propensity for abdominal fat, poor core stability
Pelvic and Genital Tension	Reduced libido and sexual dysfunction
Spinal Tension	Collapsed posture, aches, and pain
High Heart Rate	Cardiovascular problems
Digestive Tension	Gut pain and digestive problems

Table 1.3: Submissive Displays and the Unhealthy Consequences

As the exercises in later chapters will discuss, the way to reinvigorate these bodily systems is to use them to their full extent. By completely contracting the muscles involved, you can pull them out of their partially contracted state and thus out of chronic fatigue and chronic pain. The problem is that contracting these muscles when breathing shallowly risks pushing them into a cramp or spasm. However, contracting them while breathing deeply will restore their normal range of motion, reinstate their proper blood supply, and remove all manifestations of tension, strain, and trauma.

The Program Peace Method: Replace Submissive Behaviors with Assertive Ones

Now that you know what submissive displays are and how they can be so damaging, let's talk about fixing them. The goal is clear: To improve your health, you need to replace your default submissive habits with their assertive, relaxed alternatives. We'll start with a simple example.

Consider sneering. The sneer is made possible by muscles that run along the sides of the nose and lift the upper lip when contracted. Mammals sneer so that they do not bite into their lips during an attack-bite. Most mammals also sneer when threatened or uncomfortable. This is because displaying the canines is the equivalent of flashing a dagger or putting a hand on a gun.

Dominant primates rarely sneer, while subordinates do it constantly. The most socially damaged monkeys have tense, stiff sneering muscles that they cannot relax. Because they are always sneering, they always feel threatened. It is the same in humans. The tension in these muscles crushes our facial composure, making it difficult to appear calm and collected. Once I realized that my sneering muscles had painful knots in them, I developed exercises alternating between completely contracting and completely relaxing them, pairing both with diaphragmatic breathing. I also created a massage routine to release the cramps. Completely loosening the knots in my sneering muscles took me a couple of minutes a day for a few months, but it was well worth it. The once-painful, knuckle-sized knots are gone completely. I look much calmer now and feel less defensive. After completing the exercises in Chapter 9, you will, too. The next activity may capture your interest in this phenomenon.

Activity #1.3: *Fully Contract Your Sneering Muscles*

Open your mouth as wide as you can. Next reveal all your teeth as much as possible. With your top and bottom teeth fully exposed you should feel like a predator about to bite into something. Allow the sneer to fully contract muscles in your lips, cheeks, and nostrils. Even your nose should be fully crinkled. Try to hold this sneer for an entire minute. This will push many of the muscles involved into a full fatigue. After this extended full range contraction all these muscles should be able to rest more than they have in years.

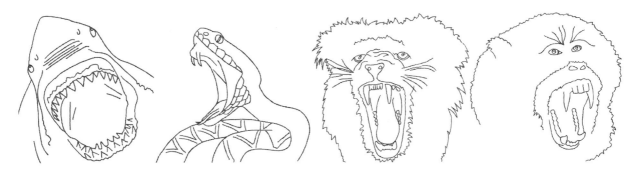

Illustration 1.4: Four animals baring their teeth.

Most people would feel very uncomfortable performing the exercise above in public. Interestingly enough, most people also feel extremely unguarded when they let their sneering muscles go lax. This is why these muscles are stuck in "sustained partial contraction." You can pull these muscles out of partial contraction by pairing both sneering and its absence with diaphragmatic breathing, which will afford your face a whole new level of composure. Each chapter in this book will guide you to combine a different set of displays, and the accompanying contractions, with proper breathing in a thorough, systematic approach. The next section explains how this approach works and why it relies on pairing both submissive and dominant displays with diaphragmatic breathing.

The Methodology: Combining Optimal Behaviors with Diaphragmatic Breathing

As shown in the figure below, breathing slowly and deeply with the diaphragm reduces your heart rate and stress response.

Diaphragmatic Breathing Decreases Stress

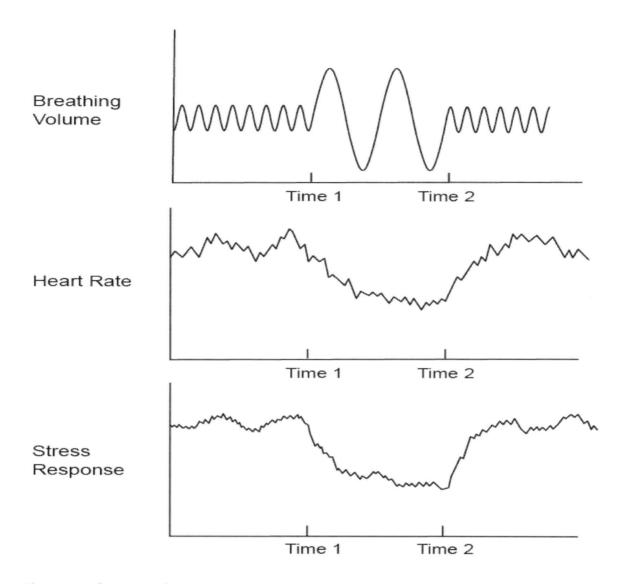

Figure 1.1: Before time 1, this person is breathing short, shallow breaths with a high heart rate and a high stress response. At time 1, this person takes two slow, deep breaths. You see a corresponding decrease in their heart rate and stress response. At time 2, they resume shallow breathing, causing their heart rate and stress levels to go back up.

Learning how to breathe deeply is not enough, however. We need to build it into the basic ways we carry ourselves, move through the world, and interact with others. The key to adopting dominant behaviors is to train your body to feel comfortable engaging in them. You can do this by practicing diaphragmatic breathing while using confident postures and displays. This will enable you to replace your long-standing associations between assertive behavior and the stress response.

As another example, consider the involuntary placement of your eyes in social situations. Looking upward, above the eye line, is a clear dominance display. This is why most people feel uncomfortable looking up in public. If you spend 30 seconds on a crowded street looking upward, you will likely become very self-conscious. Your breathing will become shallow and rapid, your heartbeat will speed up, and your stress level will increase. Here is what that looks like:

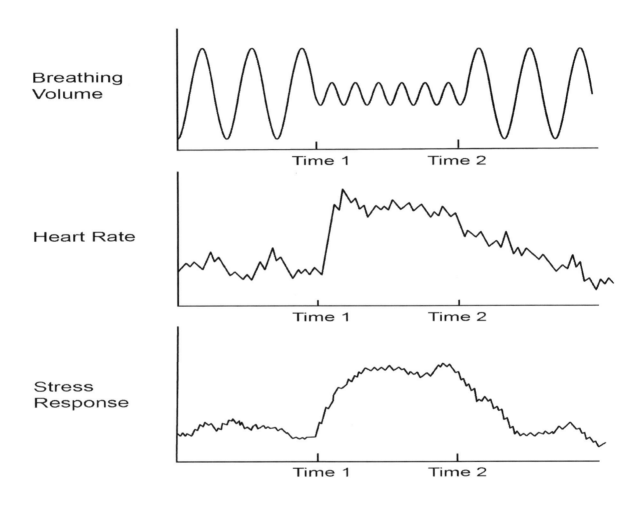

Figure 1.2: These graphs show relaxed breathing that is slow and deep until the person uses an optimal display starting at time 1. Using the display causes their breathing to become more shallow than usual, and you see a corresponding increase in their heart rate and stress response. This lasts until time 2 when they cease performing the display.

The unconscious fear of behaving dominantly keeps our body language withdrawn and demure. But there is a simple solution. If you spend a few minutes per day practicing slow, long, deep breaths from your diaphragm while looking up, then an upward gaze will stop recruiting the panicked breathing response. It will instead begin to feel natural and even occur involuntarily. You should start by practicing alone, then in public, and transition toward using it socially. Practicing for just a few minutes a day can train you to stop looking down in a few weeks. This technique can be used to make all forms of optimal body language feel comfortable and arise spontaneously.

After Exposure to Diaphragmatic Breathing Optimal Body Language No Longer Increases Stress

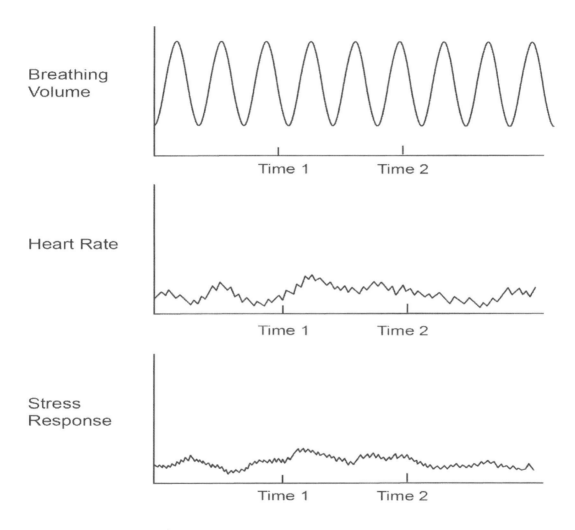

Figure 1.3: These graphs depict data from a person who has used the Program Peace method of exposing a dominant display to diaphragmatic breathing. Despite using dominant body language from time 1 to time 2, their breathing remains slow and deep, and there is no discernable change in their heart rate or stress response. Because they have calmed their body's unconscious reaction to the display, it no longer provokes fear, guilt, or stress.

The exercises in this book will first ask you to pair assertive behavioral subroutines that you would ordinarily find unnerving with paced breathing. After isolating and treating them individually, you will be asked to combine several of them together so that you can become comfortable using many assertive nonverbal behaviors at once. For instance, we will learn to breathe deeply with a calm face, upward eyes, straight neck, and relaxed vocal posture. You will also work on dissociating optimal postures from the submissive ones that often accompany them. For example, we will isolate widening your eyes from raising your eyebrows and isolate smiling from squinting and sneering.

Your brain's current records of how to hold your body correspond with remarkably high precision to where you think you fit in the hierarchy of your social group. Most people who want to be more assertive try to manipulate the environment by competing, conniving, or using power plays to change other people's perceptions of them in hopes that they will be allowed to gradually assume a more dominant role. Unfortunately, this is a stressful process that tends to compound their problems. Instead, Program Peace will show you how to transform yourself from the inside out.

The Program Peace method relies on established principles from the science of neuroplasticity. Neuroplasticity is the brain's ability to restructure neuronal connections in response to new experiences and demands. This process underlies all learning, training, and rehabilitation.[14] It is always available, so you can start at any age and practice whenever you want. Another great aspect of neuroplasticity is that it makes things automatic. With time, neuroplastic changes consolidate and stabilize, making what you have learned second nature. The exercises in this book leverage neuroplasticity to optimize your composure by exposing your brain circuits for acting like a boss to the brain circuits for feeling safe. Coactivating the neurons in these circuits will allow you to override your autopilot and make the habits of an alpha your default.

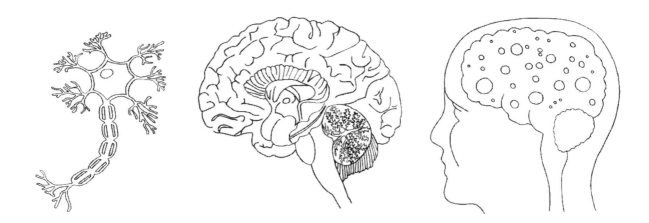

Illustration 1.5: A. A neuron; B. Cross section of the brain; C. Coactive brain regions.

Even behaviors that express positive emotions have been routinely coactivated with distressed breathing over your lifetime. Smiling is the quickest way to recruit shallow breathing in most people. We will use long, deep breathing in Chapter 10 to detraumatize your smile and in Chapter 25 to detraumatize your laugh. This book will provide you with a diaphragmatic makeover, restructuring dozens of behaviors and postures, dissociating them from the fight-or-flight response, and decoupling them from distressed breathing. By now, you may be curious to find out what diaphragmatic breathing feels like, so let's get acquainted with it using the activity below.

Activity #1.4: *A Diaphragmatic Breath*

In part one of this activity, you will exhale, and in part two, you will inhale. For each part, focus on taking exceptionally long and deep breaths to fully engage the diaphragm. Try to make each last eight to 20 seconds.

1) Diaphragmatic exhalation: Inhale completely before starting your exhalation. Purse your lips, and blow on your fingertip for as long as you comfortably can. While you slowly breathe out, pay attention to the sound of your breath and the sensation produced by the air hitting your fingertip, ensuring that both are steady and constant. Deep, long breaths with a constant flow rate are the keys to activating the diaphragm. Blow out until you have no more air left. You should notice that during the last few seconds, it is challenging to keep the stream steady. This is the aspect of the muscle most in need of retraining.

2) Diaphragmatic inhalation: Do the same for an inhalation. Take a couple of normal breaths, and then exhale completely before starting. Purse your lips and place your finger on them. This will make your breath audible. Then inhale until you cannot inhale anymore. Breathe in slowly and steadily, ensuring that the sound you make is constant and unflinching.

If you were able to make these breaths last longer than eight seconds and make your breath smoother than usual, then you experienced what engaging your diaphragm feels like. After you perform both activities a couple of times each, consider what it would take to make every breath a diaphragmatic breath.

Next is the first Program Peace exercise, which pairs a long diaphragmatic exhalation with vocalization to strengthen both your voice and diaphragm. Being able to talk for an extended period before needing to inhale is a very dominant trait. To do it, you need a strong diaphragm that can push all the way through its full range of motion, squeezing most of the air out of the lungs. On the other hand, it is very common that submissive people with tense diaphragms have to gasp after every few words they speak. Partially because they are used to being interrupted, their diaphragm is not capable of unwavering, prolonged contractions. Once you extend the amount of time you can speak on a single breath, even by a couple of seconds, you will feel and appear much more confident.

Introductory Exercise #1.1: *Prolonged Vocalization*

You are going to vocalize for as long as you can, 15 times in a row. Before each vocalization, take a full inhalation. During each following exhalation, vocalize in a deep, but relaxed register. It can be loud or soft. Choose a low note and a vowel sound such as "ah," "uh," or "om" and maintain it as long as possible. Continue vocalizing until you cannot breathe out any longer. You should be able to do this for at least five seconds, but shoot for eight or even up to 20 if you can. You might pull out the stopwatch on your phone and time yourself. Do this 15 times in a row.

This exercise is challenging for the diaphragm and the voice and can be somewhat uncomfortable because you are forcing the diaphragm to work in an unfamiliar and atrophied zone. Normally your voice is confined to a shallow range in which the diaphragm falters neurotically in response to emotional fluctuations, threatening stimuli, and interruptions. Keeping your voice steady will teach your diaphragm to contract more steadily.

If you perform this exercise five times over the course of a week, it will cease to be uncomfortable. You will get used to it quickly and find that you can do it for several minutes at a time. Because it ensures diaphragmatic motion, it should make you feel very relaxed after just a few minutes. The longer you do it, the more relaxed you will feel. It is a great exercise to use if you are feeling anxious. You can also do it around others by humming quietly with your mouth closed. Within a few weeks, your voice will be noticeably more impressive and commanding. This is a skill that leaders and lecturers develop: the ability to use the diaphragm to put sustained, continuous pressure on the voice box using fluid, uninterrupted contraction.

Not only will the exercise above strengthen your diaphragm, but it will also strengthen your voice. Let's consider a hypothetical example of how sustained diaphragmatic breathing can help rehabilitate other parts of your body. Take the neck, for instance. Imagine that you have been forced to crank your neck into an uncomfortable position, like looking up and to the extreme left for five straight minutes. Now, imagine four scenarios:

1) In the first scenario, you breathe very shallowly, as if you were frightened by something terrible. At the end of five minutes, you would likely have developed a cramp that would be painful for a few days.
2) In the second scenario, you breathe normally. You might come out of this ordeal with your neck feeling a little tight and uncomfortable, and the feeling might disappear after a few hours.
3) In the third scenario, you do your best to breathe slowly, deeply, and diaphragmatically. Breathing in this way, you might avoid neck pain entirely at the end of the five minutes.
4) Finally, in the last scenario, you breathe as you will be able to do after you spend 12 weeks completing the breathing retraining outlined in Chapter 3 of this book. In this situation, your neck would be much less likely to take on any long-term strain. Rather, it would be strengthened and toned by the five-minute effort.

Diaphragmatic breathing protects us from the negative consequences of repetitive strain, while shallow breathing makes us vulnerable to it. Shallow breathing at our desks destroys our necks and lower backs. Shallow breathing during exercise limits our potential gains and recovery. Shallow breathing while grinning destroys our smiles. Shallow breathing while socializing drives chronic anxiety. The rest of this book will guide you to pair deep breathing with a diverse assortment of different muscle activation patterns. The exercises will engage muscles in the spine, gut, throat, face, genitals, and many other locations, building strength, flexibility, mobility, and optimal tone.

The process of working through suboptimal postural habits to gradually retrain your body is emotionally cathartic and will give you an opportunity to reinvent yourself. The reprogramming you're taking on will act like a "cheat code" allowing you to "hack" into the programming of your nervous system and reset it to a lower level of stress. Each chapter resets a different bodily system. Rather than listing them here, the specific topics that will be discussed can be found in the chapter titles in the Table of Contents. The figure below illustrates the problems at hand and how they are addressed by Program Peace.

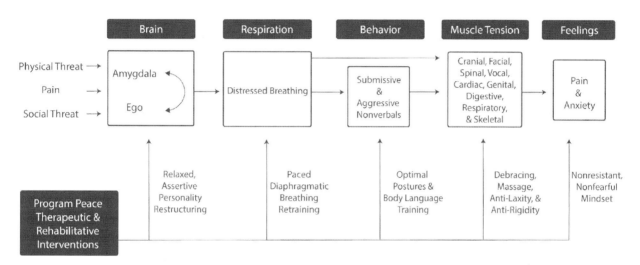

Figure 1.4: Threats are interpreted by the brain and go on to affect breathing, behavior, and muscle tension. The Program Peace exercises address these issues individually.

How This Book Is Organized

This book features over 200 activities and exercises grouped by chapter. After the description of each exercise in the book, you'll find the recommended length of time that exercise should be performed (e.g., five minutes). Also listed is the number of sessions you should expect to take to reach proficiency (e.g., four sessions per week for 12 weeks). Proficiency means you should expect to have made a considerable gain and created a self-perpetuating habit that will provide continued improvement with time. This is followed by the recommended number of sessions to maintain the ability after proficiency is reached (e.g., two times per month). Note that these details are only given for the exercises and not the activities. Activities are exploratory and intended to be completed only once.

Example Exercise #__: *Description Here*

The directions for performing the activity or exercise are in this box, including setup, steps to take, and the general parameters of the exercise.

Some exercises have a "risk of injury" warning, which means that it is quite possible to hurt yourself while doing the exercise as described. Take great care with these and ensure that you read the warning and disclaimer section in the book's Preface. Some exercises are given five stars, which means that I highly recommend them and that they are especially valuable as part of your retraining. Nearly every exercise is intended to be performed with paced diaphragmatic breathing, synchronized with a breathing metronome, as explained in Chapter 3. Alternatively, you can synchronize each exercise with the breathing pattern from Exercise 1.1.

My clients and I generally find that keeping a record of completed sessions is helpful and motivating. There are two worksheets at the end of this chapter to keep track of your initial progress. Each contains 14 key exercises and make it possible to log the number of times you have completed them. These are what I consider the book's 28 most beneficial, five-star exercises. You can complete a three-month crash course in Program Peace by performing 14 exercises two days per week over the course of 12 weeks. Each week, you can alternate between worksheets 1 and 2. Completing all 14 exercises in a worksheet takes less than an hour, and there is no pressure to complete these on consecutive days or weeks.

This book also has a companion workbook called *Program Peace: Exercise Manual and Journal*, which comes complete with daily entries and a calendar in which you can record the exercises you have completed as part of a 12-week regimen. It is not necessary, but it is helpful and can be downloaded for free from the website or purchased online as a hard copy.

Using Program Peace by Yourself and with Others

Strangers aren't the only ones who want us to use submissive displays. The people closest to us positively reinforce our endearing behavior, rewarding us for acting in non-threatening ways. They also punish assertive behavior, chastening us for acting self-assured. However, we cannot be mad at people for doing this to us because, whether aware of it or not, we do the same to others. It is an unconscious human instinct. We are constantly using body language to check and balance each other, and in doing so, we are mutually denigrated. Tearing each other down instead of building each other up is a waste of time and energy that ultimately programs our brains for sadness and our bodies for disease.

If you immediately start practicing the activities in this book in social situations, they will be feeble. People will recognize this and may attempt to punish you for being what they may interpret as rude. When I first started practicing, some acquaintances were confused by the new way I carried myself because my assertiveness was not fully fledged. For this reason, it helps to begin developing these postures alone. Start in your room, while driving, or as you take a walk. Build up to active social engagement slowly. Once it is evident that your dominant behaviors have become ingrained, people will not question them. By practicing alone, you can build yourself a stolid countenance that is so convincing that it is beyond reproach.

Alternatively, most of the exercises here can be performed with a close friend or in a group, and I encourage you to do so after first practicing them on your own. Fostering a low-stakes environment will make it dramatically easier to bring your new postures into the wider world. To this end, I recommend that you start by discussing the ideas in this book with close friends and family. You can create an understanding with your loved ones that your relationship is better off without submissive signaling. Instead of making each other weaker, you can train each other to feel comfortable and at ease in strength. Ask your roommate or spouse to walk around your home like they own the place. Tell them to expect you to do the same.

If you don't have this discussion with the people close to you, they may become disheartened, not understanding why you seem different. However, if you explain the practice to them, you can transform them whether they perform the program's specific exercises or not. When they see you relaxed, standing straight, and speaking in a powerful voice, they will find themselves mirroring you without even thinking about it.

Program Peace will give you the knowledge and exercises you need to progress to a point where you have the strength of personality to dominate everyone in your life. But you don't want to dominate people. Domination is an aggressive attempt to get someone to submit. It is abusive and will repel even your close friends and family. You simply want to be dominant. Being dominant doesn't stop others from also being dominant. It's not a competition. Domination is one-sided and aggressive, but dominance is not. So that we are clear on the difference, for the final section of this chapter, let's more clearly define aggression.

Dominant Nonverbals Make Aggression Unnecessary

A very early version of this book that I started working on in my late teens set out to describe the many costs of aggression. I saw aggression as a pitiful coping tactic that is often rewarded in the short term but, ultimately, results in negativity. I saw it as a vestigial instinct and a heuristic that people employ inflexibly and far too frequently. I felt that by living my life without aggression, I reaped many benefits. I wanted to share with others how to use diplomacy and a "nice guy" approach to navigate difficult social situations.

However, to avoid appearing aggressive, I accentuated my subordination displays and debilitated myself through intense self-handicapping. I spent so much energy placating people and repressing my personality that I became perpetually distressed. In trying to let go of aggressiveness, I had also unwittingly lost my assertiveness. But this is only because I was confusing the two.

Much of this book is about how to perceive the distinction between aggression and assertion so you can act confidently, knowing you are maintaining your ground without threatening others. What do assertion and aggression mean to you? In the animal behavior literature, the word "assertion" is constructive while "aggression" is destructive. An animal chasing down its prey is acting assertively because it needs to eat. An animal hurting another without benefit to itself is being aggressive. In mammals, the brain pathways controlling aggression, like fighting members of your species, are entirely distinct from the brain pathways for searching out and obtaining prey.[15]

For example, a cat pursuing a rat does not hiss or arch its back. The active brain areas reflect hunger rather than anger.[16] If you were to wipe out the aggression and anger systems of a carnivore's brain, it could still be a stone-cold predator. On the other hand, when a cat is aggressive toward another cat, it is almost always impelled by fear.[17] Aggression is a destructive use of force that is rooted in trauma and insecurity. If more people knew this basic neurological truth, they likely wouldn't praise aggressiveness or confuse aggression with assertion.

At its core, this book is about being assertive without being aggressive. That means being self-possessed but also kind at the same time. It is difficult. I have spent my life trying to be both but have only come close in the last few years. Many people see being "assertive" and being "nice" as two distinct modes that are incompatible or mutually exclusive. Religious leaders tell us to be nice at the expense of being assertive. Dating coaches and business gurus tell us to be assertive at the expense of being nice. Like most stressed primates, we mistakenly believe that we are forced to choose between these two options.

Because our psychological schemas for assertiveness are often conflated with those for aggression, many people find it impossible to be one without the other. This means that as soon as they start acting non-submissive, they inadvertently also start being intrusive, pushy, and unkind. They can't help it; they have never learned to make this fundamental distinction. Once you can discern between assertion and aggression, you can be powerful without malice. You can simultaneously be confident and friendly, poised and thoughtful, dominant and pure of heart. The key is exhibiting incorrigibly courageous body language while still having your intentions in the right place. Ultimately, you want to make your nonverbals ruthless, uncompromising, and unapologetic, but you want to temper this by making your words humble, considerate, and affectionate.

Mammals that don't feel threatened don't get angry. They also don't threaten others. As we will discuss in the next chapter, aggression usually follows desperation. It is a form of compensation for the inability to be calm while being assertive. In fact, in primate literature, aggression is often characterized as "submissive threat." This indicates that threats come from monkeys that feel vulnerable or are trying too hard not to be submissive. Think of the times when you have been really aggressive in the past. You felt threatened and were breathing in a shallow, distressed manner. Correct? It is the straight jacket of stress, muscle tension, pain, and breathlessness that causes us to lash out. In preparing us for confrontation, it makes us confrontational.

Learning to breathe slowly, deeply, and on long intervals will help you develop emotional maturity. Doing it in social situations will make you hardened to threats, immune to being dominated, exempt from defensive sentimentality, and unsusceptible to feeling offended. Once you use Program Peace to train yourself to breathe easily and stop sending submissive displays, you will no longer have to choose between being assertive and doing the right thing. This is because the combination of the two will come with ease.

Chapter 1: **Bullet Points**

- Submission and aggression are highly detrimental and we want to replace them with assertiveness and playfulness.
- All mammals use submissive displays to show subordination to more dominant animals. They do this to reduce social conflict over food, sex, and other resources.
- Humans use submissive displays, too, often just to be friendly.
- We commonly use suboptimal body language because we are afraid that, otherwise, we might come across as too aggressive.
- It is difficult to stop using submissive displays because they become habitual, and the people around us come to expect them.
- Your composure, posture, and breathing style are all products of your social environment.
- Ongoing submissive displays lead to muscle tension that is apparent to others. The chronic muscular strain caused by the display becomes a badge of self-perceived low status.
- As you perform the Program Peace exercises, I think you will be surprised by how much and how often you use suboptimal body language due to modesty.
- We all suffer from this to different degrees, and it causes suboptimal functioning of various muscles and organs. It also causes chronic pain, which contributes to depression and anxiety.
- Our attempts to stop acting submissive and make our behavior more dominant are fear-inducing and cause us to breathe shallowly.
- Shallow, distressed breathing is a submissive display.
- Ask yourself how the following things affect your breathing: being isolated, being shunned, being attacked, being put down verbally, being put down nonverbally, being judged.
- Using diaphragmatic breathing while practicing dominant displays and postures can make them very comfortable and make nonverbal assertiveness a new default.
- Replacing submissive behaviors with assertive ones will improve how you feel, the way others perceive you, and how you get along with them.
- Dominant animals are the most assertive, and submissive animals are the most aggressive. This should inspire us to be assertive without being aggressive. It requires that we learn to retain our composure and learn not to allow provocation or threat to affect the face, voice, spine, or breath.
- This chapter is the first step in helping you reconceptualize yourself as dominant, pure of heart, slow to anger, and not easily offended.

Program Peace: *Exercise Tracker*   **Week 1**

Date: _____ Start Time: _____ Finish Time: _____

Exercise Name		Set 1	Set 2	Set 3	Set 4
# 1.1: Prolonged Vocalization	3 mins				
# 3.1: Deep Breaths	2 mins				
# 3.3: Practicing a Smooth Inhalation	2 mins				
# 3.4: Smoothing Over Discontinuities	2 mins				
# 4.2: Wide Eyes with No Façade	5 mins				
# 4.6 / 4.7: Relaxed Frowning / Glaring	5 mins				
# 4.9: Looking Up While Talking	5 mins				
# 4.15: Watching TV Upside Down	10 mins				
# 8.2: Conserving the Calm	2 mins				
# 8.4: Freeing Up the Face	10 mins				
# 9.1: Soft Facial Percussion	5 mins				
# 10.5: A Sneerless Smile	2 mins				
# 11.3: The Slowest, Smallest Breath	1 min				
# 11.6: Pant-hooting	1 min				

Meditation (mins)	Paced Breathing (mins)	Sleep (hours)	Total Steps	Exercise (mins)	Flights Climbed	Standing (hrs)	Stretching (mins)	Self-Massage (mins)

Thoughts and Feelings:

Program Peace: Exercise Tracker   **Week 2**

Date: _____   Start Time: _____   Finish Time: _____

Exercise Name		Set 1	Set 2	Set 3	Set 4
#11.7: Isometric Contraction of the Diaphragm	2 mins				
# 12.2: Diaphragmatic Vocalization	5 mins				
# 12.9: Reading Out Loud	5 mins				
#13.8: Optimal Posture While Standing	2 mins				
# 14.1: Search Your Body for Rigidity	5 mins				
# 15.1: Anti-laxity and Anti-rigidity with Light Weights	5 mins				
# 16.1: Neck Retraction	5 mins				
# 16. 3-11: Various Neck Anti-rigidity Postures	5 mins				
# 18.1: Take a Walk with Exaggerated Posture	5 mins				
# 20.3: Diaphragmatic Fasting	5 hrs.				
# 22.2: Compressing the Internal Organs	2 mins				
#22.3: Listen to Your Heartbeat	5 mins				
# 25.1: Diaphragmatic Laughing	5 mins				
#26.1: Diaphragmatic Phone Conversation	5 mins				

Meditation (mins)	Paced Breathing (mins)	Sleep (hours)	Total Steps	Exercise (mins)	Flights Climbed	Standing (hrs)	Stretching (mins)	Self-Massage (mins)

Thoughts and Feelings:

Chapter 1: **Endnotes**

1. Cafazzo, S., Lazzaroni, M., & Marshall-Pescini, S. (2016). Dominance relationships in a family pack of captive arctic wolves (Canis lupus arctos): The influence of competition for food, age and sex. *PeerJ*, 4, e2707.

2. van der Borg, J. A. M., Schilder, M. B. H., Vinke, C. M., & de Vries, H. (2015) Dominance in domestic dogs: A quantitative analysis of its behavioural measures. *PLoS ONE, 10*(8), e0133978.

3. King, A. J., Johnson, D. D., & Van Vugt, M. (2009). The origins and evolution of leadership. *Current Biology. 19*(19), R911–R916.

4. Petersen, R. M., Dubuc, C., & Higham, J. P. (2018). Facial displays of dominance in non-human primates. In Senior C. (Ed.) *The facial displays of leaders* (pp. 123–143). Palgrave Macmillan.

5. Knowles, K. (2018). The evolutionary psychology of leadership trait perception. In C. Senior (Ed.), *The facial displays of leaders* (pp. 97–122). Palgrave Macmillan.

6. Boswell, J. (1798). *The table talk of Dr. Johnson*. C. Dilly.

7. Crozier, R. (2010). The puzzle of blushing, *The Psychologist, 23*(5), 390–393.

8. Breed, M. D., & Moore, J. (2016). *Animal behavior*. Elsevier.

9. Churchland, P. S. (2011). *Braintrust*. Princeton University Press.

10. Dunbar, N. E., & Burgoon, J. K., (2005). Perceptions of power and interactional dominance in interpersonal relationships. *Journal of Social and Personal Relationships*, 22(2), 207–233.

11. Werner, R. (2020). *A guide to deep tissue neuromuscular therapy*. Jones and Bartlett.

12. Gerwin, R. D. (2001). Classification, epidemiology, and natural history of myofascial pain syndrome. *Current Pain and Headache Reports*, 5(5), 412–420.

13. Fried, R. (2013). *The psychology and physiology of breathing: In behavioral medicine, clinical psychology, and psychiatry*. Springer Science.

14. Douyon, P. (2019). *Neuroplasticity: Your brain's superpower*. Izzard Ink Publishing.

15. Panksepp, J. (December 2000). The riddle of laughter neural and psychoevolutionary underpinnings of joy. *Current Directions in Psychological Science*, 9(6), 183–186.

16. Gleitman, H., Fridlund A. J., & Reisberg, D. (2004). *Psychology* (6th ed). W W Norton and Company.

17. Lorenz, K. (1966). *On aggression*. Methuen Publishing; de Waal, F. (2013). *The bonobo and the atheist: In search of humanism among the primates*. WW Norton & Company.

Chapter 2: **Persistent Adaptation to Chronic Stress**

"Being defeated is often a temporary condition. Giving up is what makes it permanent." — *Marilyn vos Savant (b. 1947)*

Our Bodies Compensate in Response to Suboptimal Environments

Although our bodies are capable of finding peace, they were never designed to do so. Rather, they developed to internalize environmental hardship to ensure the perpetuation of our genes. Harmful experiences cause organisms to promptly deviate from otherwise optimal body plans, restricting growth and mobility while reducing their quality of life. The focus of this chapter is to explain why we retain stress in the form of bodily trauma.

From microorganisms to monkeys, all life forms respond to stressors with innate biological programs.[1] They are prepared to alter their bodies and life strategies if they encounter adverse environments. To be clear, this is a form of non-mutational adaptation that takes place without natural selection during an individual's lifetime.[2] We all have the potential to become highly stress-adapted, and this could happen to you in a matter of weeks if you were exposed to extreme hardship. The DNA (genotype) does not change; however, the genes that are expressed change and cause the body (phenotype) to change.[3] Your genes specify the blueprint and the foundation, but the environmental circumstances influence how soundly your structure is built.

The changes bodies make allow conformation to occasional but regularly recurring environmental pressures faced by the species. These are usually stressors. Changes can be either transient or permanent and are examples of a scientific concept called *developmental plasticity.*[4] How you responded plastically to your environment results in a unique developmental trajectory. For instance, if you were a sad child growing up, you are more likely to be a melancholy adult. Certain developmental windows close early in life, but we retain a great deal of plasticity even in old age. This means that your fundamental nature (dominant, submissive, calm, anxious, etc.) is in the process of being determined even as you read this.

Developmental plasticity is any change in the body, good or bad, mediated by changes in gene expression as a response to the environment. When I say *gene expression,* I am referring to the process where the body's cells determine that a particular protein is needed, they find the gene that encodes the protein from within the DNA in the cell's nucleus and use it to build the protein. For example, when you exercise consistently, genes that encode the proteins needed for muscle tissue become highly expressed, resulting in muscle growth. That's a clear case of developmental plasticity: your body responds to exercise by building new muscle to make the lifting easier.

The same thing happens on a faster scale when your eyes adapt to darkness. Cells in the retina use the rhodopsin gene to build the rhodopsin protein necessary to see better in low light. The production of breast milk involves expressing milk proteins within the breast tissue that are not expressed before pregnancy. Tanning involves the production of the protein pigment melanin. The formation of long-term memories (neuroplasticity) involves physical changes to brain cells that necessitate protein expression. Each of the 25,000 genes in the human genome codes for a protein that performs a specific function within our bodies when needed. Some of these genes, and their proteins, contribute to anxiety.

The Tradeoffs of Adapting to Adversity

Simple single-cell organisms respond to stress (excessive heat, starvation, and abrupt chemical changes in their environment) by tweaking their body plan. Molecular cues that they pick up cause them to express genes that may otherwise remain dormant, causing changes within their cell walls to respond to the demands at hand. Even in the simplest organisms like bacteria and protists, these emergency alterations have costs. Resources are funneled toward responding to the crisis rather than to longevity and upkeep. Over time, this negatively affects the health of the microbe.

Humans also make unhealthy changes in response to bad environments. Constant muscle strain incites protein expression that changes the muscle, making it hard, inflexible, and limiting its range of motion. Shallow breathing becomes persistent because the body uses gene expression to retune the breathing apparatus to become maximally efficient at shallow breathing. The heart is similarly retuned to beat rapidly. Threat-sensing areas of the brain are reinforced after threatening experiences.[5] Stress stimulates the expression of a large variety of different proteins in organs throughout the body and brain that would not otherwise be expressed. These proteins are used in defensive structures, defensive maneuvers, and the creation of a defensive mind state. The effects of developmental plasticity can be lifelong or even multigenerational. Recent findings have found that many of the negative effects can be reversed, but the longer you wait, the harder it will be.

These changes might be useful, for instance, if your environment is filled with predators. But they can produce drastic bodily changes, especially if they are triggered early in development. This is easiest to see in non-human examples like certain species of horned beetle. The beetle's body type can vary sharply based on food availability. Visually, the two versions look very different. Even many scientists at first assumed these two morphs were from different species. When they don't have enough food, developing males become smaller and weaker and never develop their characteristic horns. Their metabolism is reduced, and they utilize "sneaky" reproductive tactics rather than the direct combat typical of their better-fed peers. This morph is adaptive—it has better reproductive success—but only in environments where food is scarce and larger beetles cannot feed themselves.[6] Outside those environments, a hornless horned beetle has no real chance to compete.

A similar thing happens to the water flea Daphnia. If exposed to the smell of their natural predators early in life, they develop a large protective covering that helps them resist being eaten. However, this armor also makes it harder to move and feed. These examples of plasticity involve fundamental tradeoffs. The same kinds of responses occur in mammals, although the effects are usually less obvious. Still, sometimes, you can visually recognize the ravages of stress in people who are extremely anxious, highly traumatized, drug-addicted, or on the bottom of the social totem pole. What these people share in common is that their stress system has been turned up too high for too long. For the beetle, the environmental cue predictive of adversity is malnutrition. For the flea, it is the smell of its natural predator. Can you guess what ours is? It is distressed breathing. Shallow thoracic breathing drives the threat system and a cascade of harmful cellular modifications that change our physical body plan.

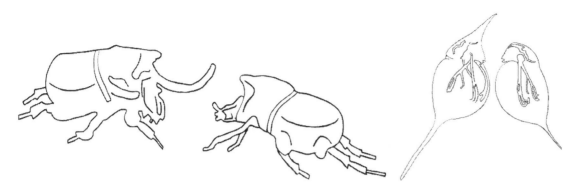

Illustration 2.1: A. Horned beetle and smaller hornless beetle; B. Water fleas with and without protective armoring

How Mammals Adapt to Chronic Stress

Decades of experiments have found that the offspring of nervous mothers are biologically programmed to also be nervous.[7] Mothers exposed to adversity before, during, or after pregnancy upregulate their babies' stress-response systems permanently. Mammals from mice[8] to monkeys[9] with stressed-out moms exhibit increased adrenal activity, which causes higher concentrations of stress hormones. Mammals with more active adrenal systems are more susceptible to stress, responding to mildly threatening events in exaggerated and inappropriate ways.

These responses often last for the animal's entire lifetime. They are a specific type of developmental plasticity called "predictive adaptive responses." The idea is that if a mother's environment is hostile, then her offspring are likely to face that same environment and ought to be prepared for it. For the same reason, rat pups born to calm mothers tend to be calm themselves. Those that received high levels of maternal care in the form of licking, grooming, and nursing show increased resilience to stress even in adulthood.[10] All mammals begin to adapt plastically to stress in the womb and continue to do so throughout life. This is why it is so important to take control of your reactions to stress: you have the power to steer yourself away from suffering.

We were all born with the capacity for unmitigated strength, consummate confidence, and unconditional dominance. Despite this, our body's cells are constantly searching for cues about predation and social competition. Upon encountering these cues, stress hormones are turned up, the respiratory and cardiovascular systems are strained, muscles grow tense, and the brain is adjusted to make us angry, fearful, and paranoid.[11] Again, these responses may result in subtle, microscopic changes or profound, visible ones. The Program Peace method aims to reverse the negative changes and create lasting, positive ones by providing your body's cells with the cues necessary to cause them to interpret their environment as advantageous.

The Sympathetic and Parasympathetic Nervous Systems

The autonomic nervous system controls the function of our internal organs. It affects the heart, lungs, various organs in our abdomen, skin, muscles, and many areas of the brain. It generally influences our organs to either prepare for stress, as in the fight-or-flight state, or for calm, as in the resting-and-digesting state. The fight-or-flight state is associated with the *sympathetic* branch of the autonomic nervous system while the "rest-and-digest" state is associated with the *parasympathetic* branch. These two systems are constantly working together to maintain homeostasis to meet organismic needs. Both are necessary for health and normal functioning. They work in unison, but at any given time, one is usually more active than the other.

The activity of the sympathetic nervous system rises when we feel stressed and lowers when we feel calm. The sympathetic nervous system becomes toxic when it is augmented by developmental plasticity. This is when the body builds stress-adapted proteins into various organ systems. This keeps a person locked in a perpetual state of stress that scientists call "hyperarousal."

Specialists describe the retuning of the autonomic system toward stress as an imbalance that equates to a "shift toward sympathetic upregulation." This is the antagonist of our story, and it is an adversary for each of us to different extents. It is important to point out that the sympathetic nervous system itself is not our enemy; the problem comes only from long-term, persistent sympathetic over-activation. This happens when fear and intimidation are regular occurrences. As you might expect, inferior and submissive mammals have greater sympathetic upregulation. For example, low-ranking baboons have the highest blood pressure, stress hormones, and heart rates.[12]

Moreover, the upregulation of the sympathetic system is almost always a ratchet, meaning that shifts toward stress are generally steady and irreversible. This is partly because many experiences coerce us to breathe more shallowly, but very few convince us that it is safe to breathe more deeply. The table below details the physiological changes associated with both branches of the autonomic system.

	Sympathetic	**Parasympathetic**
Nickname	Fight or Flight	Rest and Digest
Breath Volume	Shallow	Full
Breathing Rate	Faster	Slower
Muscles	Tense	Relaxed
Average Heart Rate	Higher	Lower
Blood Pressure	Higher	Lower
Stress Hormones	High	Low
Short-term Memory	Poor	Good
Thinking	Muddled	Clear
Emotion	Anxious	Calm
Immune System	Weakened	Strong
Social Communication	Defensive or aggressive	Receptive or assertive

Table 2.1: The Autonomic Nervous System: Sympathetic and Parasympathetic Branches

If I were to walk over to my cat and bang my fist on the counter next to him, his autonomic nervous system would react strongly, raising his sympathetic activity. This would be very apparent in the form of a full-body startle and increased defensive activity. After a few minutes, his autonomic activity would go back to baseline (but repeated threatening surprises would shift his baseline toward sympathetic upregulation). If someone were to make a loud, unexpected noise next to me, I would also experience transiently increased autonomic arousal. Humans share a common ancestor with cats 85 million years ago. This funny-looking little mammal would have shared its habitat with dinosaurs and would have had an autonomic nervous system very similar to ours. But the autonomic nervous system is much more ancient than this.

If you were to find a group of ants walking around on a tabletop, then strike the surface they were walking on, they would freeze for an instant before running about their business in a frenzy. The neural components that receive and interpret the quick blow to the tabletop are very similar in structure to our own. Mammals and insects both inherit their autonomic nervous systems from a common aquatic ancestor that lived around 590 million years ago, near the end of the Precambrian supereon[13]. Yet, we still share this same basic structure.

Not all animals have an autonomic stress system. Animals that live their lives attached to rocks, including corals, sea squirts, and anemones, have no use for it. Even some primitive mobile animals such as jellyfish also lack this system. We should consider ourselves blessed to have it. We just have to teach ourselves how to bring it under control because it is a great servant but a terrible master.

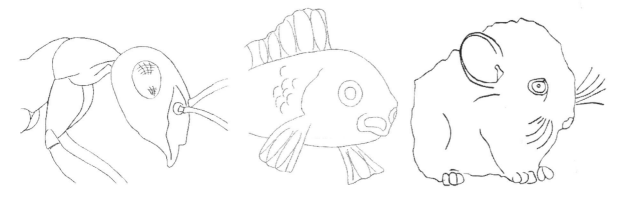

Illustration 2.2: Many orders of animals share similar stress responses and adapt to chronic stress in similar ways.

I know a man who is a psychopathic bully. He is friendly to people at first to gain their trust. Then, he says whatever he can to confuse, upset, and undermine them for his amusement. Before long, his victims are breathless, trying desperately to mount defensive arguments against his red herrings. Eventually, he points at them, laughs, and says, "This man is fighting for his life right now." We are no different. We overuse the sympathetic system during simple social confrontations as if we were fighting for our very lives.

The sympathetic system retunes our organs for intense, uninterrupted physical exertion. This might be appropriate for a person forced to defend themselves against death on a minute-to-minute basis. But none of us do this in modern times. Our stress system is set to overdrive, even though most of us sit on our butts throughout the day and the most upsetting things that happen to us are minor verbal putdowns. The likelihood of you dying prematurely is very low, but your body is operating as if it is high. Persuade your body to stop this by choosing to breathe in a new and different way: as if your survival was guaranteed.

To bring the sympathetic and parasympathetic back into balance, we must recognize that we are not fighting for our lives. This is accomplished by spending more time with the parasympathetic prevailing over the sympathetic. How can we accentuate the parasympathetic system? Relaxed deep breathing. But, as you know, maintaining a relaxed breathing pattern can be extraordinarily difficult because we overreact to minor intrusions so strongly.

Control Your Reaction to Stress by Mastering Your Startle Reflex

Your body has an inborn reflex known as the startle reaction that controls the frequency and severity of stress. Startle is a panic response to something alarming. It is initiated in the brainstem and kickstarts the sympathetic system. It lasts for a fraction of a second (between one-half and one-fiftieth of a second) and can be elicited by threatening stimuli such as loud sounds and fast-moving objects. It can also be elicited by thoughts about unpleasant subjects such as dangers or deadlines. When it happens, our heart rate increases. The next heartbeat comes early, which is a jarring experience. This is often described as the heart "skipping a beat." Adrenaline floods into the body. The breath shortens. We also gasp reflexively when startled, and this has the effect of making the breath shallower and more rapid. Repeated startle responses over weeks or months sensitize the startle pathway in the brain, which explains why anxious people are much more prone to startling.

Startling can be very subtle, in which case you may not realize that you have been startled. When subliminal startling happens continuously, it is often recognized as nervousness. The submissive person will almost always experience more frequent startling than the dominant person. Highly submissive people will startle every few seconds during social interactions. They often startle during their own actions as if to apologize for them. I used to startle whenever talking to someone. It made me come across as shaken and fear-stricken. Sadly, for some of us, startling and trembling are part of being "nice."

Startling devastates our composure. You cannot look someone in the eye with a straight face and decent posture after you have been startled. Once another animal sees that you have experienced a full-body startle, you immediately become prey. With introspection and patience, we can learn to inhibit our startle magnitude and reduce our emotional reaction to it. To do this, we must keep ourselves from overreacting when it happens. When you feel yourself startle, don't get caught up in it or let it carry you away. Instead, let it wash over you, like a wave you have ducked under. Reducing the startle reflex, despite not being acknowledged by mainstream science, is feasible. Some Buddhist monks have demonstrated significant inhibition of their startle reflex, even inhibiting almost all evidence of it.

Startle also causes the body's muscles to tense up. Some muscles, including those in the hands, feet, face, and abdomen are contracted intensely. Contractions in the back jerk frail spinal segments into unfamiliar positions. Sustained contractions from frequent startling can cause achiness and exhaustion. Much of your muscular pain is centered in muscles overworked by your startle response. This is why it is important to cultivate awareness of how startle manifests in your body so that you can ensure that you do not remain stuck in this configuration.

Aside from questions of frequency and intensity, the posture you hold when being startled is telling. When your startle posture is indicative of surrender, people and animals can see this. The way you carry yourself at the point of startle affects your default posture and comes to dictate many aspects of your personality. The full-body startle is accompanied by specific movements in mammals intended to protect certain body parts such as the neck and eyes. In human infants, the eyes blink, the face grimaces, the back arches, and the arms and legs flail out with elbows and knees bent. Adults form their startle postures over a lifetime. Many people flinch, cower, wince, slump over, flail, duck, backpedal, drop things, or buckle at the knees.

In high-level military, police, and martial arts training, combatants are drilled to assume specific fighting stances when alarmed. Through repetition, we can reshape the automatic movement pattern that is recruited. Most people startle recognizably several times every day so you should have ample opportunity to correct your startle. To begin experimenting on your own, start with Stress Adaptation Activity 2.1.

Stress Adaptation Activity #2.1: *Designing Your Startle Posture*

Imagine yourself startling. How does it feel? How do you usually move? As you imagine it, or whenever it happens to you, turn your full attention to how you respond. Inspect your actions and carriage, and try to subdue the response. Don't let yourself get caught up in the emotions it evokes. Also, don't let yourself freeze, stay loose and unfixed. What do you want as your favored startle position? Look back at Table 1.2 from the last chapter and think about how it would feel to retain these optimal displays during and even after startling.

I recommend maintaining an erect posture, a stable stance, a calm face, and steady, uninterrupted breathing. Remember that diaphragmatic breathing inhibits the startle response. How do you orient toward the stimulus that startled you? Face it head-on rather than turning away. How would your role models startle? How can you prepare or defend yourself in a respectable way without submitting, overreacting, or lashing out?

If I touch my cat unexpectedly when he is nervous, he will startle. If he's not nervous, he won't. We need to carry ourselves in a way that if something intense happens unexpectedly, we won't startle. Reducing and reshaping your startle response is an example of how you can begin to make progress in replacing anxious nonverbals with more healthy ones. The discussion of optimal postures throughout this book will help you determine what you want your startle posture to consist of.

Stress Adds Tension to Our Organ Systems

Over months or years, elevated activation of the stress response can be highly detrimental to health.[14] This is called "stress adaptation" and it reallocates the use of available resources in a way that hinders the organism in the long term. This is because most responses to stress are desperate efforts to keep the organism alive just a bit longer. The changes sacrifice long-term investments in health and biological maintenance for intense short-term expenditures. It's an ecological wager that acknowledges that the organism will likely not survive for years in the present environment but may be able to survive long enough to reproduce one last time. Our modern bodies continue to make this same pitiful wager even though it is completely unnecessary in today's environment. The sympathetic upregulation that bought our ancestors a little more time to reproduce today causes us strife, adversely impacts our health, and sacrifices longevity. Getting stuck in survival mode is antiquated and anachronistic. It can be seen as a Stone Age, or even a Mesozoic (the age of reptiles), way of remembering just how bad the environment is.

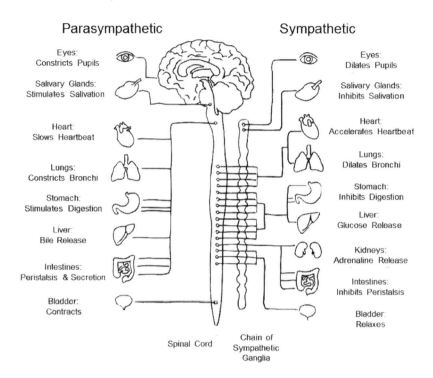

Illustration 2.3: How the parasympathetic and sympathetic nervous systems affect the organs to prepare us for either "resting and digesting" or "fight or flight."

The sympathetic branch of the autonomic nervous system revs up various organs. Each of these organs responds by overexerting itself differently. Some people hold more trauma in the stomach while others hold more in the face. Each person has a different trauma setting, for each of dozens of modules and hundreds of muscles. This gives everyone a unique pattern of strengths and vulnerabilities. Some of these modules correspond to functional structures, such as the swallowing apparatus, the muscles of urinary control, or the intestinal sphincters. Some modules may correspond to plexuses, or clusters of nerves, such as the pharyngeal plexus, the cardiac plexus, or the solar plexus.

These anatomical modules partially overlap with the ancient Hindu yogic structures called chakras. Chakras are thought to channel energy and correlate with both physical ailments and emotional strengths. Chakra-based practices are characterized as pseudoscience today because they stem from an ancient philosophy that made some assertions that turned out not to be true. However, the primary concept of the chakra has some validity. Modern medicine generally acknowledges that even the archaic descriptions of chakras bear a remarkable resemblance to contemporary anatomical descriptions of nerve clusters.

For example, consider the "throat chakra." All of us hold some degree of tension in the muscles that control the vocal tract. This traumatizes our voice boxes and manifests as a painful lump in the throat, which worsens as stress increases. It causes us to feel "choked up," diminishes vocal range, and makes the voice weaker and hoarser with age. However, we can retrain our vocal apparatus using a series of exercises designed to relax and strengthen the muscles, restoring a broader vocal range and effectively healing this chakra-like module. This is the subject of Chapter 12.

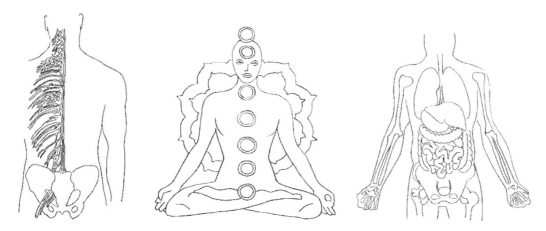

Illustration 2.4: A. Spinal nerve plexuses; B. Meditating yogi with chakras represented by circles; C. Internal organs

The extent to which our chakras have been impacted by stress and trauma determines the extent of our submissive displays and our aptitude for composure. In other words, chronic stress disfigures organs through developmental plasticity. This includes tensing the muscles behind the face (nasopharynx), retracting the genitals, and contracting the smooth muscle of the gut. The people most afflicted are more susceptible to sensations like "the jitters," a "bleeding heart," "butterflies in the stomach," the sensation of a heavy weight on the chest, and shortness of breath. These forms of chakra discomfort are the primary causes of anger, pain, shyness, introversion, and the background hum of persistent anxiety.

Most of the time, we don't notice our compromised displays, the physiological dysfunction, or even the pain they cause. Neither angry nor shy people understand that their behaviors are dictated by the discomfort that comes from unbalanced organs. Instead, and quite unfortunately, they often attribute their responses to aspects of their environment. They use violence or submission to try to change the environment instead of using self-care to change themselves. This lack of awareness allows their pain to control their behavior all the more effectively.

Each chakra-like module has its own mini nervous system, and each sends and receives messages to both conscious and unconscious areas of our brain. Our mind is continually receiving updates from these modules and has the opportunity to send instructions back to them. However, if you neglect to guide attention to the sensations, the brain develops a blind spot, or scotoma, for them, making them almost impossible to self-regulate. Program Peace will help you develop an awareness of, and control over, these different modules. We will focus on sensing where the modules are, whether you are straining them, and by how much. The program will also help you learn how to hold them optimally while breathing diaphragmatically so that you can combine them into healthful ways of being.

Often, when an individual attempts to withhold submissive displays, other signs of submission spill out despite their best efforts. When someone unintentionally emits signals that betray nervousness, psychologists call this phenomenon "tension leakage." Examples of tension leakage include a cracking voice, swallowing at inopportune times, body sway, increased blinking, trembling, fidgeting, stammering, and startling. People who show such leakage early in a confrontation are sometimes thought of as "weak" or "soft." Unfortunately, most people socialize by default in a state of moderate physiological distress just below their threshold for tension leakage. This book will also help you become aware of your tension leakage and try to persuade you not to be afraid or ashamed of it.

Stress Adaptation Activity #2.2: *Accepting Tension Leakage*

Our bodies often betray us by showing others that we are anxious. We know that other people perceive this nonverbal tension leakage and make judgments about us. Because it is embarrassing, this can add an additional layer of stress and pain. When we know that other people can see that we are choked up, or our hands are shaking, we feel we have been humbled and fear this as a type of demotion.

The next time you find yourself nervous in a social situation, don't allow other people's perceptions of your composure to throw you off or make things worse. Be a legendary warrior like Gilgamesh, Shaka Zulu, Athena, or Hattori Hanzo, who has the focus and gumption to continue unphased. Instead of being crushed by your body's demonstration of its weaknesses, let your heart shine right through them. Push through the instability without denying it, covering it up, compensating for it with anger, or being defeated by it. Learning to do this will allow you to harness the energy seeping through the cracks and transform it into excitement and power that you can reroute to your advantage.

If you had to point to places in your body and say, "My anxiety exists in the pain I feel here," where would you point? Do you think it is possible to rehabilitate that area? I think it is. Do you think it involves muscles that can be contracted? I think it does. As Chapter 1 discussed, you can heal your chakras by bringing them to fatigue. Holding the muscles involved in a firm, sustained contraction for several seconds will exhaust them. If you are relaxed and breathing diaphragmatically, muscular exhaustion leads to recuperation.

The chakra-like modules are pots that are boiling over, leaking everywhere. People engaging in tension management try to put a lid on the pot but find themselves constantly cleaning up the spillage. The exercises in this book take another route. Instead of trying to cover up the spills or hide them, they turn down the heat on the stove so that you can exhibit grace under pressure.

Even Sea Slugs Take on Trauma

One of Earth's simplest animals provides a great model for trauma. The sea slug *Aplysia californica* is a large shell-less sea snail. The Aplysia has a defensive reflex to protect its respiratory organs from damage. When the area around its gill is touched, the animal retracts the gill up into the bulk of its body. The response is so simple and reliable that neuroscientists have used it to study the cellular basis of protective reflexes.

In 2000, neuroscientist Eric Kandel was awarded the Nobel Prize for Physiology or Medicine for his research on these animals. He decided to use the sea slug in his experiments because it has very large neurons, and there are only about twenty thousand of them. Contrast this with the one million neurons in a cockroach or honeybee and the 100 billion neurons in the human brain. This simplicity, however, is no barrier to effective function. The slugs are more than capable of learning carefully about when and how much to retract their gills, and, thanks to Kandel's work, we have a clear understanding of the neural mechanisms involved.

The Aplysia's gill retraction reflex exhibits a phenomenon called *sensitization*, whereby the reflex can be strengthened by adding a painful stimulus. By shocking the animal with a small amount of electricity, experimenters cause it to startle. Pairing the shock with a touch to its gill can make its natural defensive response much more powerful. Sea slugs trained this way are constantly "on guard," withdrawing their gills more forcefully and for up to four times as long when touched. This change occurs because the slugs on high alert have generalized the negative experience of the shock to other stimuli so that even a benign, light touch elicits a powerful withdrawal.

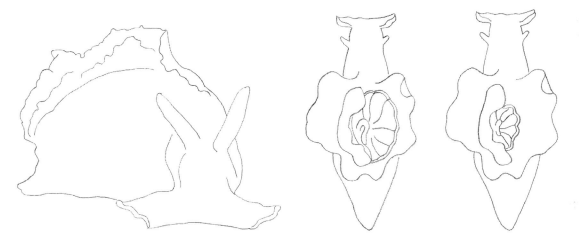

Illustration 2.5: A. Sea slug *Aplysia californica*; B. Aplysia with gill fully relaxed; C. Aplysia with gill fully retracted.

You could say the muscles and nerves involved in retracting the gill constitute a chakra. This is similar to how humans come to hold tension in muscles all over their bodies, overreact to unthreatening stimuli, and generalize traumatic experiences to everyday life. The Aplysia's gill retraction reflex is analogous to the reflexes responsible for a wide range of submissive displays, from our squinting eyes to our hoarse voices, from our suppressed sexuality to our tense diaphragms. The only real difference is that the sea slugs are traumatized by actual painful stimuli, whereas most of our trauma comes from the way we interpret social competition.

The good news here is that the Aplysia can very easily be *de*sensitized, and so can we. When the slug is touched lightly and repeatedly without being shocked, there is a progressive decrease in how far it retracts its gill. Gradually, it relearns that there is no risk associated with light touching and it becomes able to relax. Such a decreased reaction to a stimulus is known as desensitization or habituation. Slugs cannot heal their own chakras in this way. However, by simulating an optimal environment through relaxed diaphragmatic breathing, and using the right mindset, we can. Rather than researchers prodding us with electrodes, we have social contacts prodding us with provocation. This book will teach you how to desensitize your chakra-like modules to their competitive attacks.

Stress and Competition in the Dominance Hierarchy

Since the discovery of the pecking order among hens by Schjelderup-Ebbe in 1922, status hierarchy has been understood as the predominant form of social organization in vertebrates. Animals that live in social communities must actively compete in the same space for resources. When food, mates, or territory are disputed, dominant individuals will prevail over subordinates. Interestingly, a tiered social system helps the group become stable and viable over the long term. On average, it is beneficial for each member, even for those of the lowest ranks. This is because it minimizes violent competition over resources by defining the relationships among members. Dominance hierarchies improve reproductive fitness for all the animals involved by discouraging physical fighting, thereby saving time and energy and reducing the risk of injury.

Unfortunately, a stable hierarchy necessitates constant signaling. Many mammals send out submissive signals even before any direct confrontation occurs. For instance, the subordinate dog will often whimper and place its tail between its legs in response to an immediate threat. Even in the absence of any threat, it will carry its head low, tremble slightly, and adopt a restricted tail posture all the time.

In primates, being harassed or subjugated by higher-ranking individuals, even without any physical contact, is the major form of stress for many species.[15] But it is not just being dominated that is stressful. It is the compensatory response. Submissive displays activate the body's sympathetic nervous system and create continuous strain on the muscles and organs responsible for them.

Chronic Submission Turns into Social Defeat

Most animals have a nearly equal propensity to display dominant and submissive displays in infancy, and young mammals often use both interchangeably in bouts of play. However, as the animal matures, one of the two types of display becomes more frequent and more pronounced. Their experiences with victory and defeat drive this shift.[16] The term *social defeat* refers to losing a confrontation or dispute with a member of your species. This happens constantly in the wild. The more frequently you feel defeated, the stronger your submissive signaling becomes. It is anticipatory and preemptive. Animals that lose repeatedly exhibit *chronic subordination*, wearing the extent of their social defeat on their sleeves to advertise their place in the hierarchy.

Cricket fighting is a popular pastime in China and provides a perfect example of social defeat. A cricket loses a match if it is thrown from the ring, runs away from a battle, or avoids contact. Studies have found that after just one loss, a cricket can "lose its fighting spirit" and will only fight again one time out of ten.[17] Rather than engaging in actual combat, the insect will simply flee the next time it is approached without even taking the time to size up its opponent.

Other examples are just as dramatic. In experiments with mammals, the "resident-intruder" paradigm is often used. This involves placing a subordinate rat near the cage of a more dominant one. Inevitably, the dominant rat will make a dominance display, resulting in the subordinate animal being threatened and acting defeated. Sometimes, the submissive rat is placed inside the dominant rat's cage, which leads to the intruder being attacked and forced into submission. Because the cage is small and escape is impossible, the intruder will lie on its back, emitting distress calls and freezing behavior to appease the attacker. In both experimental protocols, the submitting animal's physiology is significantly changed[18].

Social defeat is a source of chronic stress in animals capable of affecting both neuro- and biochemistry.[19] In mammals, social defeat routinely leads to social withdrawal, lethargy, reduced exploratory behavior, anhedonia, decreased sexual drive, and reduced levels of testosterone in males and females.[20] In humans, it is linked to low self-esteem, feelings of depression, avoidance, anxiety, and increased levels of stress-related hormones. One of the most dramatic changes is the attenuation of the breath. You may have noticed that after a soul-crushing defeat, the most notable change is that it sucks the wind right out of you.

There is good evidence that social defeat in humans leads to poor health[21] and goes hand-in-hand with sympathetic upregulation. Low social status is a robust predictor of death and disease in humans.[22] Several large-scale public health studies have found that low socioeconomic status is strongly related to illness, disease, and mortality.[23] The lower a person's status, the more likely they are to have cardiovascular, gastrointestinal, musculoskeletal, neoplastic, pulmonary, renal, or other diseases. This association between disease and social status cannot be explained away by related factors such as age, income, health behavior, race, sex, or access to healthcare and is thought to be a direct effect of stress.[24] In places where everyone is poor, the effect is nowhere near as strong. It is the inequality that affects health, and it seems that social stress is the real culprit, as socially isolated people and those who receive less social care and inclusion have a greater risk of dying from any cause.[25]

Experiences of social defeat cause us to become preoccupied with matters of status. Male chimps are obsessed with it. They organize most of their lives around issues of rank, allowing social struggles to consume their time, energy, and mental lives. Chimps use intimidation, bluffs, isolation tactics, and obtrusive social maneuvers to challenge and undermine others and dethrone the leader.[26] Similarly, human glory-seeking behaviors, personal vendettas, crimes, and even large-scale political conflicts almost always involve efforts by individuals to improve their rank. Innate tendencies to resist social defeat form the basis of human egotism, hubris, false pride, and insecurity. The primate ego is the source of much of our existential suffering.

Our egos reflect the place in the pecking order in which we imagine ourselves. This is why the ego plays such a pivotal role in our mental lives. The ego is a neurological mechanism designed to help us navigate the primate social hierarchy while avoiding defeat. It causes us to compulsively compare our attributes to those of others and to use these comparisons to guide our use of dominance and subordination displays. After using the exercises in this book to rehabilitate your breathing and other bodily functions, I hope you feel divested of your submissive inclinations and with them your susceptibility to defeat. When this happens, you should feel that your ego expands to include others rather than exclude them.

We want to develop egalitarian relationships in which there is no vying for dominion. Don't bother subjecting yourself to the never-ending, back-and-forth game of status displays. Rise above them. To do this, you must respond to other people's aggressive and submissive displays toward you without feeling compelled to respond with those of your own. Doing so involves subduing four central mammalian instincts. This means that whether they play submissive or aggressive, you choose not to respond with either aggression or submission. You will find that virtually anything else you respond with will be perfect.

Trauma Devalues Us

"We may encounter many defeats but we must not be defeated. It may even be necessary to encounter the defeat, so that we can know who we are." — Maya Angelou (1928-2014)

This book's premise is that, due to our molecular heritage and primate ancestors' preoccupation with social competition, we are highly susceptible to becoming stress adapted. This causes us to hold various lesions in modules throughout the body. It poisons our minds and causes our behavior to be desperate, combative, and vindictive. It causes us to perceive threat when it is not intended and appraise real threat as more dire than it really is. The resulting tendencies cause unnecessary negativity that significantly impedes humanity's cultural and intellectual progress.

Stephen Hawking once argued that the human race is equivalent to "chemical scum on a moderate-sized planet." I used to think that we were scum in both senses of the world: 1) grotesque, biological waste and 2) miserable, immoral miscreants. Now, I think it is the symptoms and physical stigmata of stress that cause us to act reprehensibly. For that reason, I think that they make us scum. In my mind; however, if we can transcend our physical afflictions, we can transcend our propensity for evil. In doing so, we would also rise above our lowly biological origins.

Dominant Animals Are the Least Aggressive

What happens to an animal that reaches the top? Does an ape that becomes an alpha individual in their group become more aggressive or less aggressive? What is your guess? Many people tacitly assume that dominant individuals are more aggressive than subordinate ones. The opposite is true. When an ape or monkey is accepted as the alpha of its group, its violent tendencies evaporate. They are the most assertive while also being the least aggressive. There is no need for either violence or threat displays (except under unusual circumstances, as when a rival challenges the alpha). This is true of both males and females. It is, therefore, counterproductive for a human to act aggressively in an attempt to appear dominant. What they appear as, instead, is impetuous and foolhardy. According to primatologists Richard Wrangham and Dale Peterson:

> *The male chimpanzee behaves as if he is quite driven to reach the top of the community heap. However, once he has been accepted as alpha (in other words, once his authority is established to the point where it is no longer challenged), his tendency for violence falls dramatically. Personality differences and differences in the number, skills, and effectiveness of his challengers produce variation in how completely he relaxes. However, once males have reached the top, they can become benign leaders as easily as they earlier became irritated challengers. What most male chimpanzees strive for is being on top, the one position where they will never have to grovel. The difficulty of getting there induces aggression.[27]*

Scientific observations like this document for us that acting aggressive is a sign of weakness and self-perceived inferiority. I believe that the main reason dominant primates are not aggressive is that their own subordination signals no longer haunt them. As with apes, so also with humans: we are kept controlled by our egos and obsessed with issues of pride because we want desperately to stop having to submit. I know this was the case for me. My nonverbals were so submissive that I was embarrassed by them. I didn't want to appear weak so I would instead get angry, angry enough to cross ethical boundaries. Deep down, we know that submissive behavior is the source of much of our physical and emotional pain, so we are always seeking ways to feel confident in leaving submission behind. But the necessary confidence is elusive.

In the last chapter, we discussed how once we stop sending submissive displays, we no longer have to choose between assertion and aggression because being assertive without being aggressive will become second nature. How is this so? Imagine you were always blushing, always sneering, and that you always looked like you were about to cry. Imagine how frustrating and difficult it would be to come across as assertive. To be assertive, you would almost have to be passive-aggressive. Right? Chapter 6 will show you that the tension we hold in the muscles surrounding our cheeks and eyes keeps us continually on the verge of blushing, sneering, and crying.

Releasing the tension responsible for such displays will allow you to reach true equanimity and present you with a different option. At this point, you will have to choose between being a good person and being a bad person. You can utilize your newfound composure altruistically or malevolently. At this crossroads, I believe most people will realize that being good is the only real path because once your submissive behaviors have disintegrated, it will become clear that they were always the primary drivers for bad behavior.

I can tell you from firsthand experience because I went from one extreme to another. When I felt I was on the bottom, I was sulky, ill-tempered, and hateful. I always felt like I had something to prove. The majority of my time alone was spent planning retorts and retaliation. I experienced "other people" as a type of hell. Since being desensitized by Program Peace's exercises, I no longer feel these emotions at all. Other people are just not a source of negativity anymore.

Our ingrained bodily habits make it difficult to just stop sending submissive signals. Even if, somehow, we could leave behind our mental concerns related to status, our bodies would continue to carry symptoms of social defeat like shortness of breath, the rock in the pit of our stomachs, and the hot tension in our faces. These are spiritual burdens that will inevitably drag us back into the hierarchical fray. This book will show you how to mend these symptoms and how to lay down the burden of submission, shame, and stressful social comparison. Where do we start? With the cornerstone of confidence: "breathing easy."

Breathing Easy Will Pull You Out of Survival Mode

In most mammals, shallow breathing accompanies submission and aggression, while deep breathing accompanies dominance and assertion. A submissive chimp always greets a more dominant chimp first and does so using a sequence of short pant-grunts. These depthless pants are indicative of self-handicapped breathing. Chimps whimper when acting submissively, producing a high-pitched sound accompanied by attenuated breath. We also breathe shallowly around others, especially when experiencing social anxiety. I believe that if it were studied, researchers would find that the extent of deep, diaphragmatic breathing is an accurate predictor of social dominance, the number of offspring, quality of life, and a wide variety of other positive outcomes in primates and all mammals generally. Unfortunately, there has been extraordinarily little related research on breathing style in animals or humans.

Recent experiments have offered us glimpses into the benefits of breathing with the diaphragm. Study participants that practiced deep breathing achieved significant reductions in self-reported anxiety, stress hormones, heart rate, breathing rate, blood pressure, [28] and the activity of the sympathetic stress system.[29] It also enhances mood, oxygen levels, pulmonary function, cardiorespiratory fitness, and respiratory muscle strength, as well as parasympathetic activity. Findings like these, along with the benefits I have experienced myself, have led me to believe that the most important message that you can send your body and its cells is, "Hey, it's totally safe to breathe slowly and deeply."

The scientific community knows shallow breathing to be an indicator of stress and sympathetic over-activation. But it is rarely recognized as a submissive and conciliatory display. Recognizing it as such is important in understanding how to counteract it. We breathe shallowly to show people we are listening to them, that we are concerned and do not think of ourselves as better than them. We face strong unspoken social norms telling us to breathe shallowly. Tragically, however, it results in stress adaptation, increases our tendency to startle, creates tension in chakras throughout the body, and rewires our mind for negativity.

It is possible to escape the social pressure to breathe shallowly. We can do so by building strong, consistent diaphragmatic breathing habits, training ourselves to breathe deeply under every possible circumstance. Deep breathing in social situations breaks the link between social friction and fight or flight. It allows you to stop responding to social pressures as if they are matters of survival.

Whether you are sitting in a meeting, chatting with a friend, having an argument, or taking an exercise class, there should be only one competition that is going on in your head. Out of everyone in the vicinity, you want to have the most relaxed breathing. The only way to accomplish this is to breathe slowly, smoothly, and deeply, reducing the number of breaths you breathe per minute. Relaxed breathing will liberate you from the status hierarchy and is the only thing that you should do aggressively. The next chapter will show you how.

Chapter 2: **Bullet Points**

- Your body is a "survival machine" designed to support a competitive molecular replicator: namely, your DNA.
- Our biology prioritizes the DNA, and for that reason, our bodies are designed to sacrifice our physical and emotional well-being for the sake of survival and reproduction.
- As one example of this, we are built to adapt to stressful environments by upregulating our stress-response activity, resulting in anxiety and pain.
- Even in the modern world, everyone's stress system has been over-activated to some extent. This anxiety or "hyperarousal" results in chronic muscular, respiratory, and cardiovascular fatigue.
- Anxiety and chronic stress negatively affect every organ in the body. These organ systems are roughly congruent with the ancient Hindu system of chakras—familiar body parts that need to be rehabilitated with love and care.
- We use anxiety as a submissive display to prove to others that we are neither "too calm" nor "too good" for them.
- The overuse of submissive signals leads to the accumulation of trauma within our tissues and organs, especially the breathing muscles. The result is often chronic defeat, otherwise known as depression.
- Being nonsubmissive is not about being tougher than anyone else; it is about not wasting energy on competitive nonsense that leads nowhere.
- Dominant mammals are usually the most composed, and the least traumatized and hyperaroused. They don't feel any need to use anxiety as a form of social lubrication.
- Deep, diaphragmatic breathing is the foundation of dominant behavior because it builds unconscious self-confidence.
- You can escape the cycle of social anxiety by breathing deeper and longer breaths in social situations—fearing no one but treating everyone well.
- Through developmental plasticity (new gene expression), you want your body to make persistent, beneficial adaptations that are responses to an optimal environment.
  To do this, you must give the body the right cues to trick it into assuming that your environment is safe and full of resources. This is accomplished by breathing with the diaphragm.

Chapter 2: **Endnotes**

1.   Dewitt, T. J., Sih, A., & Wilson, D. S. (February 1998). Costs and limits of phenotypic plasticity. *Trends in Ecology & Evolution*, *13*(2): 77–81

2.   Kelly, S. A., Panhuis, T. M., Stoehr, A. M. (2012). Phenotypic Plasticity: Molecular Mechanisms and Adaptive Significance. *Comprehensive Physiology*, 2, 1417–1439.

3.   Gabriel, W. (2005), How stress selects for reversible phenotypic plasticity. *Journal of Evolutionary Biology*, 18, 873–883.

4.   Pigliucci, M. (2001). *Phenotypic plasticity: Beyond nature and nurture*. Johns Hopkins University Press.

5.   Reser, J. E. (2016). Chronic stress, cortical plasticity and neuroecology. *Behavioral Processes*, *129*, 105–115.

6.   DeWitt, T. J., & Scheiner, S. M. (2004). *Phenotypic plasticity: Functional and conceptual approaches*. Oxford University Press.

7.   Hoffman, K. M. & Trawalter, S. (2016). Assumptions about life hardship and pain perception. Group Processes & Intergroup Relations, 19(4), 493–508.

8.   Lin, K. N., Barela, A. J., Chang, M., Dicus, E., Garrett, S., Levine, M., Oray, S., & McClure, W. O. (1998). Prenatal stress generates adult rats with behavioral and neuroanatomical similarities to human schizophrenics. *Society for Neuroscience Abstracts*, *24*, 796.

9.   Schneider, M., Roughton, E., Koehler, A., & Lubach, G. (1999) Growth and development following prenatal stress exposure in primates: An examination of ontogenetic vulnerability. *Child Development*, 70(2), 263–274.

10. Talge, N. M., Neal, C., Glover, V., & Early Stress, Translational Research and Prevention Science Network: Fetal and Neonatal Experience on Child and Adolescent Mental Health (2007). Antenatal maternal stress and long-term effects on child neurodevelopment: how and why? *Journal of child psychology and psychiatry, and allied disciplines*, *48*(3-4), 245–261.

11. Sapolsky, R. M. (1996). Why stress is bad for your brain. *Science*, 273(5276), 749–750.

12. Sapolsky, 1996, "Why stress is bad for your brain."

13. Miller, T. A. (1997). Control of circulation in insects. *General Pharmacology*, *29*(1), 23–38.

14. McEwen, B. S., & Stellar, E. (1993). Stress and the individual: Mechanisms leading to disease. *Archives of Internal Medicine, 153*(18), 2093–2101.

15. Nelson, R. J. (2005). *An Introduction to Behavioral Endocrinology* (3rd ed.). Sinauer Associates; Sapolsky, R. M. (2005). The influence of social hierarchy on primate health. *Science, 308*(5722), 648–652.

16. Hermann, H. R. (2017). *Dominance and aggression in humans and other animals: The great game of life.* Academic Press.

17. Laufer, P. (2011). *No animals were harmed: The controversial line between entertainment and abuse.* Lyons Press.

18. Alcock, J. (2005). *Animal behavior: An evolutionary approach* (8th ed.). Sinauer.

19. Bjorkqvist, K. (2001). Social defeat as a stressor in humans. *Physiology and Behavior, 73*(3), 435–442.

20. Huhman, K. L. (2006). Social conflict models – Can they inform us about human psychopathology? *Hormones and Behavior. 50*(4), 640–646.

21. Allen, N. B., & Badcock, P. B. (2003). The social risk hypothesis of depressed mood: Evolutionary, psychosocial, and neurobiological perspectives. *Psychological Bulletin, 129*(6), 887–913.

22. Sapolsky, 1996, "Why stress is bad for your brain."

23. Adler, N. E., Boyce, T., Chesney, M. A., Cohen, S., Folkman, S., Kahn, R. L., & Syme, S. L. (1994). Socioeconomic status and health. The challenge of the gradient. *The American Psychologist. 49*(1), 15–24; Kaplan, G. A., & Keil, J. E. (1993). Socioeconomic factors and cardiovascular disease: A review of the literature. *Circulation, 88*(4), 1973–1998.

24. Pincus, T., Callahan, L. F., Burkhauser, R. V., (1987). Most chronic diseases are reported more frequently by individuals with fewer than 12 years of formal education in the age 18-64 United States population. *Journal of Chronic Diseases, 40*(9), 865–874.

25. Seeman, T. E. (2000). Health promoting effects of friends and family on health outcomes in older adults. *American Journal of Health Promotion, 14*(6), 362–370.

26. Stanford, C. (2018). *The new chimpanzee: A twenty-first-century portrait of our closest kin.* Harvard University Press.

27. Wrangham, R. W., & Peterson, D. (1996). *Demonic males: Apes and the origins of human violence.* Houghton, Mifflin.

28. Chen, Y. F., Huang, X. Y., Chien, C. H., & Cheng, J. F. (2016). The effectiveness of diaphragmatic breathing relaxation training for reducing anxiety. *Perspectives in Psychiatric Care*, *53*(4), 329–336.

29. Janet, K. S., & Gowri, P. M. (2017). Effectiveness of deep breathing exercise on blood pressure among patients with hypertension. *International Journal of Pharma and Bio Sciences*, *8*(1), B256–260.

Chapter 3: **Breathe Deeply, Smoothly, Slowly, and on Long Intervals**

"Regulate the breathing, and thereby control the mind." — B.K.S. Iyengar (1918-2014)

What is breathing? Breathing is the exchange of gasses used by land animals to provide their bodies' cells with the oxygen. They need that oxygen to burn food into energy. Oxygen allows cells to break down sugars derived from food and provide us with energy to move and think. Breathing takes many forms. For example, crickets simply circulate air through open tubes while fish use gills to collect oxygen from water.

In animals with lungs, breathing is called "ventilation." During the ventilatory process, air is pulled into the lungs, where gas exchange takes place. Oxygen diffuses from the air into the blood during inhalation, and carbon dioxide diffuses from the blood into the air during exhalation. When the environment requires that an animal move more than usual, its breathing rate increases so that more oxygen can be delivered to its busy cells.

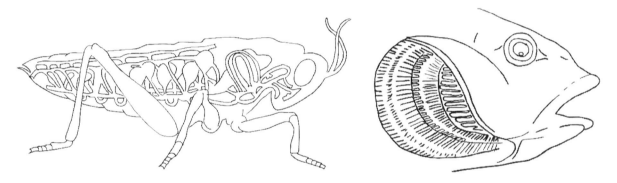

Illustration 3.1: A. Circulatory system of a cricket; B. Gills of a salmon

Mammals have muscles in the chest that act to inflate and deflate the lungs. The most important of these is a specialized muscle located beneath the lungs called the respiratory diaphragm. Other land vertebrates, including amphibians, reptiles, and the late dinosaurs exhibit a similar structure, although theirs is simpler and sits above the lungs rather than below. The mammalian diaphragm changes its behavior depending on the immediate circumstances, focusing on efficiency in safe environments but producing paranoid overexertion in threatening ones. This chapter will describe how stress causes the diaphragm to produce quick, shallow strokes, and how deliberately practicing longer, fuller breaths can reinstate its proper function.

Distressed Breathing vs. Diaphragmatic Breathing

Breathing shallowly, at short intervals, is known as distressed breathing. It is also known as defensive breathing, nondiaphragmatic breathing, or thoracic breathing. The behavior is strongly associated with stress and anxiety disorders and tends to cause nervousness and discomfort. Distressed breathing is characterized by rapid, uneven breaths, punctuated by gasps, sighs, and breath holding. It can easily become habitual, leading to serious long-term dysfunction.[1]

Distressed breathing has a reciprocal relationship with the brain's stress and threat response systems. We breathe more defensively when we are afraid, and we become more afraid when we breathe defensively. Distressed breathing is also used as a signal of submission. This is why improving your breathing will not only help you control negative thinking but also help you become more dominant. Indeed, you will find that true diaphragmatic breathing is incompatible with anxiety, social and otherwise.

People who breathe shallowly are usually unaware of the condition and do it unknowingly throughout the day. Most of us breathe by default with "bated breath." We wait for everything in our lives with abated breathing as if a judge were about to announce our prison sentence. We do this even when circumstances are normal and unthreatening. Everyone understands more or less instinctively that inhibited, irregular breathing is a source of tension and stress. This is clear from the popularity of idioms like "waiting to exhale," "sigh of relief," "couldn't catch my breath," "breath of fresh air," "give me some breathing room," and "short of breath."

Breathing patterns are contagious and often modeled. Children learn how to breathe from their parents. For this reason, children often take on the anxiety level of their parents. We perceive others' breathing patterns from their movements, speech patterns, sounds of inhalation and exhalation, and facial tension. We all alter our breathing to accommodate, or match, that of the people around us. I saw this clearly when my distressed breathing would contaminate the breathing of others.

Is your breathing unhealthy? Likely so. Imagine that you are threading a small needle with a thin thread. As you line up the thread with the hole, are you holding your breath? You shouldn't be. Experience pronounced distressed breathing firsthand by doing the following activity:

Breathing Activity #3.1: *Simulating Distressed Breathing*

Sit comfortably and focus on your breath. Time your inhalations and exhalations to last only a second each, and breathe like this for 10 seconds. Next, time each breath to last for just half a second. Continue to breathe this way for one minute or until you feel uncomfortable, whichever comes first. Now stop and observe your body and mind. How does your chest feel? How do your shoulders and neck feel? How has your mood changed? Wouldn't it be terrible to be stuck breathing like this forever?

After performing this activity, most people report uncomfortable sensations such as anxiety, panic, or tension, accompanied by increased heart rate, physical agitation, breathlessness, chest pressure, or even the feeling of starving for air. These are the typical outcomes of distressed breathing, and many of us unnecessarily subject ourselves to them daily. An anxious person will breathe at an average rate of 18 to 20 breaths per minute. A relaxed person practicing diaphragmatic breathing will breathe only five to seven times per minute.[2] Problems with diaphragmatic breathing are best conceptualized as falling on a continuum rather than as a threshold. There are no firm diagnostic criteria for distressed breathing; virtually everyone is somewhere on the spectrum.

Newborns breathe diaphragmatically, but, by age ten, diaphragmatic function is usually minimized. This is because few of us experience childhoods that our bodies interpret as optimal. The transition away from diaphragmatic breathing occurs during early childhood as we learn which environmental stimuli should be linked to concern and worry. The process is normal and prepares us to be especially cautious in specific situations. However, by the time we reach adulthood, nearly every situation recruits distressed breathing, just some more than others.[3] Distressed breathing is implicitly conditioned to occur alongside many activities and postures, and these associations are often never unlearned. That leaves us gasping when the telephone rings, holding our breath while sitting at the keyboard, and hyperventilating during everyday conversations.

We cannot immediately switch from distressed breathing to competent, calm, diaphragmatic breathing because we are held back by long-term physiological changes wrought by years of breathing shallowly. These changes involve a multitude of alterations to the muscles and nerves of the respiratory system. They cause the diaphragm to atrophy and become stuck in partial contraction. These changes are driven by gene activity, constitute developmental plasticity, and are largely responsible for the sympathetic overactivation discussed in the last chapter. Fortunately, the changes are reversible. However, you cannot pay anybody to retrain your breathing for you, and there is no pill you can take. It requires time and discipline. As with the other exercises in this book, you will find the breathwork rewarding once you start to see the results.

Many therapists, books, and self-help resources promote breathing exercises. Most of these exercises last only a few seconds, are intended to counteract panic attacks, and come with no guidelines for permanently changing breathing style. Moreover, users are often only told to "breathe deeply" or "focus on the breath" without being provided any further instructions. Simply focusing on the breath is beneficial because it prompts the individual to note when their breath is unnaturally shallow. It causes the person to think, "Wait, my current predicament is not all that bad, so why am I breathing like there is something at stake?" That is a productive first step.

Awareness of desperation in the breath is a start, but it does not address the problem at its source. Rather than simply focusing on the breath, we need to actively lengthen and deepen our breaths throughout the day to strengthen the muscles and reprogram the unconscious breathing circuits in our brainstems. Consciously overriding its injurious commands will rewire your brain and retune your entire body.

Diaphragmatic Breathing Utilizes the Respiratory Diaphragm

Deep, non-distressed breathing is controlled by the diaphragm, a dome-shaped skeletal muscle that separates the thorax (containing the heart and lungs) from the abdomen (containing the intestines, stomach, liver, and kidneys). Only an eighth of an inch thick, it extends across the bottom of the rib cage and moves air into and out of the lungs by changing shape. It moves like a plunger. When it contracts, the diaphragm moves downward, drawing in breath, resulting in inhalation. When it relaxes, it moves upward, expelling air and causing you to exhale. The diaphragm can move as much as ten centimeters, but many adults use only around one centimeter or 10% of the total range. Expanding the range of your diaphragm is essential, and I designed this chapter's exercises to do just that. But first, let's explore how to move the diaphragm at all.

Diaphragmatic breathing, also known as eupnea in the scientific literature and belly breathing in the vernacular, is an unlabored form of breathing seen in untraumatized mammals. You should be able to observe it in any young mammal resting peacefully.[4] It is easiest to spot in a sleeping infant, a kitten, or a puppy lying on its side. The animal's stomach will move up and down with each breath. How do you know whether you are breathing with your diaphragm? Your belly should move in much the same way. Use the conventional guidelines for belly breathing in the activity below:

Breathing Activity #3.2: *Belly Breathing*

Lie on your back with a pillow under your head. Place one hand on your chest and the other on your stomach. Focus on how your belly moves. Ensure that it rises with each inhalation and falls with each exhalation. When you are breathing with the diaphragm, it displaces the stomach, causing it to move up and down. On the other hand, during distressed breathing, the chest, neck, and shoulders move and the stomach remains still.

Distressed breathing makes you feel like you are growing taller and lengthening. Diaphragmatic breathing makes you feel like your belly, lower ribs, and lower back are expanding. Distressed breathing makes you feel like you are fighting to retain control over your environment. It can be hard to give up the false sense of security it provides. Diaphragmatic breathing may feel uncomfortable at first as if you are letting your guard down to an extent that is unsafe. You may find that letting your stomach rise takes courage and a bit of faith.

You should notice that that at certain points during your inhalation the diaphragm locks up and the belly stops moving entirely. Watch for these impediments. It's almost like you are trying to convince your diaphragm that it is safe to come out and play. Try different breathing styles until you find one that lets you easily and naturally keep your stomach rising and falling. It may help to place an object like a book on your belly. Give yourself several minutes to experiment.

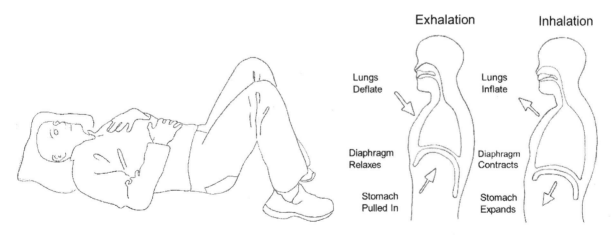

Illustration 3.2: A. Belly breather ensuring that the stomach rises and falls; B. Motion of the diaphragm during breathing.

The motion of one's stomach is the telltale sign of diaphragmatic breathing, and this method works for many people.[5] However, most instructions for diaphragmatic breathing end here. This was discouraging for me because I felt there should be a more substantial protocol. Moreover, I realized my stomach was rising and falling only because I was using my abdominal muscles, rather than my diaphragm, to suck it in and push it out. No matter how I tried to vary my approach to each breath, my stomach would not move unless I used my abdominals to move it. My diaphragm was so tense that monitoring the motion of my stomach did nothing for me. I wonder how many other people following these guidelines simply use their abdominal muscles to mimic the movement without breathing diaphragmatically.

After years of exhaustively reading the medical literature on anxiety, I became convinced that my problem lay with my dysfunctional breathing style. I was determined to correct it but couldn't find anything that explained how. I would lay on the ground for hours trying to perceive the movement of my diaphragm to no avail. The diaphragm has relatively few proprioceptive nerve endings, meaning that it is difficult to tell how much it is contracting and where it is in space. That makes it very difficult to perceive consciously, which makes the problem all the worse.

Why did natural selection hide our diaphragm from us? Perhaps, as with the heart, our genes don't trust us to know how to control the diaphragm consciously. Grievously, the body has a vested interest in keeping us from interfering with trauma's adaptive manifestations. If our environment is seemingly drastic, our genes want us to treat it as such. One of the few times we notice our diaphragms is when we have hiccups. With this in mind, try using the following activity as an alternative route to getting a feel for your diaphragm.

Breathing Activity #3.3: *Simulating Hiccups*

Fake a hiccup ten times. A genuine hiccup utilizes the diaphragm to generate force.
Pay special attention to how it feels to move the diaphragm in the form of a hiccup. As you feel the muscle contract, remind yourself that this is the muscle you want to use to power your breath.

A hiccup is initiated by a reflex arc that produces a spasm of the diaphragm (myoclonic jerk). Hiccupping involves rapid, abrupt diaphragmatic contractions. Of course, this is the opposite of how you want to breathe—i.e., slowly and smoothly. However, hiccupping helps you become acquainted with your diaphragm. Fake a few hiccups, and you will localize your diaphragm in space and sensorium. Another way to sense your diaphragm is to hold your breath for 20 to 40 seconds. You will feel a muscle between your stomach and chest pulsate. This is the diaphragm trying to jumpstart your breathing pattern.

The key to sensing and recruiting the diaphragm is teaching yourself to breathe at a smooth, continuous, and constant rate. This automatically mobilizes the diaphragm because it is what the diaphragm is specialized for and designed to do. Shallow breathing stifles diaphragmatic movement. When the diaphragm is stifled, we use other, less efficient muscles for breathing.

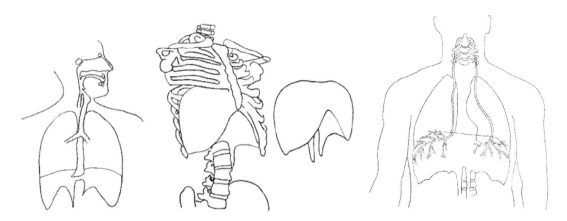

Illustration 3.3: A. Diaphragm, lungs, and respiratory airways; B. Diaphragm shown within and outside the rib cage; C. The phrenic nerves send motor commands to the diaphragm and receive sensory information from it.

Distressed Breathing Utilizes the Thorax and Clavicles

During distressed breathing, the stomach doesn't move, but the chest does. It involves pivoting the ribs around the joints where they attach to the vertebrae. The thoracic (or intercostal) muscles of the thorax perform this function. The thoracic muscles form the meat in between the bones of barbecued ribs. The external intercostals swing the ribs upward and forward, powering inhalation. The internal intercostals pull the ribs inward and downward, powering exhalation. In a nutshell, diaphragmatic breathing presses the floor of the lungs up and down, whereas thoracic breathing expands the walls of the chest inward and outward. One effect of this difference is that thoracic breathing does not fill the lower portions of the lungs with air, while diaphragmatic breathing does. Thoracic breathing is inherently shallow. It is also less efficient because it requires more work—and more breaths—to transport the same amount of oxygen into your blood.

Clavicular breathing is another form of distressed breathing that involves a shrugging of the clavicles and shoulders. It is even shallower and less efficient than thoracic breathing. It is also called upper thoracic breathing, as it only pulls air into the top third of the lungs. Clavicular breathing is a serious problem, as it can nearly eliminate the function of the diaphragm, leading to even weaker, less effective breaths.

A respiratory physiologist can measure the extent of clavicular and thoracic breathing using electromyography by placing electrodes on the muscles surrounding the clavicles and upper thorax. The electrode readout indicates how active these muscles are and, thus, how defensive the person's breathing is. You can observe this yourself by paying careful attention to the movement of your shoulders during breathing. If they move up with the in-breath, you are breathing with your clavicles. Clavicular breathing becomes especially pronounced during exercise. In general, you should never breathe with your shoulders. As Chapter 15 will explain, it is preferable to keep the shoulders still and pressed toward the floor.

During ideal diaphragmatic breathing, the thoracic muscles and the diaphragm work together with every breath. The diaphragm should lead the thoracic muscles, setting the pace and making each breath long and smooth. As in the synergy seen between sympathetic and parasympathetic branches of the nervous system, the diaphragm is supposed to work in unison with the thoracic musculature. This synergy falls apart during anxiety when the thoracic musculature and the sympathetic system take over. We have so far encountered two major antagonists in our story about chronic stress. First, we have the overactive sympathetic nervous system. Second, we have overactive thoracic breathing. It should come as no surprise that the two problems collaborate, exacerbating the detrimental effects. The resulting distressed breathing drains our energy, ties knots in our muscles, ages us prematurely, and turns us into nervous wrecks.

The critical link between emotion and stress is the breath. The fear and grief circuitry of the brain activates thoracic breathing and inhibits diaphragmatic breathing. Habitual thoracic or clavicular breathing chronically overstimulates the sympathetic nervous system, keeping heart rate and blood pressure elevated while loading the diaphragm with muscular tension. This causes sympathetic overload. On the other hand, the neural circuitry for self-soothing, mood stabilization, and the calming branch (parasympathetic) of the nervous system is linked to the diaphragm.

There is a simple explanation for this. The diaphragm is structured and situated to contract slowly and steadily to take in just the right amount of air to oxygenate the body at peace. It moves at the optimal rate to procure the proper amount of oxygen needed in a tranquil environment. However, its leisurely pace would be a hindrance to wild animals in a hostile environment.

Thoracic musculature is optimized to produce accelerated breathing during a crisis. Thoracic breathing allows mammals to actively modulate their breaths in response to fluctuations in anticipated danger. In the short run, this would have helped our prehistoric ancestors prepare for the increased oxygen requirements they would need for "fight or flight" maneuvers. Sadly, most of us live in this mode, even though we are no longer protecting our bodies from predators or club-bearing maniacs. The modern world has "tricked" our bodies into thinking that our environment is too stressful to breathe peacefully when the opposite is true.

Distressed Breathing and Social Rank

If you would like to experience pronounced thoracic/clavicular breathing, watch an internet video of a violent street fight and pay careful attention to your breath. The shallow rapidity will become apparent. You could achieve a similar effect just by watching an internet video of an argument between two people. This is because, in primates, social confrontation dysregulates breathing nearly as much as physical violence. When you feel disrespected, cheated, or compelled to explain yourself, you enter a state of respiratory distress. When this happens, people usually act at two extremes, either becoming conflict-avoidant (submissive) or quick to anger.

Respiratory distress is marked by breathing so shallow that it interferes with your speech, causing your voice to falter. You may feel like you are choking and suffocating at the same time. It is usually apparent to those around you, and most people are embarrassed when it happens to them. The truth is that awkward social encounters cause most of us to experience a state of respiratory distress throughout the day.

My experience is that most people have little interest in using breathing exercises to deepen their breath until I explain to them that deep breathing is a dominant trait. Then they become eager. Our respiratory behavior affects our social standing and how we are treated and perceived. People hear changes in the cadence and pitch of your voice that are caused by distressed breathing and use them to make judgments about your level of confidence. Breathing is one of the most common markers of social rank.

Diaphragmatic breathing retraining will make you practically immune to respiratory distress. With enough retraining, people will be able to tell that you have little susceptibility to it. When your breathing shows no signs of distress, people will not want to challenge or provoke you because they realize they will reach respiratory distress before you do. As you develop your capacity for diaphragmatic breathing, you will come to understand that the people around you are constantly fighting wars of attrition to see who will show signs of respiratory distress first.

We also breathe shallowly in a distressed manner to communicate friendliness. Because we don't want to come across as overbearing or audacious or because we want to make others comfortable, we shorten our breaths and disengage the diaphragm. In other words, we breathe in a distressed manner when we are afraid, when we are mad, *and* when we are being nice. No wonder it seems inescapable.

Stifling and Neglecting the Diaphragm

Social and environmental stress are not the only causes of distressed breathing. It can also be the result of surgery or injury. After colon surgery, a gastric bypass, a Caesarean procedure, or an appendectomy, for instance, the patient will have an incision wound on their abdomen. It is common for recovering patients to inhibit normal abdominal expansion during breathing to avoid the pain of having their injury disturbed. They learn to actively stifle diaphragmatic movement out of fear of pain or stitches bursting at the incision site. This learned pain avoidance can be long-lasting, causing the patient to neglect the diaphragm and adopt thoracic breathing as a fixed habit. Chronic shallow breathing can result, along with breathlessness and anxiety. It is uncommon for such patients to revert to diaphragmatic use even after the pain from the surgery is gone unless breathing retraining therapy is undertaken.[6] You may have never had abdominal surgery, but, to some extent, past trauma and submissive signaling have stifled your diaphragm in a similar way.

Fortunately, we have good models available for how to reinstate diaphragmatic use. The best of these is recovery from a ventilator. In situations where medical patients are having trouble breathing, a machine called an artificial ventilator can be used to move air in and out of their lungs. When a doctor takes a patient off a ventilator, they need to assess the person's breathing mechanics to ensure the breathing musculature is strong and coordinated enough to support unaided breathing.[7] Withdrawal from mechanical ventilation is known as "weaning."

Think of your thoracic breathing musculature as akin to a ventilator from which you need to wean yourself. Years of stress have caused the thoracic muscles to take control, and your diaphragm has weakened through atrophy caused by disuse. The good news is that the diaphragm can grow stronger quickly.[8] When you first start breathing diaphragmatically, it will be difficult. It will feel as if you have been taken off a ventilator; the muscles you are forcing to breathe for you are not yet up to the job. You will need to wean off thoracic breathing by training the diaphragm. I encourage you to use the exercises in the rest of this chapter to remove the ventilator of thoracic breathing and plunge headfirst into strengthening your diaphragm.

The Four Rules of Diaphragmatic Breathing

In the thick of my anxiety, I could tell that my breathing was highly dysfunctional. I used myself as a model for what not to do and slowly made inferences about how to do the opposite of my acquired tendencies. I read copiously about ventilatory mechanics and experimented with numerous breathing styles. Slowly, after ten years of research, introspection, and trial and error, I developed eight rules of diaphragmatic breathing. This chapter will address the first four, which are:

1) Breathe Deep (high volume): Breathe nearly all the way in by the end of each inhalation and all the way out by the end of each exhalation.

2) Breathe Long (low frequency): Engage in long-interval breathing, breathing in for four to ten seconds and breathing out for six to twelve seconds at a time.

3) Breathe Smooth (continuous flow): Breathe at a steady, slow, nearly constant rate during all breathing.

4) Breathe Assertively (confident): Do not permit social concerns or life stressors to conflict with the first three rules.

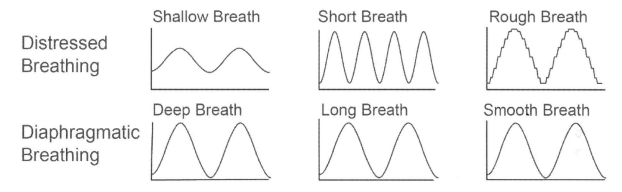

Figure 3.1: A graphical representation of the first three rules of diaphragmatic breathing. The vertical axis designates the depth of inhalation or volume of air in the lungs; the horizontal axis designates time.

A helpful way to improve your ability to monitor your breathing is to draw your breathing pattern on paper. Use the examples in Figure 3.1 to work through the exercise below.

Breathing Activity #3.4: *Draw Your Breathing Pattern on Paper*

Sit down with pen and paper. Become curious about your breath as if it is a phenomenon you have never encountered. As you observe each breath, graph it with a free hand. Make the vertical axis correspond to the depth of the breath and the horizontal axis to how long each breath lasts. In other words, volume on the y-axis and time on the x-axis. Take different kinds of breaths at different depths and frequencies. Depict each as a curve on paper in real time. Just taking a few minutes to represent your breathing in this way will increase your breath awareness, helping you better visualize and monitor your breathing.

After my personal experimentation, I was convinced that adherence to these four rules guaranteed diaphragmatic breathing. I researched these concepts to find support for them in the scientific literature. Further research brought me to the realization that certain clinicians have been using tenets remarkably similar to these for decades. For instance, psychologist Erik Peper developed an excellent system he calls "effortless diaphragmatic breathing," which consists of a large tidal volume (> 2000ml), slow respiration rate (< 8 breaths per minute), and continuous flow rate.[9] Additionally, "Resonant Breathing," "Coherent Breathing,"[10] and the "Conscious Breathing Method"[11] are similar breathing methods that I think are scientifically accurate and very helpful.

Related techniques for diaphragmatic breathing retraining have been used by relaxation and biofeedback programs for decades.[12] They have also become popular in psychiatry and clinical psychology and are now considered fundamental tools in cognitive behavioral therapy.[13] Diaphragmatic breathing, in general, is now touted as an effective, evidence-based stress reduction intervention that is low in cost, easy to use, and can be self-administered with no equipment needed.[14] You might be wondering, "How is diaphragmatic breathing defined in medicine?" It's simple. In the clinical literature, participants are considered as performing diaphragmatic breathing if sensors show that they are breathing longer and deeper (decreasing the respiratory rate while increasing the amplitude of the respiratory waveform).

Diaphragmatic breathing is well known to slow the heart rate and decrease blood pressure. It has been proven to reduce sympathetic arousal, anxiety, panic attacks, and hyperventilation syndrome.[15] It is also an effective treatment modality in pain management,[16] motion sickness,[17] breathlessness,[18] and a range of psychiatric and medical disorders.[19] For all these reasons, diaphragmatic breathing retraining is used by healthcare providers around the globe.[20] Participants in clinical stress reduction programs often report that "the breathing stuff" was the most important thing they learned.

Let's not forget that diaphragmatic breathing is also an ancient practice. Scientists and clinicians appropriated diaphragmatic breathing methods from India, where they have been used for thousands of years as part of religious and social customs. Diaphragmatic breathing is central to the practice of yoga. Yogis use long, deep inhalations and exhalations. The Buddhist form of meditation called anapanasati ("mindfulness of breathing") and the Hindu practice of pranayama ("control of breath") have both explicitly utilized the first two rules outlined above since antiquity. Yoga teachers in every tradition make it clear that the only way to control your mind is to cultivate control of your breath. These sages advocate that we never stop paying attention to it. Yogis who are masters of svarodaya, the yogic science of breathing, claim to be aware of every breath they take.

Diaphragmatic breathing has been around for thousands of years and may just be the most powerful tool in psychiatry, if not medicine as a whole. Why isn't it more mainstream? How did I finish a formal education in psychology and brain science without being introduced to it? I don't know for sure, but I think this is partly because it has never been taught correctly. Most existing breathing practices don't offer a systematic regimen to permanently increase the depth and duration of breathing. Consequently, they don't provide enough of a benefit to make a substantial difference for most people and, thus, are only used for extreme cases of anxiety. I believe the unique program outlined in this book is so powerful that it can provide substantial benefits for any user. Hopefully, by the end of this chapter, you will agree. Let us continue by looking more closely at each of the four rules.

Depth of Breath: Increase Your Tidal Range

The average adult human has a total lung capacity of five to six liters of air, but only a small part of this capacity is used during normal breathing. Nervous breathing will often involve inhalations of less than half a liter. We rarely breathe fully, and most of our breaths are confined to a narrow range. This range is called "tidal volume." When you increase your tidal volume, which is done by deliberately breathing all the way in and out, you increase your likelihood of accomplishing the other two criteria of longer interval and constant rate.

There is more than one way to deepen your in-breaths, but the exercise below is one of the most straightforward and reliable. It's based on the work of Joseph Pilates, who saw forced exhalation as the key to full inhalation. He advised his students to squeeze out their lungs as if they were tightly wringing a wet towel. Doing so improves the strength of your breathing musculature quite rapidly. Take advantage of this to increase your tidal range.

Breathing Exercise #3.1: *Deep Breaths*

Take five complete breaths. For each breath, inhale as much as you can and exhale as much as you can. To ensure that you are exhaling completely, purse your lips and blow on a fingertip, as you did in Chapter 1, until you can no longer feel your breath. Both the top and bottom of your exhalations will probably feel unfamiliar, stiff, and achy. Just one full evacuation of the lungs is often enough to kick-start diaphragmatic breathing because the resulting vacuum automatically pulls the diaphragm through its full, bottom-end range of motion.

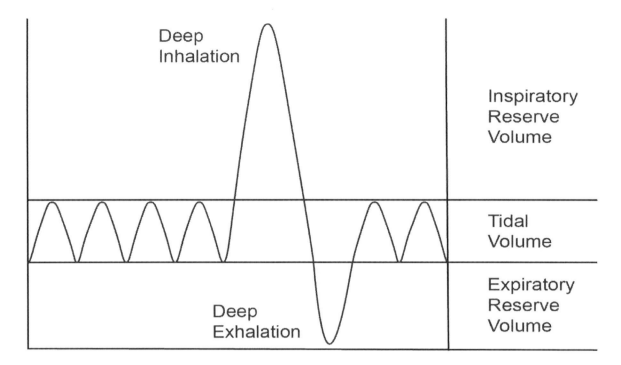

Figure 3.2: This graph shows a sine wave that indicates normal tidal volume. The increase on the fifth breath depicts a deep inhalation that extends the tidal range into the inspiratory reserve. This is followed by a deep exhalation extending the tidal range into the expiratory reserve. Regularly extending the tidal range in this way during breathing training will permanently broaden your default tidal volume and increase the involvement of the diaphragm.

Using an inspirometer while practicing Exercise 3.1 can be very helpful. An inspirometer, which you can purchase online for about ten dollars, is an instrument that allows you to keep track of exactly how much air you can breathe in (vital capacity). Using one consistently can be helpful to track your progress. You might consider monitoring your lung capacity for several weeks with an inspirometer, recording the results and watching your tidal range expand.

At first, it can feel uncomfortable when you breathe all the way in. You might cough. It might feel like your lungs are going to pop. It did for me. Within two months of performing Exercises 3.1 and 3.2, this all changed. There was nothing uncomfortable about being at either the top or bottom of my capacity, and it no longer made me cough. Before the training, it took me six seconds to inhale completely and about ten seconds to exhale completely. After training, it took me only one second to inhale completely and only five seconds to exhale completely. What is more, the maximum I could breathe in, as indicated by the inspirometer, went from 4,000 to 5,000 milliliters.

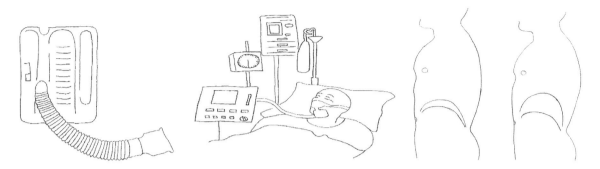

Illustration 3.4: A. Inspirometer or incentive spirometer; B. Patient on a medical respirator; C. Two chest views from the side depict a narrow diaphragmatic range versus a wide range.

The next activity will help you develop comfort while breathing outside of your normal tidal range. Focus on the uncomfortable sensations that arise. Try to reinterpret them as pleasurable. I try to associate the sensation of taking a full breath with satisfaction, satiety, and fulfillment as if each full breath offers relief and rejuvenating sustenance.

Breathing Exercise #3.2: *Breathe Outside Your Normal Range*

Start by taking a full breath in. Then, without pausing, resume breathing while remaining near the top of your lung capacity. In other words, allow yourself short, shallow exhalations but keep taking full breaths in, keeping your lungs full and your diaphragm expanded. Do this for ten breaths.

Then, do the opposite for another ten breaths. Breathe all your air out, then begin taking very shallow inhalations, alternating with full exhalations. This will force your breathing muscles to work outside of their normal tidal range, expanding into the reserve volumes and building a sense of comfort there.

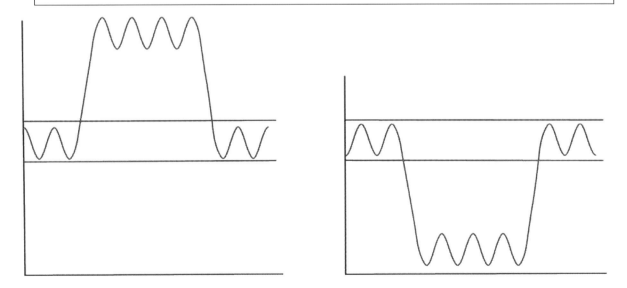

Figure 3.3: A. A graphical depiction of breathing above the normal tidal range for Breathing Exercise 2 above; B. A graph of breathing below the normal tidal range.

Length of Breath: Paced Breathing

The typical adult breathing pattern is marked by shallow thoracic breathing at a rate of 12 to 20 breaths per minute. Many people with anxiety average from 18 to 22, which means each inhalation and exhalation last only one and a half seconds. A breathing therapy technique called "paced breathing" will help you slow this down to a calmer and more grounded five to eight breaths per minute.

The goal of paced breathing is to extend your default habitual breathing rate. Imagine that you customarily breathe at a rate of twenty breaths per minute. If you practice paced breathing at a rate of five breaths per minute for several weeks, the exercise will gradually decrease your default rate from twenty down toward five. The more you practice, the closer your habitual breathing rate will come to the target rate.

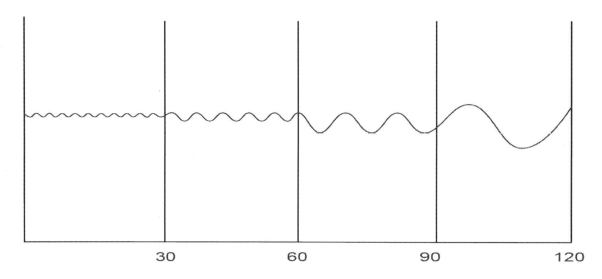

Figure 3.4: This graph displays a breathing rate of twenty breaths per minute during the first thirty seconds, then ten breaths per minute during the next thirty seconds, then six breaths per minute, then only two.

The sympathetic nervous system (fight or flight) exhibits reduced activity when a person takes fewer breaths per minute.[21] The correlation is direct and immediate. Increasing the number of breaths per minute causes sympathetic nervous system activity to spike, whereas decreasing this number causes it to plummet within one minute.[22] If you maintain a rate of five breaths per minute, heart rate and blood pressure drop, nervous sweating declines, and subjective discomfort in response to threat declines significantly.[23] There is no easier, faster way to reduce sympathetic activation and the stress it causes. I believe that the most effective intervention for life stress is paced breathing and that it should be used outside of the clinic— by everyone—on a daily basis.

I recommend using a breath metronome (sometimes called a breathing pacemaker) to aid you in pacing your breath. You can download one in the form of a mobile app for your phone or tablet. They generally cost between $1 and $5. All Apple watch users are prompted by the watch to use paced breathing daily. They are guided for one minute to take four breaths (around six-second inhalations and eight-second exhalations). This is a step in the right direction, but to retrain your breathing, it is necessary to spend several minutes per day consciously engaged in paced breathing.

I developed a free app that you can use, called Program Peace: Paced Breathing. It is available for Android and Apple's iOS. The app gives both audible and visual cues to help you time your breathing. It displays a cylinder that fills and empties in time with your target inhalation and exhalation rate. Alternatively, I offer free downloadable audio MP3 files with paced breathing cues on the Program Peace website. As another option, you can use the breath metronome videos on the Program Peace YouTube channel. My second favorite commercial app is called Breathe 2 Relax. It was developed by the U.S. Department of Defense for veterans and individuals with post-traumatic stress disorder (PTSD). Please take a minute to procure a breath metronome now.

Recommended Breath Metronomes:

1) Smartphone and tablet applications: Program Peace: Paced Breathing, Breathe2Relax, Breath Lesson, Breath Pacer, iBreathe, Breathwrk, Breathe Well, Breath Counter, Pranayama, BioBreathing, Calming Breath, Deep Breath, Essence, Tactical Breather.

2) Audio MP3 tracks: www.programpeace.com

3) Videos: The Program Peace channel on Youtube

It is very difficult to maintain paced breathing without using an external aid such as a breath metronome. In clinical studies of paced breathing, most participants quickly return to baseline in the absence of an external pacing signal.[24] You could use a clock or watch, or you could count the seconds in your head, but this quickly gets tiresome and can be extremely difficult to maintain, as it relies on unwavering focus. Unaided, most of us are unlikely to stick with paced breathing for more than a few seconds at a time. By contrast, using a breath metronome frees up your mind to attend to other things. You can do almost any activity with your breath metronome playing in the background. Having one—and familiarizing yourself with its use— is essential because the rest of this book's exercises will require that you use paced breathing.

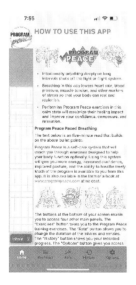 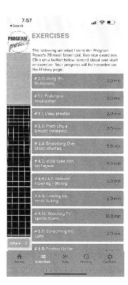 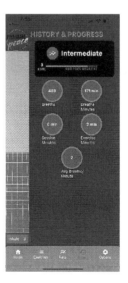 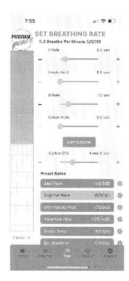

Figure 3.5: The Program Peace Paced Breathing app is free on both Apple and Android devices. It contains a breathing bar on the left side of the screen that rises on the inhalation and lowers on the exhalation.

The next step is to find a reduced "target" breathing rate that will help you slow and deepen your breath without overreaching. Try the rates in the table below for thirty seconds each until you find one that feels challenging but comfortable. For many people, the best starting point is four seconds in and six seconds out, for a total of six complete breaths per minute. This is an extremely healthy way to breathe. I want to encourage you to work up from here toward an ultimate goal of five breaths per minute, which is recommended by many experts.[25] It's fine if you want to stay higher or go lower. This standard of five breaths per minute varies slightly depending on size and age. For adults over six feet tall, the ideal rate is three to four breaths per minute, whereas for children under the age of ten it is between six and nine. Any extension of your breathing interval will be beneficial. Your goal should be to train yourself to breathe at your target rate without any sense of effort or air hunger. Be patient; this will take time. The practice should feel sustainable and good.

Inhalation (seconds)	Exhalation (seconds)	Breaths Per Minute
1	2	20
2	3	12
3	4	8
4	6	6
5	7	5
6	9	4
8	10	3.3
9	12	3
12	14	2.3
14	16	2

Table 3.1: List of Target Breathing Rates

Notice that in each row in the table above, the exhalation is longer than the inhalation. This is because when you breathe out longer than you breathe in, you activate the vagus nerve, the parasympathetic system, and the body's relaxation response.[26] The longer you can extend your exhalations, the more your autonomic nervous system will be pacified, and the more your heart will decelerate. To augment this calming effect, try to consciously relax during the exhalations. Think of every breath out as a long sigh of relief and the acceptance of a moment of peace. When you're ready to start, explore your ideal breathing pace by working through the activity below.

Breathing Activity #3.5: *Using a Breathing Metronome*

Use the chart above to find a breathing pace to work toward. If you aren't sure, 4x6 or 5x7 are good starting places for most beginners. Once you've chosen a rate, set your breath metronome accordingly and sit or lie comfortably. Follow the metronome's prompts.

Settle into a constant rate of inhalation that brings you to the top of your lung capacity at the moment just before the metronome switches to exhalation. As you breathe out, find a constant rate of exhalation that will allow you to reach near the bottom of your lung capacity just before the metronome switches back to the inhale.

Try working with the metronome for five minutes before a meeting or a date, and you will be amazed by your level of composure. Practice paced breathing for ten minutes in advance of an interview to give yourself a distinct advantage. At a party, excuse yourself for a few minutes. When you return, you will find your social equilibrium restored. It can help you relax your muscles after a workout, steady yourself after a stressful encounter, prepare for the day, or get to sleep.

Over the next few weeks, find opportunities to include the breath metronome in your daily routines. I often use it in the morning when I wake up, before I go to bed, while reading, while watching TV, while working at my desk, and during my commute. I don't use the mobile app when driving because pressing buttons on the phone can be distracting and dangerous. Instead, in the car, I listen to the breath metronome mp3s.

Whenever you are doing monotonous busywork or your attention is otherwise free to roam, you can be breathing with a metronome. Watching a movie is a chance for two hours of calming, grounding practice. It can enhance the experience, too—we usually breathe thoracically when we watch film and television because of the suspense and tension that it creates, but paced breathing will de-traumatize your psychological orientation toward even the most intense scenes. Put the metronome on silent and simply hold it in your lap or place it next to the TV, computer monitor, or tablet so that you can use it passively while you attend to other content.

Use it with headphones while walking, gardening, or in the gym. Let your use of it adapt to your routines. Regular use of a breath metronome will help you reestablish optimal breathing, and with it, an optimal life. I think that breath metronomes should be found in every classroom, in every workplace, in every therapist's office, in every yoga and Pilates studio, in every ambulance, and beside every hospital bed.

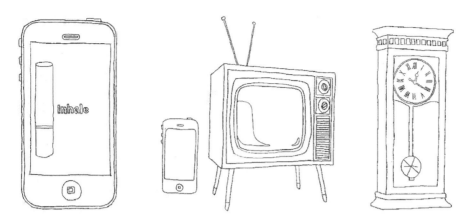

Illustration 3.5: A. Mobile phone with breath metronome application for paced breathing; B. Set your phone next to your television so that you can be cued to perform paced breathing while watching your favorite show; C. Grandfather clock with pendulum.

When you start, staying with the metronome can be tricky. If you have not yet filled or emptied the lungs before the metronome switches, go ahead and finish the breath that you are currently on. Quickly inhale or exhale the rest of the air before catching up with the metronome on the next breath. You may feel that you are getting too much air (hyperventilating) or not enough (hypoventilating). This is normal and will pass, but, if it bothers you, just choose a rate that is closer to your default. Work gradually toward a lower rate.

<u>To Avoid Getting Too Much or Too Little Air</u>

1) If you are getting too much air or feel dizzy during work with the metronome, simply breathe more slowly. You should be breathing at the same pace but inhaling less powerfully, filling the lungs a little less completely.

2) If you are getting too little air or feel faint, do just the opposite and increase the force of your in-breaths. Ensure that you breathe all the way in and all the way out. Sometimes, the metronome will be going too slowly, and you will feel air hunger. If you still feel air hunger, disregard the metronome and take a few deep breaths using whatever timing you need until you are ready to return to your target breathing rate.

Paced breathing involves a learning curve. At first, it takes a fair amount of attention to follow the metronome's cues and regulate the breath accordingly. After just a couple of hours of cumulative use, you will find that it takes almost no attention at all. This will encourage you to do it more often and allow you to combine it with numerous activities. If you're having trouble settling on a breathing rate that feels comfortable, use the table below as a rough guide. It lays out estimated breathing rates for what your target pace should be under different conditions and cardiovascular demands.

Beginner User	Experienced User	Advanced User	Inhalation Time	Exhalation Time	Breaths per Minute
Jogging	NA	NA	1	2	20
Light Exercise	Jogging	NA	2	3	12
Weights/ Walking	Light Exercise	Jogging	3	4	8
Standing	Weights/ Walking	Light Exercise	4	6	6
Sitting	Standing	Weights/ Walking	5	7	5
Lying Down	Sitting	Standing	6	9	4
NA	Lying Down	Sitting	8	10	3.3
NA	NA	Sitting	9	12	3
NA	NA	Sitting/ Relaxing	12	14	2.3
NA	NA	Lying Down	14	16	2

Table 3.2: Comfortable Breathing Rates by Experience and Level of Physical Activity

When Not Using a Breath Metronome:

1) Try to focus on your breathing frequently throughout the day, monitoring it and deciding whether it is too shallow or too fast. If so, consciously deepen your breath.

2) Catch yourself preparing to switch prematurely from breathing in to breathing out (or vice versa) before you have taken a full breath. Instead of switching, prolong the tail end of the breath in which you are currently engaged.

Advanced paced breathing at a rate of fewer than four breaths per minute can be powerfully relaxing. I should point out that it is not a comfortable or realistic default breathing rate, but training at this rate will help improve your default rate and train smooth breathing, which is the topic of the next section.

Smoothness of Breath: Breathing at a Constant Speed

The third element of healthy diaphragmatic breathing is the smoothness of your breath. This is a question of how fluidly you breathe, and it ties together the previous two elements of your practice. Paced breathing and deep breathing can still allow for too much variability on a moment-to-moment basis. This is where the flow rate of each in-breath and out-breath becomes important.

For instance, at the beginning of my practice, about halfway through each five-second inhalation, the speed of my breath would drop, leaving the second half of the inhalation weaker. After this lapse, I would try to make up for it at the very end of the five seconds by gasping. I was being lazy, holding my breath mid-count to get out of doing the work of strengthening the diaphragm. Instead, we should try to breathe at the same rate throughout each breath to keep the diaphragm engaged. This involves breathing slowly, gently, and steadily.

The biggest barrier to smooth breathing is our tendency to switch from diaphragmatic to thoracic inhalation when you near the top of your tidal range. Every inhalation begins with the diaphragm, but once using the diaphragm outside of its default range, we transition to a swift thoracic inhalation to draw in that last bit of air. Resist this instinct. Instead, try to get to the top of your inspiratory reserve using only the diaphragm by breathing slowly and gradually. Do the exercise below to practice using your diaphragm throughout the entire inhalation.

Breathing Exercise #3.3: *Practicing a Smooth Inhalation*

Exhale completely. Then, inhale as slowly as possible. Try to make the inhale last for at least eight seconds but aim for 15 to 60. Notice how this feels. It should feel natural and normal for the first few seconds until your lungs expand beyond your usual tidal range. Maintaining a slow and constant inhalation rate will become more uncomfortable as you reach the top of your tidal range. Notice the urge to switch to an abrupt thoracic gasp and resist it. Continue to inhale slowly and steadily. Take ten nonconsecutive inhalations in this way.

You experienced the impulse to switch to a rapid thoracic inhalation in the exercise above because your diaphragm is not accustomed to providing steady suction for a breath outside its normal tidal range. I think of this weakness as a diaphragmatic speedbump at the end of the diaphragm's habitual path. Forcing smooth inhalations steadily past this range will rehabilitate the muscular knot in your diaphragm responsible for this speedbump. It will also accustom your nervous system to utilizing the diaphragm more fully. Breaking down this restriction that limits your diaphragm's range of motion is unique to the Program Peace system yet integral to diaphragmatic retraining.

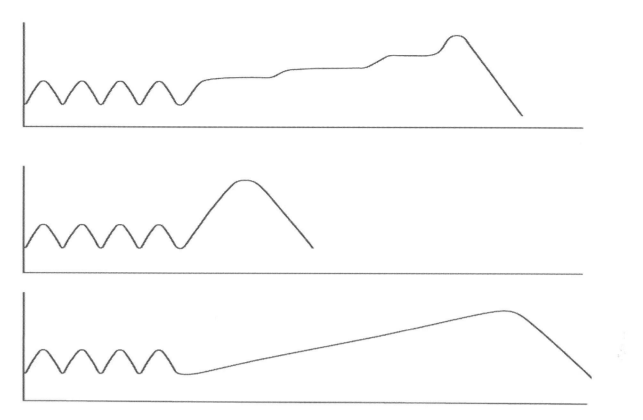

Figure 3.5: A. Each of the three graphs starts with four shallow breaths for comparison. In the first graph, the fifth inhalation is deep and long. However, the inhalation does not occur at a constant rate (the slope of the line varies). As you can see, it plateaus three times and ends with a gasp. This person is gasping and breath holding because they are uncomfortable breathing above their normal diaphragmatic range; B. The fifth inhalation in the second diagram is also very deep. However, it is short in duration, so it is basically a thoracic gasp (the line's slope is very high); C. The fifth inhalation in the third diagram shows the optimal breathing pattern of a long, deep inhalation at a steady rate (with a constant slope).

As you practice, keep your flow rate steady by imagining yourself smelling a rose, inhaling very slowly as you savor its fragrance. Or imagine that you are curled up with a small pet. Make your breathing as smooth and calm as possible to soothe it gently to sleep. Realize that hasty, quivering, jerky breaths would likely rouse and frighten it. It is interesting to note that when a cat purrs, its breathing is slow, even, and powered by the diaphragm.[27] Above, I recommended that you invest ten dollars in an inspirometer to monitor the depth of your breathing. If you do so, purchase one with a flow rate indicator. This will provide real-time feedback on how steady and smooth your breathing is.

Another option is to buy yourself a stethoscope to listen to your breathing. You can find these for around $15 online. When you put the "bell" of the stethoscope up to your mouth, you can hear tiny distortions and discontinuities in the breath—desperate little gasps. These gasps are more noticeable when you are self-doubting and are sometimes described as "fluttering" or "catches" in the breath. It sounds a bit like the voice when it "cracks." While listening to these distortions in my breath, it became clear to me that breathing, especially breathing deeply, is a struggle. It doesn't have to be.

The more slowly and fully you breathe outside of your tidal range, the more you can hear and feel these points of weakness in the breath. The technical term for them is *apneic disturbances*, and they usually last for tiny fractions of a second. They are such a basic feature of most people's breathing that they seem natural and normal, but they are suboptimal without a doubt. These disturbances are caused by weakness in the diaphragm and correspond to absences in its range of motion. They are linked to the startle response and keep you feeling on edge. As the next activity shows, you do not need a stethoscope to hear these.

Breathing Exercise #3.4: *Smoothing Over Discontinuities*

Cup both hands between your mouth and ear, creating a bridge for the sound of your breath. Your breath should sound louder, and the discontinuities in it should be more apparent. Listen for brief cessations or unevenness in the sound. Once you notice them, concentrate on modulating your breathing so that these disturbances disappear, making the breath perfectly smooth and even. The ribcage and stomach should be expanding evenly as well. Do not let the rate of your inhalation change. Each second, you should be taking in the same volume of air. Imagine that you are playing a single note on a trumpet and carefully keeping its volume steady. Try your best to ensure that the sound made is smooth, even, and progresses at a constant rate.

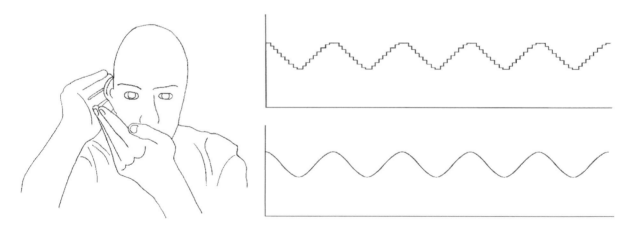

Illustration 3.6: Person cupping their hands from mouth to ear to amplify the sound of the breath; B. Depiction of a discontinuous, rough breath compared to a continuous, smooth breath.

Buddhist and Hindu practices emphasize breathing through the nose and down the back of the throat. Many meditators concentrate on the "ha" or "so" sound this produces. Creating an even sound throughout each breath will ensure that the breath is being taken in at an even rate. To do this, focus on maintaining the same sound from the beginning of each inhalation/exhalation to the end. You know you are breathing diaphragmatically if the sound of your breath is not changing. Other ways to make sounds that you can monitor for constancy include breathing as if you are fogging up glass, making a hissing sound with your tongue, a "haaaa" sound with your voice, a buzzing sound with your throat, or a glottal sound with your vocal folds. Many meditators use mantras to accomplish this. Using a stethoscope, cupping your hands, or making a sound of some kind all accomplish the same thing. So, perform Exercise 3.4 using any of these methods.

I was concerned the first time I heard my breath amplified by a stethoscope because I immediately recognized that these irregular pauses and gasps were unhealthy. The irregular pauses are magnified by adversity and are responsible for the sensation of respiratory distress. Breathing is strained whenever a single inhalation pauses, slows, or speeds up. When someone is stressed, you can often hear them straining for more breath, as multiple rapid gasps or shudders will punctuate the inhalation. The gasps occur when one is continuing to inhale despite their body's inclination to "switch" to exhalation. The weakness in the breath tells us to stop taking a full inhalation and go back to exhaling prematurely. This is the same mechanism that causes us to breathe shallowly, and that creates the diaphragmatic speedbump. This phenomenon of fighting against oneself for breath is sometimes called *paradoxical breathing*.

We are constantly modulating the rate of each breath from second to second, depending on our level of air hunger and transient stress. We may alter the rate of a single breath many times. This is not ideal. Tell yourself that you will stick with the same rate for the entirety of each breath. If you need to change the rate because you need more air, change at the beginning of the next inhalation or exhalation, but not during an actual breath. One helpful way to assist you in this is through breathing exclusively through the nose, which we will discuss in Chapter 11.

Imagine that your breath is an accordion that you have spent your life thrusting and thrashing in a distraught, feverish way. Imagine now playing the accordion by moving your hands very slowly and continuously stretching the accordion out to its full length and then gently pressing it closed, over and over.

People who perform intricate manual work, or marksmen who shoot targets, find that holding the breath helps steady the hands. Once you reprogram your breath to be continuous and smooth, breath-holding is no longer necessary to keep you from shaking. As you paint an eyebrow on that tiny face on your canvass or take aim at a distant target, you will find yourself smoothing out your breath rather than holding it.

Distressed breathing progresses like an automobile that is alternating between stalling and redlining. You want your breathing to be like a reliable car, engine purring, on a smoothly paved freeway, with the cruise control on.

Breathe Assertively

So far, we have covered methods for breathing smoothly, deeply, and at longer intervals. The fourth rule is to breathe assertively. We usually breathe as if we don't have any faith in our breath. A thoracic breather knows that a negative thought could interrupt the breath at any time by prematurely turning an exhalation into an inhalation or vice versa. This causes them to breathe not only shallowly but cautiously and hesitantly as if they are tiptoeing. It also keeps them from breathing efficiently because they are not taking advantage of inertia. If a breath proceeds steadily, it can capture its own momentum, resulting in reduced effort. During hesitant, unsteady breath, the breathing musculature is constantly building and then losing momentum.

Model your breathing on the motion of a pendulum or some other uninterrupted, inevitable oscillating process. Something that moves with certainty. Each stroke of a pendulum fully captures its momentum until gravity reverses the swing. Any pendulum would be useless if it slowed or stopped midway. Picture your diaphragm stroking up and down in a slow but unfaltering, unagitated way. Breathe out with certain knowledge that you are not going to switch prematurely to a gasp. Commit to each breath steadfastly.

To feel comfortable breathing with confidence, you will need to be willing to let the people around you hear your breath. You must not be afraid of being heard or noticed. Instead, be proud of how your breath does not waver, falter, or hesitate. Don't think that people will hear it and be offended. Breathe decisively and audibly if necessary, for all to hear. Breathing assertively is the demonstration of true aplomb. Start by using your imagination.

Breathing Exercise #3.5: *Uninterrupted Inhalation*

Take a deep, long, smooth breath all the way in. Make the inhalation last as long as you comfortably can, preferably from five to 20 seconds. Do this eight times, imagining each of the distress-provoking scenarios below in turn. As you do this, don't let the upsetting aspects of the scenario interrupt or cause discontinuity in your inhalation.

1) Someone says something to offend you.
2) You realize you forgot your phone.
3) You notice you misplaced your wallet.
4) You pass by a stranger while walking down the street.
5) You hear a car backfiring or an ear-piercing siren.
6) You notice someone looking at you out of the corner of your eye.
7) You tell someone what you expect of them.
8) You are rudely awakened by a loud alarm.

Many people who are widely admired and described as charismatic are merely assertive breathers. The self-taught dog behaviorist, Cesar Millan, is one such person. He is widely known for his *Dog Whisperer* television series, in which he works with aggressive and abused dogs. In 2009, *The New York Times* attributed his success to his sense of equanimity, describing this as, "a sort of uber-balanced mien."[28] Millan calls it "calm-assertive energy" and says that he approaches dogs as a pack leader.[29]

There is good reason to believe that Millan's effect on dogs derives from his breathing. Throughout the episodes of his TV series, his breathing remains calm, constant, and resolute despite repeated problematic encounters with both the dogs and their owners. Cesar Millan and people like him have an autonomous breathing pattern that is not susceptible to being stopped short by the behavior or misbehavior of others. Dogs are in tune with how the status hierarchy is conveyed through breathing. I think the dogs know there is nothing they can do to disturb his breathing, so they listen to and respect him. Millan's techniques work as well on abused and subordinated dogs as on aggressive and intractable ones.

Respiratory rates, and fluctuations in them, constitute a language that all mammals speak. Try sitting near your cat or dog, breathing calmly, and then suddenly switch to short, quick, loud breaths. The animal will become concerned, appear nervous, and adopt your breathing pattern.

If, instead, you breathe slowly and deeply, they are likely to relax, yawn, and start stretching. If you breathe slowly and deeply while training or correcting them, they will heed you.

Health practitioners often need to assess their patients' respiratory rate, the number of breaths (inhalation-exhalation cycles) taken within 60 seconds. The method a doctor or clinician uses to measure the respiratory rate of a child, an animal, or an adult can affect the measurement. Simply handling an animal will increase its respiratory rate, giving a false reading, unless the animal is handled very gently, in which case its respiratory rate may fall. Using a cold stethoscope to measure respiratory rate in a child will increase their respiratory rate, whereas other less "obtrusive" methods (like counting the number of times the chest rises) may not.

Clinical texts refer to the "invasiveness" of different methodological procedures for assessing respiration. A doctor that acts either domineering or too accommodating can raise it. Different aspects of our environment are constantly "invading" our respiratory dynamics. Don't allow your breathing rate or depth to be dictated by banal occurrences in your environment. Confidence starts with assertive, uninterruptable breathing.

The Connection Between the Breath and the Mind

Feelings of pain and frustration are compounded by shallow breathing. Pride, vanity, and guilt are also ramped up by distressed breathing, and I will focus on these relationships in later chapters. Shortness of breath makes us feel like we are suffocating. In such a state, we can't help but think negative thoughts. Once you have internalized the four rules and are breathing deeply, smoothly, and at long intervals, it will become clear to you that the mental bondage chaining us to our ego and the social hierarchy is severed when breathing diaphragmatically.

The discomfort from shallow breathing magnifies many addictive behaviors by making us feel desperation. Our breathing becomes shallower when we are hungry, thereby strengthening our cravings for food. People use the phrase "I'm starving" when they notice that their hunger is affecting their breathing. Similarly, many people turn to cigarettes, alcohol, and anger when they feel their breathing affected by unfavorable life circumstances. When people use drugs to change their emotional state, they are really changing the state of their breathing.

One can transform disordered breathing into quasi-healthy breathing in minutes using barbiturates, sedatives, or opiates. However, that effect is short-lived, and the inevitable withdrawal symptoms actually accentuate disordered breathing. By contrast, metronome-aided paced breathing kicks in faster than drugs or alcohol and makes you a stronger person rather than a weaker one. Over time, expect paced breathing to vastly increase your distress tolerance and your capacity for emotional regulation.

After I started practicing paced breathing, I experienced a process of self-re-creation. At the end of this process, I had a new aura, a new persona, and a new relationship with others. The change within me elicited a different set of reactions from the people I encountered. Strangers initiated pleasant conversations with me. Individuals in crowded, public spaces were polite and, at times, even kind. I was more easily accepted in groups and committees. I found that children and animals approached me without hesitation. However, it made some adult males uncomfortable. People who are competitive with you may assume at first glance that your undaunted breathing pattern is a façade. But, even after a brief interaction, they will realize you are not faking it.

You can't feign the poise made possible by diaphragmatic retraining. Distressed breathing, on the other hand, is a signal to predators that you are in panic mode. When someone "smells fear," they are actually sensing distressed breathing. It tempts bullies to close in for the kill and tends to intensify arguments into fights. Diaphragmatic breathing does the opposite by broadcasting assertive, noncombative calm. Diaphragmatic breathing safeguards you from violence, whereas thoracic breathing invites it.

Many people only breathe easy in social situations in which they are with someone they feel they can patronize and talk down to. We should be breathing easy no matter who we are with. What people think about you, how they are judging you, and their current level of displeasure should not be a factor in the equation that determines your ease of breathing. I used to try to breathe more shallowly than everyone else around me to be polite. This quickly becomes dangerous to your health. You may not feel comfortable with how secure you appear to others when you breathe slowly and diaphragmatically. You may feel there is incongruence between it and your level of attractiveness, strength, or socioeconomic status. I'm writing to promulgate the idea that there is never incongruity among these things.

A part of us is afraid that breathing calmly around others is the ultimate insult. We are afraid that the other person will become angry if s/he sees us breathing too deeply. We breathe the most shallowly around the most dominant people in our lives. This is partly because when we breathe deeply, our emotional reactivity decreases and our facial response time is delayed. Our faces become calmer and may appear less attentive. You might feel that this makes you look distant or disconnected.

You will notice that you breathe at long intervals during a conversation, that your face goes blank and non-expressive. We need to get over the fear that someone will see us and think that we look too calm. As Chapter 7 will discuss, there should be no such thing as looking too calm. The best way to train this is to try to retain diaphragmatic breathing during all social encounters. It will become sincere with practice. Don't let outside influences or internal fears about them perturb your optimal breathing pattern.

Breathe Diaphragmatically in Public

Diaphragmatic breathing in public is truly transformative. When you first try it, it will reveal your tendencies for agoraphobia and social anxiety. Within a few minutes, you will start to overcome them. Here's what to do. Take your breathing app with you to a restaurant, coffee shop, café, picnic table, or bench in the park. Then, using headphones, listen to your breath metronome's auditory breathing cues to practice paced breathing. You will gradually feel yourself letting go of social uneasiness. As this new attitude becomes your default, you will lose your apprehension about potentially negative social outcomes, making your outward appearance more assertive and less defensive. Other people will see in your face that you are not afraid. You will start to appraise the vast majority of people as harmless. Instead of being a potential assailant or judgmental critic, each person will become just another face.

> **Breathing Exercise #3.6:** *Diaphragmatic Breathing in Public*
>
> Use your breathing metronome or paced breathing app in a public place (with headphones if necessary). Good options include parks, libraries, malls, and the block you live on. If you are moving, notice how you feel obliged to shorten your breaths when you

> pass by someone. If you are seated, notice the same when they approach you. In either case, resist the instinct and continue paced breathing. Notice how you feel like other people are judging you for being "too calm" and realize how ridiculous that is. Alternatively, try recruiting a friend to paced breathe with you.

Breathe Diaphragmatically While Speaking

Once you've become familiar with breathing diaphragmatically in public, try it in conversation. This is more difficult. Many of us become short of breath during social encounters, especially when public speaking. I used to fully inhibit my diaphragm as soon as I began speaking. At first, I tried workarounds, like taking intermittent breaks from conversation to regain my composure. But that was socially disruptive. What you want is to learn to breathe deeply and diaphragmatically while speaking. This isn't easy because you must formulate what you want to say and simultaneously focus on monitoring your breath.

The best way to start is to read aloud while breathing diaphragmatically. It will likely be uncomfortable at first because we all normally speak within a very narrow tidal range. The trick to calming your speech is to prolong your speaking time and ensure that anxious gasps do not punctuate it. The following exercise will guide you through the process (note that it does not use a breath metronome).

Breathing Exercise #3.7: *Diaphragmatic Speech*

Sit down with a good book. Take a slow, full breath in and then start to read aloud. Keep reading until you have no breath left to exhale. Pause as you breathe in for five to ten seconds, and then resume reading. Repeat this cycle for five minutes or for as long as you like. To do this, you have to stop reading out loud for several seconds during the inhalations—do so patiently. You should find that you inhale for somewhere between five and 10 seconds and that you speak/exhale for between six and 20 seconds. Try to keep your voice at the same volume and pitch even when you approach the end of your exhalation. It helps to speak in a calm, friendly voice. If you speak loudly and deeply while doing this activity, your voice will become louder and deeper with time. This exercise will make your extemporaneous speech balanced and collected.

Find your limit—how long you can read without inhaling—and then repeat that level of performance over and over. To determine where that limit is, try reading the remainder of this paragraph without breathing in. Continue until you cannot possibly speak another word. There should be a few seconds at the end where your voice changes appreciably and it becomes very uncomfortable to speak. Your voice will begin to waver and lurch. You will sound like someone in extreme respiratory distress, and it may even start to feel like you just got punched in the chest. If you work on Exercise 3.7 in this manner for only a few minutes every day, you will, in short order, alleviate this impediment and any related discomfort.

Breathe Diaphragmatically During Exercise

Another effective way to strengthen your diaphragm is to pair diaphragmatic breathing with a cardiovascular workout. Try taking a short jog, focusing on the sensations you feel when alternating between inhalations and exhalations. You are likely alternating far too quickly. Try blowing nearly all the way out and breathing nearly all the way in with each breath. This can feel uncomfortable but is extremely healthful.

Ironically, many people breathe shallowly while exercising because they are concerned they will not get enough air if they breathe too deeply. The sensation of elevated heart rate makes you want to take tiny breaths. Ignore the panic signals from your heart and ensure that you breathe in and out near full capacity. As long as you are breathing heavily, you are getting plenty of oxygen. When you persist in an exhalation, even when you feel your heart beating hard in your chest, you are restructuring your unhealthy breathing patterns and breaking through the trauma that underlies them. Don't bother using your breathing metronome during cardio, just make sure you are taking full breaths. Use the next exercise to get you going.

Breathing Exercise #3.8: *Diaphragmatic Jogging*

Take a light jog, well within your comfortable limits for cardiovascular exercise. As you run, begin extending your inhalations and exhalations. Focus on the effort involved in doing so and on the accompanying sensations. Instead of panting at a rate of multiple inhalations per second, try to breathe in for one to three seconds, and then breathe out for two to four seconds. Once you get a feel for it, use this technique for all forms of aerobic and anaerobic exercise.

Breathe Diaphragmatically While Eating

There's one other daily activity that deserves specific attention. It is surprisingly difficult to follow a breath metronome while eating a meal. Attempting it makes us aware of just how entangled our appetitive drives are with distressed breathing. The first time I tried it, I realized that distressed breathing had created a starving, ravenous creature inside of me. The activity below offers a puzzlingly difficult challenge that should pique your interest in the benefits of diaphragmatic breathing. The last two activities do not require the use of a breath metronome, but this activity, like most of the activities in this program, is greatly improved by using one.

Breathing Exercise #3.9: *Diaphragmatic Eating*

Set your breath metronome at your preferred rate. Find space by yourself and set your meal in front of you. Start paced breathing. Attempt to slowly consume the entire meal while breathing at your pre-set rate. Notice how aspects of the biting, chewing, and swallowing are frenzied. Slow everything down and pay attention to how your body responds. This may be frustrating because you are accustomed to shallow, short-interval breathing while eating. After a few meals, though, it will start to feel normal.

Generalizing Diaphragmatic Breathing

For many people, distressed breathing is pervasive and affects every aspect of daily life. This book aims to help you develop just the opposite: an ingrained habit for deep, diaphragmatic breathing that you practice every waking moment. As Chapter 1 explained, this new habit will desensitize your stress system by pairing experiences that are normally stressful (and linked to thoracic breathing) with diaphragmatic breathing instead.

I was partially inspired to create a system based on this concept by my experiences in the yoga studio. Hatha yoga revolves around yoking various stretches and poses with calm breathing. Since developing the present program, I have found that this concept is not even new in the clinical arena. It is a little-known technique called "generalization of diaphragmatic breathing."

Some therapists use diaphragmatic generalization to help clients associate peaceful breathing with distressing thoughts and other activities such as standing, sitting, and walking. Forming those associations ensures that proper breathing predominates in most life situations.[30] Yoking relaxed breathing to various activities in this way can be considered a form of systematic desensitization.

Systematic desensitization is a psychological method used to help people overcome phobias and anxieties. It is a popular form of exposure therapy that uses counter-conditioning (a Pavlovian process) developed by South African psychiatrist Joseph Wolpe. The idea is simple:

If the source of the person's anxiety is discovered (i.e., spiders), the person is trained in relaxation techniques (i.e., reappraisal, breathing, and muscle relaxation exercises) and then guided to use these techniques while they are exposed to increasing levels of fear-inducing stimuli. They might progress from talking about spiders to looking at pictures of spiders, then to videos of spiders, and finally to holding real spiders. Their fear of spiders is thus brought to extinction by gradual exposure. This cognitive-behavioral therapy technique is considered one of the most effective in clinical psychology today.[31] It is used to help people become comfortable with all kinds of stressors, including things like elevators, dogs, knives, and public speaking.

As the last three exercises have illustrated, you can apply the same principle to the simplest of behaviors. If you can maintain diaphragmatic breathing while you gradually and systematically perform actions that would normally increase your breathing rate, you can habituate to these stressors and reprogram the way your breathing system relates to them. Taking this a step further, you can even desensitize yourself to your attempts at assuming dominant or optimal postures that would normally cause you to breathe shallowly.

The rest of this book's exercises are intended to be performed with paced diaphragmatic breathing, guided by a breath metronome. This is done to make every nonsubmissive posture a safe and fun "place to be." Having spent more than ten years pairing hundreds of different activities with diaphragmatic breathing, I am sharing the ones that benefited my clients and me the most. Below is the fundamental diaphragmatic breathing exercise that I would like you to combine with every other exercise and activity in the remainder of this book (please note that Exercise 1.1 from Chapter 1 can be used as an alternative to breathing with a metronome).

Breathing Exercise #3.10: *Paced Breathing to Combine with Exercises*

Set your breathing metronome to your target breathing rate, which for most people should be at least four seconds in and six seconds out. Follow the metronome's prompts. Breathe deep, full breaths. If you can, breathe through your nose. Breathe slowly, smoothly, and at a steady rate. Breathe assertively.

Here's a way to quickly and easily get a sense of just how powerful generalized diaphragmatic breathing can be. I am going to ask you to do a deep backbend without paced breathing, and then again with it. Lie down on your stomach on a carpet, bed, or soft surface. Then, use your arms to lift your torso off the ground while your legs and hips lie flat, performing a gentle "upward dog" pose. Notice how shallow and irregular your breathing becomes when you do a backbend? Lie back down and imagine what it would take for you to improve your upward dog. Lots of time and effort, right? Years of yoga training? Not quite.

Spend five minutes practicing the paced breathing method in Exercise 3.10 above. Now, try the upward dog again. The position should be easier to hold and less stressful to perform. Your back should feel supported and safe, rather than exposed and vulnerable, and you should have a sense that you are stretching and strengthening your lower back rather than straining it. The reason this works so well is that diaphragmatic breathing affects muscles directly. Chapter 5 will address how distressed breathing makes muscles throughout your body close down with tension, while diaphragmatic breathing makes them receptive to being toned.

Every time you repeat a breathing exercise, you make innumerable cellular and molecular improvements to the function of your muscular, nervous, and respiratory systems. These beneficial alterations accumulate. As a bonus, all the mental work involved in learning to incorporate the diaphragm into your breathing is saved to procedural memory—in other words, routinized—which makes diaphragmatic breathing easier in the future.

Conclusion

After six months of paced breathing, I decided to try belly breathing again. This is the activity in which one places a hand on the chest and another on the abdomen to check for natural movement of the stomach with breathing (outlined in Activity 3.2 in this chapter). Before I started, there was nothing I could do to use my breath to raise my abdomen. Only half a year later, my abdomen rose and fell on its own with every breath. To get your diaphragm back in the groove, work toward the following goals:

1) Belly breathing: once you've been pace breathing for a few months, every breath should move your belly.
2) Aim to iron out all the apneic disturbances in your breath by breathing right through them, slowly and smoothly.
3) You want deep inhalations and exhalations that reach the very end of their range to feel comfortable.
4) Work toward increasing the target breathing rate you picked for yourself earlier in this chapter.

Your goal should be to progress to the point where you are training somewhere in the vicinity of five breaths per minute (5x7). Once you have trained here comfortably for around a dozen hours, you will be belly breathing. Spending time practicing at a much lower rate, such as 10x12, is slower than optimal for everyday breathing but amounts to a form of cross-training that will help strengthen you overall.

To accomplish these goals as quickly and efficiently as possible, I recommend spending at least 20 minutes each day practicing paced breathing with a breath metronome. That may sound like a lot, but it is easy. You can do it while you watch TV. In the coming chapters, we will talk a lot more about the breath and introduce four more tenets of optimal breathing.
In Chapter 11, we will return to the material from this chapter and view it from the perspective of hyperventilation and nasal breathing. In the next chapter, though, let's put what you have learned about paced breathing to work and pair it with exercises intended to rehabilitate the windows to the soul: the eyes.

Chapter 3: **Bullet Points**

- The brain's fear and grief circuits are tied to distressed breathing. They inhibit the diaphragm, causing breathing to become rapid and shallow.
- The more traumatized a mammal is, the less its diaphragm moves with each breath. The animal instead recruits other muscles to power breathing and the diaphragm atrophies.
- Disuse due to stress reduces the diaphragm's range of motion and causes it to become stiff.
- Most people breathe in a narrow diaphragmatic range. This range narrows further as stress increases. You want to expand your diaphragm's range of motion by breathing more deeply.
- To engage the diaphragm fully, follow these four rules: (1) breathe deeply, (2) breathe at long intervals, (3) breathe smoothly, and (4) breathe assertively.
- Breathing slowly, deeply, and smoothly forces the diaphragm to contract evenly, increasing diaphragmatic strength, coordination, and range of motion.
- It is common for people with anxiety to have inhalations that merely last one second and exhalations that last only two seconds.
- To rehabilitate our breath, we should practice breathing at least three seconds in and five seconds out (3x5). To make this your default breathing rate, it helps to practice breathing at even longer intervals. Performing paced breathing at 5x7 and working toward 10x12 will accomplish this.
- Weakness in the diaphragm is apparent in the form of tiny gasps or unevenness in the breath, called apneic disturbances, which are associated with the startle response.
- You can iron out apneic disturbances by breathing smoothly at a slow and even rate.
- Breathing assertively involves making sure that social concerns do not interfere with the first three rules. You want to breathe deeply, smoothly, and at long intervals while you are socializing.
- Using a breath metronome daily is essential to developing a strong diaphragmatic breathing habit because it will allow you to train yourself to follow the four rules while you focus on other tasks and activities.
- Monitor your breathing carefully during conversations; don't let it become shallow.
- Your breath should be a tiny but continuous sip of air that never pauses and always proceeds at a steady rate.

Program Peace: *Paced Breathing Session Tracker*

Starting Date: _____   Ending Date: _____

You can use this page by placing a check inside each box after you complete five minutes of paced breathing. There are 120 boxes for a total of 600 minutes. This equates to two, five-minute sessions a day, five times per week for 12 weeks. Once you have checked every box you will have completed the goal outlined in Exercise 3.10 and should be well on your way with diaphragmatic retraining.

Chapter 3: **Endnotes**

1.   Meuret, A. E., & Ritz, T. (2010). Hyperventilation in panic disorder and asthma: Empirical evidence and clinical strategies. *International Journal Psychophysiology.* 78(1), 68–79; Lum, L. C. (1987). Hyperventilation syndromes in medicine and psychiatry: A review. *Journal of the Royal Society of Medicine.* 80(4), 229–231.

2.   Ravinder, J., Crawford, M., Barnes, V. A., & Harden, K. (2015). Self-regulation of breathing as a primary treatment for anxiety. *Applied Psychophysiological Biofeedback, 40*(2), 107–115.

3.   Hamasaki, H. (2020). Effects of diaphragmatic breathing on health: A narrative review. *Medicines* (Basel), *7*(10), 65.

4.   Lippincott, W. & Wilkins (2006). *Stedman's medical dictionary* (28th ed). Julie K. Stegman.

5.   Farhi, D. (1996). *The breathing book: Good health and vitality through essential breath work.* Henry Holt.

6.   Ford, G. T., Whitelaw, W. A., Rosenal, T. W., Cruse, P. J., & Guenter, C. A. (1983). Diaphragm function after upper abdominal surgery in humans. *The American Review of Respiratory Disease, 127*(4), 431–6.

7.   McConville, J. F., & Kress, J. P. (2012). Weaning patients from the ventilator. *New England Journal of Medicine, 367*(23), 2233–2239.

8.   Levine, S., Nguyen, T., Taylor, N., Friscia, M. E., Budak, M. T., Rothenberg, P., Zhu, J., Sachdeva, R., Sonnad, S., Kaiser, L. R., Rubinstein, N. A., Powers, S. K., & Shrager, J. B. (2008). Rapid disuse atrophy of diaphragm fibers in mechanically ventilated humans. *New England Journal of Medicine, 358*(13), 1327–35.

9.   Peper, E. & Tibbetts, V. (1994). Effortless diaphragmatic breathing. *Physical Therapy Products. 6*(2), 67–71.

10. Elliot, S., & Edmonson, D. (2008) *Coherent breathing: The definitive method, theory, and practice.* Coherence Press.

11. Olsson, A. (2014). *The power of your breath. The secret key to reshaping your looks, your body, your health, and your weight.* Anders Olsson.

12. Gevirtz, R. N., & Schwartz, M. S. (2003). The respiratory system in applied psychophysiology. In M. S. Schwartz & F. Andrasik (Eds.), *Biofeedback: A practitioners guide* (3rd ed., pp. 212–244). The Guilford Press.

13. Hazlett-Stevens, H., & Craske, M. G. (2009). Breathing retraining and diaphragmatic breathing techniques. In W. T. O'Donohue & J. Fisher (Eds.), *General principles and empirically supported techniques of cognitive behavior therapy* (pp. 166–172. John Wiley & Sons.

14. Hopper, S. I., Murray, S. L., Ferrara, L. R., & Singleton, J. K. (2018). Effectiveness of diaphragmatic breathing on physiological and psychological stress in adults: A quantitative systematic review protocol. *JBI Database of Systematic Reviews and Implementation Reports*, *16*(6), 1367–1372.

15. Gervitz & Schwartz, 2003, The respiratory system in applied psychophysiology.

16. McGeary, C. A., Swanholm, E., Gatchel, R. J. (2014) *Pain management. The encyclopedia of clinical psychology*. John Wiley & Sons.

17. Stromberg, S. E., Russell, M. E., & Carlson, C. R. (2015). Diaphragmatic breathing and its effectiveness for the management of motion sickness. *Aerospace Medicine and Human Performance*, *86*(5), 452–457.

18. Borge, C. R., Mengshoel, A. M., Omenaas, E., Moum, T., Ekman, I., Lein, M. P., Mack, U., & Wahl, A. K. (2015). Effects on guided deep breathing on breathlessness and the breathing pattern in chronic obstructive pulmonary disease: A double-blind randomized control study. *Patient Education and Counseling*, *98*(2), 182–190.

19. Vranceanu, A., Gordon, J. R., Gorman, M. J., & Safren, S. A. (2016). Behavioral medicine strategies in outpatient psychiatric settings. In T. Petersen, S. Sprich, & S. Wilhelm (Eds.), *The Massachusetts General Hospital handbook of cognitive behavioral therapy* (pp. 243–257). Springer.

20. van der Kolk, B. A., Stone, L., West, J., Rhodes, A., Emerson, D., Suvak, M., & Spinazzola, J. (2014). Yoga as an adjunctive treatment for posttraumatic stress disorder: A randomized controlled trial. *Journal of Clinical Psychiatry*, *75*(6), e599–565.

21. Lichstein, K. L. (1988). *Clinical relaxation strategies*. Wiley-Interscience.

22. Elliott, S., & Edmonson, E. (2006). *The new science of breath: Coherent breathing for autonomic nervous system balance, health, and well-being*. Coherence Press.

23. Gervitz & Schwartz, 2003, The respiratory system in applied psychophysiology.

24. Clark, M. E., & Hirschman, R. (1990). Effects of paced respiration on anxiety reduction in a clinical population. *Biofeedback and Self-regulation*, *15*(3), 273–284.

25. Brown, R. P., & Berbarg, P. (2012). *The healing power of the breath: Simple techniques to reduce stress and anxiety, enhance concentration, and balance your emotions*. Shambhala Publications; Gervitz & Schwartz, 2003, The respiratory system in applied psychophysiology.

26. Bae, D., Matthews, J. J. L., Chen, J. J., & Mah, L. (2021). Increased exhalation to inhalation ratio during breathing enhances high-frequency heart rate variability in healthy adults. *Psychophysiology*, *58*(11), e13905.

27. Remmers, J. E., & Gautier, H. (1972). Neural and mechanical mechanisms of feline purring. *Respiration Physiology*, *16*(3), 351–361.

28. Wallace, A. (2009, October 11). Whispering to Rottweilers, and to C.E.O.'s. *The New York Times*.

29. Millan, C., & Peltier, M. J. (2006). *Cesar's way: The natural, everyday guide to understanding & correcting common dog problems*. Random House.

30. Peper & Tibbetts, 1994, Effortless diaphragmatic breathing.

31. McGlynn, F., Smitherman, T., & Gothard, K. (2004). Comment on the status of systematic desensitization. *Behavior Modification*, *28*(2), 194–205.

Chapter 4: **Hold a Steady, Upward Gaze with Wide Eyes**

"The soul, fortunately, has an interpreter—often an unconscious but still a faithful interpreter—in the eye."
— Charlotte Brontë (1816-1855)

Eyes are essential for animals to perceive their surrounding environment and were among the first organs to evolve, even predating the development of gills and lungs. The vast majority of animals have eyes. Even some single-celled organisms have eyespots or patches of light-receptive proteins. However, mammals are one of only a few classes of animals that use their eyes to communicate.

Mammals visually inspect other animals' eyes for social cues, often determining where the other animal is looking, what its mental state is, and whether the other animal is returning its gaze. Humans, more than any other animal, use the eyes to communicate intention and emotion. How you look at others and how you use your eyes affects you on a deep psychological level. By modifying the involuntary patterns of your gazing behavior in the ways described in this chapter, you can foster your sense of well-being, improve the quality of your relationships, and ensure your social interactions are positive and empowering.

This chapter focuses on four ways that subordination unconsciously impoverishes our eyes' posture: 1) squinting, 2) raising the eyebrows, 3) looking down, and 4) avoiding eye contact. All four are relatively simple to change with the application of consistent effort. As you read on, you'll come to understand both how these behaviors can be harmful and why it is worth investing your time and energy in changing them.

Open the Eyes Wide and Refrain from Squinting

Many mammals appraise the intent of other animals by the wideness of their eyes. Widened eyes are intense and bold, communicating fearlessness. Squinted eyes are defensive and associated with either attack or submissiveness. For instance, you may notice your dog or cat squinting slightly and looking at the floor after brief eye contact. They do this to demonstrate unobtrusiveness. Humans squint in social situations for much the same reason—it communicates propriety. However, when squinting happens too frequently, the muscles take on tension. Chronic squinting, like shallow breathing, is another example of a suboptimal display that has the potential to reduce our standard of living.

Squinting is controlled by the orbicularis oculi—rings of muscle (technically, "sphincters") that encircle the eyes and open and close the eyelids. Of all the muscles on the surface of the human body, the orbicularis oculi display the most conspicuous evidence of cumulative strain. This is because the skin surrounding the eye is unusually thin and easily reveals discoloration, creasing, inflammation, and the accumulation of fluid. These conditions are caused by chronic squinting and lead to purple rings, dark circles, and bags under the eyes. The muscle fibers of your orbicularis oculi have become tonically contracted, maintaining a squinting posture throughout the day without you being aware. The solution to this postural eye strain is to train yourself to widen your eyes so that they squint less frequently and to a lesser degree.

The activity below will ask you to position yourself in front of a mirror with your eyes as wide as possible. You will realize that it is not easy to keep them wide and that your lower eyelids become tense as your thoughts drift to other topics. That's the force of habit reasserting itself. Your eyes are accustomed to squinting by default due to the actions of lower brain centers. You may even notice that they twitch involuntarily when you think negative thoughts. Squinting acts as an anchor in the face that recruits wincing.

Once you have observed the habitual tension for yourself, you are ready to start changing it. Your goal is to stop overusing the orbicularis oculi muscles and, instead, start relying on the underused levator palpebrae superioris instead, which opens the eyes wide. After completing the exploratory activity below, you should notice that your eyes look wider and friendlier for several hours.

Eye Activity #4.1: *Watching the Lower Lid*
Sit or stand in front of a mirror with your eyes as wide open as possible. Ideally, you should be able to see your entire iris and a bit of white border above and below it. If you can't, set this as the goal. You should notice two tendencies: 1) Your lower lid will tremble and tighten, revealing a tendency to revert to squinting; 2) Your eyebrows will raise on their own. Your job is to keep your eyes wide and your brow fully lowered and limp for five full minutes. You should notice that performing this activity is much easier when using a breath metronome.

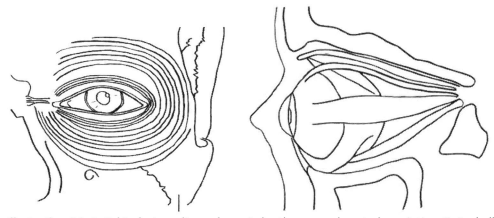

Illustration 4.1: A. Orbicularis oculi muscle encircles the eye and controls squinting; B. Eyeball in the eye socket. Eye movement is controlled by ocular muscles surrounding the eye. Eye wideness is controlled by the levator palpebrae superioris above it.

A friend once said to me, "See these bags under my eyes? I never had these before. I spent two years partying: staying out late, smoking cigarettes, doing drugs, and drinking. They developed abruptly. And even after I stopped partying so hard, they never went away." Most of us have creases under our eyes, and I had only seen them get worse with time, so I assumed that the change in my friend's appearance was permanent. But his comments did start me wondering about the underlying biological reason for changes in the skin around our eyes. It took me years to realize that the problem is caused by muscular strain from excessive squinting and years more to confirm that it is completely reversible. Chapter 9 will show you how to massage the muscles of the eyes and forehead, which is necessary to fully release the muscles and erase the dark circles. But this chapter will help you change how you use the muscles surrounding your eyes during daily life, which is arguably more important.

At first, you may feel these eye exercises are driven by vanity, which is uncomfortable for most of us, but at a certain point, you will realize that your real motive is inner bravery. Reducing the appearance of eye strain is merely an aesthetic side effect of widening your eyes. Far more important are the effects on emotional prosperity. It is well documented that negative emotions generally cause squinting and that positive emotions cause eye-widening.[1]

Squinting itself is never an emotionally neutral activity. Squinting is the continual elicitation of the defensive blink response, which evolved to protect the eye from damage. Animals squint unconsciously when they feel the safety of their eyes is in jeopardy. (Imagine pushing your way through face-height tree branches, for instance. You will feel your eyes instinctively narrow.) That is why most mammals squint when fighting or when they anticipate a fight erupting. Heavy squinting is a form of trauma that maintains a defensive eyelid posture and disinhibits the blinking reflex. Mammals that feel threatened blink hard and fast, whereas mammals that feel safe blink very slowly. Practicing a few slow blinks will help you widen your eyes and develop a calmer blinking pattern.

Eye Exercise #4.1: *Slow Blinking*

Blink ten times very slowly. Blink another ten times as slowly as you can. The calmer a mammal is, the slower it blinks. However, most people have no awareness of or capacity for slow blinking until they practice it.

As you might have guessed, the startle response and distressed breathing both heighten squinting. They are all part of the same neurological circuit. Allowing unconscious brain centers to maintain tension in the eyelids sends messages to other threat centers in the brain, communicating that the current environment is potentially threatening to the eyes. This is ironic because, in today's world, our eyes are rarely threatened. In the ancestral past, it was adaptive for anxiety and fear to potentiate squinting, but today, work and relationship stress are practically never indicative of impending damage to the eyes.

Your stress response also spikes when you widen your eyes during social situations. If you were hooked up to a machine that measured your sympathetic nervous system activity, it would spike every time you opened your eyes all the way. Wide eyes give us a sensation of showing off, and that, in turn, makes us breathe shallowly in an attempt not to be too forward or noticeable. Exercise 1 overrides this by asking you to pair paced breathing with widening the eyes. Performing the exercises herein will make it so that your body becomes accustomed to having the eyes wide without breathing shallowly.

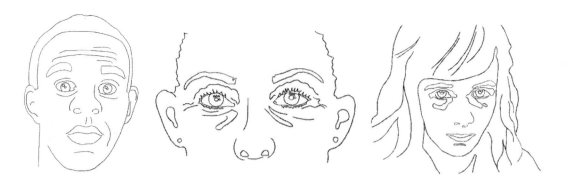

Illustration 4.2: Man raising eyebrows; B & C. Women with apparent strain in the orbicularis oculi.

Eye Exercise #4.2: *Wide Eyes with No Façade*

Do one or both of the following two things. 1) spend ten seconds gently rubbing your eyelids and upper cheeks to stimulate blood circulation, or 2) spend ten seconds squinting tightly. Both actions will potentiate squinting.

Next, spend five minutes within four feet of a mirror trying to make your eyes as wide as possible while keeping your brow relaxed. Drop your social façade and just look into your own wide eyes. It is okay if you look insane or demented. After a couple of minutes, you may feel you are staring into your soul. You should feel comfortable looking at everyone this way. This will reset your eyes to a wider aperture and diminish your overreactive, superficially pleasing veneer. Once you have the coordination, you can achieve it without a mirror. Consistent practice will lead to continued improvement.

Like rubbing the eyes and squinting them tightly, crying also encourages squinting to linger. When most people cry, they look sad, their eyes become puffy, and they continue to squint for hours afterward. However, this is not a necessary part of crying. Immediately after the next time you cry, sit in front of a mirror breathing diaphragmatically, and widen your eyes for five full minutes. For the rest of the day, your eyes will feel light, carefree, and wide instead of compressed and miserable. The reason for this is that crying actually involves deep squinting and a full healthy contraction of the orbicularis oculi rather than the continuous partial contraction that usually takes place. This sends blood to the muscles and makes them more responsive to efforts at widening. As we will discuss in depth in later chapters, one of the best ways to get a muscle to relax is to contract it to fatigue it and then give it a chance to rest fully.

This means that crying is good for you as long as you help yourself recover in a healthy, emotionally uplifting way. That fits with its functional purpose. Humans are the only animals that cry, and biologists have hypothesized that it might serve a communicative function that asks for help and elicits altruistic behavior from others.[2] It has also been characterized as a reliable signal of appeasement and vulnerability because, by blurring our vision, it handicaps aggressive or defensive actions.[3] I think that, more than anything else, crying serves to fatigue the respiratory muscles and the facial muscles (especially the ones involved in squinting and sneering), enabling them a period of respite afterward.

Relaxing the orbicularis oculi will look and feel artificial at first. A few weeks of concerted effort combined with diaphragmatic breathing will fix this, making it your new default state. When I first attempted to stop squinting, I looked absurd. I appeared like a sickly drug addict that had been startled or like an uptight person trying too hard to appear calm. At times, I felt my face was a leering death mask. It took several weeks for the rings under my eyes and the general sleepless appearance to fade. With time, the cheeks and the areas under the eyes began to look less puffy, lose their discoloration, and appear healthier. When you are alone, shoot for a "bug-eyed" look. Soon, it will pass for normal. Once it does, do it in public. When you realize that your eyes remain wide open when speaking to others, you know you have gotten the hang of it. Once you do, going back to squinting will feel like glaring.

Many military personnel and people suffering from PTSD have a tense look that is centered around the eyes. Pictures taken before and after warzone deployment illustrate this dramatically. Many martial arts instructors and students squint, often have one eye more affected than the other, and have dark circles under their eyes. This is because walking into a martial arts studio without squinting sends the signal: "I am not afraid." Unfortunately, this sign of bravery is one that many people are too conscientious to allow themselves to make. This is also a case of art following life. The most heinous villains in cartoons and storybooks are portrayed with dark creases under their eyes. On the other hand, people who are candidly carefree and cheerful are often portrayed as wide-eyed. Many children look this way naturally, and their appearance is mimicked by artists and animators trying to create an impression of innocence, angelic virtue, or even naïveté. It usually works, as in the case of many Disney characters, because what we perceive are eye muscles with no signs of cumulative strain. If a person's eyes don't advertise a history of defensive posturing, we subconsciously assume that they can negotiate the world without defensive thinking. Common phrases in the vernacular, like "sensitive eyes," "gleam in the eye," "sparkling eyes," "light in the eyes," or "twinkle in the eyes," describe this effect. Bring the brightness back to your eyes by living with your eyes wide all the time.

Eye Activity #4.2: *Techniques to Widen the Eyes*
1) Open your eyes wide and keep them there. Now, raise your eyebrows for a fraction of a second and widen your eyes even further in the same moment. Subsequently, allow your eyebrows to relax while keeping your eyes just as wide. This will help you "reset" eye wideness.
2) Gently pull down on the skin just below your eyes, exposing the underside of both eyelids to the air, and open your eyes as wide as you can. Hold the position for a few seconds and then let go.
3) Looking to the far right or left side of your visual field can help widen the eyes. Hold this "side-eye" posture for several seconds. As you move your eyes back to the center, the eyes may go back to squinting again. Don't let them. It is possible that, like me, you have repressed looking to one side with wide eyes due to a natural fear of giving people the "side-eye." Don't be.

4) Practice widening your eyes while looking down. You can do this while watching TV in a reclining position from a couch, armchair, or bed. Notice your tendency to squint while you do this and, instead, make your eyes as wide as possible.

5) Practice micro-squints. Start in front of the mirror with your eyes wide open. Fix your gaze on your lower lid, and practice briefly making the smallest squint you can and then releasing it. Your lower lid should move less than a millimeter. Repeat this twenty times. Developing this subtle control will help you build awareness of the unconscious muscular contractions involved in squinting.

Think of actors with especially wide eyes. Your eyes can look just like theirs. The actors you're thinking of may not have earned their ocular posture, having just fallen into it due to favorable or lenient early environmental circumstances. By following the neural reprogramming exercises in this chapter, along with the muscle massage and compression exercises in Chapter 9, you can earn it. In fact, all the exercises from Program Peace zero in on optimal microhabits that you may not have fallen into but you can, instead, earn through repetition.

Another aspect of the squinting problem worthy of our attention is squinting while sleeping. Many people sleep with their faces screwed up tight, their teeth clenched, and their eyelids clamped together. To determine whether you fall into this category, start by asking yourself this: *What state are my eyes in when I wake up?* Most of us clench them shut during the night, contracting the entire ring of the orbicularis oculi, from the cheeks to the eyelids. This amounts to hours and hours of low-grade, repetitive strain.

To avoid nighttime muscular strain in your face, you will need to close your eyes with the upper lids rather than the lower ones. This involves contracting the inner palpebral portions of the orbicularis oculi (which perform eye blinks) as well as the ciliary portions (which control the rims of the eyelids). To do this, you need to learn how to contract those muscles and then strengthen them with consistent practice. If your upper lids are not strong enough to close the eyes on their own, the lower lids will rise to meet them, introducing the strain you are trying to avoid. Most of us have weak upper lids, which is why we end up squinting whenever we close our eyes.

When you squint during sleep, your eyelashes are swallowed up by your lids and the skin around the eyes will wrinkle. However, if you close your eyes using your upper lids, your eyelashes will be fully visible and your eye area will be smooth. Every night before sleep, practice shutting your eyes very tightly using only the upper lids. I think of this as "eyes wide shut." When you start to use your upper lids, the muscles may flutter and waver because they are weak. This will subside with time. Repeat the exercise until the muscles develop the tone they need for the action to become second nature. Enjoy the more relaxed sleep that results.

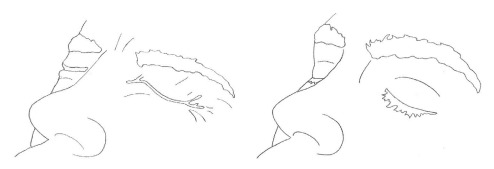

Illustration 4.3: Eyes closed by straining the lower lids; B. Eyes closed by modest contraction of the upper lids.

Eye Exercise #4.3: *Stop Squinting in Your Sleep*

Spend two minutes closing your eyes using only the upper lids. Do this without squinting and while keeping the lower lids wholly relaxed. During the second minute, tightly clench the upper lids to exercise the muscles and help them develop tone. Perform this exercise while looking upward to make it harder. Also, spend a few seconds alternating between using the upper lids and the lower ones to isolate and dissociate the two actions.

One common problem with eye-widening exercises is dry eyes. You will find that the outer periphery of the eyeball, which is normally covered when you squint, feels dry when exposed to the air. This is normal and happens only because the area is not used to being uncovered. Don't let the dryness keep you from widening your eyes for prolonged periods. You can use eye drops a few times a week and then gradually transition off them. Another helpful option is to use the following simple technique to naturally stimulate your tear glands to lubricate your eyes.

Eye Activity #4.3: *Lubricating the Eyes by Stimulating the Tear Glands*

When your eyes begin to feel dry, keep them open for several more seconds until you are forced to blink. Once you do, close them tightly using only the upper lids. Keep them closed and wait for them to start stinging. That stinging sensation is the stimulation of your underused lacrimal glands and tear ducts. It is the feeling of secreting tears. Most of the time, you open your eyes when they sting, ending the secretion process. Instead, embrace the stinging, breathe through it diaphragmatically, and wait for your eyes to produce their natural aqueous lubrication. Doing this frequently will increase the natural moistness of your eyes and allow you to widen them further.

If you perform these exercises, you will gradually develop the ability to keep your eyes open wider. Bright light is another hindrance. The next section will address how to keep your eyes wide even outside on a sunny day.

Expose Your Eyes to More Sunlight

Most people wince and squint heavily in both direct and indirect sunlight. Living most of our lives indoors, we get far less exposure to the sun than our ancestors did. We have become acclimated to dim environments, which causes heavy squinting when we finally make it outside. You may have noticed that people with full-time outdoor jobs, such as gardeners and construction workers, often have no trouble keeping their eyes wide when standing in direct sun.

The good news is that squinting in the sun is merely a habit and one that can be completely unlearned with practice. After performing the following exercises, you will be able to comfortably be outdoors with your eyes completely open. The most basic exercise is to increase your exposure: try to position yourself in just the right amount of indirect sunlight to let you bask in it wide-eyed. After a while, you'll be able to expose yourself to brighter and brighter light without squinting.

Eye Exercise #4.4: *Wide-Eyed Sunlight Exposure*

Go outside during the day and find a place in the shade where you can comfortably open your eyes all the way. Make sure that you aren't squinting or raising or lowering your brow. Remain wide-eyed for at least five minutes. The next time you practice, try to find a place that is a little bit brighter.

Eye Exercise #4.5: *Sunlight Through Closed Eyes*

Allow yourself to sit or lie in the sun with the sunlight hitting your face. Close your upper lids without squinting. The sun should be hitting your eyelids. It should be very bright, and you should be seeing red. (Make sure never to look directly at the sun itself, even with your eyes closed.) Breathe diaphragmatically. Remain in the sun for a full minute. Over time, practice will allow you to tolerate more sunlight and improve the look of your eyes, making them healthier, calmer, and wider. You might consider performing this exercise from behind a window or car windshield to partially reduce your exposure to UV rays.

Studies have shown a significant relationship between depression and diminished exposure to sunlight. The opposite is also true: increased exposure to sunlight may ameliorate some forms of depression and even common malaise.[4] Traditional forms of light therapy, which use bright artificial lights, have shown great promise. I believe that this therapy is efficacious because it teaches patients to become comfortable, without squinting and tightening the face, in the presence of bright light. Unfortunately, this form of clinical therapy does not explicitly address squinting. However, you can, and using the sun, you can do it at no cost. Pairing bright light exposure with diaphragmatic breathing while remaining wide-eyed could help make you a "brighter," happier person.

It can be hard to maintain your new wide-eyed facial posture in social situations. One way to support your practice is through the strategic use of sunglasses. If the sun is making you squint, put them on. If you enter a social situation in which you know you are likely to squint, put them on. Then, with the sunglasses on, open your eyes as wide as possible. This will train you to feel comfortable keeping your eyes wide while speaking to and interacting with others. By the time you choose to take the sunglasses off, your eyes will be large and peaceful.

Refrain from Chronically Raising the Brow

The next thing to focus on is the position of your eyebrows. Most of us cannot widen our eyes without raising the brow, and many people squint automatically when they let their eyebrows relax. This is because widening the eyes is not submissive while raising the eyebrows is, and we are conditioned by social experience to balance one with the other. We offer submissively raised brows as a peace offering to compensate for wide eyes. The problem, of course, is that in doing so, we are simply trading one form of tension for another.

The biological details are interesting. The eyebrows are raised using a contraction of the frontalis muscle, which controls the movement of the forehead. Among many mammals—and primates especially—it is an appeasement display, while lowering the eyebrows in a frown is a display of dominance. The frown uses the procerus muscle to pull down the inner brows, which are then drawn together by the corrugator supercilii. Together, those two movements induce furrows in the lower forehead.

Evidence regarding the social effects of eyebrow posture is compelling. The brows are generally raised in primates low in the hierarchy and lowered in those high in the hierarchy.[5] Raised brows correlate with the "tendency to flee" during disputes among human children. People rate pictures of models with lowered brows as more dominant than models with relaxed or raised brows. Monkeys seem to feel the same way. Rhesus monkeys submissively avoid the gaze of humans with lowered brows but gaze at humans with raised brows for prolonged periods.[6] The question is: Why are raised eyebrows subordinating? Researcher Caroline Keating offers one possible explanation:

Some expressions characterizing the dominance encounters of nonhuman primates involve eyebrow position. Generally, the brows are lowered on dominant or threatening individuals and raised on submissive or receptive individuals. Theorists have speculated on the evolutionary origins of facial gestures. Darwin believed that many expressions evolved from "serviceable associated habits" or preparatory responses associated with attack, defense, locomotion, or changes in visual or respiratory functioning. Several current theorists agree. Selective pressures apparently shaped certain elements of preparatory or supportive responses into displays that reflected the original impetus of the behavior. Thus, submissive brow raising may have evolved by originally aiding the visual scanning of animals in threatening circumstances. Because lowered brows protect the eyes from physical harm and facilitate near-focusing during attack, perhaps this behavior evolved as a dominance gesture by forecasting physical aggression.[7]

It is thought that our propensity to raise and lower our brows may derive from ear movements used by our ancestors before they lost muscular control of their ears. Many specialists believe that raising the eyebrows is a throwback to the ear retraction reflex that pulls the ears backward. Ears back is a submissive display seen in most mammals.[8] In contrast, lowering the brow likely originates from ear protraction, which pushes the ears forward and is an assertive display in many mammals. Like direct eye gaze, ears forward communicates that the sensory apparatus is focused on assertive or predatory action. Stated simply, the animal chasing has it ears forward, the animal being chased has its ears back.

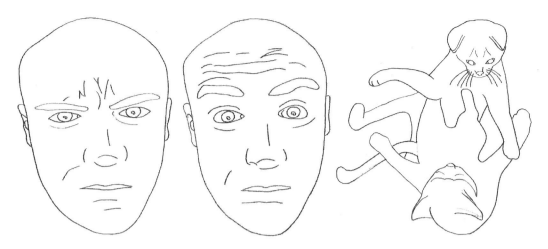

Illustration 4.4: Eyebrows lowered; B. Eyebrows raised; C. Cat on top with ears forward, cat on the bottom with ears back.

Whether you are raising or lowering your eyebrows, doing so too frequently for too long will lead to muscular strain and psychological tension. As we will discuss in Chapter 8, the optimal posture is neutral eyebrows and wide eyes. Again, this involves relaxing the frontalis and the orbicularis oculi and lightly and infrequently contracting the (eyelid-widening) levator palpebrae.

Practice Frowning and Glaring to Increase Nonverbal Dominance

You should make an effort to become comfortable frowning and glaring. Body language experts agree that frowning, measured by the decreased distance between the eyebrows and the pupils, is strongly associated with dominance and leadership.[9] Unfortunately, many of us are afraid to frown because frowning in a social situation involuntarily recruits the stress response. You can conquer that reaction using the next exercise.

Exercise 4.6 reduces eyebrow raising and increases the size and tone of the frowning muscles. Someone who appears accustomed to frowning (i.e., who does it spontaneously and effortlessly) comes across as someone who has spent a lot of time being in charge. When you start using your new frown around people, don't use it to intimidate but rather to express empathy or resolve. Do it the way the king of the jungle, an empress, or a superhero might do it.

Eye Exercise #4.6: *Relaxed Frowning*

Spend five minutes frowning as hard as you can while engaging in paced breathing. Holding a firm contraction in the procerus may feel very awkward and may even sting, but it will reprogram you not to be afraid to use this highly dominant display. Keep your eyes wide, the rest of your face relaxed, and your breaths coming in deep and long.

Most of us have grown up afraid of giving someone else the "evil eye," so we have stricken this contraction from our repertoire and left a "glaring omission" in our ability to emote using our eyes. The glare is a temporary and intense contraction of the squinting muscles. Glaring is considered dominant[10] because you generally must be authoritative to get away with it. Let's not use it to threaten people. Use it very briefly to demonstrate concentration, conviction, or valor. You might choose to do this exercise, as well as the previous exercise, in front of a mirror so that you can combine them with eye contact while monitoring your face.

Eye Exercise #4.7: *Relaxed Glaring*
Spend five minutes glaring as hard as you can while engaging in paced breathing. Squint your eyes tightly so that the opening is tiny and you can barely see through your eyelashes. Hold this contraction and try to keep it from wavering or trembling. As you do so, you might pretend that you are confidently leading a large group of people through a snowstorm or a sandstorm. Holding a firm contraction in the part of the orbicularis oculi that contracts the eyelids will help you develop its strength and coordination. Take a 10-second break every few dozen seconds so that you don't push the muscles into persistent contraction.

When I was in junior high school, my Dad asked me, "Jared, why do you always look timid and afraid in your yearbook pictures? Try not to make that face anymore, tiger." At the time, I had no idea what he was talking about. I do now. I constantly raised my eyebrows and squinted (but never frowned or glared) so that I would appear friendly. Used briefly, eyebrow raising can communicate curiosity and engagement, but I overused it without giving the muscles any rest. It appeared affable in the short run but caused my face to become very tense and age rapidly in the long run. Use a brief eyebrow raise as an olive branch, but do not use extended eyebrow raises that go on for more than just a few seconds. Those are white flags.

Look Upward

The stress that overtook me at age 17 caused me to lose the hair on my head rapidly. Ashamed of my bald spots, between the ages of 17 and 32, I wore a hat seven days a week. For 15 years, the brim of a baseball hat blocked the sky from my view, training me not to cast my eyes upward. My whole behavioral repertoire involved looking down. Then, when I turned 32, I shaved my head and stopped wearing hats. Suddenly, I became aware that I had developed a behavioral blind spot for the entire space above me. That revelation galvanized me to train myself to look up.

We have all learned to habitually cast our gaze downward. We often do this to avoid eye contact, all the while signaling submission, disinterest, or fear. The vast majority of us do this customarily, even when alone. Most people's nervous systems are so conditioned to looking down that they do it even when they dream. How dismal.

Most of us have grown up in an environment that discourages us from looking up in the presence of others. Other people's reactions to our upward gaze have communicated to our unconscious brain systems that we should avoid looking up for fear of reprimand or reprisal. The subject matter that makes a person glance at the floor is very telling and provides a window into their insecurities. More than this, looking down is neurologically tied to depression and anxiety through numerous brain pathways. It is another habit that stifles our soul on a neurological level.

To overcome this, we can do two things: 1) train our nervous system to look upward through practice, and 2) build the ocular muscles responsible for lifting the eyes. The exercise below is a great way to determine whether the muscles responsible for looking up (superior rectus), have atrophied from disuse.

Eye Exercise #4.8: *Strengthening the Muscles that Allow You to Look Up*

Close your eyes and use your index fingers to press your upper eyelids and eyelashes down, pinning them against the top of your cheeks. Refrain from squinting. Next, look straight up for several seconds. Then look up and to the left, then up and to the right. Keep at it for 30 to 60 seconds. It will likely burn and feel uncomfortable in the muscles around your eyes. If it does, then you know they have atrophied and can be strengthened by repeating this exercise. Simply repeating the exercise on five different days should vastly reduce any burning and help tone these muscles.

I used to look at the floor unconditionally when speaking. I would look at the ground around my feet during most conversations. Somehow, I didn't understand that this was a primary reason I couldn't keep a conversation going. Try to stop looking down when you talk to people. People who are more severely affected can start looking at waist height, then shoulder height, and so on. Work toward being able to keep your gaze up around the height of your head. Once that starts to feel comfortable, work on looking up during conversations above the shared eye line.

It is generally discourteous to look directly above another person's head, so look off to one side. As you look up during the conversation, you might be concerned that the other person will become puzzled or suspicious of this. If you are not accustomed to looking up, are not used to breathing deeply when doing it, or if your ocular muscles are weak, the other person will likely be able to tell that it is unnatural for you. Again, the only way for it to look natural is for you to practice.

People look up for many different reasons.[11] With the head facing down, it can be coy and suggestive. With the head neutral or facing up, it can communicate boredom. Looking up when someone walks into a room can be interpreted as a sign of disdain or disregard. This is why people roll their eyes. Eye rolling is a nonverbal statement of superiority exclaiming, "*That* is beneath me." You don't want to adopt an upward gaze with these as your motives. Some people look up when they are thinking. Others do it to recall something from memory. Use these as motives. Pretend that you are using the ceiling or sky as a canvas for your imagination to paint pictures of the topic of conversation. Looking up appears natural to others when you use the upper visual field to imagine things in the mind's eye. Encourage others to do it with you.

Eye Exercise #4.9: *Looking Up While Talking*

Simulate a conversation, or have an actual phone conversation, while looking upward. As you listen and speak, make certain your gaze does not drop below your eye line. Keep your eyes wide, and your eyebrows relaxed. Become aware of your tendency to look down. Instead,

---

> alternate between looking at things around the same level as your eyes and things that are higher than them.

There will be ample opportunities to practice during daily life. When you are standing at the register ordering fast food, look up at the menu on the wall calmly with wide eyes, even if the cashier is looking directly at you. Feel comfortable doing this while in line before you order or even after. As you pass a stranger on the street, feel comfortable looking up. While you do so, keep your head up, too. Gaze at the buildings, signs, telephone wires, and clouds. If you need to, remind yourself that looking up is your right. Your eyes are yours to use as you wish. As an added benefit, looking up naturally widens your eyes by engaging the levator palpebrae superioris muscles.

Eye Activity #4.4: *Take a Walk with Wide Eyes and an Upward Gaze*

Take a walk around your block with your eyes all the way open. Try to look at the ground as little as possible. Then, walk around the block again, this time without looking below the horizon. Do it a third time, now without looking below your eye line. It may help to focus your gaze on roofs, streetlights, or treetops. Finally, try walking around the block with your nose high in the air—that will compete with, and override, your tendency to point it at the floor. Notice how all of this feels, especially in your face, neck, and shoulders. See whether you can replicate that feeling in daily life.

Improve Your Eye Contact Skills by Looking at Your Eyes in the Mirror

When I first started trying to make concerted eye contact with myself in a mirror, it was uncomfortable. It became apparent that eye contact with others was awkward for me because eye contact with myself was awkward. After spending time holding my own gaze, I realized that instead of looking myself directly in the iris or pupil, I usually looked around the eyes rather than directly at them. Then, I found that I was doing the same thing when I made eye contact with others. Sometimes I looked at a person's cheeks, nose, mouth, or ear, other times off into the space to the side of their head. I felt astounded when I realized that I virtually never looked anyone straight in the eye.

The most interesting thing about this is what would happen if I tried to sustain eye contact with myself in the mirror. I could only look into my iris for a mere second or two before my eyes would flinch or dart away. This was caused by reflexive startle and was, therefore, unconscious and hard to resist. It happened because my brain areas devoted to controlling eye movement (such as the frontal eye fields and the superior colliculi) were not acclimatized to continual eye contact. My eyes were retreating out of fear.

Everyone's eyes autonomously flinch away from eye contact to different extents. They do so more when stress levels are high, and the extent to which they do it is another marker of social rank. Some of our worst social experiences, when threats forced us to avert our gaze, have traumatized the unconscious motor systems that control the eyes. We should all try to break this neurological reflex to glance away from eye contact because it stunts our social growth.

Do you make direct and sustained eye contact with the characters on television? If not, then you probably have an aversion to making eye contact, as I did. Make a concerted effort to always look the characters onscreen straight in the eye. Many of us must force ourselves to start taking simple steps toward building up a tolerance for eye contact, which will help you develop a preference for it.

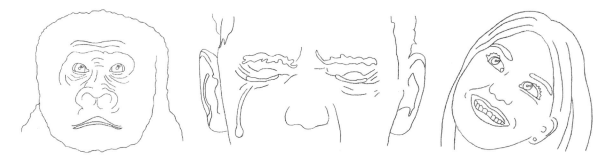

Illustration 4.5: A. Gorilla with wide eyes; B. A boy squinting and crying; C. Woman looking up and smiling.

The best way to desensitize yourself to eye contact is to spend prolonged periods looking into your own eyes in a mirror. Notice and resist the impulse to glance away. You will achieve results quickly. After pairing the exercise below with diaphragmatic breathing for one week (five minutes a day), you should be able to make unwavering eye contact with yourself and feel calm while doing it. After practicing it for a few weeks, you can do this with anyone. Now, I only look away when I choose to. I also have a different relationship with myself now. Not only do I feel more confident, but I also feel more trustworthy.

Eye Exercise #4.10: *Making Eye Contact with Yourself*

Sit in front of a mirror and make eye contact with yourself for five minutes. Look straight into your irises or pupils. Do not raise your eyebrows and keep your eyes wide open. Start at a typical conversational distance, one to four feet from the mirror itself. Later, try it from other distances, from one inch to 10 feet. Try to maintain a tranquil and confident expression, and breathe long, deep breaths guided by a breath metronome. Ensure that you maintain steadfast contact with your irises throughout each smooth inhalation and exhalation. I thought that one of my eyes was smaller than the other, but this exercise proved to me that I was merely squinting my left eye harder and within a few sessions this asymmetry was healed. After you have practiced this alone several times, try maintaining eye contact in this way with a friend.

One of the best times to practice is right after you wake up when the tension in the muscles surrounding your eyes is most apparent. Performing the above eye-contact exercise in the morning will help you settle your eye posture into a positive, healthy mode early in the day, making it easier to keep your eyes wide throughout the day. You might also want to try it right before meeting someone on whom you want to make a good impression. Breathing usually becomes shallow during eye contact. If you can breathe diaphragmatically during sustained eye contact with yourself, you will be able to do it with other people. This is because most of the subcortical circuits involved don't know the difference between looking yourself in the eye in a mirror and looking someone else in the eye. People will be surprised by how easy it is for you to sustain wide-eyed eye contact and impute saint-like qualities to you.

Make Your Assertive Eye Contact Friendly

Socially dominant wolves stare freely and casually at their packmates, but those packmates never stare at the dominant animal.[12] The same is true with monkeys. Momentary eye contact with a dominant individual causes them to perform a submission gesture as an apology.[13] These patterns also pertain to apes. For example, chimps avoid eye contact during confrontations and physical struggles, and subordinate chimps make much less eye contact when they are around their dominant peers. Chimps may charge at an individual from another group if it makes eye contact. Staring between unfamiliar apes is often interpreted as a threat signal. Even an unfamiliar human staring at a primate often elicits an attack response. However, chimpanzees and gorillas from the same group frequently share gazes and use their eyes for communication, much like us.[14] Familiar chimps that are similar in rank make concerted eye contact under normal conditions, especially when making up after a fight.

Of course, eye contact behavior among humans is far more variable than among primates, with sizeable cultural differences in the frequency and significance of different ocular behaviors. In many cultures, direct and prolonged eye contact is seen as a challenge or a test of nerves, so everyday eye contact tends to be brief. In America, averting the eyes is interpreted as a lack of confidence, certainty, or truthfulness[15] while sustained eye contact is taken to indicate sincere interest, forthrightness, and attentiveness.[16] In the American context, people who make more eye contact are seen as more competent, likable, and trustworthy overall.[17] In general, the longer eye contact is maintained, the greater the intimacy levels.[18] Positive feelings toward another person generally increase as the length and frequency of a mutual gaze increase.[19] This instinct seems to be built into us. We are born expecting and craving eye contact. Infants prefer to look at faces that engage them in mutual eye contact[20] and cry less when exposed to them.[21]

As a child, I made minimal eye contact with my parents, teachers, and classmates. I didn't want to challenge anyone, I didn't want to make any waves, and usually, I just wanted to be left alone, so avoiding eye contact worked for me. Also, most of my life, I felt like an ugly person, and I thought that by initiating eye contact, I was forcing someone to look at an ugly face. Most people have this worry to some degree. If you do, get over it. Also, keep in mind that refusing eye contact can be domineering, as when the alpha chimpanzee refuses to make eye contact or even look at some of their "subjects." Release any unkind tendency you may have to avoid eye contact with people you may think are ugly or "beneath" you.

Throughout my adolescence and young adulthood, I paid little attention to eye contact in general, and because I did not attend to it, I was clumsy with it. The next two exercises helped me tremendously. Making more frequent eye contact has opened doors for me, allowing me to meet new people, prolong conversations, build rapport, and prove to others that I am not a pushover. On the other hand, it also sometimes has the effect of making the person I am talking to feel uncomfortable, giving them the lurking suspicion that my eye contact is a way to assert myself. That trade-off seems to be intrinsic. There is no way to avoid sometimes appearing overbearing. All we can do is work toward healthy eye-contact habits even if they sometimes make people uncomfortable.

I spent years trying to figure out how to make eye contact in a way that is welcoming and not domineering. I eventually concluded that eye contact comes across as affable when it appears as if it takes no thought. However, it takes lots of experience for eye contact to become genuine and uncontrived. After some trial and error, I came across the following rules of thumb:

1) Make as much eye contact with others as they make with you. You might want to look away first, but then, when you reinstate eye contact, feel secure that it is now their turn to look away. Keep in mind that rigidly keeping track of every glance takes away from the natural flow. Take turns, be fair, but don't sell yourself short.

2) The more expressive you are, the longer you can maintain your gaze without upsetting the other person. If you gesture with your hands, raise your brow momentarily, or build a slow-growing smile, you can maintain your gaze without coming across as intense. If you can get yourself to feel trust, respect, or even love for others, your eye contact will become trusting, respectful, and loving. This is, perhaps, the most powerful and endearing way to make eye contact.

3) Do not look down when you look away from the other person's eyes. When you look at the floor after making eye contact, it can be taken as a sign of defeat and often interrupts the flow of the conversation. Rather than looking down, try to look to the side of the person at the eye line. This will make them feel that you are listening, have remained engaged, and are ready to reinstate eye contact.

4) Look someone in the eyes and wait until their eyes meet yours to start talking. If done in a friendly manner, this can motivate someone to connect with you. When in a group, take the time to look each person in the eye while you talk.

5) Many experts in nonverbal communication recommend trying to make eye contact about 60% of the time during a conversation.[22] Be sensitive, however, to how the other person is responding to your extended eye contact. They may feed off it or actively avoid it.

6) I think it is profitable to discuss eye contact with friends and acquaintances. I have told several friends: "I have been trying to make more eye contact recently. I want you to be comfortable with this. How do you feel about the dynamics of our eye contact?" I have even gone as far as saying things like: "Let's work together on using more eye contact so that we can get better at it."

The following exercise combines several tactics into one larger practice to help you develop reflexes around a healthy, assertive social gaze that communicates to others your bold eye contact is a positive form of social engagement.

Eye Exercise #4.11: *Well-Functioning Eye Contact Behavior*

Sit a foot or two in front of a mirror, staring into your pupils. Perform the following while engaging in paced breathing:

1) Widen and then relax your eyes every few seconds.
2) Deftly move your gaze between your two eyes without breaking eye contact. Try to alternate from one pupil directly to the other. Try doing it rapidly dozens of times.
3) When you blink during contact, immediately reinstate eye contact without ever looking away. Try using the slow blink you worked on earlier in this chapter.
4) Break eye contact by raising your gaze above your eye line, then reestablish eye contact.
5) Raise your eyebrows in a friendly way, then let them lower completely. Do not compensate for lowering your brown by squinting.

In apes and monkeys, dominant individuals stare down subordinate ones.[23] The state of affairs is similar for humans. The visual dominance ratio (VDR) is a concept used in psychology to quantify eye contact behavior between people in a conversation.[24] A person's VDR is calculated by taking the percentage of time that one spends looking into another person's eyes while speaking and dividing that number by the percentage of time that person spends looking into another's eyes while listening.

VDR = (% eye contact while speaking) / (% eye contact while listening).

This means that if you make about the same amount of eye contact while speaking that you do while listening, your VDR is roughly 1. If you make more eye contact while speaking, your VDR rises above 1, which is dominant. If you make most of your eye contact while listening (and look away when you speak), it drops below 1. Usually, a high VDR indicates that you think what you have to say is important.

Studies have shown that when people speak to their peers and colleagues, they have an average VDR of around 1. When they speak to experts or high-status individuals, their VDR drops, and when they speak to people lower in status, their VDR rises. For example, when individuals in the military speak to someone of higher rank, their VDR goes down; when they speak to someone of lower rank, it goes up. The same has been shown to occur in the corporate hierarchy as well as in fraternities and sororities.[25]

The upstanding, genteel strategy is to aim for a VDR of around 1.00 with everyone regardless of their status. However, I was unable to achieve a VDR higher than .20 because I found it extremely difficult to maintain eye contact as I formulated my sentences. Making eye contact would leave me tongue-tied. Years of subordination made it so that I just didn't have the processing capability to do both things at once. The exercise below cured this. Use the training exercise below to raise your VDR quotient.

Eye Exercise #4.12: *Using the Telephone in Front of a Mirror*

When you speak to someone on the phone, sit or stand in front of a mirror and make constant eye contact with yourself. As you listen and speak, make eye contact with your reflection in the mirror, keeping your eyes wide and your eyebrows relaxed. Notice your tendency to look away while you are formulating your sentences. Perfect your ability to produce and deliver your speech while maintaining unbroken eye contact with yourself.

Try to use eye contact to show the other person that you are curious about their facial responses to the topic of conversation. This will keep them engaged. It has been my experience that most people find eye contact that comes across as interested in them to be validating and endearing. Finally, the last major benefit of increased (positive) eye contact is that you learn so much more when you look at people than when you look away. It makes you better at processing emotions and will increase your empathy quotient.

It was easy to help my cat become more comfortable with eye contact. First, I would hold him gently so that he was facing me in a way that allowed him to rest and be still. I would position my face close to his and make eye contact with him while petting him for reassurance. While breathing calmly, I would look into both his eyes for just under a minute. I would feed him afterward. This dramatically increased the frequency at which he sought eye contact. He even began to seek it out when he wasn't hungry. Like most cats, his normal pattern had been to squint, look down, or break eye contact when looking at me. To help counteract that, I fostered his ability to make sustained contact by not staring him down, instead looking away about half the time. To help him stop squinting, I also gently massaged the orbits of his eyes.

The results were noticeable quite quickly. Within a few weeks, he stopped squinting and his eyes were wider all the time. He now actively seeks wide-eyed eye contact from everyone. That, in turn, seems to have increased his social intelligence. This is probably because he is now exposed to more information from people's faces as he interacts with them. I watched my cat become more personable and noticed a real increase in the strength of our bond. Studies back this up, reporting that extended eye contact between a dog and its owner increases the secretion of oxytocin, a neuromodulator involved in social connection, in both animals.[26]

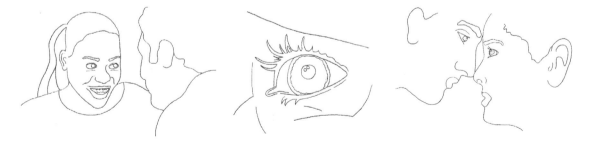

Illustration 4.6: Friends talking with eye contact; B. Eye, iris, and pupil; C. A couple making intimate eye contact.

From kindergarten through college, I could not hold eye contact with my female classmates. Unbeknown to me, this was likely the main reason why I had so much trouble talking to girls. Most of the boys in my elementary classes had the same problem, at least to some extent. There was one boy though who spent every recess with the girls. They all adored him, and I never understood why. I also never understood why he would idiosyncratically roll his eyes up into his head every few minutes. I get it now. He would roll his eyes to engage the muscles that widen the eyes. The wide eyes are part of what allowed him to keep sustained eye contact with the girls. His eyes were as wide as or wider than theirs. Because he looked neither offensive nor defensive, the girls welcomed his gaze. There are reciprocal relationships between having wide eyes, looking up, and making eye contact. If you can widen your eyes and make looking up comfortable using the exercises above, you will find that others will seek out eye contact from you.

Use Sensory Deprivation to Unmask Neurotic Activity

Most of us are afraid that fixing our gaze on anything will make us look too calm. We keep our eyes busy to make others feel comfortable. Take a minute now and observe yourself looking around. You should be able to sense pressure to keep glancing neurotically. This comes from a form of anxiety in the eye motor centers that act below the level of conscious awareness. The restlessness makes it difficult for you to maintain eye contact and to fixate on anything if other people are watching you. The best way to retrain this nervous habit is to become more comfortable anchoring your gaze without worrying about how you may appear to others while doing it.

Eye Exercise #4.13: *Sustained Gaze*

Spend two minutes staring at a single point. Notice any impulses to glance away and gently override them. You might try to keep your eyes fixated on a single feature of the wall or ceiling, or you might try to keep your gaze limited to a circumscribed region of space like a light fixture. If you're having trouble, cut out a picture of a face from a magazine and tape it to your wall or ceiling to gaze at contentedly. Allow yourself to feel free to space out like a child absorbed in a daydream. Don't be concerned about looking dazed or stupefied and don't worry if this level of ocular relaxation causes your eyes to cross for a few moments.

Sensory deprivation can help uncover baseline neurotic tendencies. Let's start with sight. Tracking your ocular behavior in complete darkness will make it clear how much of your eye movement is high-strung and unnecessary. The best way to do this is to wait until nighttime, turn off all the lights in your home, and lie down on the floor of a closet or bathroom. Do whatever you can to make this area completely dark. You may need to put up curtains or drape some towels over the cracks. Being in pitch blackness makes it easier to feel absolutely certain that no one can see your face, expressions, or eye movements. Think back to the way your submissive signaling diminished when you took that walk around the block while pretending to be invisible. Complete darkness allows you an even greater degree of invisibility and anonymity. No one and nothing can be offended by how relaxed you appear because you truly are invisible. Take the opportunity to relax fully and open your eyes very wide without compunction.

In absolute darkness, I feel like a slimy, gelatinous sea slug that has been removed from all danger. I can feel the squinting contraction release in the same way that the sea slug we discussed in Chapter 2 releases its gill. The complete vacancy of visual stimulus will desensitize you and provide your eyes with the experience they need to grow wide. This phenomenon is also a bit like eyestalk extension in snails. When you touch a snail, its eyestalks retract. The eyes invert within the eyestalks and travel down toward the head. This action blinds the snail but is an essential defensive reflex meant to protect the eyes. After several seconds, when the snail starts to feel safe again, the eyes slowly evert, the eyestalks reach full length, and the eyes pop out at the top. Use the exercises above to develop fearless, wide eyes and fully extend your "eyestalks."

In absolute darkness, you will also be able to see phosphenes, which are colored shapes that are produced by your visual system. These may take the form of dots, stars, lines, static, circles, or various other shapes.[27] This visual activity will be accentuated if you lightly rub your eyes. The phosphenes represent a type of background noise that is usually not noticeable yet always ongoing. When the lights are on, phosphene activity is put to work, helping you make perceptual distinctions. When the lights are off, that activity hits a stumbling block, amounting to a low-level form of hallucination.

I believe these phosphenes can play a role in driving anxious thought. Notice when they flash abruptly, and calm your reaction to this. You may notice that they flare when you look straight, keeping you from maintaining a fixed gaze. You may also notice that they burst in the corner of your eye. When they flash like this in the periphery of your vision, I believe they may be reminding you to scan for potential threats that are to the side of you or behind you. When I first started doing this, the phosphene activity appeared sinister and frightening. I even saw flashes of scenes from horror movies. This all contributed strongly to the feeling of being unsafe in the dark.

This may have also been the case for my cat Niko. He cried like a kitten in the dark closet the first few times, but now he will join me of his own volition. Notice your reactions and try to bring peace to your conscious and unconscious responses to the phosphene activity by pairing the experience with diaphragmatic breathing. After doing Exercise 4.14 twice for five minutes, I never again saw any frightful apparitions. I strongly recommend that you use this technique to free the background activity of your visual system from unnecessary negativity.

Eye Exercise #4.14: *Vision in Complete Darkness*

Lie down on the floor in a pitch-black room. Keep your eyes as wide as possible and observe your eye movements. Practice looking in different directions and sustaining your gaze at different points with the eyes wide and eyebrows relaxed. You will notice your eyes dart around in the dark. They will display an intense, agitated tendency to move quickly on their own without any conscious deliberation. Simply observing this and practicing sustained gazing in utter blackness will allow you to reduce the intensity. Nonjudgmentally monitor the visual activity (colored phosphenes), the eye movement activity, and the feelings that come from being in utter darkness. Use this method to dismantle your fear of the dark.

I recommend buying noise-reducing earmuffs to use in your dark closet. With the earmuffs on, you will be able to hear the background activity of your auditory system just as darkness reveals the background activity of your visual system. For most of us, background auditory function takes the form of a ringing or buzzing in the ears, which is known as tinnitus.[28] When I first heard the hissing sound, amplified by the earmuffs, it was very upsetting. I abhorred it.

Many people feel this way, which is unfortunate because some degree of tinnitus is always there, whether we are conscious of it or not. I found that the practice of breathing diaphragmatically and listening to my tinnitus gradually reduced its volume and made it far less emotionally disquieting. Paced, diaphragmatic breathing will quickly help you come to peace with being alone, in complete darkness, with nothing but the background noise of your own visual and auditory systems. This will make it so that their default settings do not haunt you during everyday life.

Conclusion

The final exercise puts several of the routines from this chapter together into a single routine that you can perform while watching television.

Eye Exercise #4.15: *Watching TV Upside Down*

Lie on the floor, on your back, with your head near the TV and your feet away from it. Watch a movie or television program upside down so that you are looking straight up at the screen. Your eyebrows should be visible but out of focus, just below the bottom of the TV's border. Do not allow your brow to raise. Keep your eyes wide and your face relaxed. Try to maintain constant eye contact with the characters on the television. Place your breath metronome next to the TV so that it can guide you in paced diaphragmatic breathing. Remain this way for the duration of a TV show or movie.

Afterward, look in a mirror. You should notice that your eyes look fuller, happier, and calmer. Watching inverted video is also a challenge for your brain's visual systems and may build cognitive and perceptual skills.

Some of these exercises may seem strange, forced, and almost comical. Remember, though, that when you perform them, you are coactivating behavioral subroutines not ordinarily coactivated together because of social constraints. By pairing these with diaphragmatic breathing, you reeducate your nervous system to treat them as safe, making that combination of subroutines possible. The more you do it, the more probable it is to arise spontaneously in the future and, eventually, become a fixed part of your personality. You will rarely have the opportunity to make prolonged eye contact, looking up with wide eyes, breathing diaphragmatically in the course of everyday life. To build optimal behaviors into our repertoire, we must create artificially ideal worlds in which to practice.

The next chapter widens our focus. Behaviors like squinting, looking down, and glancing away all have muscular components to them. Chapter 5 discusses repetitive muscular strain in detail and considers the panoply of negative effects on us. This will set the context for the rest of the book, which will guide you to overcome it.

Chapter 4: **Bullet Points**

- Squinting, eyebrow raising, looking down, and gaze aversion are forms of trauma that fracture our composure but can easily be rehabilitated.

- Widening your eyes, relaxing your brow, looking up, and practicing a fixed gaze have many benefits and will literally change your perspective on life.

- Squinting is defensive and intended to protect the eyeballs. On a fundamental level it is a sign of defensiveness or submission. Deliberately widening the eyes can end excessive squinting and is especially easy to do when breathing long, deep breaths.

- Raised eyebrows are analogous to the action of moving the ears backward in other mammals. This action is performed by an animal being chased so that it can hear its attacker behind it. It is submissive and so should not be strained for long periods.

- Eyebrows lowered is analogous to ears forward, which is the posture for an animal chasing another. This should not be strained, either. However, becoming comfortable lowering your eyebrows into a full frown will increase your nonverbal dominance. The same goes for glaring and the side-eye.

- Looking down is submissive and doing it habitually weakens the muscles that allow us to look up. Looking upward above the horizon more often strengthens your ocular muscles and conditions your nervous system to stop casting your gaze toward the floor.

- Social trauma has caused us to become afraid of fixing our gaze on anything, especially another's eyes.

- Making prolonged eye contact with yourself in a mirror or simply gazing calmly at points in space will train your unconscious visual control systems to be comfortable maintaining a fixed gaze.

- After making eye contact, look at or near the eye line rather than below it.
- Looking at characters on the TV straight in their eyes will strengthen your ability to look real people in the eyes.

- Speaking to someone on the telephone while making sustained, wide-eyed eye contact with yourself in a mirror will strengthen your face-to-face rapport with others.

- Spending time in complete darkness while engaging in paced breathing will help you make your visual system's default activity less chaotic and frightening. Using sound-reducing earmuffs can do the same for your default auditory activity.

- Watching TV upside down can reinforce looking up and eye-widening

Chapter 4: **Endnotes**

1. Pease, B., & Pease, A. (2004). *The definitive book of body language*. Bantam Books.

2. Lutz, T. (2001). *Crying: The natural and cultural history of tears*. Norton.

3. Hasson, O. (2009). Emotional tears as biological signals. *Evolutionary Psychology*, *7*(3), 363–370.

4. Even, C., Schröder, C. M., Friedman, S., & Rouillon, F. (2008). Efficacy of light therapy in nonseasonal depression: A systematic review. *Journal of Affective Disorders*, *108*(1–2), 11–23.

5. Keating, C. F. (1985). Human dominance signals: The primate in us. In S. L. Ellyson & J. F. Dovidio (Eds.), *Power, dominance, and nonverbal behavior* (pp. 89–108). Springer-Verlag.

6. Keating, C. F., & Keating, E. G. (1982). Visual scan patterns of rhesus monkeys viewing faces. *Perception*, *11*(2), 211–219.

7. Keating, 1985, Human dominance signals.

8. Chevalier-Skolnikoff, S. (2006). Facial expression of emotion in nonhuman primates. In P. Ekman (Ed.), *Darwin and facial expression: A century of research in review* (pp. 11–90). Malor Books.

9. Trichas, S., & Schyns, B. (2012). The face of leadership: Perceiving leaders from facial expression. *The Leadership Quarterly*, *23*(3), 545–566.

10. Carney, D. R., Hall, J. A. A., & LeBeau, L. S. (2005). Beliefs about the nonverbal expression of social power. *Journal of Nonverbal Behavior*, *29*, 105–123.

11. Tubbs, S. (2009). *Human communication: Principles and contexts* (12th ed.). McGraw-Hill.

12. Hermann, H. R. (2017). *Dominance and aggression in humans and other animals: The great game of life*. Academic Press.

13. Sapolsky, R. M. (2005). The influence of social hierarchy on primate health. *Science*, *308*(5722), 648–652.

14. Gomez, J. C. (1996). Ostensive behavior in great apes: The role of eye contact. In A. E. Russon, K. A. Bard, & S. T. Parker (Eds.), *Reaching into thought: The minds of the great apes* (pp. 331–151). Cambridge University Press.

15. Cruz, W. (2001). Differences in nonverbal communication styles between cultures: The Latino-Anglo perspective. *Leadership and Management in Engineering*, 1(4), 51–54.

16. Sadri, H. A., & Flammia, M. (2011). *Intercultural communication: A new approach to international relations and global challenges*. Continuum International Publishing Group.

17. Knapp, M. L., & Hall, J. (2010). *Nonverbal communication in human interaction* (7th ed.). Cengage Learning.

18. Knapp & Hall, 2010, *Nonverbal communication in human interaction*.

19. Hogan, K., & Stubbs, R. (2003). *Can't get through. 8 barriers to communication*. Pelican Publishing Company.

20. Farroni, T., Csibra, G., Simion, F. & Johnson, M.H. (2002). Eye contact detection in humans from birth. *Proceedings of the National Academy of Sciences*, 99(14), 9602–9605.

21. Lohaus, A., Keller, H., & Voelker, S. (2001). Relationships between eye contact, maternal sensitivity, and infant crying. *International Journal of Behavioral Development*, 25(6), 542–548.

22. Van Edwards, V. (2017). *Captivate: The science of succeeding with people*. Penguin Random House.

23. Chance, M. R. A. (1967). Attention structures as the basis of primate rank orders. *Man*, 2(4), 503–518.

24. Dovidio, J. F., Ellyson, S. L., Keating, C. F., Heltman, K., & Brown, C. E. (1988). The relationship of social power to visual displays of dominance between men and women. *Journal of Personality and Social Psychology*. 54(2), 233–242.

25.   Dovido at al., 1988, The relationship of social power to visual displays of dominance.

26. Nagasawa, M., Mitsui, S., En, S., Ohtani, N., Ohta, M., Sakuma, Y., Onaka, T., Mogi, K., & Kikusui, T. (2015). Oxytocin-gaze positive loop and the coevolution of human-dog bonds. *Science, 348(6232)*, 333–336.

27. Tehovnik, E. J., Slocum, W. M., Carvey, C. E., & Schiller, P. H. (2005). Phosphene induction and the generation of saccadic eye movements by striate cortex. *Journal of Neurophysiology*, 93(1), 1–19.

28. Baguley, D., McFerran, D., & Hall, D. (2013). Tinnitus. *The Lancet, 382*(9904), 1600–1607.

Chapter 5: **Recognize Muscular Tension and Dormancy**

"You translate everything, whether physical or mental or spiritual, into muscular tension."
— *F. M. Alexander (1869-1955)*

"Suppose you're interacting with an abusive boss. Without realizing it, you hold some part of your body still in order to manage your behavior during the confrontation. Tension in your jaw, throat, or shoulders keeps you from lashing out and losing your job. Tension in your hips or feet keeps you from storming out of the room. Similar tensions may arise when you deal with a relative's expectations of you or during a disagreement with a friend."
— *Mary Bond (b. 1942)*

This chapter discusses a form of trauma that transforms muscles on a cellular scale: repetitive strain. The first half of the chapter introduces the concepts of bracing and persistent muscular tension and explains how to recognize them in your own body. The second half dives into the social and emotional aspects of muscle tension, laying out the relationships between long-term strain, pain, breathing, and submissiveness. Exercises are offered throughout to aid you in recovering from your bodily tension.

Recognizing Excessive Muscular Tone

It can be difficult to recognize the physical sensations of muscular strain. We become so accustomed to the pain and discomfort that they become effectively imperceptible, the same way we stop noticing unpleasant smells. It often takes a significant shift for us to notice how our bodies really feel. This happened to me after I strained my shoulder skateboarding. After the accident, a doctor prescribed me a dozen pills of meloxicam, a nonsteroidal anti-inflammatory drug (NSAID) with analgesic effects. After my first dose, I spent a few hours trying to analyze the effects of the drug. My muscles felt looser, and this quickly put me to sleep.

I woke up in the middle of the night to feel my hamstrings burning intensely, but they had not been stretched or exercised recently in any unusual way. It took me a few minutes to realize that this pain was their normal baseline condition. The strain had simply been unmasked by the NSAID drug. I had become utterly accustomed to the fact that this tension went to bed with me every night. I quickly realized that the problem was widespread. My hamstrings were chronically strained from overzealous exercise, but so were my hips, lower back, shoulders, and neck. That night, as I focused on gradually relaxing these body parts, I began to realize just how much I had been clenching them in a bizarre, contorted way.

This experience made me think of a lesson that my mother taught me. In my twenties, I developed a condition called plantar fasciitis that causes pain in the soles of the feet. She shared the method that she used to cure her plantar fasciitis, saying something along these lines: "Jared, it's a medical disorder, but it comes from tension. You must be curling your feet into 'fists' at night. Right now, you are unconscious of this tendency, but it is possible to create awareness. Each evening before you go to bed, focus on the sensations in your feet and tell yourself that you plan to let the tension release and remain released as you sleep. Don't allow your feet to remain clenched all night." I had painful plantar fasciitis for a full year, yet after two nights of following her instructions, meditating closely on the sensations of tension, the pain in my feet was gone. Right there, lying in bed, I saw the connection and realized that this same lesson applied not only to my heels, but to my hamstrings, my heartache, my headache, and my whole body.

Tone, Hypertonia, and Hypotonia

Muscle tone, also referred to as residual muscle tension or tonus, is a continuous and passive partial contraction found in all skeletal muscles. It is often conceptualized as the muscles' resistance to passive stretching during a resting state. Muscles receive continuous innervation from the nervous system ensuring that, even in rest, they remain in a semi-active default state. Thus, there is no complete rest in living muscle tissue.

Both extensor and flexor muscles are constantly kept activated, which helps us maintain muscle readiness. For instance, your bicep (a flexor) and triceps (an extensor) are both always in a state of partial contraction. They complement and support each other, no matter how much you try to relax them. Muscles on opposite sides of a joint contract in unison to stabilize the joint. This kind of antagonism occurs all over the body. It is beneficial and necessary.

Muscle tone is normal, but it can become too intense under certain conditions and begin to cause harm. Excessive tone is referred to as persistent muscle tension, muscle spasticity, or hypertonia. Hypertonic muscles can be found in crucial places throughout our bodies and are sources of chronic pain, stiffness, and premature frailty for every adult on the planet.

The cause of excessive muscular tone and the accompanying pain we experience is multifactorial. Hypertonia can be exacerbated by bad habits, wear and tear, genetic risk factors, and injuries such as car accidents and falls. However, most of the preventable muscular pain that we suffer is derived from a low-energy injury to the tissues known as repetitive strain. A repetitive strain injury is caused by repetitious tasks or by sustained awkward positions. Almost any job, profession, or chore you can imagine involves monotonous contractions through which muscles are subject to continuous or near-continuous strain. While repetitive strain may occur intermittently, its effects build up over years, resulting in chronic conditions.

Longstanding instances of muscular tension develop pathways in the nervous system that reinforce and perpetuate them. Simultaneously, an array of cellular changes takes place within muscle cells themselves, forcing them to contract permanently, forfeiting strength and flexibility. By becoming accustomed to such burdens, we force ourselves to carry them unknowingly. This is how we come to feel the weight of the world on our shoulders. We are all hauling an invisible, intangible load, forcing dozens of muscles throughout our body to push and pull against absolutely nothing.

Refrain from Muscular Bracing

Excessive tension in any posture is called muscular bracing, and it is pervasive. We brace muscles all over our bodies every day. Squinting and the raising and lowering of the brow discussed in Chapter 4 are also forms of bracing. Mostly, we brace as a reflexive response to things that make us worried or uncomfortable. Due to the false sense of security it can afford, some researchers have termed it "muscular armoring." Bracing is intended to prepare us to quickly initiate offensive or defensive movements as when we protect the neck by keeping the shoulders raised. Small amounts of temporary bracing are healthy and can be helpful during rough and tumble play, contact sports, falls, or collisions. Unnecessary bracing, however, keeps the body "on guard" and rigid. Thus, when you need to move, you are forced to overcome your own resistance, forfeiting grace and coordination.

Keeping our muscles tense makes us feel in control but is a dysfunctional coping tactic. People generalize bracing from physical challenges to intellectual and social ones. This is why some experts refer to instances of bracing as "neurotic holding patterns." For instance, we tense during social encounters, especially confrontational ones. People tense their bodies during standardized tests, social gatherings, and public speaking. This hinders their performance by interfering with productive efforts and by causing discomfort and autonomic stress. As we will discuss in Chapter 22, the sensation of fear in your gut and the sensation of having your heart in your throat are also manifestations of chronic bracing.

Imagine that you are standing alone in a strange, dark parking lot with nothing nearby to grab ahold of. You hear someone yell, "Brace yourself!" What pose do you strike? Whatever pose you imagined is likely one that you commonly adopt during stress and startle. The muscles responsible for this pose are the ones you brace most often, and so they are likely currently in the process of becoming locked up. Explore this a little further using the first unbracing activity below.

Relaxation Activity #5.1: *Making a Claw*

Tense all the muscles in your hand, making it into a stiff claw. Curl your fingers so that all fifteen knuckles are partially bent. Keeping your hand in that formation, see whether you can tense it even further. Keep it tight as you open and close it five times.

Now, use your imagination. Try to feel what would happen to your hand if you were forced to hold it like this for a week straight. It would become immobile, inflamed, and excruciating. Consider how often you tense your hand in daily life. Has it already taken a toll? Going forward, work on undoing that tension. Try to notice the claw whenever it materializes and allow it to revert to a soft, lithe hand.

You also want your hands to be strong, so contracting their muscles firmly is necessary. The important thing is that you allow them to relax deeply after you stop using them. Make a very firm claw and then let it relax five times in a row. How you respond to the discomfort involved in the effort makes all the difference. Don't allow the discomfort from the contraction to influence you to keep bracing. Rather, plunge into the deeper level of relaxation that is available after you have brought the muscles to fatigue.

There are cyclical relationships between stress, bracing, and arthritis.[1] Some specialists refer to forms of bracing as "prearthritic postures." Joints can only be braced for so many years before they become inflamed and degenerative. My mother has osteoarthritis in her hands. Some of her knuckles are larger and more deformed than others. She firmly believes that the most affected knuckles are those that she braced more during stress over decades. An extreme example is the "raised-arm babas" of India. These are men who, for spiritual reasons, have decided to always raise one arm in the air. Over the years, their shoulders become stiff as a board and completely useless. As you look over the table below, think about which bracing patterns you use.

Internal	Facial	Postural
Tightening the Jaw	Squinting the Eyes	Raising the Shoulders
Constricting the Throat	Raising the Eyebrows	Bracing the Lower Back
Sucking the Tongue	Straining the Smile	Hunching the Neck
Constricting the Nasopharynx	Straining the Sneer	Neglecting the Glutes and Abs
Straining the Vocal Folds	Pursing the Lips	Bracing the Shoulder Blades
Shallow Breathing	Tightening the Cheeks	Clenching the Hands and Feet
Abdominal Tensing	Drawing Down the Corners of the Mouth	Tilting the Pelvis to One Side

Table 5.1: Common Forms of Bracing that Compromise Muscle and Cause Pain

Bracing belongs to a more general category known as *dysponesis*, or the misdirected use of energy in the musculoskeletal system, of which unnecessary tensing of the muscles is just one example.[2] This wasting of energy is destructive. For example, dentists and orthodontists make particular note of jaw clenching, teeth grinding, and tongue tension because those movements push the teeth out of their optimal alignment. In Chapter 13, we will discuss how bracing the back pushes the spine out of alignment. Muscular bracing is a factor in almost all joint disorders and is responsible for carpal tunnel, temporomandibular joint disorder, tennis elbow, and countless others. I believe that most chronic injuries, despite the fancy and distracting terms used by physicians, start with tension caused by bracing.

One way a mammal remembers that it just glimpsed a predator is by crouching down and becoming very tense. We often use muscular tension to keep something in mind. When I need to remember something, or when there is an urgent need to do something that cannot be done right away, I become tenser. The specific part of my body necessary to carry out the task is often where the tension manifests. For instance, I will try to remind myself to write down a thought by tensing my fingers as if I were gripping a pencil. Recognize when this happens to you and try not to use tension as a mnemonic aid.

We tend to be negligent of excessive increases in muscle tension even when we are performing simple tasks. We tighten muscles that are not involved in what we are doing and then keep those muscles tight even after we finish. If the action is built into your job or daily routine, you can start by improving the ergonomics of your workspace or taking more regular breaks. You can also teach yourself to selectively calm muscles that you are not actively using for the task at hand. The key is to constantly and creatively alter your body posture so that unused muscles are engaged and overused muscles are given a break.

> ## Relaxation Activity #5.2: *Monitor Your Bracing During Teeth Brushing*
> The next time you brush your teeth, notice the movements in your hand, arm, shoulder, neck, face, and torso. Are you tensing muscles or expending energy that you don't need to? For instance, you might be gripping the toothbrush too tightly, flexing heavily at the elbow or shoulder, locking your jaw, or craning your neck to one side. Do you alter your posture and vary the repetitive motions to give your muscles breaks? Use this activity as an example that you can extend to all your daily chores and rituals. Generalize this experience to as many other activities as possible, including writing with a pen, typing with a keyboard, or holding a phone, tablet, book, remote controller, or steering wheel.

Microbreaks Allow Muscles the Short Rests They Need

Not all muscle tension is bad. After all, there is no way to exercise without tensing your muscles. But bracing is very different from healthy exercise because it does not include tiny rest periods called "microbreaks." Sometimes, all our muscles need is a few seconds, or even just a few fractions of a second, without being held taut. When the electrical activity of muscle is tracked with electrodes, these moments of downtime show up as "electromyographic gaps"— brief intervals during which the muscles slacken and relax. They are essential.

For example, every step you take involves significant exertion as you push off against the ground. However, as one leg takes over, the other is given a break during the time it takes to swing it forward again. That respite allows the muscles to "regenerate" and prepare for the next step. If you didn't have this microbreak after every step, walking more than a few hundred meters would be difficult. In much the same way, all the muscles in your body require microbreaks.

Without momentarily reverting to a relaxed baseline tone, muscles cannot replenish and unwanted processes ensue. You have probably noticed the difference between fatigue caused by sustained bracing (hyperfatigue) and fatigue caused by exercise that contains microbreaks. The former aches and is unpleasant while the latter is both soothing and exhilarating. Indeed, the most important factor in building healthy muscle is to allow it to relax. The more relaxed your muscles are at rest, the more quickly they recover from exercise. This is why relaxed muscle responds dramatically to training, whereas tense muscle responds sluggishly. Whenever you are not using a muscle, allow it to go limp. It almost seems slothful, but it's not; it's the way you should live your life.

Intermittent breaks and rests can help you disrupt long periods of unnecessary rigidity. Naps can work wonders in this regard. During sleep, and especially during REM sleep, changes occur in brain signaling that cause vastly reduced muscle tone, known as atonia. This is one reason why short (10- to 20-minute) naps can be so invigorating. Short naps can also restore alertness, mental performance, and learning ability.[3] As you nap, you are even giving your heart a brief rest, which may be why naps have been associated with reduced coronary mortality.[4] Just remember that naps of 30 minutes or more often lead to sleep inertia, impaired alertness, and tiredness. When you feel depleted, after the gym, after an upsetting episode, or whenever you start to feel stiff and sore, set your phone's timer for 20 minutes and allow yourself a recuperative power nap. Even if you don't fall asleep, just giving yourself a few minutes to lay down during the day provides a reprieve that can be highly beneficial in the long term.

Why don't we allow ourselves the microbreaks that our bodies call for? Often, it is due to social pressures. Propriety and intimidation related to the status hierarchy cause us to brace, then feel guilty about relaxing. Chronic submissive signaling disallows you from claiming the microbreaks that your muscles need. When at a dinner date or in a board room, we don't give our neurotic holding patterns a single second of downtime. Well-composed people give various muscles involved in social displays microbreaks. In fact, we can conceptualize composure as skill in microbreaking. Of course, even our breathing muscles require microbreaks.

Unbrace Your Exhalation with the Passive Exhale

Diaphragmatic bracing is the central feature of distressed breathing and a core symptom of trauma. Remember Activity 5.1, in which you held your hand like a claw and kept it tight as you opened and closed it? This is exactly what you are doing with your diaphragm when stressed. This kind of bracing could be an excellent exercise for the diaphragm if it only lasted for 30 seconds at a time, but we tend to do it for hours or days at a time. Continuously over-tensing the diaphragm and other respiratory muscles reduces their strength and range of motion, resulting in rapid shallow breathing.

The inbreath requires muscular contraction, but the outbreath does not. It is not necessary to do any muscular work during exhalation. The positive pressure of air in your lungs is enough to create the force. This effortless return of the diaphragm to its resting position is called elastic recoil. The air naturally wants to be pressed out of your lungs as it would from a deflating balloon. Unfortunately, most of us keep our breathing muscles tense during exhalation, and this ensnares us in a state of fight or flight. Stopping this requires awareness and practice. To perform a passive exhalation, all you need to do is let your breathing go limp while you are exhaling. After a minute or two of practicing this, you should actually be able to feel the diaphragm simmer down.

Relaxation Exercise #5.1: *Unbracing the Diaphragm While Exhaling*

Perform paced breathing for five minutes. Take full inhalations, and when you start each exhalation, let go of the diaphragm completely. Every exhalation should be a completely passive form of freefall throughout which all the breathing musculature is relaxed. Imagine the leisurely descent of a parachute. You are not doing any work at all, and it should proceed at its own pace. The air should be oozing out of your nostrils on its own. Once you practice this for five minutes, you should be able to tell that you were holding your diaphragm like a tense "claw" during your exhalation before. Allowing the diaphragm to go limp during the exhale is extremely important for its health because, just like all muscles, it needs periods of inactivity to regenerate. Because you never stop breathing, its only chance for such a microbreak is during the exhalation.

Imagine that for some reason you are responsible for driving a car up and down a low-grade hill, over and over again. For a while, you keep the engine on during the descent, but since the descent lasts for a few minutes, you realize that you can turn the engine off, put the car into neutral, and just let it coast without having to touch the brake, the accelerator, or the wheel. This is what a passive exhalation should feel like. After you finish your inhale, just take the keys out of the ignition.

Your inhalation is also braced; it is just much harder to notice. An inhalation requires the contraction of the diaphragm down into the gut to create the vacuum that draws air into the lungs. But this contraction is often braced beyond what is necessary, like the opening of a tightly clenched hand. This bracing impedes belly breathing and pulls the air into your upper chest. If you can interrupt it during an inhalation, you will feel your belly coming uncoupled from the bottom of your rib cage. The passive exhale will help you with this uncoupling. As you learn to sense your diaphragmatic tension during the exhale, you can teach yourself how to lessen the unnecessary tension occurring during the inhale. Once you have done this, your breathing will become much more efficient and less labored.

It is worth mentioning that aside from bracing the inhale during the exhale, many of us also brace the exhale during the inhale. This is when we keep the thoracic muscles responsible for exhalation clenched while breathing in. This is also completely unnecessary. Spend some time trying to notice these effects in your own breathing.

After performing the passive exhalation for a few days, a sense of irritation in your chest will dissipate. When this discomfort and inflammation is totally gone, you will feel a profound sense of relief. The passive exhalation is so important that I consider it the fifth tenet of optimal breathing. Expect it to increase the benefits you get from paced breathing. The passive exhale is such a fundamental routine that it is actually a reflexive response that all mammals use after a stressor has come and gone. Can you guess what it is?

Once a stressful episode has resolved, all species of mammal exhibit "deep spontaneous breaths." They inhale very deeply so that they can then exhale passively to reset and restore equilibrium in their autonomic nervous system. We know this as sighing. Even mice sigh, and I believe that, like us, they do it to provide the diaphragm with a microbreak. However, if you provide your diaphragm with a microbreak during every exhalation, you won't feel the need to sigh anymore. The trick is to learn to exhale limply even after a shallow inhalation. Sighing is very frequent in people diagnosed with panic disorders. I used to sigh constantly, but after diaphragmatic retraining, I rarely catch myself doing it anymore. Master the passive exhalation because it is highly de-traumatizing.

Persistent Muscle Tension Creates Trigger Points

Excessive muscle tension and the absence of microbreaks eventually produce "knots" that can be felt under your skin. They occur all over the body. They are often palpable, raised nodules tender to the touch, producing a dull, aching pain when pressed firmly. In the medical literature, these knots are referred to as trigger points, trigger sites, or spasms, and they cause reductions in muscle mass, flexibility, strength, and endurance.[5] They are hyper-irritated spots in taut bands of skeletal muscle fibers created by chronic muscle overload. They usually involve a local contraction in a small number of muscle fibers within a larger muscle bundle.[6]

Many scientists refer to these knots as "myofascial trigger points." The "myo" is derived from the Greek word for "muscle" while "fascial" refers to the tough outer lining that keeps muscles in place (fascia is a type of connective tissue that forms a continuous scaffold around all the muscles and tendons in the body). Myofascial trigger points are small patches of muscle and fascia that pull together in an isolated spasm. They are different from whole-muscle spasms like a charley horse or cramp, which are more transient, have a sudden onset, and involve hard contraction of the entire muscle. Although they can contribute to cramping, trigger points are different in that they are long-lasting, have a gradual onset, and involve partial contractions in small portions of the muscle.

In addition to their immediate detrimental effects on muscle function, trigger points often cluster together and pull on tendons and ligaments, causing joint problems and "deep" pain. The tension they cause at joints can result in clicking, popping, and grating sounds. Over time, they can contribute to bone spurs, pinched nerves, and arthritis.[7] Trigger points can be seen in greatly magnified pictures of muscle tissue like the one below. They look like bunched-up distortions in a web-like matrix.

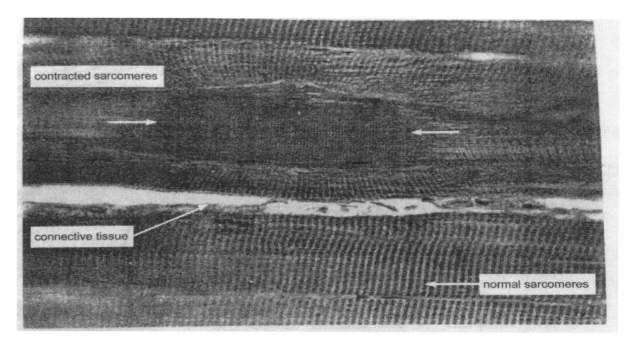

Figure 5.1: Knot of partially contracted sarcomeres in the muscle fiber from the leg of a dog at 240x magnification. Compare with the normal sarcomeres above and below it. This knot looks like an active contraction but has no electrical (EMG) activity and is, thus, stuck in partial contraction. Reprinted with permission from Simons and Stolov (1976).

Dr. Janet G. Travell, MD (1901-1997) is generally recognized as the leading pioneer in trigger point diagnosis and treatment. It has been said that she "single-handedly created this branch of medicine."[8] Travell, who was the White House physician during the Kennedy and Johnson administrations, emphasized that trigger points are demoralizing and devastating to quality of life. She called them the "scourge of mankind." Advanced-stage trigger points are the worst. They usually present in clusters, are the most painful, and involve highly warped muscle fibers with large numbers of molecular aberrations. In reality, most people are practically covered in trigger points from old injuries, bad posture, poor workout techniques, and bracing.

Muscle Tension Develops at the Molecular Level

To better understand trigger points, we need a little more background on muscles themselves. Muscles are composed of fibers, which are themselves made of smaller fibers. The thinnest of those hold sarcomeres, in which contraction takes place. A sarcomere is a microscopic structure built from two kinds of filament-like molecules: actin and myosin. Actin and myosin form interdigitating strands that can be activated. When active, they move past each other, quickly creating contractile force.

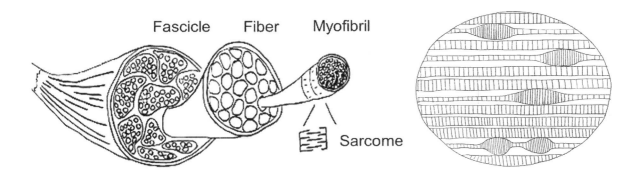

Illustration 5.1: A. Muscle made of fibers, containing sarcomeres; B. Microscopic view of contracted sarcomeres in a muscle myofibril. An actual trigger point may contain dozens of these tiny knots.

Millions of sarcomeres must contract to perform even the smallest movement. After they contract, the sarcomeres relax when their actin and myosin strands are uncoupled from each other and pull apart. In healthy muscle, actin and myosin wait patiently in a relaxed, decoupled state until an impulse from the nervous system tells them to pull past each other again. In unhealthy muscle, they are stuck. Many specialists believe that trigger points start to form when overuse causes actin and myosin to become fixed in an interlocked position. This interlocking puts the muscle into a static state of *contracture*, in which the strands no longer separate and relax.

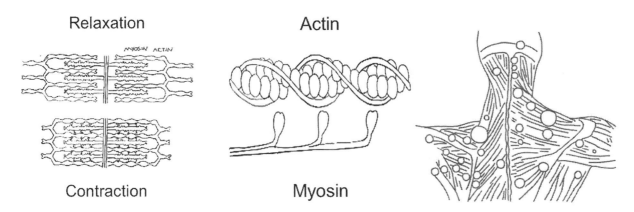

Illustration 5.2: A. Relaxed sarcomere on top and a contracted sarcomere on the bottom with actin and myosin visible; B. Myosin curls like a finger, pulling on actin and allowing them to slide past each other to create muscular movement; C. Human neck and shoulders covered with clusters of trigger points.

Trigger points originate from a few different sources: (1) sustained low-level contraction, 2) sudden muscle overload, (3) "eccentric" contraction when a muscle stretches and contracts simultaneously, and (4) gross trauma or injury to the muscle. Regardless of the cause, trigger points slow blood flow to the muscle and cause oxygen deprivation at the affected site. The reduced blood flow then causes sarcomeres to contract further, constricting the surrounding capillaries. Capillaries normally supply the muscle with blood, so when they constrict, it leads to reduced circulation or *ischemia* that impairs many cellular processes.

Without blood flow, chemical waste products from muscular activity start to accumulate. Eventually, the waste stimulates pain receptors in nearby nerve endings, sending pain signals to the brain.[9] Active trigger points demonstrate an unusual biochemical mix not seen in healthy tissue. It is an acidic milieu containing increased levels of proinflammatory, contractile, and pain-causing substances. And remember, we draw our very breaths with muscles that are affected by these symptoms.

Muscle Shortening and Scar Tissue

A muscle can change its resting length to adapt to the length at which it is habitually used or positioned. Muscles usually become shorter due to prolonged contracture. This is known as *adaptive muscle shortening* and places the muscle in a state of partial contraction. It is another pervasive clinical finding that affects every person who has ever lived.

People confined to long periods of sitting exhibit debilitating shortening of the lower back and hip muscles, especially the hip flexors. Similarly, wearing high-heeled shoes causes prolonged plantar flexion of the foot, which results in adaptive shortening of the soleus muscles. Constant squinting shortens the muscle fibers of the orbicularis oculi, narrowing the eyes. Straining the sneer causes the muscles that lift the top lip to shrink, making the face appear hideous. When the muscles in your knees and ankles shorten, they leave you vulnerable to sprains and tears. Holding a hunched neck posture leads to shortening of the sternocleidomastoid and other muscles in the front of the neck, making it very difficult to stop hunching because the decreased length of these muscles pulls the head down. As Chapter 19 will explain, bracing the muscles surrounding the genitals may play a role in sexual dysfunction. There are examples of adaptive muscle shortening in muscles all over our bodies.

The pressure from prolonged contracture pulls on tendons, straining them and distressing the joints when they move. Next, ligaments and joint capsules retract. These changes perturb nerve endings within the muscles and joints, causing deep-seated pain. Muscle shortening also increases wear and tear, contributing to inflammatory and degenerative changes such as tendonitis, fasciitis, bursitis, and osteoarthritis. Many different tissue types are damaged by strain, including articular cartilages, connective tissues, tendons, fascia, menisci, ligaments, and spinal disks.

Adaptive muscle shortening can be made worse by the accumulation of *scar tissue*. Scar tissue is a very tough, inflexible, fibrous material that binds itself to strained muscle fibers, attempting to draw the damaged fibers together. The result is a bulky mass of stiff tissue surrounding the site. In some cases, it is possible to feel and even see this mass under the skin. When scar tissue adheres to muscle fibers, it prevents them from sliding back and forth properly, limiting the flexibility of a muscle or joint.

Scar tissue tends to shrink and deform the surrounding tissues, diminishing strength and making the body feel heavy. It tends to adhere to nerve cells, leading to chronic pain. Existing research has found that scar tissue is weaker, less elastic, more prone to future re-injury, and up to 1,000 times more pain-sensitive than normal, healthy tissue. This results in chronic pain that, under most circumstances, lasts a lifetime. In people who brace the most, these effects create visibly apparent postural distortions.

Excessive Tension is Debilitating and Constrains Your Physique

Muscles encumbered by trigger points and adaptive shortening can be conceptualized as *dormant* muscles. This is so because they are difficult to recruit, don't move with the rest of the body, and are starved of blood. Dormant muscles cannot recover adequately after a workout and are resistant to growth and strengthening because they can never fully relax, and thus can never fully heal. As long as they are under constant self-imposed strain, they will continue to grow harder, more fragile, and decrepit. Scrunched-up muscles crumple your body and cause it to buckle under every movement.

Pregnancy itself does not necessarily adversely affect a woman's physique. Rather, it is the months of prolonged bracing, absence of postural variety, and limited range of motion that can accompany the later stages of pregnancy for some women that have prominent, long-lasting effects. Moreover, although some of the natural variation in physique between humans is due to exercise, genetics, and exposure to testosterone, much of it can be attributed to differences in dormant muscle that arose due to bracing during stress.

You have significant untapped reservoirs of muscle in your body that correspond to areas you brace and have been bracing for decades. For example, think about the hunch you probably have in your neck. Starting at birth, you had a natural tendency to straighten the cervical vertebrae in your neck, stacking them in a straight line. That straight-necked, upright posture is optimal. But social pressures can affect how we carry our heads and necks; the less safe, stable, or welcoming your childhood environment was, the more you were conditioned to hunch over, communicating modesty or submission. The standard submissive neck posture is to stoop over, jut your chin out, and tilt your head back. All of those changes reduce your height and help you appear guarded. But they also introduce a slant in your neck, which is an inefficient way of stacking vertebrae against the force of gravity. The excessive tension that develops leads to the proliferation of trigger points, and those, in turn, cause muscle dormancy in your neck, shoulders, and chest, and from there on down the spine.

Chapter 13 will detail exactly how to reclaim your neck and regain its flexibility and full range of motion. But the neck is just one example of a reservoir of muscle that has been suppressed that you can tap into. These reservoirs can be found all over our bodies. Take your clothes off and look in the mirror. Any body parts that don't appear nubile and supple have great potential. If all of our muscles were brought completely out of dormancy, we would have the physiques (if not bulk) of elite athletes.

Injuries Lead to Muscular Bracing

Injuries contribute to and interact with bracing. After getting hurt, individuals often try to avoid experiencing pain by tensing the area surrounding the site of injury. When someone sprains their ankle, they unintentionally contract many muscles in the ankle, setting it in a fixed, defensive position. This is intended to protect the injury. In fact, it is known as "splinting" because it acts as a splint to immobilize the joint. Unfortunately, it also deprives the muscles of the rest, oxygen, and nutrients they need to heal. As a result, splinting worsens the pain in the long term by overtaxing the muscles involved. This happens partly because we tend to breathe extremely shallowly whenever we injure ourselves (because as you know, shallow breathing causes bracing). This is why, whenever I experience an injury, I pull out my breath metronome immediately.

Injuries almost always result in some form of persistent muscle tension. Even major medical procedures can contribute. *Iatrogenic pain* is a term referring to pain caused by medical treatment and is especially common with the use of braces, slings, casts, and surgeries. Immobilizing a broken forearm with a cast can easily lead to frozen shoulder syndrome, in which a group of deltoid muscles is barred from moving through its normal range of motion as tension gradually mounts.

I had a melanoma removed from my shoulder blade in my mid-teens, and I recently found that I have a series of muscular knots under the scar from bracing the area. My brother received a large shot in the quadriceps during his appendectomy 20 years ago, and he says the same area troubles him often. Think conscientiously about past injuries, medical procedures, and other forms of trauma, identifying how they might be causing you to brace or tense muscles even today.

Stress and muscular tension also make us more susceptible to physical injury because tense muscles fail and tear under excessive force, whereas relaxed ones are more resilient. The muscles strained by sitting in a fixed position at a computer for eight hours a day are the most susceptible to damage from a fall or car accident. Thus, injury can lead to bracing, and bracing can lead to re-injury.

Tense muscle tissue can be conceptualized as an injury or as a trauma even if there was no precipitating accident. The word "injury" is defined as physical damage to a biological organism. The word "trauma" is defined as an abnormality in an organism's tissues usually caused by injury. By these definitions, any form of persistent bracing, and the trigger points stemming from it, are both injurious and traumatic. Unfortunately, once they get bad enough, they can poison us emotionally.

The Link Between Tension, Pain, and Negative Emotion

"These mountains that you are carrying, you were only supposed to climb." — Najwa Zebian (b. 1990)

Physical pain is an adaptive, evolved mechanism. The pain from a cut or burn informs us that our bodies are suffering damage. It gives us built-in motivation to withdraw from the source of harm and learn to avoid it in the future. But what about muscular pain, also known as myalgia? In contrast to physical pain, myalgia has more to do with restricting movement. It compels us to refrain from specific motions that might be damaging or harmful—it tells us not to over-stretch a strained muscle, not to bend a weakened joint too far. It also tells us when we approach the limits of our healthy range of motion, giving us important feedback about what our bodies can and cannot do. This would have restricted aging hunter-gatherers from movements that had proven necessary and probably also helped them save energy.[10] Due to the negative emotions it creates, however, muscular pain is destructive to our well-being.

Suffering is not abstract or conceptual. It is embodied in the pain circuits of your nervous system. *Nociceptive pain* is pain caused by the activation of pain receptors known as nociceptors. Nociceptors respond to either thermal (e.g., heat or cold), chemical (e.g., inflammatory), or mechanical (e.g., crushing or tearing) sources of harm. They come in three general types: visceral (organ), superficial (skin), and deep somatic pain (muscle). Deep somatic pain is triggered by the activation of nociceptors in ligaments, tendons, bones, blood vessels, fascia, and muscles. It is dull, aching, and difficult to localize. Strangely, we become so accustomed to it that we don't consciously notice its presence until a painkiller takes it away. Drugs like heroin and ecstasy induce intense euphoric states, largely by alleviating this pain.

Long-term bracing of our body parts and "chakras" causes deep somatic pain that poisons our minds. The toxicity is especially apparent in extreme examples, such as people with chronic pain. People living with long-term pain of any kind frequently display psychological disturbances and exhibit elevated levels of hysteria, depression, and hypochondriasis (the "neurotic triad"). Chronic pain patients also generally have low self-esteem[11] and higher-than-average levels of anxiety, fear, and anger.[12] In fact, somatic pain is known to interact with *psychogenic* pain, which arises from social rejection, defeat, heartbreak, and grief. These two forms of pain comingle and exacerbate one another.[13] There is no telling how much the undiagnosed chronic pain from our muscular tension desecrates us emotionally.

The experience of pain is transformed by paced breathing. Try it the next time you feel either physical or psychological pain. It takes all the edge off. One of the quickest and easiest ways to create massive amounts of non-damaging pain is to submerge an arm or leg in ice water. Without paced breathing, this is excruciating for the two to five minutes it takes for the body part to go numb. For me, it is usually so bad that I end up pulling my body part out of the water 4 or 5 times before I go numb. The discomfort is so intense that I practically involuntarily retract my limb. With paced breathing, however, the pain is tolerable and I have no inclination to pull it out of the ice. When we allow pain to control our breathing rate, we also allow it to control our behavior.

Pain signals from nerve endings in tense muscles bombard our brains throughout the day. Those signals are relayed to brain areas involved in fear and grief, such as the insula, the anterior cingulate cortex, and the amygdala. These brain centers integrate pain input from anatomical landmarks all around the body to help compute the appropriate level of pained reactions: stifling, agitation, rage, dread, submission, and distressed breathing. Thus, we become tense, breathe shallowly, then respond to the ensuing discomfort with more tension.[14] This cycle is depicted relative to other concepts we have addressed thus far in the diagram below.

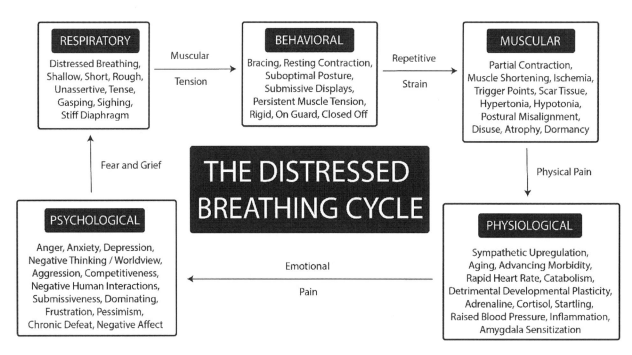

Figure 5.2: Distressed Breathing Cycle

We feel like the emotional pain we experience originates from the content of our thoughts. But this is backward. Negative thinking is driven by the inability to take a full breath and by preexisting pain in our muscles and related tissues. These are the ultimate causes of our persistent background unease. Our thinking becomes oppositional only when it is imbued with pain. Tense muscles are leeches latched on to our souls. I believe that trigger points in our faces, spines, and internal organs are the physical embodiment of melancholy, world-weariness, ennui, and angst.

Don't Let Your "Pain-Body" Control You

Spiritual author Eckhart Tolle has elaborated on a concept he calls the "pain-body." According to Tolle, the pain-body is the accumulation of negative life experiences that create affective pain and discomfort.[15] Tolle discusses how it is intrinsically tied to the ego and how environmental circumstances that assault our pride amplify the pain-body and its negative effects on our behavior. He advises that people "live in the present moment" so that they can recognize when the pain-body shifts from being dormant to being active. When it becomes active, it makes us act in desperation, distorting our interpretations and judgments and causing us to do things that we later regret. I believe that his assessment is correct and that a considerable proportion of the pain-body corresponds to deep somatic pain from the cumulative effects of muscular bracing. I also believe that the pain-body becomes active when latent trigger points become active.

Specialists traditionally categorize trigger points as either active or latent. An active trigger point is painful, whereas a latent trigger point is not. Latent trigger points, which are far more numerous, generally cannot be felt unless deep pressure is applied. Latent trigger points can be activated by muscular strain, especially after an abusive workout, a sudden shock, or a long car ride. Alternatively, they can be activated by shallow breathing, which is why facial tension, headaches, and back pain coincide with stress. Consider the unpleasantness of public speaking, for example. As we stand in front of a room of people with our eyebrows raised, our eyes squinting, our neck tense, our shoulders elevated, our stomach in knots, our vocal musculature taut, and our back stiff, latent trigger points in all those muscle groups become active. The resulting pain derails us, undermining our presentation and diluting our message. When latent trigger points become active, we become an inferior version of ourselves.

The pain can also provoke us to lash out. Even rats exhibit pain-induced aggression. If you place two rats on a metal grid through which they receive an electric shock, they will attack each other ferociously when the shock is delivered.[16] Hundreds of similar studies suggest that mammals have a tendency to displace aggression, reallocating blame for their physical pain toward other nearby animals.

This is consistent with Tolle's account. He explains that the pain-body is born of and enticed by pain. In his words, it is a "psychic parasite" that wants to provoke pain in others and then "feed on the ensuing drama." He says that people's pain-bodies possess them, causing them to do bad things that they would never otherwise do, and that they react to the pain-bodies of others with either revulsion or aggression.

I believe that we constantly provoke one another's pain-bodies (and latent trigger points) to establish social hierarchy by determining who has been debilitated more by chronic stress. Do we all do this constantly? Yes. Are we evil for doing it? No. Remember, competing for social dominance is an innate system for determining which animal has priority over resources. It is a highly preferable alternative to actual violence and represents the mammalian brain's imperfect attempt at creating order. A considerable step toward becoming free of this evolutionary design flaw is to unburden yourself from the cyclic relationship between distressed breathing, bracing, and pain. Use Exercise 5.2 to start breaking the cycle.

Relaxation Exercise #5.2 *Desensitize Yourself to Pain*

The next time you feel angry, anxious, lonely, sad, or any negative emotion, try to find the root cause of it in the form of your bodily pain. Once you localize it in your body, take its power away by recognizing it for what it is. Use the following concepts to help you.

To overcome our pain-bodies, we must change our relationship with pain. Our aversion and oversensitivity to discomfort are exactly what drive it. When pain makes us brace or breathe shallowly, we are fighting against it and making it worse. The way we bear our suffering should be dignified. Accept it with courage and grit. The unease we manufacture when we wallow in pain braces trigger points that keep us tense. Instead, like a warrior, we need to be tolerant and nonreactive in response to internal discomfort.

The pain you feel is not you. It is just an annoying buzzer going off in the background reminding you that you have been going too hard on your body. This should cause you to ease up on your body rather than go harder. Recognize the limited validity of the discomfort and develop the ability to tune it out of your experience. Disidentify from it. Don't allow it to flip your thoughts from positive to negative. Don't allow it to make you attack others.

> You will find that the raw, agonizing buzz of anxiety will fall away if you breathe as if you weren't in pain. By breathing slowly and deeply while focusing on the subtle stinging reverberating throughout your body, you will learn to unbrace. This will heal you.

The Link Between Distressed Breathing and Muscular Tension

Scientists have documented that average muscle tension, especially tension in trigger points, increases during transient stress. Muscles will tighten up during a paper and pencil examination or during and after watching a horror film. The same is true for more chronic sources of stress, like long-lasting personal or work-related stress. Stress, and more specifically heightened arousal of the sympathetic nervous system, increases the risk of repetitive strain injury—especially during repetitive tasks.[17] This means that if you are stressed while sitting at the computer for hours, your body is fast at work, cementing your computer posture into your joints.

Stress causes bracing via distressed breathing. Numerous brain pathways connect shallow breathing to muscle tension.[18] This is a hardwired connection that prepares mammals for physical conflict. As our breath becomes shallow, we brace more in preparation for fighting.[19] Relaxed breathing, by contrast, causes us to brace less and experience less pain. So, unbrace your diaphragm and let your outbreaths become passive and limp.

Since childhood, my hands used to hurt and cramp after just a few minutes of uninterrupted writing or drawing. Since I started breathing diaphragmatically, however, my hands do not hurt or cramp even after an hour of pushing a pencil. When I do manual labor all day with friends, they all tell me the next day that their bodies are sore, but I notice that mine is not. This is because the way that I breathe now, after diaphragmatic retraining, is conducive to microbreaking. As you pursue the five tenets of diaphragmatic breathing described thus far, you will find similar examples in your own life.

Find Calm Through Visual Imagery

Imagine finding yourself alone on an inflatable raft following a nasty shipwreck. Your mind is racing, playing out the worst possible scenarios. You glance at the few remaining tins of food, realizing there is no way to know how many days you will be out on the open sea. The thought of starvation brings on a wave of panic and bodily constriction. Then, you hear a voice in your head: "Conserve your energy or you are going to die." Imagine at that second, you have an epiphany. You recognize panic as an energy consumer that will only increase your caloric requirements. You realize that you needed a life-and-death experience to see how your familiar neuroticism is simply a metabolic state that can be adjusted. "Wow," you say. "I've been carrying this frenetic tension for so long, but I can just let it go."

Picture yourself laying your head down on the plastic surface of the raft and making a concerted effort to placate your hectic reactivity. Let your body descend to an absolute minimum of activity. Your face goes lax, your heart beats slowly but steadily, you are breathing just enough to get adequate oxygen, and every muscle you aren't currently using unwinds. You let yourself be still as the rhythm of the ocean lulls you. Now, this was an extreme example, but it was meant to help you see that stressing out on a survival raft is counterproductive.

Similarly, your baseline level of stress today is almost certainly out of proportion to your immediate physical challenges.

There is no need to return to that raft. That was an intentionally provocative example. Instead, come up with positive imaginary. In mine, I am a man foraging on a sub-Saharan savannah 200,000 years ago, well before humanity split apart into distinct races. I am moving and working constantly, but at the same time, I am impossibly calm, cool, and level-headed. Most importantly, this version of me allows every muscle in his body to go lax unless it is needed for a particular motion. With hunger and nutrition major concerns, it would have been imperative for our ancestors to conserve metabolic activity, doing only what is required. So, this Jared walks and talks with incredible ease. His stride is fluid, his face is placid, and his posture is perfect yet effortless. I would like to encourage you to spend some time creating similar mental imagery that is compatible with calmness.

Stress raises metabolism in the short term, and activation of the sympathetic nervous system can double our resting (or "basal") metabolic rate. But it does so only for a few hours. Over weeks and months, chronic stress actually leads to a lowered metabolism and everything that comes with it, including weight gain, visceral fat, elevated blood pressure, cardiovascular disease, diabetes, and other health risks. One of many reasons for this is that, as you read earlier, when you start bracing a muscle, it burns a lot of energy, but if you keep bracing it, it shortens physically so that it doesn't have to burn energy to remain in contraction.

Scientists distinguish between *catabolic* states, in which energy is burned for movement, and *anabolic* states, in which energy is stored and used to construct necessary molecules like proteins. The parasympathetic system uses anabolism during periods of rest to build the body back up, leading to revitalization. The sympathetic system uses catabolism to burn energy for fight or flight. Catabolic breakdown that goes on too long consumes our energy stores, including important proteins, leading to depletion and corrosion. When we become stuck in anxious, stressed, or hyperactive states, catabolic pathways within our cells become overactive and place huge, unnecessary demands on our body's other systems. Stress even burns away muscle, making it harder to stay fit and lean. We are lumbering cellular survival machines burning ourselves to the ground because we are stuck in overdrive. You need to let your body relax so that you can stop burning parts of the ship.

If you need a role model for this kind of calm, look to those who naturally breathe with their diaphragm: toddlers. I have been fortunate enough to spend time babysitting my friends' children. One day with an imperturbable two-year-old girl was especially transformative for me. She was so sweet and pacific that my high-strung personality seemed likely to scare her. So, as we passed blocks back and forth, I worked on getting closer and closer to her level of wide-eyed peacefulness. Now, I often pretend that it is my responsibility to be a calming influence on others the way she was for me.

Some people don't want to be calmer. They enjoy being energetic and intense. The truth of the matter is that being energetic and being calm should be two sides of the same coin. Without the ability to dole out microbreaks, exhilaration turns into exhaustion in a matter of minutes. If a person cannot balance intensity with periods of rest, then they will burn out like a sprinter running a daily marathon.

Never Be Afraid of Being Too Calm

One of the greatest barriers to relaxation is the instinct to keep alert, on edge, and ready to act. Some people are afraid that becoming too calm will result in tragedy. It is true that increasing the output of the stress system might indeed help you fight or take flight if your challenges are immediate and very severe. However, if you don't know when the challenge will arise, then you are better off relaxing completely. This is because a chronically activated sympathetic stress system becomes a detriment in a matter of hours.

For instance, if you were convinced that someone or something was going to threaten your life in the next few minutes, maybe you would need to activate the sympathetic stress system. This is because it just might free up enough energy or accentuate a reaction that saves your life. However, if you have no grounds for assuming that a physical threat could take your life in the next hour, then you are better off turning the stress system all the way down and allowing your muscles and mind the rest they need to stay strong. Even a mixed martial artist would benefit from being as calm as possible up until minutes before entering the ring. So, stop holding your breath, stop clenching your diaphragm, and allow yourself to let go of the suspense.

Very few of us have life-threatening challenges. Most of the challenges we stress over are far from life or death and do not depend on adrenaline or split-second timing. Given our body's design and the nature of our modern challenges, the best strategy by far is to develop a relaxed, low-energy disposition. Know that even when you are calm, you can still be strong, quick, and nimble. Let this knowledge validate your confidence in relaxation.

Relaxation Activity #5.3: *Stay Limp Until You Spring into Action*

We tend to brace because we are preparing ourselves to spring into action. We have a deep inner fear that if we relax too much, we will not be able to react in time when something bad happens. Ironically, stress leads to startling, trembling, and excessive bracing, all of which interfere with our ability to produce effective physical responses. With this in mind, imagine the scenarios below and envision your entire body remaining completely relaxed up until the point at which you must react.

1) You are an actor in a play, waiting for your cue to come on stage.
2) You are a professional basketball player leisurely dribbling down the court, with just three seconds before you will make a fast break toward the basket for a dunk.
3) You watch your friend accidentally knock over a glass, and you prepare to catch it in midair.
4) Someone is yelling at you and is about to strike at your face.
5) You are a football player resting on the ground briefly between plays.

6) You are sitting patiently in your boss's office waiting for them to start your annual performance review.
7) You are reclining with your phone on your chest. The ringer is on high volume, and you are expecting an important phone call at some point in the next five minutes.

Don't think of resting as something you have to earn, and never feel guilty for taking downtime. We are animals. Breaks are not a reward; they are a necessity.

Bracing Is Submissive

Another reason we are afraid to let go of our bracing patterns is that we use them as submissive displays. During an encounter or confrontation, the less dominant individual will brace more. It is a visible proclamation that exclaims, "Look, I'm wasting energy, handicapping myself during this encounter. Don't attack me; I'm not looking to fight." When we engage in this "social paralysis," we strain many muscles and drastically restrict their range of motion. The more serious the situation, the stiffer we become.

Submissive people adopt tight, symmetric stances, often pinning their arms tightly to their sides. They minimize the amount of space that their bodies occupy by collapsing themselves inward as much as possible and then freezing in place. When you brace your muscles in this way, you submissively close yourself off from the world. Dominant postures, on the other hand, emerge naturally when bracing is at a minimum. Once you stop bracing, you take up space. Dominant people appear the least stifled in their body movements. Their motions are fluid and open. This is why expanding your range of expressive movement will help you convey dominance. So will asymmetry, openness, and repose in your body and limb positions.

Relaxed physical bearing and relaxed body language are highly characteristic of dominant primates. Dominant monkeys and apes are even-tempered and collected, while subordinate animals are uptight and agitated.[20] Of course, none of us want to think about dominance and status when trying to relax. Still, it should be reassuring to know that your unbraced and relaxed posture is the antithesis of inferiority in primates. Whether you are at a party, at work, or passing time with friends and family, be the most carefree, laid-back, slack-muscled monkey you can be.

Find Calm Through Corpse Pose

Another way to confront tension is through physical relaxation techniques. An indispensable one is "corpse pose," or shavasana. Corpse pose is a recumbent yoga pose in which you lie on your back and focus on the total relaxation of your muscles. Although the name is a little morbid, it drives home the reality that you must embrace some aspects of death to truly rest. You must retire certain defensive muscular contractions that are intended to keep you alive. While lying down in shavasana, focus on retiring all the defensive contractions that you use while upright, including those that keep you from falling while walking. Most people take those contractions to bed with them every night; this is a chance to let them go.

Relaxation Exercise #5.3: *Corpse Pose*

Assume corpse pose, lying on your back. You can lie straight or with your arms out at 90-degree angles and your legs spread at about 45 degrees. Try your best to completely relax every muscle. Scan your entire body for muscular tension of any kind. Become a fresh cadaver with no trace of rigor mortis. Become a carcass resting in peace. Become a limp pool of flesh.

> After the first two minutes of corpse pose, you will feel your neck and lower back start to writhe. Focus closely on this tendency to twist about. Try to remain still. Notice the discomfort that stillness creates in your muscles and how it makes you want to squirm, toss, and turn. By inhibiting your tendency to squirm, you quell the bracing patterns. Building comfort with complete motionlessness will greatly enhance your composure.

When I began practicing it, I found corpse pose to be a chore. I was so restless that trying to lie still was stress-inducing. Paced breathing changed my experience completely. As you confront individual pockets of tension, the long, slow breaths dismiss and discharge them one after the other. A week of practicing paced breathing while in corpse pose for just five minutes a day is profoundly transformative. A hot bath can do much to reduce muscle tension and increase blood flow,[21] so use corpse pose while soaking. Epsom salts, aromatherapy, candles, and a breath metronome may help. I believe that diaphragmatic breathing and corpse pose similarly enhance cold body therapy, also known as cryotherapy, in which cold air, ice packs, or ice baths are used to reduce pain and tension.

There are numerous muscles in our bodies that we simply do not know how to relax. Our necks and hips are full of them. We toil all day without giving these muscles even a few seconds to regenerate. Use corpse pose to provide that time. At least three times per day, lie down wherever you happen to be, and replenish. Eventually, work toward a walking corpse pose, and then imagine extending that same kind of utter relaxation to all your waking movements.

Find Calm Through Relaxation Training and Unbracing

As we have discussed, most people are entirely unaware of the tension they carry in their muscles, even though it causes them pain.[22] One way to develop awareness is by engaging in bidirectional control. Bidirectional control, or increasing and then decreasing muscle tension, is used to treat many disorders that are made worse by bracing. When you find a posture that you brace within, let it go, then incrementally bring it back and let it go again. The more familiar you become with specific instances of bracing, the better you will be at noticing them, interrupting them, and bringing them to rest.

When you first find and relax a particular bracing pattern, you may notice yourself breathing more shallowly. This is because bracing gives us a false sense of protection and security, and when we interrupt it, we feel naked and unguarded. Re-bracing the area puts us back into our comfort zone. The only way to circumvent this pattern of escape and relapse is to practice unbracing while overriding distressed breathing with paced diaphragmatic breathing. The unbracing protocol below will guide you through the process.

Unbracing Protocol

1) Recognize a pattern of tension that you brace within. It might be in the face, neck, tongue, eyes, jaw, hands, arms, legs, back, shoulders, stomach, etc.
2) Spend time discovering how to brace it further and how to bring it into a full contraction. Explore the muscle's range of motion and degree of freedom.
3) Use bidirectional control to relax it, tense it, then relax it again. Use this method to gradually identify the most relaxed resting state that you can achieve.

4) Notice that when the muscle is unbraced, underlying pain and discomfort become apparent. Deep, slow breathing will become more difficult than usual. Focus on the discomfort involved as you continue to breathe diaphragmatically. The discomfort will slowly subside. This is what it feels like to heal trauma.

Bidirectional control and the unbracing protocol can be used in conjunction with "progressive relaxation," a tool developed in the early 1920s by Edmund Jacobson. In progressive relaxation, different muscle groups throughout the body are relaxed one at a time. As a therapeutic exercise, it has been shown to lead to reductions in neuromuscular tension, breathing rate, and sympathetic activity.[23] I recommend that you search online for guided progressive relaxation exercises and videos. You might also try searching for a similar practice called "body scan." Make a record of the videos that you like and practice them weekly. We need to delve into this inner space if we are to bring peace to it. Below is a progressive relaxation exercise that you can combine with the unbracing protocol above.

Relaxation Exercise #5.4: *Progressive Relaxation for Bedtime*

Lie down in bed and assume one of your typical sleeping postures. Hold each of the following 12 forms of bracing with moderate to high intensity for 10 seconds, then let them go utterly. Release the muscles abruptly and enjoy the feeling of limpness. Allow the relaxation to develop for at least 10 seconds.

1) Flex or curl your feet, and let go.
2) Bending at the knees, pull your heels up toward your butt to engage your hamstrings, and let go.
3) Arch your lower back, and let go.
4) Use the muscles of your pelvic floor to pull your thighs together, and let go.
5) Tilt your hips to one side, then the other, and let go.
6) Raise your shoulders, and let go.
7) Flex your biceps, and let go.
8) Tighten your hands without making fists, and let go.
9) Brace your neck in different directions, and let go.
10) Squint your eyes, and let go.
11) Press your tongue firmly against the roof of your mouth and suck, and let go.
12) Finally, assume the spinal position you would be in if you were in an atrocious amount of physical pain. Hold that position, and let go.

Throughout the book, we will build on this concept of forcing a partially contracted muscle to contract completely and then letting it relax. Chapter 14 will detail how this can be used to reverse all the partial contraction and pain in your body using a technique that I call "anti-rigidity training." As discussed in that chapter, this involves using physical poses that activate underutilized joint configurations. It narrows in on poses that ache and cause the joints to crack. Once you find these achy configurations in your body, you will work on contracting the muscles involved to full fatigue. It feels like a good stretch, but it is much more than that.

The process of holding the contraction outside its normal range of motion encourages blood flow, unlocks trigger points, and elongates muscles to their optimal length unlike anything else—aside from massage, that is.

Massage Counteracts Partial Contraction and Dormant Muscle

Despite the growing recognition that muscle tension causes most common pain, targeting the trigger points that cause it is not part of mainstream medical education. Physicians, psychiatrists, and psychologists rarely consider muscular dysfunction despite it being a major contributor to a wide variety of diseases and disorders. The medical establishment has found that it is more profitable to direct funding toward pharmaceuticals, medical devices, surgeries, and other medical procedures than toward massage and the manual compression of trigger points. This is true, even though there is overwhelming support for the concept of trigger points and the use of massage in resolving them from distinguished medical institutions such as the American Pain Society.

I am generally aligned with and fond of the modern medical establishment, but its neglect of bracing, repetitive strain, and trigger points is unacceptable. Today, many experts worldwide recognize that muscle pain may be the biggest cause of disability and loss of productivity in the workplace. Nonetheless, clinicians focus on major surgery and on masking muscle pain with drugs rather than less invasive, safer, and more effective solutions that are already known. We can't expect doctors to solve all of our problems. We need to let the doctors off the hook and take responsibility for our muscles into our own hands.

Physically massaging trigger points with firm pressure breaks them up, allowing blood and oxygen back into the muscle. Massage is thought to be the least invasive, most cost-effective, and safest way to reinstate circulation and reverse the self-sustaining contraction that maintains them. The next chapter will explain precisely how to perform compressive massage on your own muscles.

Trigger point massage and anti-rigidity are easy to do and work wonders. However, there is a simple explanation for why you and everyone you know aren't already using these techniques regularly. The body only allows muscle groups to open up if the person is breathing diaphragmatically. This means that these two techniques don't work nearly as well for people who have not undergone diaphragmatic retraining. However, combining long breaths with massage, achy poses, and contraction into the most painful muscles in my body liberated my neck, shoulders, hips, and lower back from a state of stinging rigidity. After reading Chapters 6 and 14, you will have all the knowledge you need to do this for yourself.

Chapter 5: **Bullet Points**

- Tense muscles with excessive tone burden us. Their tension develops from extended periods of uninterrupted use. This prolonged use is known as repetitive strain or persistent muscle tension.
- Much of the muscle tension that we experience comes from unnecessary bracing. Bracing is largely involuntary but is avoidable because we can become aware of it.
- Rest and microbreaks give strained muscles the downtime they need to regenerate.
- Deprived of breaks, overused muscles become ultra-fatigued. But, given the proper microbreaks, the same muscles could have been healthy and toned.
- Long-term strain changes our muscles physically, leading to adaptive muscles shortening, scar tissue, and the formation of trigger points.
- Adaptive muscle shortening is a form of partial contraction in which a muscle can neither rest nor contract completely. The fact that the muscle is shorter can distort posture and proper skeletal alignment.
- We have partially contracted muscles in the face, vocal tract, spine, abdomen, genitals and other areas.
- Muscles that have been in partial contraction for years go dormant. Dormant muscles limit movement, promote frailty, and lower metabolism. They are atrophied, weak, inflamed, surrounded by fat deposits, susceptible to injury, and, worst of all, painful.
- Most people have unknowingly allowed muscles in the crux of their necks and lower backs to become completely dormant to the point where they are immobilized and can hardly be contracted at all. If they happen to contract fully, as during a fall or when lifting something heavy, it would be painful and would result in injury.
- We brace our breathing muscles, including the diaphragm, when we are nervous. This can push them into partial contraction. To unbrace the diaphragm, allow your exhalations to become passive. This involves doing no work during the exhalation and letting the breathing muscles go limp. The exhalation provides a brief opportunity for all the breathing muscles to relax and receive a microbreak.
- Pain signals sent to our brain from tense muscles overwhelm our emotional lives. They cause the "pain-body" to flare up, heightening aggression, ego, and competition for status.
- Muscular tension is a fundamental medical and biological problem. Due to its relation to stress, it is responsible for a wide range of downstream pathologies and health issues.
- Several studies have shown that relaxing the muscles of the body reduces anxiety.
- Distressed breathing results in muscle tension and increased bracing. Chronic distressed breathing results in copious dormant muscle.
- Diaphragmatic breathing reduces excessive muscular tone, allowing muscles the microbreaks they need to regenerate. This makes it so that the repetitive strains of everyday life strengthen our muscles rather than weaken them.
- Your body has learned to be tense, but you can teach it to let go of the tension.

- Unbracing, which can be accomplished by allowing muscles to go limp, is an acquired skill that can rehabilitate your entire body when combined with diaphragmatic breathing.
- Corpse pose involves lying on the back and focusing on full-body relaxation.
- Progressive relaxation involves systematically scanning over the entire body, tensing muscles, then completely releasing them.
- The most dominant primates are the least affected by bracing and brace the least during confrontation and opposition. So, unbrace.

Chapter 5: **Endnotes**

1.   Reser, J. (2009). Does rheumatoid arthritis represent an adaptive, thrifty condition? *Medical Hypotheses*, *74*(1), 189–194.

2.   Whatmore, G. B., & Kohli, D. R. (1968). Dysponesis: A neurophysiological factor in functional disorders. *Systems Research and Behavioral Science*, *13*(2), 102–124.

3.   Rajiv, D., & Harjyot, S. (2007). Good sleep, bad sleep! The role of daytime naps in healthy adults. *Current Opinion in Internal Medicine*, *6*(6), 91–94.

4.   Androniki, N. (2007). Siesta in healthy adults and coronary mortality in the general population. *Archives of Internal Medicine*, *167*(3), 296–301.

5.   Alvarez, D. J., & Rockwell, P. G. (2002). Trigger points: Diagnosis and management. *American Family Physician*, *65*(4), 653–60.

6.   Alvarez & Rockwell, 2002, Trigger points.

7.   O'Sullivan, S. (2007). *Physical rehabilitation*. F.A Davis Company.

8.   Davies, C. (2001). *The trigger point therapy workbook: Your self-treatment guide for pain relief*. New Harbinger.

9.   Shah, J. P., Danoff, J. V, Desai, M. J., Parikh, S., Nakamura, L. Y., Phillips, T. M., & Gerber, L. H. (2008). Biochemicals associated with pain and inflammation are elevated in sites near to and remote from active myofascial trigger points. *Archives of Physical Medicine and Rehabilitation*, *89*(1), 16–23.

10. Reser, J. (2009). Does rheumatoid arthritis represent an adaptive, thrifty condition? *Medical Hypotheses*, *74*(1), 189–194.

11. Wall, P. D., & Melzack, R. (1996). *The challenge of pain*. Penguin Books.

12. Bruehl, S., Burns, J. W., Chung, O. Y., & Chont, M. (2009). Pain-related effects of trait anger expression: neural substrates and the role of endogenous opioid mechanisms. *Neuroscience & Biobehavioral Reviews*, *33*(3), 475–91.

13. Eisenberger, N. I., & Lieberman, M. D. (2004). Why rejection hurts: A common neural alarm system for physical and social pain. *Trends in Cognitive Science*, *8*(7), 294–300.

14. Pluess, M., Conrad, A., & Wilhelm, F. H. (2009). Muscle tension in generalized anxiety disorder: A critical review of the literature. *Journal of Anxiety Disorders, 23*(1), 1–11.

15. Tolle, E. (2005). *A new Earth: Awakening to your life's purpose.* Penguin Books.

16. Azrin, N. H., Rubin, H. B, & Hutchinson, R. R. (1968). Biting attack by rats in response to aversive shock. *Journal of the Experimental Analysis of Behavior, 11*(5), 633–639.

17. Aras, A., & Ro, O. (1997). Workload when using a mouse as an input device. *International Journal of Human-Computer Interaction, 9*(2), 105–118; Buckles, P.W. & Devereux, J. J. (2002). The nature of work-related neck and upper limb musculoskeletal disorders. *Applied Ergonomics, 33*(3), 207–217; Veiersted, K. (1993). Sustained muscle tension as a risk factor for trapezius myalgia. In R. Nielsen & K. Jorgenson (Eds.), *Advances in industrial ergonomics and safety.* Taylor & Francis.

18. Gevirtz, R. (2006). The muscle spindle trigger point model of chronic pain. *Biofeedback, 34*(2), 53–56.

19. Travell, J., & Simons, R. (1983). *Myofascial pain syndrome: The trigger point manual.* Williams & Wilkins.

20. Mehrabian, A. (1971). Verbal and nonverbal interactions of strangers in a waiting room. *Journal of Experimental Research in Personality, 5,* 127–138; Reynolds, V., & Reynolds, F. (1965). Chimpanzees in the Budongo Forest. In I DeVore (Ed.) *Primate behavior: Field studies of monkeys and apes* (pp. 368–424). New York: Holt, Rinehart and Winston.

21. Fioravanti, A., Cantarini, L., Guidelli, G. M., & Galeazzi, M. (2011). Mechanisms of action of spa therapies in rheumatic diseases: What scientific evidence is there? *Rheumatology International, 31*(1), 1–8.

22. Shumay, D., & Peper, E. (1997). Healthy computing: A comprehensive group training approach using biofeedback. In G. Salvendy, M. J. Smith, & R. J, Koubek, (Eds.), *Design of computing systems: Cognitive considerations* (pp. 555–558). Elsevier; Stein, C., Schafer, M., & Machelska, H. (2003). Attacking pain at its source: New perspectives on opioids. *Nature Medicine, 9*(8), 1003–1008.

23. Ditto, B., Eclache, M., & Goldman, N. (2006). Short-term autonomic and cardiovascular effects of mindfulness body scan meditation. *Annals of Behavioral Medicine, 32*(3), 227–234.

Chapter 6: **Release Tense Muscle with Massage**

"The mind, which before massage is in a perturbed, restless, vacillating, and even despondent state, becomes calm, quiet, peaceful, and subdued after massage. In fact, the wearied and worried mind has been converted into a mind restful, placid, and refreshed." — Thomas Stretch Dowse (1809-1885)

The Power of Massage to Alleviate Tension Insanity

The benefits of massage are most apparent in cases in which muscular tension is so extreme that it becomes debilitating. Let us start with an especially vivid example from my own life. It involves a close friend who suffered psychotic episodes during which he became highly delusional. His breakdowns were so severe that he had to be hospitalized on three separate occasions. He had previously been diagnosed with schizophrenia as well as bipolar disorder, conditions that were precipitated by harmful life circumstances. His mother had recently died of cancer; his father had been murdered years before; he faced frequent bullying from hardened, streetwise men; he had gone through a harsh breakup, been homeless for months, and drank large amounts of caffeine every day.

In the days leading up to hospitalization, his thinking became severely deranged. He would become convinced that his friends were saints and that he was an angel responsible for preventing a coming apocalypse. Twice his state regressed to the point of *catatonia*, which has also been called "tension insanity." Catatonia is a rare form of "psycho-motor immobility" in which a patient holds rigid poses, performs stereotyped, repetitive movements, and often cannot speak.[1]

On the first occasion, he was found by a mutual friend who called me to ask for help. When I arrived, I found our buddy standing rigidly, shaking, with a pained expression plastered on his face. He would not sit or lie down and had been standing for two straight days. He did not respond to speech or any form of communication. He squinted heavily. The circles under his eyes had become much darker than usual. He made no eye contact and stared vacantly at the floor. He was normally a conscientious person, but by the time I arrived, he was urinating and defecating in his shorts. When I checked his breathing, I found that each breath he took lasted about half a second and his tidal range was minimal.

Most worrying of all was his physical bearing. Although he was only 25, his posture was that of an old, sick man. He looked fragile, and the tension in his neck and back seemed excruciating. Having lost all concern for self-presentation, he looked as if he had been standing in a cold shower for hours. All his muscles were braced. I recognized his tortured posture as a direct expression of his pain-body, the suffering we all carry and attempt to conceal. At that point, I realized that if I were in a catatonic state, my postural deformities would similarly rise to the surface.

His catatonia made him very difficult to help. There was nothing we could do to move his rigid frame down the stairs and into the car. When we tried to carry him, he shook and moaned violently, and it became clear that he would need to relax if he were going to get to the hospital. So, I began massaging him. I started with his neck, then moved on to his shoulders and back. His back felt crooked, the curvature unnatural and deformed. But we rapidly made progress: at first, his spine resisted my efforts, but every minute he loosened up a little more, and within ten minutes, he was crying with relief. After 30, he was able to hobble to the car and sit down inside it.

On our way to the hospital, he uttered his only full sentence of the day: "If I calm down, I will die." Experts consider catatonia to be a vastly reduced state of consciousness. Yet, from this state, he was able to verbalize perhaps the most entrenched albeit delusional conviction that all humans have. I did my best to explain to him why this was an irrational and self-defeating belief. I will spend the rest of this book attempting to convince you of the same. The main takeaway of this chapter is that massage can convince your body that relaxation does not come at the risk of death.

Getting to the hospital, though, was not the end of his struggles. For that visit alone, which turned out to be just the first of three, he owed more than $100,000 in medical bills. I asked him what the doctors did for him that cost so much, and he told me that they restrained him in a bed and gave him drugs for two weeks. (He wound up dependent on those drugs and had to be weaned off them slowly and painfully.) It is not clear what benefit the medicines and doctors provided, other than removing him from his stressful environment. Certainly, they conferred no long-term benefit.

I believe that a year of weekly, hour-long, deep-tissue, full-body massages would have largely rehabilitated him. At $50 per massage, this would have cost less than $3,000. If this had been his treatment, I think he would have had a much better chance at real, lasting recovery. If he had received $100,000 worth of massage therapy, this would have bought him 2,000 massages. That equates to an hour-long massage every week for 40 years. If I had been in charge of his health, I know how I would have invested the money.

After reading this chapter, you will know how to massage yourself for free. This will complement and reinforce the other Program Peace techniques you are using to promote your overall health.

Use Compression to Remove Trigger Points, Scar Tissue, and Muscle Shortening

Recent estimates indicate that around 98 percent of the atoms in the body are replaced every year. Despite this constant remodeling, the body unfortunately preserves its muscle tension. It does this because it treats tension as an essential form of memory. Our organism trusts and values the specific pattern of trauma distribution across our various limbs, organs, and body parts because that pattern is a historical record telling us exactly how best to be defensive. We were pre-programmed to conserve our tension, increase it as necessary, and die with it—but not to reverse it.

Modern medicine has no cure for muscular tension. There is no pill you can take to remove its physical manifestations. Compared to many other diseases and disorders, there is very little active biomedical research on curing muscular strain. Some researchers attempt to treat trigger points with injections, therapeutic ultrasound, or transcutaneous electrical stimulation, but none of these have yet proven very effective. I think basic and preclinical research on the issue should be given the highest priority in medicine, especially because persistent muscular tension is a contributing factor to many mental and physical diseases. Molecular pharmacologists will eventually develop a drug that completely eradicates muscular strain, but it will take decades for such a panacea to surface. Our bodies and minds don't have decades.

That leaves us with non-clinical treatment options for the time being. Massage combined with diaphragmatic breathing is by far the best therapy available, and I recommend starting your practice immediately. I have been using physical compression for years to rouse dormant muscles all over my body. Before I began, I was covered in muscles that were painful to compress. Applying even light pressure almost anywhere stung. Now, all of these spots have become painless even when subjected to significant pressure.

Massage is effective for straightforward reasons. Compression forces the muscle to relax and allows it to reset to a lower level of tone. It feeds slack into the injured muscle, reversing muscle shortening and reducing mechanical deformation at the joint. It breaks down trigger points as well as deposits of calcium. It accelerates venous blood drainage and lymphatic clearance. Compression breaks up adhesions between muscle fibers and disintegrates scar tissue, freeing the fibers to slide past each other again. It is unclear exactly what compression does at the level of actin and myosin, the microscopic proteins discussed in the last chapter that form the structure of individual muscle fibers. Many researchers believe that it detaches strands of actin from myosin after they have become stuck together, allowing them to function freely again.

Specific conditions that are consistently and successfully treated with manual compressive therapy include headaches, back pain, neck pain, shoulder pain, carpal tunnel syndrome, shin splints, sciatica, TMJ, fasciitis, tendonitis, and many other soft tissue inflammatory disorders of the joints.[2] Given the prevalence of those conditions and the general level of muscular tension that most of us develop over lifetimes of bracing and social submissiveness, self-applied trigger point massage is a necessary life skill.

Focus Compression on Tender, Achy Muscles

One of the most studied therapies for combatting trigger points is a form of compression called soft tissue therapy, also referred to as "soft tissue mobilization" or "myofascial release." The practice involves pinning down and squeezing an area of muscle with hard pressure for several seconds. The idea is to press firmly into soft tissue, including skin, fascia, periosteum, and superficially and deeply located muscles. The best locations for applying pressure are the trigger points themselves, which you can detect with your fingers. They often feel like a small length of partially cooked pasta or a slender worm under the skin. Most professional masseuses describe muscles with multiple trigger points as having a "crunchy" or "spongy" quality.

Muscles with trigger points are also easy to identify because they are tender to the touch. In contrast, healthy muscles don't elicit a pain response under pressure. Tenderness should be your operative diagnostic criterion. Concentrate your efforts on any tender mass you find. Apply pressure, dig, and release. Use your knuckle, fingertip, the heel of your palm, or elbow to get in as deep as possible to break down the scar tissue and fibrous adhesions. The tip, side, or first knuckle of the thumb can be particularly useful. You want to compress tender muscles all over your body.

You can use a tool to avoid straining your hands or to apply pressure more easily to hard-to-reach areas. Pictured below are the implements that I use to perform compression on myself. You can find an eyebolt in any hardware store, and the other tools can be found easily online, if not at your local sporting goods store. Aside from my own hands, the Index Knobber, shown at the far right of the picture below, is my tool of choice.

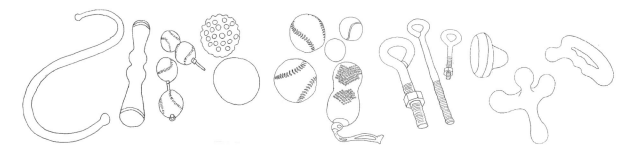

Illustration 6.1: Tools for compression: A. Thera Cane™; B. Backknobber™; C. Baseballs attached with drilled holes and metal screws; D. Spiked massage ball; E. Foam therapy ball; F. Softballs; G. Squash ball; H. Tennis ball; I. Yoga Therapy Balls™ in sack; J. Three sizes of eyebolts (1″ x 8″; 0.75″ x 12″; 0.5″ x 6″); K. Knobble™; L. Jacknobber™; M. Index Knobber™. You can also place tools on the floor, such as a hard water bottle, rolling pin, racquetball, barbell, pipe, or wooden dowel, and push your body into them.

The benefits of compression have to do with muscles' need for *microbreaks*, which we have discussed previously. The muscles that feel tender when subjected to deep compression have not had the breaks they need to remain healthy. Compression gives them a much-needed respite, reestablishing blood flow and permitting full regeneration. The muscle may feel warm afterward as fresh blood rushes to areas that are normally neglected. To send fresh blood into an area, you first need to squeeze existing blood out by performing something called *ischemic compression*.

It is helpful to visualize the effects. As you massage, imagine that you are pressing into pale, pink tissue that has lost most of its blood supply. Envision the muscle turning white as you compress it and the remaining blood is squeezed out. Then, as you release, imagine fresh red blood flooding into the area. Imagine that this redness dissipates in a few seconds but that the muscle stays more brightly colored than it was before. Of course, all of that is quite literally happening. Compression creates the cellular events necessary to express the genes required to build new blood vessels. This renewed blood supply brings the muscle "back to life." Below is an overview of the steps involved in the Program Peace compression routine.

Compression Protocol

1) Breathe. Use the tenets of diaphragmatic breathing throughout your massage practice. This will help ensure that your muscles remain relaxed even during discomfort. If compression becomes particularly painful, take a deep breath in, then breathe out slowly through pursed lips to extend your exhalation.
2) Pressure. Find a muscle that is tender when compressed. Press firmly on the muscle with the tip of a finger, knuckle, or tool for between five and 30 seconds. On most areas of the body, you can apply between five and 15 pounds of pressure. To gauge this, imagine a dumbbell of a given weight resting on top. Use less pressure on more painful or delicate areas. Release, reposition centimeters or millimeters away, and repeat.
3) Movement. Some practitioners recommend sliding a finger, thumb, or tool down the length of the muscle. They use deep, firm strokes that move in the direction of the muscle fibers. Others recommend stroking across the muscle repeatedly, like strumming a guitar string. Try to develop skill at both. Either way, you want to pin the skin down and slide it over the muscle rather than slide your fingers over the skin. You can also simply press into an area of tenderness rather than stroke it. If I can find a taught,

sore band of muscle, I will often nestle my knuckle in on one side of it and press rhythmically for minutes at a time.

4) Intensity. On a scale of one to ten, aim for a tolerable pain level of six or seven. Light massage at a pain level of two or three can also be beneficial but will take much longer to have an effect. At a six or a seven, the pain you feel should be mixed with pleasure. It should "hurt good" but should not be enough to make you squirm, brace, or breathe shallowly.

5) Attention. Once you release the muscle, pay attention to how its level of bracing has diminished. You may feel insecure or exposed now that you are no longer bracing. Note the automatic tendency to either resume bracing or breathe shallowly. Resist both urges, continuing to breathe deeply while keeping the area relaxed. This will encourage the muscle to reset to a lower level of tone.

6) Follow up. The next day, if the muscle is bruised or hurts when contracted, it is a sign that you pushed too hard. However, if it is slightly sore to the touch, then you made substantial progress. This soreness should disappear with just a few minutes of additional massage. After the soreness subsides, wait a few hours for it to come back and compress it again with the same degree of force. Repeat this process until the muscle no longer hurts to compress. Depending on the muscle's size and the severity of the tension, this could take days, weeks, or months.

Percuss Your Tender, Tense Muscles

The steady, consistent pressure of compression therapy can be complemented by percussive massage. "Percussive" here means "hitting" or "striking." Many professional masseuses routinely use slapping, beating, and pummeling, which are all examples of percussive massage. This approach is similar to the "tapotement" technique in Swedish massage and certain shiatsu regimens. It was documented to have been used in ancient Japan when children massaged their elders after long days bending over in the rice fields. Because the children's fingers were not strong enough to perform a kneading motion, they balled up their hands and struck the sore muscles with their fists. The Japanese term "mago no te" was used to describe this type of massage, which translates to "grandchild's hands." The protocol below details a related method that I'll refer to as "percussion."

Percussion Protocol:

1) Use a knuckle, fist, palm heel, baseball, or softball to repeatedly strike dormant, achy muscle. For even deeper muscle work, use a tool like the Index Knobber to strike.

2) Use force and speed similar to what would be appropriate for conventional clapping/applause. Strike the muscle firmly and repetitively like a sewing machine or a woodpecker. Strike at a rate of roughly three to five times per second, rising one to three inches above the skin between strikes.

3) Concentrate this pummeling action on a tender area of muscle just an inch or two in diameter for 10 to 45 seconds.

I percuss my neck, shoulders, back, arms, legs, knees, and ankles firmly all over with objects ranging from baseballs to knuckle-sized tools weekly. I recommend percussing your entire body with a hard implement. If you don't have any of the tools below, don't hesitate to start just using your knuckles or palm heel. Using percussion is one of the fastest and least painful ways to erode trigger points and reanimate dormant muscle.

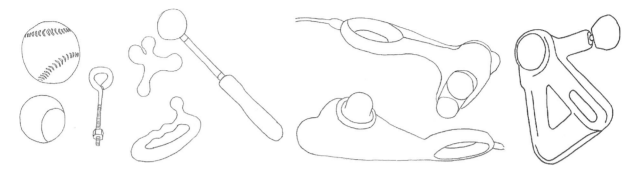

Illustration 6.2: Tools for percussion: A. Softball; B. Tennis ball; C. Eyebolt (.5'' x 6''); D. Jacknobber™; E. Index Knobber™; F. Bonger™; G. Brookstone vibrating massagers; H. Theragun™.

Vibration

I strongly recommend that you spend around $100 on a handheld vibrating massager. Using it on your neck and head should give you the chills and make your body tingle, a clear sign that it is sorely needed. Use it wherever it feels good. Vibration tends not to work as well on trigger points as compression or percussion. However, even just one minute per day of vibratory stimulation will alleviate bracing and increase circulation. When used before bed, it can promote better sleep. Also, use it on tender muscles after massage. Doing so can encourage the well-worked muscles to relax further, which helps the massage do its work.

Delocalized Pressure

Aside from targeting small, localized areas of tissue with compression and percussion, it can be therapeutic to provide firm pressure to larger areas. This is a form of delocalized pressure that compresses, but also stretches, many muscles at the same time. This occurs when someone presses firmly into a large area of the body. Thai masseuses walk on the body to provide this kind of relief. Delocalized pressure pushes various muscle bracing pattern configurations outside their normally restricted range, which can have long-lasting positive effects. It will give your joints, including those in the spine, more play and articulation.

Massage Activity #6.1: *Delocalized Pressure for the Spine*
Perform the following activity on a friend, then have them perform it on you. Have them lie down on their stomach on a bed or the floor. With your hands side by side, press into their spine with the heel of both palms for two seconds at a time. Start by pressing lightly 20 times as you move from the top of their neck to the bottom of their sacrum. Do this again with medium firmness. The person receiving the pressure should focus on how the normal, braced posture of their spine is being bowed in a different direction and thereby freed from unnecessary rigidity. Afterward, they should perform ten sit-ups to neutralize

any backward tension that has been created. Ideally, everyone should have this done to them every night before bed.

Cautions to Take with Massage

Several key pieces of advice are essential for practicing compression and percussion safely. Neither technique should ever damage tissue, nor should they bruise, scrape, or even irritate the skin. Avoid using compression on a recent injury, broken skin, or broken bones.

No matter the circumstances, medical professionals advise against compressing the following body parts: the eye, the inguinal ligament, the xiphoid process, the trachea, the median nerve near the carpal tunnel junction, the sciatic nerve, and the coccyx. Also, never massage a pulse. Many arteries accumulate plaque, and massaging them can dislodge that plaque and cause blood vessel occlusion. Additionally, avoid pressing or pinching lymph nodes.

Certain illnesses can also make massage a risky activity. If you have the following health conditions, consult your doctor before receiving or self-administering massage: aneurysm, atherosclerosis, cancer, congestive heart failure, coronary artery disease, peritonitis, or polycystic kidney disease. Other conditions that are usually contraindicated for massage include fever, cirrhosis, pitting edema, blood clots, deep vein thrombosis, embolism, fainting, uncontrolled high blood pressure, intestinal obstruction, lymphangitis, myocarditis, rheumatoid arthritis, tumors, seizures, and tuberculosis, among others.

Getting Results from Self-Massage

Applied properly, the pressure of compression and percussion should involve only dull pain. On one hand, if the muscle doesn't ache when you press into it, you are applying too little pressure and will not release the stored tension. On the other, the muscle should never hurt after you have stopped compressing. If it does, you have applied too much pressure or found an area that would best be avoided. Although compression feels like it causes pain, it would be more accurate to say that it reveals where pain already exists in your body. I believe that the level of discomfort you feel when compressing a tense muscle is proportionate to the subliminal pain signals that it sends your brain throughout the day.

It almost seems unfair that to rid ourselves of pain, we must endure it even more intensely. But there is an optimistic perspective on soft tissue release. The muscular strain that you endure today is the product of years or even decades of tension. And yet, many muscles can be largely rehabilitated in just a handful of five-minute sessions. After that initial period of regular massage, less than one minute per month can be sufficient to maintain these results. This suggests that every minute of soft tissue release reverses weeks or even months of strain. Additionally, keep in mind that if you choose not to release your muscles, you are allowing them to become tenser, raising your levels of stress and anxiety and perpetuating chronic pain and autonomic imbalance.

It is vital to appraise soft tissue therapy positively. It is "invasive" in some ways, but you want your body to embrace the sensations that you feel rather than reject them. The key is to self-soothe and trigger your natural relaxation response. To that end, it is imperative to use diaphragmatic breathing. Many specialists agree that deep breathing helps the muscle spindles receive the message to stop contracting.

There is a wealth of massage instructions and tutorials on the internet. Simply Google "how to massage." Or, if video instruction appeals to you, YouTube it. I also recommend using other guides on muscle release such as Jill Miller's *The Role Model* and Clair Davies' *The Trigger Point Therapy Workbook*. As a baseline, the exercises that follow highlight a few of the areas that I think are essential to compress and percuss.

Massage Exercise #6.1: *Compression of the Hand Web*

Use one hand to grab and pinch the web of the other hand. Firmly squeeze the area between the thumb and forefinger. Spend time becoming acquainted with the tight, painful bundles of muscles and release them with firm compression. Repeat with the other hand. Continue to compress your entire hand, searching for any achiness or tenderness.

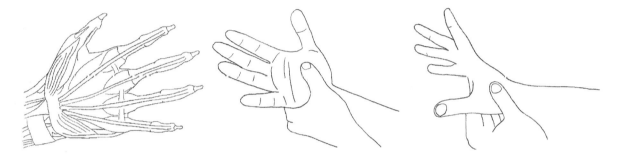

Illustration 6.3: Hand massage.

Massage Exercise #6.2: *Compression of the Foot Arch*

Step firmly on a tennis ball, pressing the ball into every area of the underside of the foot. Concentrate on the arch, but press the ball into the heel and along the ball of your foot as well. You might also try standing on the corner of a stair. Also, use the tip of your thumb to press into sore areas. After about two minutes, you should notice that compressing it becomes much less painful and that your foot feels limber and pliant. You could buy million-dollar orthopedic shoes and still not get even a fraction of the relief you can attain from a couple of hours of soft tissue foot massage.

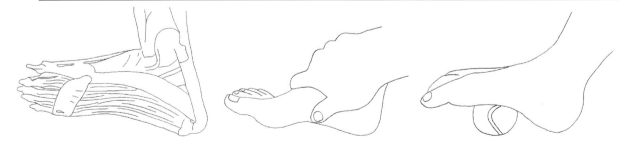

Illustration 6.4: Foot Massage.

Massage Exercise #6.3: *Compression of the Temporalis*

The temporalis muscle assists in chewing and covers much of the temporal bone on the side of the head. Use your knuckles to make small circular motions all along the belly of this large muscle. Also, try watching TV lying down on one side with your temporal muscle pressed into a softball. Releasing this muscle will reduce the low-grade perpetual headache that so many of us carry. When you work on massaging the temporalis, it is also worth compressing the cheekbones, jaw, and the three auricular muscles surrounding each ear.

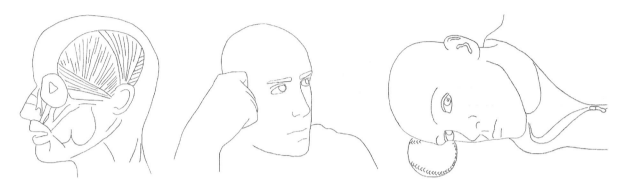

Illustration 6.5: Temporalis massage.

Massage Exercise #6.4: *Compression of the Sternocleidomastoid*

Use one hand to grab and pinch the sternocleidomastoid as pictured below. It helps to turn the head to one side. Firmly squeeze the length of the muscle from the clavicle up to just below the ear. This muscle is a major structural support for the neck, and when it is tight, it hunches the head down and forward. It also plays a role in clavicular breathing, so releasing it will help soothe your breath.

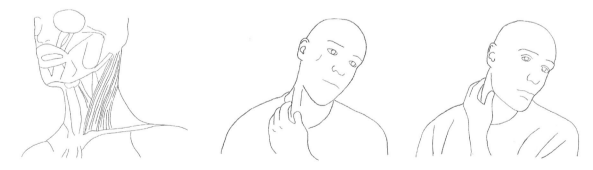

Illustration 6.6: Sternocleidomastoid massage.

Massage Exercise #6.5: *Compression of the Occipitalis*

Apply deep pressure to the occipitalis muscle and the neck muscles directly below it. Lie down and rest your head on a baseball, eyebolt, or index knobber to compress these muscles. Releasing the occipitalis will help reduce your low-grade headache and straighten the back of your neck.

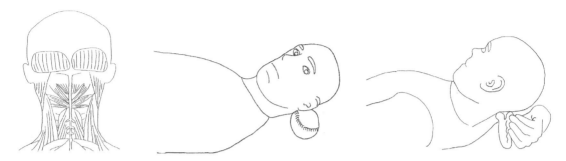

Illustration 6.7: Occipitalis massage.

Massage Exercise #6.6: *Compression of the Neck*

The front, sides, and back of the neck contain a dense array of muscles. Reach your hand into the air above your head, bend your elbow, and press the tip or knuckle of your thumb into each of the areas of your neck. Identify sore spots and concentrate on them. Alternatively, use a tool like a squash ball, Index Knobber, or eyebolt.

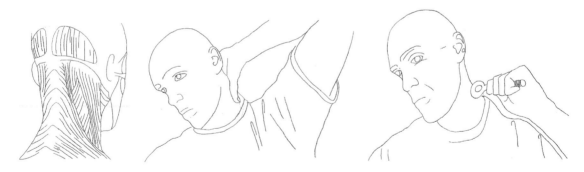

Illustration 6.8: Neck massage.

Massage Exercise #6.7: *Compression of the Corrugator Supercilii*

Place your elbows on a tabletop or bed to steady your hands. Then use the first knuckles of your thumbs to press firmly into the small muscles under each eyebrow. There are several layers of different muscles here, but you will know when you find the corrugator supercilii because it will be the most painful. The feeling of pressing on it directly will probably take your breath away, even with just a few pounds of pressure. Consistent massage will release all that pain.

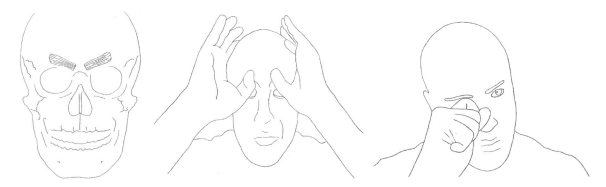

Illustration 6.9: Corrugator supercilii massage.

The results of even these simple exercises can be profound. Let's look at the corrugator supercilii muscle in Exercise 6.7, for example. It is the muscle that creates the frown, which it does by lowering the eyebrows and pulling them together. Scientists regard it as the principal muscle in the expression of suffering.[3] This means that humans, primates, and other mammals unconsciously contract their corrugator supercilii muscles when experiencing great pain. What do you think it means for this muscle itself to be stuck in painful, partial contraction? I think it means that it has come to perpetuate the condition of suffering. Realizing this strongly motivated me to compress mine until they were absolutely painless. In total, the process took me about an hour, divided into several short sessions spread over a month. It was time well spent as it released my perennial frown and changed my outlook on the world.

Below are several other easy-to-use massage techniques that should help kickstart your search for soreness and a personal routine. Other chapters in this book will specifically address massage of the face (9), neck (16), and lower back (17).

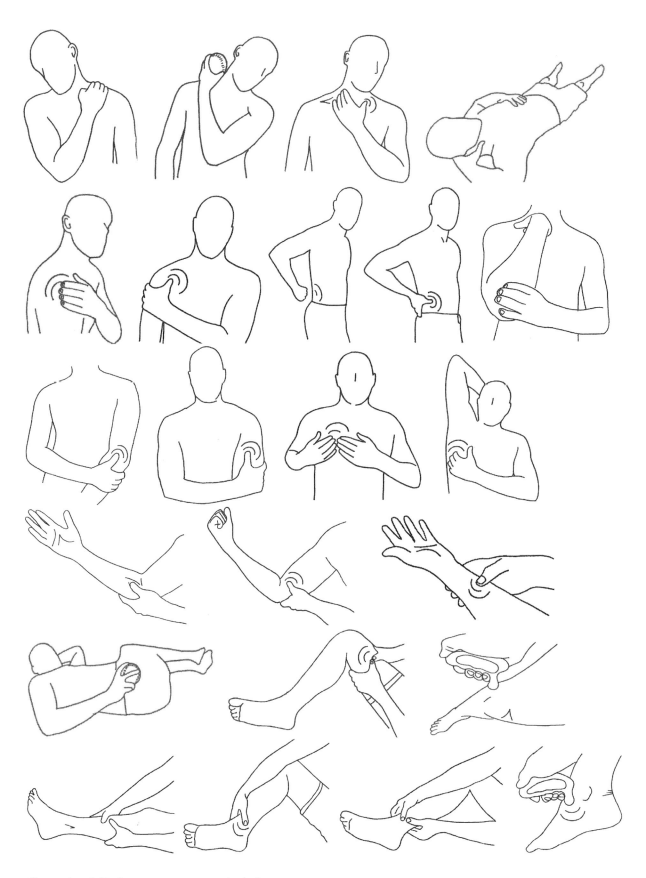

Illustration 6.10: Easy-to-use massage techniques.

The health benefits of self-massage are both real and noticeable: compression increases circulation, improves joint health, relieves muscular injuries, shortens recovery time, and reduces muscle fatigue. Aesthetically, self-massage can accentuate muscle mass, reduce the deposition of fat, improve the appearance of cellulite, and contour, tone, and firm the skin. I have released muscles all over, and it has helped me feel as though I have an entirely new body. I am stronger, more flexible, faster, and more graceful. Results are cumulative. It should be everyone's objective to release every painful muscle in the body. Finding them and learning how to compress them skillfully is a challenge, of course, and one of the best ways to start learning is to receive professional massage.

The Benefits of Professional Massage

Getting expert help can be the perfect introduction or complement to a self-treatment routine. If the option is available, I strongly recommend that you invest a significant proportion of your disposable income for the next few years on deep tissue massage. Receiving quality deep tissue massages will relieve pent-up tension in large portions of your body, curbing sympathetic hyperactivity and activating pain-gate control. It has even been shown to reduce depression and trait anxiety[4] and reduce generalized anxiety disorder symptoms.[5] What is more, it temporarily reduces blood pressure and heart rate and stimulates the production of the brain chemicals involved in pleasure and satisfaction, such as endorphins, oxytocin, and serotonin.[6] Raising the levels of these substances in your brain has recursive beneficial effects on happiness, confidence, and outgoingness.

I had my first massage at age 27. I came out of the studio angry, convinced that the masseuse had pressed too firmly on my shoulder. By the time I got to my car, I had a bad cramp in my deltoid that stayed with me for a full week. The cramp formed for three reasons: (1) I didn't ask the masseuse to reduce the excessive pressure, (2) I was a full-on thoracic breather at the time, and (3) I defensively contracted the muscle into a tight ball as it was being massaged. Massaging a muscle too intensely, especially when it is contracted, will make the muscle worse rather than better. It is important to remember that unlike in self-massage, the professional masseuse cannot feel what you experience as they press. They need your active feedback telling them when to press harder and when to press softer.

This bad first experience, which was my fault, dissuaded me from returning. Reading about the scientific benefits of massage five years later persuaded me to give massage another chance. By this time, I was practicing diaphragmatic breathing, which helped me accept, rather than brace against, the most intense parts of the massage. This second experience made me a convert.

At first, the masseuses I saw marveled at how tight my muscles were. Several voiced concern for my well-being after feeling my neck and shoulders. They would say things like: "This isn't good, are you okay?" I was even told by several masseuses that I had the worst muscle tension they had ever seen. But that feedback started to change within the first year of weekly deep tissue massages. By the end of the year, each new masseuse I worked with commented that they had never seen anyone able to take such deep pressure. It just didn't hurt anymore, and it hasn't since. I attribute this entirely to the consistent practice of diaphragmatic breathing.

Deep tissue massage should be uncomfortable at times but should not cause excessive pain or induce protective spasms. When a masseuse presses too hard on a trigger point, other trigger points throughout the body will briefly flare up in response. Encourage them to press hard but never to the point where the pain causes you to tense up in other areas, such as your face, neck, or back. To this end, concentrate on holding a relaxed "corpse pose," allowing your body to go completely limp.

Most importantly, you will know that the massage is too hard if it makes you breathe shallowly or brace your diaphragm. As mentioned above, you should be practicing diaphragmatic breathing throughout the massage. Employing paced breathing is ideal. To do this, locate the breath metronome MP3 audio tracks available from my website, upload them to your phone, and play them during the massage (you may want to put the track on repeat to keep your hands free and turn off the screen of your phone to conserve battery life). Diaphragmatic breathing will keep your muscles from fighting against the forced relaxation. This has the added benefit of reducing the extent of soreness afterward.[7]

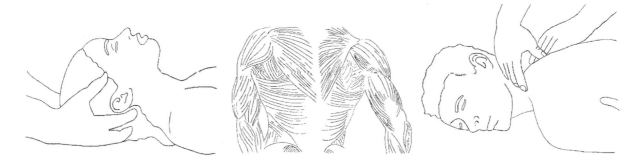

Illustration 6.11: A. Massage of the temporal muscles; B. Skeletal muscles of the back; C. Neck massage.

Most masseuses, whether they realize it or not, specialize in treating the muscles of respiration. This is because any muscle of the torso can be seen as a muscle of respiration. After all, every one of them either mobilizes or stabilizes breathing motions. Remember how we said that breathing with the muscles surrounding the thorax and clavicles is especially unhealthy? Any decent massage of the neck, shoulders, or back will release those muscles, helping diminish the strain responsible for thoracic and clavicular breathing. Also, you will find that during a relaxing massage, your breathing becomes diaphragmatic on its own and that the activity of your sympathetic stress system plunges. Stress and anxiety cannot remain chronic if you give yourself intermittent, restorative breaks in the form of professional massages.

Receiving regular professional massages will teach you how a good massage manipulates muscle, making it easier to give yourself or others effective massage later on. You will also quickly learn where on your body the muscles are dormant so that you can compress them yourself. Additionally, massage conditions dominant traits such as not flinching or pulling away when touched, relaxing completely around others, and being comfortable while in close physical contact with people you don't know well. These traits will add to your overall sense of ease and confidence in the world around you.

Massage Activity #6.2: *Visualization During Massage*

Every time you get a massage, spend some time noticing what the masseuse is doing to your body. Note the tempo, the pressure, and the locations they focus on. Notice what areas are sore and how they respond to pressure. Pay particular attention to the technique the masseuse uses, what body parts they employ and how. Visualize what the masseuse is doing to you and visualize yourself doing the same to your muscles (or those of others). Spending time picturing yourself giving the massage will make you a fantastic masseuse in no time.

Due to reductions in chronic tension and an increased blood supply, after a high-quality deep tissue massage, you will find yourself able to jump higher, run faster, and bench press more. You will have more energy, better endurance, and exercising will be more pleasurable. To help capitalize on those improvements, I strongly recommend exercising before a deep tissue massage. Afterward, you want to stretch and exercise the muscles that have been released, but you don't want to overload them. You do not want to go to a batting cage, lift heavy weights, spar, or load up a moving truck. Do these things before a deep tissue massage, but not after.

Most importantly, massage will allow you to flex into and exercise within positions that were previously barricaded. You will find that you can contract portions of muscles that were once completely unavailable. They become available because the massage gives them a temporary blood supply, allowing them to flex like healthy, active muscle tissue is supposed to. Subsequent chapters (13-18) will detail how to combine massage with exercise to reopen musculoskeletal obstructions.

I recommend trying as many different masseuses as possible. Almost any massage is going to be of value, but only a certain percentage of masseuses are worth your time and money. Your goal is to find the masseuses in your vicinity who are best at searching out and pressing into the aching, tense parts of your body. This does not necessarily mean paying top dollar. The most helpful massages I have received myself were not the most expensive ones. The Chinese acupressure studio in the mall near my home is consistently the best. In my experience, traditional Chinese massage has excellent biological validity. They know where trigger points are and how to compress them firmly while slightly varying the location of pressure every few seconds. I also stand by Thai massage, medical massage, sports massage, active release technique, osteopathic manipulation, myofascial release therapy, and trigger point therapy. With a skilled practitioner, each of those schools can lead to extremely positive outcomes.

Tension Insanity: Excitement

Having reviewed the most important ways in which touch can heal, let's return to the story that opened the chapter. That was not the only time I found my friend in crisis. Nor was it the worst.

The third time I had to take my friend to the hospital was the most dramatic. Homeless again, he had spent a few weeks with some mutual friends. One of them was another transient who harried and browbeat him constantly. After less than a week of this abuse, his speech was accelerated and the things he said came primarily from resentment and frustration. One day, I was looking after him along with a woman he was dating. We watched his mental state slowly devolve over just a few hours, and by nighttime, his behavior was delirious. He was pacing and ranting in a state of purposeless volatility. In the episode I described at the beginning of this chapter, my friend was in a state of *catatonic stupor*. This time, his condition was *catatonic excitement*, commonly cited as one of the most dangerous mental states in psychiatry.

Patients in a state of catatonic excitement are completely impulsive and exhibit bizarre, non-goal-directed hyperactivity. My friend was storming around restlessly, pointing, yelling, and making wild accusations, raving about a new topic every two sentences. It took me 20 minutes of this to realize that even though he was on his feet and talking, he was barely conscious. His nonsensical, incoherent ranting seemed inexhaustible. He wouldn't let anyone touch him and started yelling when any of us came near him or made eye contact. He repeatedly jabbed his finger into the chest of a common friend while screaming. As soon as he made a violent physical overture toward his girlfriend, I quickly but gently used a wrestling takedown to bring him to the floor. I knew that using physical force with a person with a mental health condition is unethical, but I reacted to protect the others. I spoke to him in a friendly, authoritative way and massaged him firmly. I kneaded the muscles along his spine for a half-hour until he started weeping in relief. Remarkably, our friends were able to talk him into going back to the place he dreaded the most. I can't imagine that any intervention other than massage could have helped him relax enough to make that choice willingly.

It was his third admission to a psychiatric hospital in two years. After four days there, he was expelled for fighting with other patients. I spent hours searching streets near the institution before I found him shivering in the rain. He was frenzied, rambling madly, with a swollen lip and a gash over his eye. All his medications had been stolen from him and he was "crashing down" as the prescribed drugs cleared from his cerebral circulation. Withdrawal from the sedatives and antipsychotics caused his sympathetic stress system to go berserk. I realized that no matter what we did, he would seek out and engage the most upsetting aspect of any scenario I put us in.

So, we avoided stimulation. I checked us into a hotel in a quiet neighborhood and spent three days with him, working hard to remain as calm and as boring as possible. To avoid overstimulating him, I hid my phone and took the room's television down to the front desk. At that time, he could only fathom what was physically in front of him, so because there was no television in the room, he didn't miss it. Instead, I brought a few board games for us to play. I spent most of the time trying to be the perfect combination of nondominant and nonsubmissive. He tried to dominate me, he tried to act submissive toward me, and I ignored these so as not to reinforce either.

During that time, I also practiced many breathing exercises with him. He said he liked them, but he was so restless that he could only concentrate on them for a few seconds at a time. He did not have the attention span necessary for paced breathing. For this reason, every half hour I asked him to take one long, slow inhalation and one complete exhalation while blowing on his finger. He said it made him sleepy. Calming our anxiety with proper breathing can make us drowsy, but only at first. Many people assume that becoming sleepy is an unavoidable part of relaxation. It is not. Performing the diaphragmatic breathing exercises in Chapter 3 over several weeks will prove to you that relaxation sharpens attention in the long run. The next chapter will discuss the biology of how becoming calmer, paradoxically, makes you more alert. After coaching him to take many steady, full breaths in a row, I took him to get a massage.

We went to an 80-pound woman who gave hour-long, full-body massages for $20 at a storefront on Hollywood boulevard. She had to be more gentle than usual because he could barely stand even mild pressure. I glanced at him and saw him shuddering, convulsing in what I took as the ecstasy of the woman's touch meeting the agony of his pain-body. He started moaning, and when she asked whether she should continue, his reply was, "Please." A few minutes later, he started sobbing and didn't stop for the remaining 45 minutes. The other people at the parlor didn't even complain about all the noise he was making because they could tell what he was going through.

A couple of hours after his massage, he looked bright, fresh, and reinvigorated. His appearance contrasted starkly with his appearance described at the beginning of this chapter. It was abundantly clear that various chakra-like modules were finally given the break they needed to begin restoration and regeneration. This included muscles that were never even touched by the masseuse. His face, voice, heart, diaphragm, and gut had the brief respite they needed to recharge. All because his inner animal was given 60 minutes to forget about its interminable fear of death.

Having never had a massage, he said it was the best experience of his life and asked when we could go again. Of course, his case is an extreme example. Most of us don't carry this amount of trauma or have such deeply rooted pain bodies. But massage, be it professional or self-administered, is among our most effective and accessible means of treating both.

Spend Time Rubbing and Caressing

Personal grooming (or preening) is widespread in animals and is a hygienic behavior aimed at extracting foreign objects from the body's surface. It is done to remove insects, ectoparasites, leaves, dirt, and twigs. Social grooming is common in mammals and involves stroking, scratching, massaging, licking, and gentle biting of another animal. Even animals such as birds, horses, bats, lions, and insects groom each other. Apes and monkeys groom one another daily, and the consequent trust and bonding are critical to group cohesion. Grooming plays a role in establishing alliances, is imperative for reconciliation after conflict,[8] and is one of the main ways that primates reduce stress and tension.[9]

In humans and other mammals, gentle, well-meaning touch stimulates the release of beta-endorphin. This natural analgesic attaches to the same brain receptors as morphine, heroin, and other drugs derived from the opium poppy.[10] Synthetic opioid street drugs increase the traumatic load on our bodies by leading to extreme withdrawal. But increasing the levels of natural endorphins produced by your brain does not and may be among the healthiest things you can do. It increases overall well-being. Grooming, massaging, rubbing, cuddling, and caressing all have this effect. This is partially responsible for the fact that primates with the most grooming relationships tend to be healthier on average.

Do dominant primates groom a lot or a little? What would be your guess? In fact, they groom others the most. Because the dominant primates usually have the highest circulating endorphin levels, they typically do not need to be groomed to relax but are the most willing to groom others. Most humans do not regularly rub or massage others. Do you? I think that many people are apprehensive about being affectionate because they are concerned that their manual skills are not good enough, or they worry about the social aspects of the interaction. More than anything, they don't want to have their efforts rejected. But much of this is a question of familiarity and repetition—you can't get good if you don't try. A little bit of time and practice will allow you to pass that apprehensive barrier and feel at ease touching and rubbing other people. As with other skills we've discussed, you can develop the ability on your own before perfecting it with others.

Massage Exercise #6.8: *Rub and Caress an Inanimate Object*

Find a pillow or similar object to rub, caress, or massage. Know that the pillow will not judge your efforts, allowing you to caress it in the most loving way that you are capable. Imagine you are humbly trying to gain experience and work toward caressing a real person. You might pretend to be finger painting a beautiful, cursive, abstract composition using a slow, soothing cadence. Think "slow hand," not "heated rush." Alternate between touching firmly and very tenderly. Try to touch the object in the way you want to be touched and know that you can experiment with new flourishes and rhythms without someone critiquing you. If you do this while practicing paced breathing, you will find that your hands do not hesitate—the indecision and fumbling will be absent, quickly making you into a pro. With enough practice, your loved ones will never want you to stop touching them and you will develop a "healing hand."

When you find the opportunity, practice stroking and caressing another person in a smooth, rhythmic, and doting way. Alternate between using your whole hand and the tips of your fingers. Don't hesitate or pause and try to keep your fingers from skipping along their skin. Rather, maintain fluid contact. Lightly squeeze their skin between your fingers and tug at it gently. You can rub their entire body, alternating between pressing and caressing. This kind of positive physical touch can work wonders for your spouse, children, or pets.

Caress, like vibration, does not release hypertonic muscles in the same way that compression or percussion does. It undoes tension through relaxation by significantly reducing conscious bracing. However, if the person being massaged feels uncomfortable, they may actually brace more, like a pet that doesn't want to be picked up. Many people cringe and reject touch due to past physical trauma. As the one doing the touching, it is your responsibility to touch them in a way that causes their bracing to subside. Affectionate, attentive, and flowing movements will do this.

Try rubbing or caressing your significant other as you listen to music. It can help coordinate and sensualize your movements. Rubbing and massaging the scalp is one of the best ways to release endorphins. One way to approach this is to start by pressing the tip of your thumb firmly into their upper neck and then the occipital muscles on the back of their head. Sensually depress, release, and reposition once every two seconds. Use your thumb to stroke firmly over the hair shafts around the nape of the neck, making a crackling sound, and stimulating the copious nerve endings in the area. Massaging the entire scalp in this way, rubbing it rhythmically with all ten finger pads, can be intensely pleasurable. Try lying next to your partner, nestling against them, and fondling their arms, back, and shoulders. You might lie on your back and have a significant other lie on top of you, stomach to stomach, so that you can rub their neck, back, bottom, and legs with both hands.

It is known that in primates, the grooming animal enjoys levels of pleasure chemicals that are comparable to the individual being groomed. It is the same in humans. Stroking your cat or dog releases endorphins, reduces heart rate, and drops blood pressure in the pet as well as in the human doing the petting.[11] Without question, massaging and caressing someone else is the most pleasurable, stress-reducing, and bonding activity I know of. I believe that many people feel unsated because they mistakenly seek this form of satisfaction from kissing and sex, which simply don't provide it. One look at the pervasiveness of grooming in primates convinces me that our bodies are biologically prepared for, and expectant of, being rubbed and caressed. We are doing ourselves a disservice by not doing it regularly.

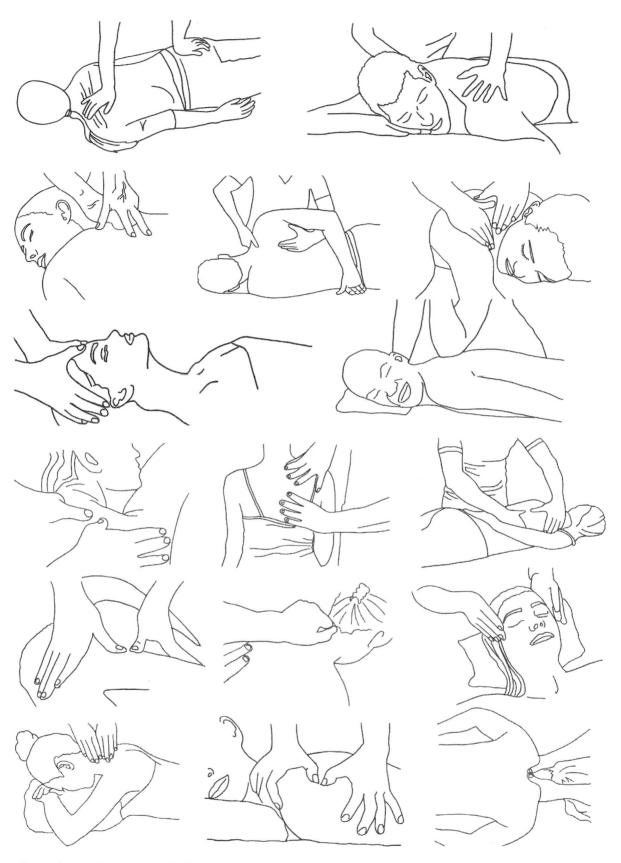

Illustration 6.12: Massage techniques.

Conclusion

Psychologists have long been puzzled by the fact that people who experience windfalls, such as winning the lottery, do not stay happy for long. Humans tend to return to a stable set point for subjective well-being and life satisfaction within a short period following major positive or negative life events. This phenomenon has been called the "hedonic treadmill."[12] You can increase the speed as much as you want on a treadmill, but you won't get anywhere. In life, you can accumulate as many riches and accolades as you want, but it likely won't make you any happier or more peaceful. A good deal of psychological research has been devoted to grappling with this issue because it seems inherently unsettling. If fulfilling our lifelong dreams and ambitions does not reduce our pain, what will?

Well, massage will. Trigger points keep us tethered to the hedonic treadmill. Winning the lottery does nothing to remove years of built-up tension in our bodies. However, breathing retraining, compression, percussion, and caressing do precisely that. They alleviate pressure and pain. They give us long-term, renewable increases in the levels of pleasure-causing chemicals in our brains. They bring us closer to other people and help us learn to be more comfortable with them physically.

You probably know someone in their nineties who has terrible posture. They would be spry and dexterous if only they had enjoyed a monthly deep tissue massage throughout their life. Many people assume that frailty, muscle pain, and loss of muscle mass are simply inevitable concomitants of aging. They are not. They are merely the cumulative toll of continuous tension.

To help reverse the effects of long-term muscle strain, I recommend creating a monthly budget for deep tissue massage. For the first several months, spend as much of your discretionary income on it as possible. Then, transition into doing it yourself. Recruit your friends, family members, and partners to practice massage with you. Whether you do it yourself or practice mutual massage with a loved one, it is a free way to rapidly increase your wellbeing.

Chapter 6: **Bullet Points**

- Massage can repair tense, painful muscles all over the body. It works by forcing partially contracted muscles into a resting state, which allows them to regenerate, heal, and receive fresh blood and nutrients.
- Pressing firmly into tender, achy muscle provides ischemic compression, which forces the blood out of the tissue and then, when released, increases blood flow.
- Muscles that are sore when compressed are the most in need of massage.
- All the muscle soreness in your body can and should be removed by massage.
- Performed regularly, compression will restore proper length and tone to the muscle, increasing its range of motion, strength, and regenerative capacity as well as reducing tension and pain.
- There are key areas of the body that, when massaged, can recover providing tremendous benefits.
- Muscle compression is most effective when used with diaphragmatic breathing.
- Percussion is another massage modality that involves gently but rapidly striking a muscle. Vibration is a third modality that uses a vibrating, electric massage tool.
- Massage also improves posture, athleticism, muscular endurance, coordination, flexibility, and mobility.
- Learning to massage yourself is awkward at first. Achieving the ability to do it effectively may take months but is a skill worth investing time in. Getting professional massages can help the learning process.
- Grooming in primates is vital to stress reduction, social cohesion, and well-being. You can achieve the same positive outcomes by making time to affectionately massage, rub, and caress those closest to you.

Chapter 6: **Endnotes**

1.   Burrow, J. P., Spurling, B. C., & Marwaha, R. (2020). Catatonia. In *StatPearls*. StatPearls Publishing.

2.   Braun, M. B., & Simonson, S. J. (2008). *Introduction to massage therapy*. Lippincott Williams & Wilkins.

3.   Fridlund, A. J. (1994). *Human facial expression: An evolutionary view*. Academic Press.

4.   Moyer, C. A., Rounds, J., & Hannum, J. W. (2004). A Meta-analysis of massage therapy research. *Psychological Bulletin*, *130*(1), 3–18.

5.   Rapaport, M. H., Schettler, P., Larson, E. R., Edwards, S. A., Dunlop, B. W., Rakofsky, J. J., & Kinkead, B. (2016). Acute Swedish massage monotherapy successfully remediates symptoms of generalized anxiety disorder: A proof-of-concept, randomized controlled study. *The Journal of Clinical Psychiatry*, *77*(7), e883–91.

6.   Fritz, S. (2016). *Mosby's fundamentals of therapeutic massage*. Elsevier Health Sciences.

7.   Weerapong, P., Hume, P. A., & Kolt, G. S. (2005). The mechanisms of massage and effects on performance, muscle recovery and injury prevention. *Sports Medicine*, *35*(3), 235–256.

8.   Smuts, B., Cheney, D., Seyfarth, R., Wrangham, R., & Struhsaker, T. (1987*). Primate societies*. University of Chicago Press.

9.   Schino, G., Scucchi, S., Maestripieri, D., & Turillazzi, P.G. (1988). Allogrooming as a tension-reduction mechanism: A behavioral approach. *American Journal of Primatology*, *16*(1), 43–50.

10. Keverne, E. B., Martensz, N. D., & Tuite, B. (1989). Beta-endorphin concentrations in cerebrospinal fluid of monkeys are influenced by grooming relationships, *Psychoneuroendocrinology*, *14*(1–2), 155–161.

11. McConnell, P. (2003). *The other end of the leash: Why we do what we do around dogs*. Ballantine Books.

12. Frederick, S., & Loewenstein, G. K. (1999). Hedonic adaptation. In D. Kahneman, E. Diener, & N. Schwarz (Eds.), *Well-being: The foundations of hedonic psychology* (pp. 302–329). New Russell Sage Foundation.

Chapter 7: **Think Peacefully**

"Never, in his brief cave life, had he encountered anything of which to be afraid. Yet fear was in him. It had come down to him from a remote ancestry through a thousand lives. It was a heritage he had received directly...through all the generations of wolves that had gone before. Fear!—that legacy of the Wild which no animal may escape... So the gray cub knew fear, though he knew not, the stuff of which fear was made." — Jack London (1876-1916), White Fang

In my twenties, I would phone my parents every week, and they would ask how I was doing. I would tell them that everything in my life was going fine but that for some reason my stress was insufferable, that I was in a state of endless panic, and could feel the devastating effect it was having on my body and mind. I was taking graduate courses in clinical psychology and was very familiar with the Western approach to anxiety. Reading numerous books and articles gave me insight into my condition but no relief from it.

It wasn't until I discovered Eastern and Stoic contemplative/meditative perspectives on stress that I found a way to start to counteract the damage that my tormented mind was inflicting on my body. I think you will find that these perspectives are intertwined with the content from the preceding chapters and that, used together, they will help you tame the unnerving impulses emanating from your brain's unconscious fear centers.

The Brain Circuits Responsible for Fear

Neuroscientists have identified seven primary emotions common to all mammals: care (nurturance), play (social joy), seeking (expectation), lust (sexual excitement), rage (anger), fear (anxiety), and grief (sadness).[1] These emotions correspond to specific subcortical brain circuits. Each is embodied in a mechanistic device made of brain cells that sits below the level of the conscious cerebral cortex. Both the emotions and the brain areas responsible for them are highly conserved in all mammals and even extend to certain species of birds and reptiles. In their book, *The Archaeology of Mind*, pioneering researchers Jaak Panksepp and Lucy Biven explain how these genetically hardwired emotional systems, often referred to collectively as the limbic system, reflect ancestral memories with adaptive functions.

Each emotion is an information processing tool built-in to animals, rather than having to be learned by them. They each steer the progression of thought in a different direction to ensure the animal is responding to its environment with the right behaviors. The fear and grief circuits respond to hardship and, despite being intrinsic to survival, are one of the primary drivers of psychological pain in mammals. At this point, you shouldn't be surprised to learn that they are the emotions most closely tied to status conflict. As such, they elicit muscle tension and distressed breathing. This chapter will focus on how you can interrupt this elicitation by taking control of your thought process.

In newborn mammals, the fear system is only activated by a few things. These are instinctually fear-provoking stimuli and include pain, sudden movement, falling, suffocation, and loud noise. Mammals are afraid of these things by nature because they are predictive of death. After experiencing such stimuli, fear is generalized to the things that the animal has found can be associated with them.[2] For instance, newborn rats are not afraid of their natural predators, such as cats, ferrets, and foxes. However, due to their strong instinctual fear of these predators' odors, they learn to become afraid after being exposed to them. In fear learning experiments, rats can easily be trained to become frightened of a variety of neutral contextual stimuli (like Kleenex or sand) that were coincidentally present during their exposure to instinctual fear stimuli. For example, the smell of a ferret can make a rat deathly afraid of a toilet paper roll.

We, too, overgeneralize our fears. Horror movies are an apt example. They are horrible for our minds because they activate and strengthen our fear circuits. They cause us to associate instinctual fears with all kinds of neutral concepts far beyond the stereotypical hockey players, dolls, dark alleys, clowns, and old houses. Do scary movies further sensitize everyone's fear circuit, or can some people watch them without repercussions? While I know it's possible to have such good posture, composure, and breathing that watching a horror flick desensitizes you to fear, I'm certainly not there yet.

When scientists surgically place electrodes directly into the brain's fear system (lateral and central amygdala, anterior medial hypothalamus, and periaqueductal gray) and stimulate it electrically, this incites an ominous, objectless fear, making the animal afraid of everything it encounters. Animals freeze at low levels of current and take precipitous flight at higher levels. When the same areas are stimulated in humans, they make comments such as "I'm scared to death," "Somebody is now chasing me. I am trying to escape from him," and "I feel an abrupt feeling of uncertainty just like entering a long, dark tunnel."[3]

Repeated stimulation of the fear center, whether through experiences or electrodes, cause rats to become constitutionally inhibited, skittish, and timid. These rats engage less in play, feeding, sex, and grooming. Repetitive activation of the fear circuit is a surefire pathway to social defeat. When the fear system is activated, every nuance of your body language tells a potential predator that you are unstable and will make an easy lunch. The same body language tells potential competitors that they have the advantage over you. Clearly, the fear system can be insidious, and you don't want its neural connections to strengthen or spread.

The Brain Circuits Responsible for Grief

The grief system is separate from the fear system. Just as the predation and aggression systems are dissociable (as discussed in Chapter 1), grief and fear involve distinct neural pathways. They even use different chemicals and respond differently to drugs. Electrical stimulation of brain regions containing grief circuitry shifts people into a state of desolation and despair that lifts rapidly when the current is turned off. The general anatomy of the human grief system (anterior cingulate, dorsomedial thalamus, and periaqueductal gray) overlaps extensively with the system responsible for separation calls in other animals.

Baby mammals and birds emit distress vocalizations when separated from their mothers. These are reflexive cries generated by the activation of their grief system made to help their mother locate them in space. We usually subdue the impulse to cry out, but much of our psychological pain involves the arousal of these same areas. Can you find the lost baby animal inside of you now? Can you feel the stress of the last week and how it puts pressure on your voice box as if you wanted to cry out and be rescued? Baby animals stop crying out, and their grief system shuts down as soon as their mother finds them. Our grief system can remain operative for years at a time. Of course, this leads to repetitive strain of the vocal tract, which Chapter 12 will show you how to overcome.

When baby monkeys are separated from their mothers for even just a few hours, they experience grief that can affect them for the rest of their lives. Some primatologists force these separations in "adverse rearing" experiments so that they can study the factors involved in risk and resilience to mental illnesses such as anxiety. Monkeys that have been separated from their mothers repeatedly develop chronic despair. As adults, they tend to have fewer social alliances, less social support, fewer grooming partners, impaired social skills, and reduced social competence.[4] They are poor at finding sexual partners, make deficient parents, and are less affiliative and more aggressive toward their peers.[5] They are also consistently more subordinate and inhabit rungs lower in the social hierarchy.[6] These things are also often true of monkeys that have been neglected, abused, or orphaned. Allowing ourselves to wallow in a state of grief, loneliness, or discontentedness results in the same outcomes.

The emotions of fear and grief intend to keep us safe and from finding ourselves isolated. In most people, however, their signals are too intense and have stayed on for too long. Unchecked, fear and grief maintain a negative state of mind that cripples us socially and mutilates our reality. We need to convince the baby mammal in the center of our brains that we are not desperately trying to find our mother, that we are not lost, that we are not missing anything or anyone, and that we are exactly where we are supposed to be.

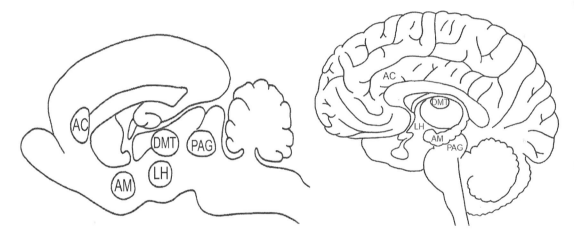

Illustration 7.1: A. Guinea pig brain cross-section; B. Human brain cross-section. Both illustrations show the fear system [amygdala (AM), hypothalamus (H), and periaqueductal gray (PAG)], and grief system [(anterior cingulate (AC), dorsomedial thalamus (DMT), and periaqueductal gray (PAG)]. Note that even though these two brains are not shown to scale, the relative size of the emotional areas is smaller in humans, and this reflects our capacity for deliberate emotional regulation.

Common to both the brain's fear and grief systems is a panic center called the amygdala. This structure is tied to the sympathetic nervous system and acts to elevate muscle tension, blood pressure, stress hormones, and heart and respiration rates. The amygdala ensures that threatened animals respond to negative situations with energy. Its messages about fear override ongoing processing elsewhere in the brain and cause us to refocus our attention on threat. Many of our most negative behaviors occur when this subcortical nucleus assumes control over the brain's higher cognitive centers in what is commonly referred to as an "amygdala highjack."

Like the fear and grief systems that it potentiates, the amygdala is always active. It is constantly running its information processing algorithms, though usually at a low level. Brain scans show that the amygdala's activity level rises when we feel threatened.[7] It is more active at rest in people with anxiety or depressive disorders and less active in those who report being happy and well adjusted. We can never be certain what will set it off, and we often are not even aware when it has been activated (for more on the amygdala, see Chapter 19).

The amygdala, and by extension the fear and grief systems, work on the smoke detector principle. Just like smoke detectors, they are calibrated to be so sensitive that they are liable to go off by accident. They are set this way because a few false alarms are tolerable if it ensures that we can recognize real peril when it arises. In terms of reproductive success, it is better to overreact to a non-threat than to underreact to a true threat.[8] This is a reasonable predisposition for wild animals but an irrational one for modern humans. Today, we tolerate constant false alarms of the fear and grief systems even though we are rarely confronted by physical threats. This vestigial hair-trigger mechanism is the reason we are predisposed to negative thinking.

The Negativity Bias, Fear, Grief, and Default Mode

"What we are today comes from our thoughts of yesterday, and our present thoughts build our life of tomorrow: our life is the creation of our mind." — Buddha (c. 563 BCE-483 BCE)

Humans are a special type of biological survival machine. Unlike viruses, bacteria, protists, fungi, plants, and most animals, we think. We are capable of simulating environmental situations so that we can predict the probable outcomes of our actions. We use these simulations to learn about and make sense of the events around us. In a perfect world, these models would always be cheerful and productive. Unfortunately, our brain's threat centers influence us to model negative things so that we can respond appropriately when negative scenarios arise. This tendency to focus on the bad is often referred to as the *negativity bias.*[9]

The negativity bias makes us more likely to focus on a negative piece of information such as a criticism than a positive one such as a compliment.[10] It results in superstitious, nonreflective fretting that rarely leads to insight or progress. Also, negative thoughts can be triggered rapidly but tend to linger for long periods. This is probably related to the poor rebound effect for diaphragmatic breathing, in which a minor threat can force a mammal to breathe shallowly within a single second, after which it takes several minutes for the breathing to return to normal.

Lamentably, rosy glasses don't contribute to reproductive success in most ecological scenarios. Further, animals that don't worry have poor survival outcomes. Studies that look at fish, mice, or primates that are bred or experimentally altered to become fearless show that these animals are great at acquiring resources but are the first to be eaten.[11] On the other hand, the most anxious animals avoid predators and stay safe. However, they are not very productive (or reproductive) because they are constantly hiding and cowering. So, it was good for our ancestors to be somewhere between fearful and fearless. But what about today? What about you? Would you benefit from being fearless?

For thousands of millennia, our forebears were hunted, mauled, and devoured by monsters. These included saber-toothed cats, cave lions, cave hyenas, dire wolves, short-faced bears, five-meter-long snakes, giant lizards, and towering, flightless "terror birds." However, anatomically modern humans employing expertly fashioned spears, clubs, axes, and knives were able to turn the tables. For the last 200 thousand years, we systematically drove these giant beasts of prey to extinction.[12] We killed off many of these "Cenozoic megafauna" for food. In so doing, we made nearly the entire surface of Earth free from predators. In the last 10 thousand years, humans have replaced brutal disputes with courtroom judgments and "every man for himself" with legal rights. Compared to our ancestors, we should feel invulnerable. Our world is far safer now. Our genes and brains just don't know it yet.

Humans today have virtually no natural predators. We fight among each other less than ever before, and cannibalism is finally out of fashion, but our brains' fear and grief systems are still fully operational. The human brain is the pinnacle of evolution on Earth and the most complex object in the known galaxy, yet it is routinely preoccupied with unsubstantiated fear, vindictive anger, regret, victimization, resentment, and status anxiety. When you experience these emotions, thank your brain for trying to protect you but know that they are vestiges from a treacherous, anarchic past. Anxiety involves a tradeoff. The table below lists several similar tradeoffs discussed in this book.

Common Behaviors	Implications for Hunter-Gatherers	Implications for Modern People
Chronic Stress	Caution and apprehension of danger. Motivation to struggle, fight, and survive.	Unhealthy bodily effects. Unnecessary psychological discomfort and woe.
Anxiety	Enhanced awareness of potentially fatal threats.	Exaggerated fear responses to nonfatal threats.
Depression / Defeat	Accepting the dominance of other group members.	Loss of confidence, drive, and ambition.
Submissive Behavior	Pacifying those who might harm you. De-escalating conflict.	Generating superfluous tension, trauma, and heartache.
Dominating Behavior	Elevating yourself in the social hierarchy.	Putting others down and making them angry.
Anger / Aggression	Healthy self-promotion and protection.	Negative interactions and social isolation.
Competitiveness	Drive to attain food and mates at the expense of others.	Competition with friends and coworkers is unnecessary and divisive.
Defensiveness	Self-protection and healthy suspicion of others.	Unnecessarily high paranoia or fear of others' intentions.
Impulsivity	Drive to quickly attain food and other resources.	Diminished capacity for patience, discipline, and goal setting.
Addictiveness	Quick to repeat behaviors that have positive outcomes.	Quick to become addicted to drugs, alcohol, etc.

Table 7.1 Behavior that was adaptive in our ancestral past is now maladaptive.

Our proclivity for chaotic and destructive thinking is largely involuntary. This is because, in most people, the brain's fear and grief centers have been recruited to be an integral part of the "default mode network." When we think about unfavorable social scenarios while under sympathetic upregulation day after day, we deeply etch the threat centers into our wiring. This makes it so that antagonistic conflict runs on autopilot. The default mode network is active during self-referential thought but is turned off whenever our attention turns to a task or distraction.[13] For many of us, the only time we have a reprieve from negative thoughts is when a diversion, such as the television or social media, drowns out our inner voice.

Many individuals with severe PTSD extrovert only when they talk about their trauma. They may be reticent and withdrawn most of the time but come alive when relating stories about being accosted, bombed in a rice paddy, or abused as a child. I, too used to only become lively when I spoke about the bad things that happened to me. I would pick the most negative topic possible and use it to whip myself into a frenzy. This made most of my conversations with friends (interactions that are supposed to be uplifting) incredibly draining. My tendency to talk about unsettling events was reinforcing my social anxiety. Next time you are with a friend, try not talking about anything irksome or disagreeable and watch how cool it helps you become.

Many of us define ourselves in terms of how tough or unique our problems are. This is due to our inherited tendency to become addicted to trauma. During fearful episodes, the brain secretes opioid chemicals that temporarily alleviate the sensation of pain. This "fear-induced analgesia" is the reason why some of us are, paradoxically, addicted to fear. We find it thrilling. This is why we can become addicted to scary movies or to focusing on negative events. It is like an animal in a cage that engages in self-injurious behavior just to stay stimulated. Almost all monkeys caged alone develop self-biting, self-slapping, and head-banging tendencies. Analyze the perverse gratification you get from thinking and talking about negative things. Isn't this something you could live without?

Thinking Activity #7.1: *Imagine Not Talking About Stress*

Analyze your tendency to talk and think unconstructively about things that incite strong negative emotions. What if you cut this out completely? Imagine not telling others about anything negative, traumatic, or fear-inducing ever again. Imagine never griping, criticizing, or discussing situations in which you feel you have been wronged. Imagine never talking about anything related to your misfortune, mistreatment, or your ego being bruised. Imagine not dragging yourself and others down with stories about hostile interpersonal interactions. Could you do it? How might this change you?

Hopefully, you can see how these types of conversations are draining you. Try going for a whole month without talking about anything stressful. By the end of the month, just see whether you have more positive energy.

Confiding in others in a relaxed, supportive environment can be highly therapeutic. However, inundating others with negativity just winds us up further. Mulling over upsetting scenarios rather than desensitizing you, usually just sensitizes you to them further. Let us differentiate between what sensitizes us and desensitizes us.

Be Nonjudgmental, Nonresistant, and Nonattached

"Accept whatever comes to you woven in the pattern of your destiny, for what could more aptly fit your needs?" — Marcus Aurelius (121-180)

It is possible to prune the fear and grief centers from your brain's default network. By intentionally reframing our experiences, we can remodel the existing biological connections and reprogram our thinking. Even the simplest popular notions about managing negative thinking can be applicable. Use these: "it's not that bad," "mistakes make me better," "don't fight reality," "everything is temporary," "this too will pass," "let's find the silver lining," "everything happens for a reason," "I learn from my mistakes," "time heals all wounds," or "I never mind." Reframing bad experiences solders resilience into our brain's circuitry and cuts out the elements that do not serve us.

The following are three especially powerful perspectives that come straight from Eastern philosophy that have helped me reframe my circumstances and rewire my worldview: nonjudgment, nonresistance, and nonattachment.

Thinking Activity #7.2: *Nonjudgment, Nonresistance, & Nonattachment*

Spend five minutes imagining what it would be like to completely embrace the following perspectives.

1) Nonjudgment: You are nonjudgmental when you make a conscious choice not to criticize. Most people judge everything that they come across. This is immature. Instead of judging something, dispassionately recognize it for what it is and move on without stamping it with your approval or rejection. You can suspend your judgment on everything from nuisances to catastrophes.

2) Nonresistance: Always accept what is going on at present as if you have chosen it. Nonresistance is choosing to accept the things you cannot change. We are constantly resisting. Not only is this often futile; it is also extremely disheartening. Give yourself a break from opposing your environment and let things take their natural course. This is not resignation or inaction. We can't fix everything at once, so it is best to learn to coexist with the things that are bothering us as we consider the best ways to rectify them. Accept everything that happens. Stoic philosophers called this the art of acquiescence. Nietzsche called this amor fati: a love for all that fate unfolds.
So, I've been asking you to become nonsubmissive, but I am also asking you to fully surrender to everything you cannot change.

3) Nonattachment: We all have unhealthy emotional attachments to things that we can easily lose. These attachments set us up for disappointment and emotional pain when we do lose them. Even if we don't lose them, we live in fear of losing them. Imagine what it would be like never to fear loss. Imagine losing everything that you love and yet still being at peace. Relinquish property, friends, family, past achievements, and every form of physical possession. Imagine giving up these things and yet still being happy. If you are afraid of losing something, you are insecurely attached to it and can never truly love it. True joy only comes from things, or aspects of things, that can never be taken away.

These three perspectives are very powerful because they force us to reanalyze our predicaments from a viewpoint inconsistent with ego, status, or defeat. This is why they are also incompatible with distressed breathing and persistent muscle tension. Due to our "experience-dependent neuroplasticity," mental states become mental traits. Thus, using these concepts to reconceptualize your world will weaken the influence of fear and grief and hardwire your brain for peace.

Meditate to Calm the Mind

"Would you have a great empire? Rule over yourself." — *Publilius Syrus (85 BCE-43 BCE)*

The next few sections discuss meditation and meditative techniques you can use to ease your mind and body. Meditation is an internal effort to self-regulate the mind. During meditation sessions, participants sustain attention toward breathing, bodily sensations, emotions, and thoughts. When they find their attention has wandered into phobias and compulsions, they are supposed to acknowledge this and then let go of them to refocus on the breath or empty the mind.[14] Calm inaction and desireless patience result in the domestication of the brain's barbarian emotional systems. Repeated failures in the first several sessions are lessons in humility and patience. Adopting a consistent meditative practice will lead you to develop self-mastery of thought—the most real and lasting power.

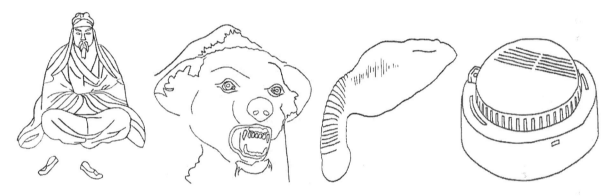

Illustration 7.2: A. Meditator; B. Rabid dog; C. Blood sucking leech; D. Smoke detector.

Siddhartha Gautama, also known as the Buddha, spent six years meditating on his suffering in an attempt to understand peace. He finally concluded that suffering is not caused by either misfortune or divine punishment but rather by thought patterns.[15] This led him to teach others that suffering derives from craving and dissatisfaction and that the only way to stop suffering is to stop wanting more and to stop wanting to impress others. Complete control of the mind is known in Buddhism and Hinduism as nirvana. The literal translation of nirvana is "extinguishing the fire"—the fire of worry, yearning, and longing. Nirvana is also defined as serenity, salvation, heaven, or an indestructible sense of well-being in which ego, hatred, and greed have been overcome. Many spiritual masters think of nirvana, and true enlightenment, to be the end of emotional suffering. I believe it is attainable for everyone.

Meditate by Watching the Thinker

"There is nothing either good or bad, but thinking makes it so." — *Shakespeare (1564-1616)*

"If you don't like something, change it. If you can't change it, change your attitude." — *Maya Angelou (1928-2014)*

We feel like we control our stream of thought, but we don't. Most of our thinking is directed by reflex-like impulses beyond our supervision. Trying to control the parade of associations is much like trying to control a dream. Our desires and discouragements are endless because they don't stem from our objective reality but the state of our default network. We ruminate about negative circumstances in a pitiful and inefficacious attempt to change individual thoughts about them for the better, but instead, we must change our overall thinking pattern. To start this process, observe your thoughts as if you were an outsider.

Thinking Activity #7.3: *Watching the Thinker*
Spend five minutes seeing thoughts as what they are: opinions. Identify negative considerations as worries and let them go without elaborating on them. Ask yourself: "I wonder why I had that last thought." Then ask yourself: "I wonder where my thought will turn to next." Never be afraid of what your next thought will be and rest secure in the assumption that it will not have the power to cut short your next long, deep, smooth inhalation.
Dwelling on problems without a constructive intention to amend them is self-punishment. Recognize that rumination about your perceived station in the status hierarchy may feel like an objective observation but that is usually a distortion of reality. Question the legitimacy of your irrational and self-critical thoughts. Don't take them seriously. Smile at the voice in your head as you would at the antics of a child. Disidentify with it.

In life, bad things are inevitable. Just don't absorb them. Don't hold them in your face, stomach, or heart. Let the pain pass right through you. Just because it would upset others or would have upset you in the past doesn't mean you should let it upset you now. Ask yourself: "Do I hold my amygdala's panic button out for the world to press?" Ask yourself honestly whether you want to be a victim of your life's events or a prisoner in your mind. If you think that weeping or throwing a tantrum over misfortune is ineffectual, realize that internal suffering is, too.

When someone honks at us, our heart rate rises. After an argument, we have a headache. When we are mistreated, we can't sleep. When someone challenges us, our jaw contracts and our stomach churns. What do all these things have in common? Mental perseveration. We can't stop thinking about unpleasant encounters. By continuing to mull over these incidents, you maintain the tension. But, if you bar yourself from searching for justifications to launch a counterattack, you can return to homeostasis in seconds.

Our struggle with peer politics is Kafkaesque in the sense that it is at once mundane, senseless, inescapable, and unresolvable. We keep struggling with the ramifications of the pecking order even though finding some semblance of control of it is impossible. There is no solace or understanding to be reached in perseverating on it. Just because they say it doesn't mean it's true. Not responding is not a loss. Getting the last word is meaningless. Thinking about just how wrong what that person did is will not change anything.

When you find yourself engaged in negative thinking, imagine yourself: 1) dropping it like it is a scalding item that you don't want to be burned by, or 2) placing it on the ground like a heavy box of rotten food. Either way, walk away from it like the unnecessary burden that it is. Pain isn't optional, but holding on to pain is. When you simulate negative scenarios in your mind, your brain and body operate as if what you are imagining is really occurring. You tense up and carry the fight around with you. But, if you can think of taking such misfortunes "philosophically" without suffering, you can protect your chakra-like modules from unnecessary strain.

Meditate Mindfully

"Who sees all beings in his own self, and his own self in all beings loses fear.... When a sage sees this great unity and his self has become all things, what delusion and what sorrow can ever be near him?" — Upanishads

"Breathe. Let go. And remind yourself that this very moment is the only one you know you have for sure.
Oprah Winfrey (1954)

Mindfulness is a meditative practice that has grown out of the Buddhist tradition. A person who is meditating mindfully attempts to become aware of their surroundings, thoughts, and actions without being critical.[16] For beginners to achieve a state of mindfulness, they must concentrate on ruling out all distractions and focus on being present in their current experience. Someone familiar with this practice can remain in a state of mindfulness throughout most daily activities. I think of all the activities and exercises in this book as meditative practices that are best done mindfully.

Medical researcher and author Jon Kabat-Zinn helped popularize the modern mindfulness movement.[17] Kabat-Zinn has influenced many medical treatment centers around the world to use mindfulness meditation to help their patients counteract psychological stress, pain, and illness. He conceptualizes mindfulness as a state in which one is aware of and focused on the reality of the present moment, accepting and acknowledging it without being frustrated by thoughts about or emotional reactions to it. One of the key elements involved in achieving mindfulness is to reside in "the now," in choiceless awareness. Nonjudgment, nonresistance, and nonattachment are fundamental to living mindfully.

Thinking Activity #7.4: *Living in the Present Moment*
Spend a few minutes immersed in the here and now, simply experiencing your senses. Allow yourself to live entirely in the moment as if you have chosen it and everything about it. Notice when you find yourself worrying about the future or regretting the past. When your mind wanders toward misgivings or social stressors, just redirect it back to your present experience: what you are seeing, hearing, and feeling right now. Don't even anticipate future moments; be content in the one that you are in presently. This present Instant is the only

time that you will ever have for peace. Keep reminding yourself to already be whole, content, and happy within it.

As we discussed in Exercise 5.2, notice the pain you feel within your body in the present moment. Acknowledge its intensity and location nonjudgmentally and with nonresistance. Don't let the discomfort make you irritated with the present or push you out of the present. Next, try to find pleasure in the present moment. It *is* there. Start training your mind to notice the faint impressions of pleasure so that you can develop the capacity to dwell within them.

In therapeutic settings, mindfulness has been shown to alleviate stress and accentuate self-efficacy and confidence.[18] Consistent mindfulness has even been shown to increase gray matter in brain areas involved in subduing emotions, including those that inhibit the amygdala.[19] Peer-reviewed articles published in a wide variety of established scientific journals have yielded data evincing that mindfulness techniques have demonstrated substantial clinical benefits for individuals suffering from a variety of mental and physical disorders. Meditation training is used to palliate anxiety, fibromyalgia, chronic pain, cardiovascular disease, addiction, bipolar disorder, insomnia, intractable depression, and many others.[20] For these reasons, substantial US federal funding has been used to produce mindfulness programs and workshops in schools, prisons, hospitals, military bases, and veterans' centers.

Thinking Activity #7.5: *What Would You Like to Think About?*

We are free to think about whatever we want to. We only have to realize this freedom. What would you like to do with your thoughts and inner voice? For the next two minutes, turn your thought to whatever you choose. Don't concern yourself with worrisome, inane things and don't allow your past thoughts and default network to determine where your mind goes next. When you know you have made a contentious or unproductive association, cut the chain. Go back to the last branch and pick up where you left off. Take responsibility to censure, edit, and rewrite the endless string of associations. How can you use your thought constructively? What are some positive questions you can address? Imagine what you are going to do tomorrow to make your day more productive. Continually ask yourself the "magic" question: "How can I make this better?"

Living in the moment is what dominant mammals do. They are not bothered by past failures or worries about the future. They are not concerned that things will suddenly go wrong. They believe that they have what it takes to handle any situation or confrontation. They trust that their instincts and first reactions will solve any problem. The winner's mindset is meditative in this sense. As a winner, approach everything in your life confidently as if you intend to succeed before you even start.

Anxiety Increases Mental Focus but Only in the Short Term

When you relax, you lose a degree of mental speed and intensity. This is because, during stress, brain chemicals such as dopamine, noradrenaline, and cortisol accelerate the brain's processing speed. On the order of seconds to minutes, they can improve performance on a variety of mental tasks.[21] Everyone knows this implicitly, and many people are afraid to relax because they don't want a lapse in their processing ability. However, on longer periods (from hours to months), these same chemicals wreak havoc on mental function. When stress hormone levels remain high for several days, the brain starts to remodel its architecture, compromising concentration, learning, and memory.[22]

As we have discussed, the most potent source of stress for primates is social conflict. Mammals that are socially stressed release stress hormones that preside over a host of negative neurobiological alterations.[23] The birth of new neurons (neurogenesis) is suppressed, connections between neurons (dendrites) atrophy, neural learning (synaptic plasticity) is impaired, and cell death (apoptosis) increases.[24] As illustrated in the figure below, the brain cells of socially defeated mammals show significant deterioration.

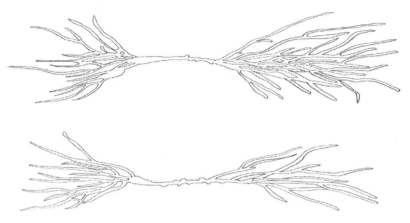

Illustration 7.3: A. The neuron on top is a normal neuron from a tree shrew. It has expansive connections to other neurons; B. The neuron on the bottom comes from a tree shrew that has been exposed to 28 days of domination by a member of its species. The reduction in dendritic branching is quite apparent. These changes can be reversed if this shrew's stress hormone levels are reduced.

Two of the most pivotal brain areas for high-level thought, the prefrontal cortex and the hippocampus, are damaged the most in humans and other mammals by the stress hormone cortisol.[25] Stress is physically destructive to the brain cells in these areas. The damage reduces learning ability, problem solving, creativity, impulse control, and long- and short-term memory.[26] Like muscle cells, brain cells perform well under acute stress but falter under chronic stress.

Anxiety and nervousness create a distracting form of mental noise. People with anxiety disorders exhibit slower reaction times in complex cognitive tasks, which is thought to derive from noise in the individual's information processing stream. Stress causes attentional deficits and instability in basic cognitive operations. When you meditate, try to quiet this mental noise with proper breathing, zero reactivity, and nonjudgmental awareness of the pressure on your mind to keep switching between neurotic thoughts and impulses.

Contrasting with the cell damage done to higher-order processing areas, brain cells in the amygdala and the brain's fear centers are strengthened by cortisol and chronic stress.[27] This heightens fear learning and intensifies fearful memories. I have written articles about how these detrimental brain changes may be adaptive for wild mammals, allowing them to switch from a controlled/attentive processing strategy to an automatic/preattentive one.[28] Becoming disinhibited, impulsive, and opportunistic in an adverse prehistoric setting may have been adaptive. In modern times, however, the cognitive repercussions of excessive stress not only decrease our quality of life but also impair our ability to function professionally.

Mental Relaxation Leads to Mental Clarity in the Long Term

After years of stress, my mind was always racing. I could tell that my thoughts were fragmented. I became all too aware that chronic stress was causing not only problems at work and in my relationships but also mental illness. My working memory declined steeply, and I began to experience perceptual aberrations. It got so bad that I even experienced minor auditory hallucinations. You can read more about these experiences on my blog.

I felt that being on constant high alert was protecting me, but it was maiming me. As you allow yourself to relax, you may feel in your gut that you are not vigilant enough or notice that your response times are delayed. For years, I was afraid of becoming too calm. I was worried that I wouldn't jump to the right conclusion or be able to talk fast enough to communicate properly. I could tell that using adrenaline spikes helped me find words, speak quickly, and put together complex sentences. I was afraid that being calm would make people think I was dim-witted or discourteous. One of the biggest steps toward becoming stress-free was realizing that I don't need fevered anxiety to keep me alert or friendly.

Thinking Exercise #7.1: *Falling Asleep Among Friends*

Take an extreme example of relaxation: sleepiness. Most of us don't allow ourselves to be sleepy around others. I was so socially hypervigilant that I was completely unable to fall asleep or even become drowsy even in the company of friends. If you work on being able to feel tired or even fall asleep right in front of other people, you will reduce your social hypervigilance. The next time you are among friends or family, try to nod off. It proves to others that you are not afraid of them or what they might do to you once you are unconscious. It demonstrates to them that you see them as allies and that you wouldn't attack them if they fell asleep. Most importantly, it proves to your biological system that completely lowering your guard among friends is not taking a risk.

When cortisol levels lower for weeks or months, the cerebral cortex exhibits a remarkable capacity for healing. Many of the cellular changes of stress that compromise intelligence reverse completely. Mammals in low-stress conditions produce large amounts of beneficial neurochemicals and brain growth factors.[29] The absence of stressors stimulates neural stem cell proliferation in the learning areas of the brain.[30] As you know from Chapter 2, the relaxation response, which can be induced by meditation and breathing practices, is characterized by a distinct gene transcription profile.[31] This means that relaxation results in the expression of an entirely different set of genes designed to build the mind and body up, as opposed to tearing it down.

When you start operating without stress, you will feel dull for a few days. However, after a few weeks and months of living at this calmer level, you will find yourself regaining mental aptitude. I feel my memory and attention are better than they have been in over a decade. I attribute this to meditation, mindfulness, and, once again, to diaphragmatic retraining.

Diaphragmatic Breathing and Unbracing the Mind

"If a man's mind becomes pure, his surroundings will also become pure." — Buddha (c. 563 BCE - 483 BCE)

Judging, resisting, attaching, and craving make us tense and cause us to breathe shallowly. Shallow breathing and muscle tension are preparatory. Because they keep us on guard for negative occurrences, we can't help but think negative thoughts. When you start breathing diaphragmatically, you are sending your body a signal that nothing bad can happen. Diaphragmatic breathing allows us to coexist with our thoughts peacefully, and it is the most reliable way to find rest in the present moment. Many clinical researchers agree that breathing diaphragmatically fills the mind with unprovocative content.[32] It disconnects you from the fear, grief, and startle systems of the brain that seek out desperate, last-ditch tactics.

Diaphragmatic breathing is a core component of most meditative practices, especially mindfulness. Mindfulness practitioners notice the sensations arising from the stomach and chest and listen to the sound of the air as it passes through the nostrils. Focus is placed on taking longer, steadier breaths and on the abdomen's movement to ensure that the diaphragm is engaged. To this end, practitioners often think about the word "rising" when breathing in and the word "falling" when breathing out. Some visualize inhaling positivity and exhaling negativity. To promote belly breathing, they also imagine that the air they breathe enters the navel, fills the stomach, and then exits the navel. If one becomes distracted from the breath, they acknowledge this nonjudgmentally and return to focused breathing. Mindfulness is also commonly combined with progressive relaxation and episodes of scanning the body for the tension we experienced in Chapter 5.

"Being aware of your breath forces you into the present moment—the key to all inner transformation. Whenever you are conscious of the breath, you are absolutely present. You may also notice that you cannot think and be aware of your breathing. Conscious breathing stops your mind. But far from being in a trance or half asleep, you are fully awake and highly alert. You are not falling below thinking, but rising above it." — Eckhart Tolle (b. 1948)

The quote above reaffirms the thinking of many spiritual leaders. They know that breath awareness helps us refrain from gasping and shallow breathing. However, mere breath awareness is not enough to shift you into a parasympathetic state. Paced breathing is much more effective in this regard. Paced breathing allows you to permanently lengthen, deepen, and smoothen your breath, which does much more to rectify your thought patterns. Moreover, once the functioning of your diaphragm is improved, you don't have to worry about staying aware of your breathing or constantly living in the now. Diaphragmatic retraining makes it so that you don't have to hide from the past or future or retreat to the present moment just to stop negative thinking.

Before I started paced breathing, my internal monologue was full of argumentation. I often could not stop myself from playing out the most dismaying and socially awkward events in my head. I constantly fought people in my mind, saying spiteful things that I would never say in real life. I would practice ridiculing people that had wronged me in an attempt to provoke an altercation. I was trying to fine-tune my angry personality to be convincing, quick-witted, and sharp-tongued. I was practicing hate.

This had been going on for years, but it ended very abruptly. Only one month after I started paced breathing with a breath metronome, my inner speech lost its violent negativity. I no longer had any "hot buttons" for people to press, and I felt nothing that anyone could say could make me lose my cool. Years of meditation, breath awareness, and living in the present moment led to modest gains. My entire ethos was transformed by only a single month of paced breathing 20 minutes a day.

Sustained Firing and Reconsolidation

When a thought shortens your breath, it is given priority. Upsetting thoughts stimulate the release of the brain chemical dopamine. Dopamine then amplifies the thought's vexing aspects by causing the neurons involved to fire for longer periods. This extended cellular activity is a phenomenon in neuroscience known as *sustained firing*.[33] Thus, dopamine makes sure that the subjects we deem important (either because they are rewarding or punishing) are kept active in mind longer. Whether you are excited about something going well or worried about it going wrong, dopamine causes the emotional elements of the situation to be retained in the stream of thought. Because the relevant brain cells keep firing, you can't help but think about those elements for a while.[34]

The thoughts that upset us are lasting due to our neurochemistry. However, when you don't allow upsetting thoughts to decrease the length of your breath (as when paced breathing), the startle doesn't happen, the dopamine doesn't surge, and the activity of the neurons that code for the upsetting aspects of the thought is not sustained. The thought enters and then quickly exits the mind without feeling compelling. Any time you recognize a disturbing thought forming, focus on prolonging the breath and eliminating the discontinuities. This will negate the thought and make it (and others like it) less likely to revisit you in the future. Lucky for us, this won't diminish dopamine's response to positive thoughts, which works via a different mechanism.

When you practice paced breathing, pay attention to your train of thought and notice how your mind refuses to cling to worry. An alarming idea that would usually capture your attention now seems inconsequential. This will permanently alter how you feel about that topic by physically changing its memory trace in the brain. "Consolidation" is the name for the complex brain processes responsible for turning a fleeting experience into a long-term memory. "Reconsolidation" is the name for the re-evaluative process that occurs whenever a memory is recalled.[35] Emotional reconsolidation happens each time something is remembered[36] and it can be either positive or negative.

Psychotherapists coax patients into remembering and talking about their past traumas, trying to get the patient to reprocess the memory in a better light, reconsolidating it in a way that is not as troublesome[37] When one speaks to a friendly therapist seated in a comfortable chair, that safe environment reframes the traumatic memory. Similarly, every memory you recall during a paced breathing episode will be retrieved in a more relaxed affective context. Memories that are normally retrieved under sympathetic dominance are now being retrieved and reconsolidated under parasympathetic dominance, systematically desensitizing you. This is how paced breathing rewires the default mode network, deflates fear and grief, and reconstructs personhood.

Prolonged Diaphragmatic Breathing Reconsolidates Traumatic Memories

I recommend that you try engaging in paced diaphragmatic breathing for two full hours. It will heighten parasympathetic activity, placing you into a peaceful mental and physiological state. Every thought you have in this state will be reframed and reconsolidated as harmless. After my first hour of uninterrupted paced breathing with a metronome, I could tell everything my mind turned to was cleansed with peace.

You may find some psychological roadblocks. Many people start to panic when their senses tell them that they are "too calm." However, if you keep breathing to the metronome, you will pass through these blockages. The first time I set out to do this, my mind unconsciously and vividly recalled three of the most traumatic incidents of my life within the first hour. One was a disagreement with a group of friends, one was a time of personal embarrassment, and one was a situation that led to a violent attack. These memories made me desperately want to switch back to distressed breathing.

It was almost as if my brain was saying: "Jared, you are calmer than you have been in years right now. Is it safe to be this calm? Remember these terrifying circumstances that upregulated your cardiovascular stress system? Is there a good reason to relax in the face of these past challenges? How do you you know these threats will not recur?" I tried to reassure my body that it was okay to sink below these arousing scenarios. All I had to do was keep breathing to the metronome. Those three harrowing incidents never bothered me again.

Thinking Exercise #7.2: *Prolonged Diaphragmatic Breathing*

Perform two hours of paced breathing guided by your breath metronome. Set your breath metronome at a moderate interval that will be easy to maintain for two hours. You might want to start with 5:7 or 6:9. I use 8:10 or 10:12. Because you will be performing this for two hours, you do not need to inhale or exhale completely; just make sure that you are taking relatively deep breaths. Monitor your body and mind as you achieve a new level of alertness and relaxation.

The first few times, do this while lying down, sitting, or relaxing. Later, try it while stretching, reading, or even while watching a movie. You might perform this prolonged paced breathing session in an area that would otherwise cause stress, such as an empty auditorium where you plan to give a speech or in your dining room where you plan to entertain guests. Pair it with anything you want to calm your body's response to, including fear, foreboding, pain, nausea, loathing, or, as we will discuss in Chapter 20, hunger.

You might want to combine extended diaphragmatic breathing with a venting session. You could do this during psychotherapy, during a talk with a friend, or in writing. The subjective intensity of negative emotions diminishes when feelings are put into words[38] and studies show that there is something highly therapeutic about putting these words on paper. Writing about past hardships has demonstrated powerful clinical benefits.[39] It is called *writing exposure therapy*. The emotional sting is thought to be extracted when a person reconsolidates and recontextualizes negative memories in this way.[40] You should find that writing or speaking about past adversity while paced breathing brings resolution and finality to lingering woes.

Thinking Exercise #7.3: *Writing Therapy*

Spend 10 minutes writing about past difficulties. These can be the most traumatic incidents in your life or just ongoing frustrations. Express your deepest feelings about your fears, griefs, guilts, insecurities, and any other malignancies subverting your thought. Confront the vexations head-on, eye to eye, by describing them in detail. You might also write about how these issues make you feel, how they have affected you in the past, and how you plan to address them in the future.

Don't worry about grammar or sentence structure. You can save your work, but you don't have to if you don't want to. Just write for the entire 10 minutes while paced breathing. If you don't have time to write, have this conversation verbally with yourself. Speak to yourself authentically and compassionately with the focus on consoling your fear and grief systems. Negotiate armistice and find closure using paced breathing as your impartial arbitrator.

Conclusion

The mind is the master controller of an intricate multidirectional communication system linking the brain, immune system, heart, lungs, and all the body's organs. The physical health of these parts is largely determined by your mental outlook and your outlook is determined by your breathing pattern. Most people operate on the unconscious assumption that we need shallow breathing, muscular tension, and the accompanying panicked thoughts to stay safe, come across as intelligent, be socially appropriate, avoid rejection, and remain occupationally productive. This is rarely true, even in the short run.

Chapter 7: **Bullet Points**

- The fear and grief centers of our brains have been recruited as part of the default network. This makes negative thinking exceedingly difficult to stop.
- Disengage from fear and grief by repeatedly envisioning yourself as nonjudgmental, nonresistant, and nonattached.
- Learn to reframe stressors, live in the present moment, and recognize thoughts for what they are: just thoughts.
- The worst-case scenarios that we worry about so much rarely come to pass.
- Recognize that many of your concerns are just defensive pessimism disguised as practicality.
- Negative thinking is a trance. Snap yourself out of it.
- Acute stress may give you a slight, temporary, advantage in some immediate situations, but chronic stress is a disadvantage in all situations.
- Keep in mind that the calmer you are, the better prepared you are to respond to adversity.
- Recognize that you do not need anxiety to be alert, cogent, and socially functional.
- Negative thoughts broadcast unhealthy biological signals to the entire body. The more airtime you give to negative thinking, the unhealthier you will become.
- Stressed thinking causes important brain areas, like the hippocampus and PFC, to physically degenerate, whereas the absence of stress causes them to flourish.
- Don't let the downsides of stress as described here cause you to fear stress or anxiety. You might even find that your anxiety calms if you allow yourself to feel free to be as anxious as you want.
- Prolonged paced diaphragmatic breathing strips negative thoughts and memories of their ability to abduct your train of thought.
- There is no good reason to be reprocessing insecurities from months or years ago. If you have already made an effort to compensate for them, let them go.
- Try being "dead calm," first by yourself and then with others.
- Minimize replaying or imagining negative social scenarios, especially confrontational or violent ones.
- Be very calm when you model social interactions in your head.
- Be very calm in social situations. Retain complete composure. Make being calm a priority in your life, eclipsing the fear of appearing rude or unsophisticated.
- Expect that the most relaxed version of you has what it takes to resolve any scenario.
- The dominant monkey is not stressed because it believes in its ability to deal with whatever new hardship comes along. It trusts that it doesn't have to overthink things to react adeptly to any circumstance.

PROGRAM PEACE Self- Care Exercises to Reprogram Your Mind and Body

Classic Stoic Quotes

"Choose not to be harmed—and you won't feel harmed. Don't feel harmed—and you haven't been." — Marcus Aurelius

"What ought one to say then as each hardship comes? I was practicing for this, I was training for this." — Epictetus

"The trials you encounter will introduce you to your strengths. Remain steadfast... and one day you will build something that endures: something worthy of your potential." — Epictetus

"On the occasion of every accident that befalls you, remember to turn to yourself and inquire what power you have for turning it to use." — Epictetus

"Here is a rule to remember in future, when anything tempts you to feel bitter: not, 'This is misfortune,' but 'To bear this worthily is good fortune.'" — Marcus Aurelius

"You don't have to turn this into something. It doesn't have to upset you." — Marcus Aurelius

"We suffer more often in imagination than in reality. You want to live but do you know how to live? You are scared of dying but tell me, is the kind of life you lead really any different to being dead?" — Seneca

"It is not the man who has too little, but the man who craves more, that is poor." — Seneca

"The chief task in life is simply this: to identify and separate matters so that I can say clearly to myself which are externals not under my control, and which have to do with the choices I actually control. Where then do I look for good and evil? Not to uncontrollable externals, but within myself to the choices that are my own." – Epictetus

"The happiness of your life depends upon the quality of your thoughts." — Marcus Aurelius

"Constant misfortune brings this one blessing: to whom it always assails, it eventually fortifies." — Seneca

"If you are pained by any external thing, it is not this thing that disturbs you, but your own judgment about it." — Marcus Aurelius

"Do not indulge in dreams of having what you have not, but reckon up the chief of the blessings you do possess, and then thankfully remember how you would crave for them if they were not yours. — Marcus Aurelius

Classic Quotes from the Buddha

"We are shaped by our thoughts; we become what we think. When the mind is pure, joy follows like a shadow that never leaves."

"If you light a lamp for somebody, it will also brighten your path."

"The whole secret of existence is to have no fear."

"Pain is certain, suffering is optional."

"Thousands of candles can be lit from a single candle, and the life of the candle will not be shortened. Happiness never decreases by being shared."

"It is a man's own mind, not his enemy or foe, that lures him to evil ways."

"We are shaped by our thoughts; we become what we think. When the mind is pure, joy follows like a shadow that never leaves."

"There is nothing so disobedient as an undisciplined mind, and there is nothing so obedient as a disciplined mind."

"Your worst enemy cannot harm you as much as your own unguarded thoughts. The secret of health for both mind and body is not to mourn for the past, worry about the future, or anticipate troubles, but to live in the present moment wisely and earnestly."

"To keep the body in good health is a duty...otherwise we shall not be able to keep our mind strong and clear."

"If the problem can be solved why worry? If the problem cannot be solved worrying will do you no good."

"A man is not called wise because he talks and talks again; but is he peaceful, loving and fearless then he is in truth called wise."

"Even as a solid rock is unshaken by the wind, so are the wise unshaken by praise or blame."

"Holding on to anger is like grasping a hot coal with the intent of throwing it at someone else; you are the one who gets burned."

Chapter 7: **Endnotes**

1.   Panksepp, J., & Biven, L. (2012). *The archaeology of mind: Neuroevolutionary origins of human emotion*. Norton & Company.

2.   Öhman, A. (2000). Fear and anxiety: Evolutionary, cognitive, and clinical perspectives. In M. Lewis & J. M. Haviland-Jones (Eds.), *Handbook of emotions* (pp. 573–593). The Guilford Press.

3.   Panksepp & Biven, 2012, *The archaeology of mind*.

4.   Nelson, E. E., & Winslow, J. T. Non-human primates: Model animals for developmental psychopathology. *Neuropsychopharmacology, 34*(1), 90–105.

5.   Winslow, J. T. (2005). Neuropeptides and non-human primate social deficits associated with pathogenic rearing experience. *International Journal of Developmental Neuroscience,* 23(2-3), 245–251.

6.   Bastian, M. L., Sponberg, A. C., Suomi, S. J., & Higley, J. D. (2003). Long-term effects of infant rearing condition on the acquisition of dominance rank in juvenile and adult rhesus macaques (Macaca mulatta). *Developmental Psychobiology, 42*(1), 44–51.

7.   Bzdok, D., Laird, A., Zilles, K., Fox, P. T., & Eickhoff, S. (2012). An investigation of the structural, connectional and functional sub-specialization in the human amygdala. *Human Brain Mapping, 34*(12), 3247–3266.

8.   Nesse, R., & Young, E. (2000). Evolutionary origins and functions of the stress response. In G. Fink (Ed.), *Encyclopedia of stress* (Vol. 2, pp. 79–84). Academic Press.

9.   Baumeister, R. F., Finkenauer, C., & Vohs, K. D. (2001). Bad is stronger than good. *Review of General Psychology, 5*(4), 323–370.

10. Vaish, A. T., & Grossman, W. A. (2008). Not all emotions are created equal: The negativity bias in social-emotional development. *Psychological Bulletin, 134*(3), 383–403.

11. Carlson, N. R. (2012). *Physiology of behavior*. Pearson.

12. Burney, D. A., & Flannery, T. F. (2005). Fifty millennia of catastrophic extinctions after human contact. *Trends in Ecology & Evolution, 20*(7), 395–401.

13. Horn, A., Ostwald, D., Reisert, M., & Blankenburg, F. (2013). The structural-functional connectome and the default mode network of the human brain. *NeuroImage*, *102*(Pt. 1) 142–151.

14. Walsh, R., Shapiro, S. L. (2006). The meeting of meditative disciplines and western psychology: A mutually enriching dialogue. *American Psychologist*, *61*(3), 227–239.

15. Billington, R. (2002). *Understanding Eastern Philosophy*. Routledge.

16. Creswell, J. D. (2017). Mindfulness interventions. *Annual Review of Psychology*, *68*, 491–516.

17. Kabat-Zinn, J. (1991). *Full catastrophe living: Using the wisdom of your body and mind to face stress, pain, and illness*. Delta Trade Paperbacks.

18. Gu, J., Strauss, C., Bond, R., & Cavanagh, K. (2015). How do mindfulness-based cognitive therapy and mindfulness-based stress reduction improve mental health and wellbeing? A systematic review and meta-analysis of mediation studies. *Clinical Psychology Review*, *37*, 1–12.

19. Hölzel, B. K., Lazar, S. W., Gard, T., Schuman-Olivier, Z., Vago, D. R., & Ott, U. (2011). How does mindfulness meditation work? Proposing mechanisms of action from a conceptual and neural perspective. *Perspectives on Psychological Science*, *6*(6), 537–559.

20. Sharma, M., & Rush, S. E. (2014). Mindfulness-based stress reduction as a stress management intervention for healthy individuals: a systematic review. *Journal of Evidence Based Complementary and Alternative Medicine*, *19*(4), 271–86; Gotink, R. A., Chu, P., Busschbach, J. J., Benson, H., Fricchione, G. L., & Hunink, M. G (2015). Standardised mindfulness-based interventions in healthcare: An overview of systematic reviews and meta-analyses of RCTs. *PLOS ONE*, *10*(4), e0124344.

21. Foy, M. R., Kim, J. J., Shors, T. J., & Thompson, R. F. (2005). Neurobiological foundations of stress. In S. Yehuda & D. I. Mostofsky (Eds.), *Nutrients, stress, and medical disorders*. Humana Press.

22. Liston, C., McEwen, B. S., & Casey, B. J. (2009). Psychosocial stress reversibly disrupts prefrontal processing and attentional control. *Proceedings of the National Academy of Sciences*, *106*(3), 912–917; Sapolsky, R. M. (2003). Stress and plasticity in the limbic system. *Neurochemical Research*, *28*(11), 1735–1742.

23. Reser, J. E. (2016). Chronic stress, cortical plasticity and neuroecology. *Behavioral Processes*, *129*, 105–115.

24. Sapolsky, R. M. (2005). The influence of social hierarchy on primate health. *Science, 308*(5722), 648–652.

25. Roozendaal, B., McEwen, B. S., & Chattarji, S. (2009). Stress, memory and the amygdala. *Nature Reviews Neuroscience, 10,* 423–433.

26. Cohen, S., Janicki-Deverts, D., & Miller, G. E. (2007). Psychological stress and disease. *JAMA, 298*(14), 1685–1687.

27. LeDoux, J. (1996). *The emotional brain: The mysterious underpinnings of emotional life.* Simon and Schuster.

28. Reser, J. (2007). Schizophrenia and phenotypic plasticity: Schizophrenia may represent a predicitive, adaptive response to severe environmental adversity that allows both bioenergetic thrift and a defensive behavioral strategy. *Medical Hypotheses, 69*(2), 383–394; Reser, J. E. (2016). Chronic stress, cortical plasticity and neuroecology. *Behavioral Processes, 129,* 105–115.

29. Day, J. J., & Carelli, R. M. (2007). The nucleus accumbens and Pavlovian reward learning. *Neuroscientist, 13*(2), 148–159; Martinowich, K., & Lu, B. (2008). Interaction between BDNF and serotonin: Role in mood disorders. *Neuropsychopharmacology, 33,* 73–83.

30. Haglund, M. E. M., Nestadt, P. S., Cooper, N. S., Southwick, S. M., & Charney, D. S. (2007). Psychobiological mechanisms of resilience: Relevance to prevention and treatment of stress-related psychopathology. *Development and Psychopathology, 19*(3): 889–920; Kandel, E. R., Schwartz, J. H., & Jessell, T. M. (2000). *Principles of neural science* (4th ed.). McGraw-Hill.

31. Dusek, J. A., Otu, H. H., Wohlhueter, A. L., Bhasin, M., Zerbini, L. F., Joseph, M. G., Benson, H., & Liebermann, T. A. (2008). Genomic counter-stress changes induced by the relaxation response. *PLoS One, 3*(7), e2576.

32. Philippot, P., Gaetane, C., Blairy, S. (2002). Respiratory feedback in the generation of emotion. *Cognition and Emotion, 16*(5), 605–607.

33. Goldman-Rakic, P. S. (1995). Cellular basis of working memory. *Neuron, 14*(3), 477–485.

34. Seamans, J. K., & Robbins, T. W. (2010). Dopamine modulation of the prefrontal cortex and cognitive function. In K. Neve (Ed.), *The Dopamine Receptors* (pp. 373–398). Humana Press.

35. Ecker, B., Ticic, R., & Hulley, L. (2012). *Unlocking the emotional brain: Eliminating symptoms at their roots using memory reconsolidation.* Routledge.

36. Hardt, O., Einarsson, E. O., & Nader, K. (2010). A bridge over troubled water: Reconsolidation as a link between cognitive and neuroscientific memory research traditions. *Annual Review of Psychology*, *61*, 141–167.

37. Centonze, D., Siracusano, A., Calabresi, P., Bernardi, G. (2005). Removing pathogenic memories: a neurobiology of psychotherapy. *Molecular Neurobiology*, *32*(2), 123–132.

38. Lieberman, M. D., Inagaki, T. K., Tabibnia, G., & Crockette, M. J. (2011). Subjective responses to emotional stimuli during labelling, reappraisal and distraction. *Emotion*, *11*(3), 468–480.

39. Baikie, K., A., & Wilhelm, K. (2005) Emotional and physical health benefits of expressive writing. *Advances in Psychiatric Treatment*, *11*(5), 338–346.

40. Pennebaker, J. W. (1997). Writing about emotional experiences as a therapeutic process. *Psychological Science*, *8*(3), 162–166.

Chapter 8: **Reprogram Facial Tension**

What is a face? To answer this question, we must also consider heads and brains. The brain, head, and face are located together because we evolved from worm-like creatures.[1] As worms move through mud, it is helpful for them to analyze new soil along the way. The head and its various sensory organs are placed in the front of the animal to relay information about the immediate (and impending) environment. This is why the mouth, tongue, nose, eyes, and ears are grouped so close together. A face is a cluster of sensory organs, and in mammals, its appearance offers insight into intentions and well-being.

Fish, amphibians, and reptiles cannot make facial expressions and can only open and close their eyes, nose, and mouth. Unlike mammals, these animals do not have muscles that attach to the skin of the face. Therefore, their facial skin is immobile and essentially devoid of expression. The facial muscles of mammals act as sphincters, constricting the area they circumscribe (eyes and mouth) or as tractors, pulling at their attachments (cheeks, brow, chin). These various muscles bring the faces of mammals to life, allow communication, and when contracted, alter the animal's outlook on its environment.

The facial muscles of mammals interact extensively with unconscious areas of the brain. Many specialized neurological modules send output to and/or receive input from the facial muscles. These include the fear and grief systems, and this is how stress is able to act as a puppeteer for our facial expressions. When the facial muscles are chronically activated by negative emotions, they undergo repetitive strain. As we will see in this chapter, the partial contraction of facial muscles has numerous harmful repercussions. Most mammals have little awareness of their facial tension and, like a puppet, almost no capacity to exercise deliberate control over their facial muscles. This chapter will focus on how to develop those capacities.

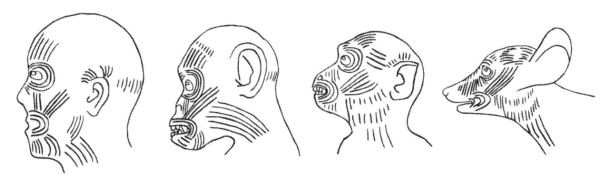

Illustration 8.1: Facial muscles of A. human; B. Chimpanzee; C. Macaque monkey; D. Mouse.

Refrain from Subliminal Grimacing and Frowning

I woke up one morning an hour before my alarm clock sounded. I realized I was too roused to get back to sleep, so I practiced a few yoga poses and laid back down to meditate. I was doing so concertedly, concentrating on abating my chaotic thinking patterns. I turned my attention to the recurring waves of negativism crashing on the shoreline of my consciousness. I was trying to methodically break them up by examining the sensations involved. After several minutes of this, the turbulent waters in my mind went still. It took me a minute to realize how I was able to do this. I was slowly relaxing a low-grade, persistent grimace from my face that I must have learned to ignore many years previously. This grimace that afflicts all of us is subtle and barely perceptible in a mirror. I stayed in bed for a full hour, trying to keep the contorted expression from repossessing me. As soon as my mind wandered, the tension around my eyes and nose would resurface, and my contentious thoughts would return.

We are constantly bracing our facial musculature. This causes repetitive strain, trigger points, muscle shortening, and the development of stiff, achy dormant muscles in the face. Though this has not been thoroughly investigated scientifically, I imagine that the pain messages sent to our brain's emotional centers from strained facial muscles are particularly tormenting. Spend some time contemplating this and attempt to bring awareness to the feeling of grimacing.

Facial Exercise #8.1: *Observe Your Facial Wincing and Grimacing*

Lie down in complete comfort and concentrate on the tone in your facial muscles. Try to relax your face completely and notice how the scowl returns on its own. Each time you notice it, allow your face to turn placid again. Notice how your expression is affected by your thoughts and vice versa. Focus on the areas that seem to tighten the most in response to negative thinking. As with the progressive relaxation exercise from Chapter 5 proceed from the top of your face to the bottom, taking notice of any tension in the brow and around the eyes, cheeks, nose, lips, and then the chin. The more time you spend doing this, the more aware of your scowl you will become and the better you will be at controlling it. After a few weeks of facial awareness, grimacing will feel uncomfortable and unnecessary, like reopening a wound.

You might be a little skeptical. You might not believe that the source of your mental hardship is your frown. Nevertheless, imagine a diminutive monkey. Imagine this monkey was horrendously traumatized as a baby and ever since has trod around with a wry wince on his little face. Just imagine how this would affect his inner world, his encounters with others, and their impressions of him. He would inevitably perceive things as more adverse than they are due to the powerful interrelationships between bodily expression, emotional condition, and social feedback. Monitor your face carefully the next time you are speaking on the phone. Are you unwittingly using expressions of pain and subordination?

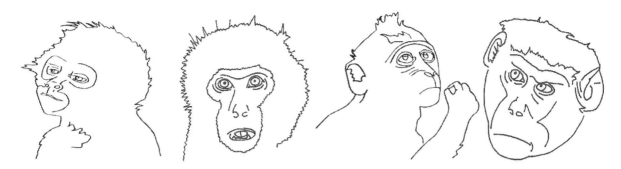

Illustration 8.2: A, B, C, & D. Monkeys wincing.

The "facial feedback hypothesis" holds that facial movement and emotional experience constantly interact with each other below the level of conscious awareness.[2] Charles Darwin was among the first to suggest this. He wrote: "The free expression by outward signs of an emotion intensifies it. On the other hand, the repression, as far as this is possible, of all outward signs softens our emotions. (...) Even the simulation of an emotion tends to arouse it in our minds."[3] Multiple concurring studies have supported this view.[4] For instance, people asked to hold a pencil between their teeth (forcing them to smile unconsciously) report better emotions during this episode than control groups that held the pencil between their lips. Botox injections have been shown to decrease negative affect by reducing tension in the eyes and forehead.[5] Individuals who have had Botox injections exhibit decreased activation of brain areas that process negative emotions such as the amygdala.[6] Frowns tie you to aversive mental states. This suggests to me that a frown burned in from years of repetitive strain anchors you to them.

Breaking My Nose Damaged My Facial Composure

A few days after discovering the wince on my face, I had a cup of coffee and bedded down in my closet for three hours in a search for the source of tension in my mind. I was in total darkness, wearing noise-reducing earmuffs, in corpse pose, with my breath metronome. I went into the experience believing that some repeating thought pattern maintained my restlessness. I waited for this pattern so that I could observe it and figure out how to interrupt it. However, the substrate of this pattern was not psychological as I expected. Instead, it was, again, facial.

I must have been ignoring the sensation for 15 years, but it was clear and unmistakable when it finally reemerged into consciousness. Lying in the dark, I felt a tingling sensation in the muscles surrounding my nose. I realized that these muscles were highly contracted. The muscles involved included the procerus, the nasalis, and the *levator labii*. For the first time, I could tell that even when I thought I was relaxing my face, these muscles were still in overdrive. All at once, I felt practically like I was hanging from the ceiling, suspended by chains with a meat hook piercing the bridge of my nose.

It took an hour of meditative thought and exploration even to notice. However, once I became aware of the sensations around my nose, they were impossible to ignore. Within a few more minutes, I realized that these sensations were the consequence of having my nose broken inside a McDonald's at age 17. The blow had shattered my nasal bone in several places and fractured my septum and maxilla. It split my nasalis muscle into two parts, and it must have also affected the nearby musculature and nerves. I realized that this injury had entrenched my wincing.

For the first several minutes, I had no voluntary control over these nasal muscles. I eventually "found" the muscles by trial and error over the course of an hour. Actually, I first had to learn to clench the muscles before I could learn to relax them. Each time I actively tightened or relaxed the muscle, it would tingle and feel numb due to the nerve damage. Of course, my experience was extreme, but we all hold our faces in a fixed expression of emotional trauma.

Having my nose broken damaged my nasal muscles and nerves and gave my face a dull, inattentive look that I tried to compensate for by keeping my nose and eyes tight. Especially in social situations, I attempted to make up for the hypotonia with hypertonia to bring some life and energy back to damaged facial expressions. This made my social interactions neurotic. The unremitting wincing compromised my composure and social standing, resulting in sympathetic upregulation.

Coincidentally, this type of damage also happened to my cat, Niko. The little guy approached a bird's nest, and a protective mother bird dove down and pecked him between the eyes, creating a deep gash down to the bone. Niko's face looked dim for at least a month because his brow and nasal muscles had been injured. He looked disfigured for a few weeks, but eventually his eyes returned to their former state. Luckily, unlike me, Niko did not try to compensate for the damage by bracing. This is why he didn't experience any lasting effects.

Much of our facial tension comes from attempts to compensate for appearing haggard, unattractive, or inattentive. Sometimes, we use our facial tension as an outward apology for our appearance. It often says: "Hey, believe me, I know that I don't look so great right now." Telling myself the following helped me: "I know that I'm 'ugly' at times. I'm not afraid or ashamed of appearing grotesque, and in that I retain dignity. There is no reason to apologize for my unsightliness with a grimace." How do you brace your face when you feel ugly? Identify it and stop it.

Submissive Mammals Have More Facial Tension

Of course, facial bracing also comes from our perceived place in the status hierarchy. More dominant people and primates don't just brace their bodies less; they also brace their faces less. By contrast, the least dominant primates have permanent appeasement expressions plastered on their faces.

Introverted and shy people tend to become tense in social situations. Their chakra-like modules develop tension quickly, and they exhibit various forms of the energy-wasting behavior discussed in Chapter 5. They quickly start to squint, sneer, and hold tension all over the body. Social pressures add up fast, and after just a few minutes of interacting with others, the introverted person starts to feel drained, exhausted, and like they want to escape. Many introverted people fake being extroverts until their trigger points have gone from latent to active, then they feel spent and try to get away from the crowd so that they can relax and refuel. I know this behavior pattern well. It was my social reality for years.

Chapter 5 discussed systematically removing extraneous bracing efforts from daily activities. Activity 2 from Chapter 5 asked you to notice your bracing habits while you brush your teeth. Now you must do the same thing for socializing. How do you tense your face unnecessarily when talking to others? How does it extend down your neck and into the rest of your body? If you systematically eliminated the bracing from all your chakra-like modules during conversation and socialization, you would become the most adept extrovert ever.

You could work a room full of people without ever tiring. Using the exercises in this book, along with self-awareness and diaphragmatic breathing, you could make *this* your social reality.

Facial Tension and Personality

There is a perpetual clenching, squirming, and cringing going on behind our faces that robs us of our facial poise. The muscles tighten when we are at the gym, when embarrassed, or when the phone rings. We should see this as gratuitous affectation. Micrometabolic studies of the anatomy of your facial musculature would reveal that some facial muscles hold more tension than others. Everyone has a different pattern of tension involving different parts of the face. These patterns are as distinct as fingerprints. Some people may have tighter lips and others tighter foreheads. Even the three auricular muscles surrounding the ears hold tremendous tension in some people but not in others.

Young infants' faces show high base rates of random combinatorial activity, enabling parents to shape a repertoire of conventional displays.[7] Infants more or less unconsciously assess the feedback that people give them and alter their facial patterns accordingly. Trial, error, and trauma program young children to brace their eyes, cheeks, and jaws in certain ways. This, in turn, distributes tension to different anatomical areas and results in a unique pattern of chronic muscular contractions.

I believe that these distinct patterns have strong associations with different features of personality. For instance, I am convinced that people who hold trigger points and shortening in the muscle between the eyebrows (the procerus, which causes the brow to furrow into a frown) are more keenly possessed by anger. These people wear a low-grade menacing glower that can contaminate their minds. Any form of facial tension tarnishes our thinking to some degree.

Have you ever noticed that a friend's face can change drastically if they go through a prolonged period of grieving? Again, this is due to tension, and without massage, it will never totally reverse even after the person's reason for mourning subsides. I believe that the blow to the face I experienced as a teenager made me an inveterate sneerer. Similarly, the pea-sized knot that I had one centimeter below each eye made me a perpetual squinter. Where do you hold your facial tension?

Facial Activity #8.1: *Warming the Face in a Hot Shower*

The next time you shower, turn the heat up (not enough to hurt) and place your face under the showerhead. Allow your face to heat up for a full 60 seconds. After a minute, turn the water off completely and focus all your attention on your face. This is the perfect time to try to contract and relax your facial muscles because heated muscles work differently on a cellular level in a way that you are not accustomed to. You will notice how the tension is amplified and that it contorts your face. You have about a minute to analyze the experience before it cools enough that the sensations end. This will pinpoint what you should be trying to relax.

You can also use a facial mask to get instant biofeedback about the tension in your face.

Facial Activity #8.2: *Using a Facial Mask*

Facial masks are usually made of clay, mud, creams, or paper cut-outs. They are marketed as products that improve the appearance of the face. People who use them claim they hydrate the skin and remove excess oils. They also happen to be a powerful form of biofeedback that should be taken advantage of by women and men alike. After the mask begins to dry, it sticks to your skin, making any movement that your face makes highly noticeable. You will sense resistance from the mask from any facial stress that you hold. Using a facial mask and trying to minimize any facial tension while employing a breath metronome can be an immensely powerful, healing experience. It will teach you to breathe easily while expressionless.

Master Expressionlessness and Own Your Face

The most important step in relaxing the facial muscles is to learn how to make a face with absolutely no expression. To do this, you must allow your face to go dead by turning your face off at the source. At first, this will look off-putting and very unattractive. Expressionlessness is the visage that many of us try to avoid making because it can convey exhaustion and disdain. Withholding your customary facial bracing can make you look evil, cruel, or irate. I was inspired to try expressionlessness after seeing my friend with schizophrenia on tranquilizers and sedatives. The physical ravages of stress and heavy facial bracing were more apparent than ever because they were contrasted with his complete facial limpness. He looked "burned out" and completely out of touch with reality. We all fear the social consequences of looking that way. But our face can never truly rest unless we do.

The strange truth is that this hideous non-expressive face is actually the most beautiful version of you waiting to emerge. The ghastly aspect is only due to the incongruity between the relaxation and the trigger points. Once the trigger points are gone, the relaxation will look natural. Practicing expressionlessness using the exercises in this chapter will get rid of the active trigger points, and using the facial massage techniques in the next chapter will get rid of the latent ones.

Working on your expressionless face will be difficult at first. You have to teach yourself to turn off each portion of your face individually. It will help to focus on relaxing the muscles around your eyes, relaxing your cheeks, and allowing your jaw to gape and go slack. Think of it as an extension of corpse pose—a corpse face. Focus especially hard on maintaining it when you are by yourself and before you go to sleep. You want to sleep every night as if every muscle in your face, jaw, and throat are paralyzed. How you look at yourself in the mirror is also decisive. When we look in the mirror, we usually don our customary "social mask." Instead, ensure that your expression is not tense and that you don't grimace, sneer, squint, or raise your eyebrows.

When you look at the ground, your face is capable of becoming very calm. It is easy to be calm when looking down because you are not challenging anyone when your gaze is below their eye line. However, when you look up again, this calmness disappears in fear of offending someone. In the next activity, don't let it disappear.

Facial Exercise #8.2: *Conserving the Calm*

Look down at the ground by lowering your eyes and head toward the floor. Next, try to look "completely relaxed." It may take a few seconds for you to configure this. Then, try to maintain this same face as you look up. It will be challenging at first, but keep working on it. This should be your default facial posture. You may want to try this a different way: Lie down, close your eyes, and make the face you usually make during sleep. Then sit up straight with your eyes open wide, wearing the exact same "sleeping" face. For this to work, you must completely let down your customary guard.

We walk around with tense faces because we are concerned that if someone sees our expressionless face, they will assume we are angry. But when actually affronted, we feel entitled to be able to drop all formalities. Many people are only expressionless when angry. I noticed this one day when I became outraged, and suddenly, all the social facial tension I had been trying to let go of disappeared on its own.

Facial Activity #8.3: *Feigned Anger*

Pretend a friend informs you that some other people said something derogatory about you that you do not deserve. For the first time in a long time, you don't care what anyone thinks about the way your face looks at the moment. You are mad. You are full of righteous indignation. Allow yourself to appear so cold, sullen, and uninviting that it makes bystanders shiver. You want a carnivorous look that says: "I'll eat you." Don't make an angry face, just allow your anger to drain all pleasantries from your face. Feel this, absorb it. Now strip the negativity from it, and make it your own.

The indignation and anger you used in the exercise above are negative emotions, so don't use them too often. Boredom is less extreme and almost equally as helpful. If you ever feel the need to regain your repose, pretend you are bored.

Facial Exercise #8.3: *Feigned Boredom and Tiredness*

Spend a minute looking exceptionally, invariably bored. Next, try looking overtired and sleepy, as if you have been up for five days straight. Then spend a minute looking both bored and tired, but with wide eyes. This instantly transforms boredom into a type of calm interest. Next, while maintaining the calm elements of this expression, move toward a face that exhibits compassion or, perhaps, an appreciation of beauty. Finally, work in a smile and turn the expression into one of happiness. Return to indignance, boredom, or sleepiness as needed to reset your face, capture the expressionlessness from it, and channel that into your calm, happy face.

After you spend a few months pairing expressionlessness with diaphragmatic breathing, you will have alleviated much of your facial tension. While working on expressionlessness, you may have to deaden your smile and some of the light in your eyes. However, after a short hiatus, when you reemploy many of your old expressions, you will find that they are unadulterated by the pained tension that previously accompanied them. It is akin to breaking an unhealthy system into its component parts and removing the unhealthy ones to build it back up anew.

Facial Activity #8.4: *Expressionless Running*
The next time you run, jog, or exercise aerobically, concentrate on maintaining an expressionless face. It takes practice to relax the face during physical exertion, but it will make it much easier to stay relaxed when you are not exerting yourself. While exercising, focus on keeping your eyes wide and otherwise allow your entire face to go limp. Think of this as your "game face."

At first, it will be uncomfortable to stay calm while keeping a straight face. You may notice that you easily break into a nervous smile, a spontaneous laugh, or a blush. This is because when you start out trying to look expressionless, your body will compensate by adding tension in other areas. Facial expressionlessness will cause you to unconsciously tighten your neck, constrict your vocal folds, or speed up your heart. Notice this. It is often a balancing act so that when you relax one aspect, another tightens up. This happens because your body keeps combinatorial records of the postures that are safe to have all at once. You have to create new, healthier records where all the optimal postures are being used together simultaneously.

We don't feel comfortable socially when our faces are at rest, so facial rest is usually paired with distressed breathing. Taking on an expressionless face generally causes us to breathe shallowly, squint, and look at the floor. At first, it will be hard to do it while maintaining eye contact. But this is all reversible. Practice expressionlessness with paced breathing, wide eyes, and looking upward, along with the fixed gaze exercise from Chapter 4. The more you can breathe diaphragmatically while maintaining a non-expressive face, the more natural and healthy-looking it will become.

Use Expressionlessness in Social Situations

We use facial tension to communicate things like: "Sorry for interrupting you," "I may be wrong about this," or "I hope you like me." Thus, the tension becomes an integral part of our social self-presentation. When you remove it, you must radically rethink your social deliveries. Your very personality will change. When allowing your face to be calm, you have to come to grips with the fact that some people won't like the way you look and will question why you have allowed your face to be so lax. At first, I took expressionlessness too far. I stopped smiling at service employees, I treated other people like robots, I stopped connecting with people emotionally, and I had the appearance of deadness. Avoid this. Use it alone, use it in public, but don't take it too far, especially in the company of friends.

Although you may try to present a completely calm face, you probably still look defensive. This is because you assume that other people will interpret your expressionless face as competitive, and you make a preemptive negative face. This keeps it from being truly calm. All you must do to ensure a socially sensitive expressionless face is to widen the eyes and breathe diaphragmatically. Trust that taking long, deep, slow breaths will wipe away the negative aspect. Welcome looking like a doe in the headlights, acting like you are imploring someone, or appearing naïve. Don't be afraid of playing the part of an inquisitive toddler with puppy-dog eyes. Sometimes, the most powerful countenance is that of a fun-loving child.

An authentically calm face is actually endearing. Chapter 4 discussed how subordinate apes avoid eye contact and how direct looking can be a threat signal. Expressionlessness can change this. When a chimpanzee gazes at another that is not using any apprehensive signals (such as pursing the lips, frowning, or glaring), it does not appraise it as threatening. Expressionlessness free from negativity will make your eye contact more inviting, opening social doors for you.

Allow me to offer some words and phrases that may help guide you in finding your new look. Ultimately, you want to imbue your expressionlessness with a cool, elegant, urbane sheen. I am not talking about being distant, detached, aloof, or unsociable. Rather, think about these words: dispassionate, collected, imperturbable, unflappable, unruffled, serene, free from agitation. You want a sedate disposition stemming from self-discipline. You want temperate self-assurance that suggests indifference. You want an easy casualness even under heavy provocation.

You might also try to incorporate a look of stoic decorum. I find the definition of the word "stoic" to be inspiring: "a person who can endure pain or hardship without showing their feelings or complaining." When I started focusing on appearing stoic, suddenly, I lost the tough guy shtick because stoicism is not a competition. It is an internal discipline. Make your appearance resigned to drama with no trace of protest. Create your own calm facial expression that you truly believe is warm and positive. If you believe it, it will come across as clear as day. The ultimate extension of this is to make your facial expressions and eye contact emanate a relaxed loving kindness.

Social Disapproval of Your Expressionlessness

I remember when I first started forcing myself to walk on the sidewalk with an expressionless face. I was genuinely worried that someone driving by would become infuriated with me because my face was too calm. I was concerned that someone would literally see my face through their windshield from 20 to 30 feet away, pull their car over, and try to fight me over it. I had to overcome delusions like this before I could let my face tranquilize. Do you? Start making this expressionless face alone in your room so that social concerns don't start to manipulate your facial muscles without your awareness. Next, try it walking around your home or neighborhood. Slowly work up to being in a store, a restaurant, or other public place while sporting your new calm demeanor.

When used during conversation, people will question the authenticity of your expressionlessness, thinking that it is artificial. One thing they will do is stare at you while you are looking at something else. Bullies do this often. They will leave their gaze on you, thinking that if they look long enough, you will revert to a more submissive facial posture. They anticipate you will look down, lower your chin, raise your eyebrows, or squint your eyes. Don't submit to their visual inspection of you. By under-reacting to them, you will show them that it is not a ruse.

Bullies will also show false tension in their faces or pretend to lose their composure to bait you into doing the same. Once you follow their cue, they instantly revive their composure to make you look stupid. Many people do this. Most of them do it half-consciously. It is a manipulative ploy.

Demonstrate a psychopathic indifference toward other people's interpretation of your calm facial posture. When they see your expressionlessness and respond with a deadpan look of their own, don't judge their version negatively, even if it looks smug. Instead, act as if you are glad to see that they are trying to be as calm as you are. It is not your responsibility to sink to the level of the other person's demeanor. Instead, make it your responsibility to pull them up to your level.

We are already accustomed to receiving disapproving nonverbal feedback from others when we let our faces relax. Many of us had parents who would become outraged if our face was too calm, thinking that we were being flippant, sarcastic, or obstinate. I have seen many children look afraid to appear calm around their parents. Kids learn by trial and error to make pained expressions to defer to parents and teachers. This kind of early environmental feedback makes us feel defensive whenever we sport a calm look.

Despite being a decent father in many respects, I have a friend who is often too dictatorial with his young daughter. To assuage his wrath, she squints, curls her top lip, pouts, and pleads with him in a high voice. Daily. Her brow wrinkles in a half-circle from furrowing and raising the eyebrows at the same time. There is no telling how many other internal chakras she strains to "buy mercy."

Other parents spoil their children, sparing their chakra-like modules but causing them to be undisciplined and disrespectful. A good proportion of beautiful and composed people were spoiled as children. Some parents can instill discipline and reverence without traumatizing, and this takes an incredible amount of parenting skill. This is the best kind of parent to be, but also the best kind of friend to be.

When people see you are stolidly composed, they will assume you are likely to mistreat them. When you are kind to them, they will be surprised because they assume the only thing holding most people back from acting abusive is their lack of composure. Usually, the person with more composure acts more abusive. This is normative and commonly accepted. As your composure improves, you may have to fight the urge to take advantage of others. You may have the impulse to be rude, scornful, or otherwise exploit your privileged position. If you are not a bad person (and, dear reader, I am sure you are not), as your composure improves, you will become less offensive. This is because you will find you have less to act defensive and oppositional about.

The Effect of Tension on the Body During Development

We have discussed how taking on facial and bodily muscle tension is an evolved strategy that communicates submissiveness to avoid being challenged and attacked. There are numerous similar strategies involving body plan changes even just in primates. For example, male orangutans are capable of exhibiting a pronounced developmental hiatus when they reach the females' size. What happens next varies. Some males go on to develop into full adult body size, along with other mature characteristics such as facial flaps. In contrast, other males will enter a prolonged period of physical juvenility (arrested growth and development) but otherwise full sexual maturity.

Environmental feedback determines whether male orangutans enter this prolonged juvenile phase or not. If their environment stifles their serotonin and testosterone levels, they are more likely to put off full maturity for a few years to avoid competing with the fully mature males.[8] Fascinatingly, suppression of maturity in orangutans is seen even in males that consider themselves subordinate to a human groundskeeper. If the keeper is replaced or the orangutan successfully challenges the keeper, the orangutan will quickly develop its cheek pads and full size.

Male gorillas do not mature into a full silverback for three to eight years after reaching sexual maturity. Some take much longer than others. This gives them more time to develop skills and relationships before they attempt to become an alpha male. This phenomenon in orangutans, gorillas, and many other animals is called sexual bimaturism.[9] It is evident in humans as well. Males hit puberty two years later than girls. This is widely thought to delay the age in which men are thrust into stressful and potentially dangerous competition with older, more dominant, sexually active males.

A similar process may be going on with our bodies and faces. The combination of distress and repetitive strain may program muscles all over the body to become weak (hypotrophic) to display our place in the pecking order. In other words, the tension keeps us from being as muscular and healthy as we could be. I previously thought that most of the variability in beauty and robust body type was explained by genes. I thought alpha animals attained their status by a stroke of genetic luck. Now, I am convinced that much of it comes from environmental feedback and developmental plasticity. Bad social environments influence children to strain their faces while good ones encourage children to relax them. Tension alters our physiognomy. Over months and years, some people look depleted and sickly while others look handsome and brawny. Most of us passively allow the environment to determine how this plays out. The Program Peace exercises can help you actively optimize it.

Remember from Chapter 5 that muscles that do not rest cannot heal. Relaxed muscles are capable of full recovery and thus are more responsive to exercise. Now that your facial muscles are capable of resting fully, they are capable of becoming more muscular.

Facial Exercises That Will Make a Relaxed Face Robust

Use the exercises in this section to contract your facial muscles beyond their normal range and out of partial contraction. To do this, flex them as hard as you can while breathing diaphragmatically. Some of the muscles are involved in superiority displays, others in inferiority displays, but I recommend pairing them all with proper breathing to unlink them from the sympathetic stress system. This will make the superiority displays indubitable and the inferiority displays playful rather than subordinating.

Diaphragmatic generalization will reduce the activation threshold for these muscles, encouraging them to contract spontaneously, effortlessly, and more frequently. This will free up previously frozen contractions and help you become more expressive. Exercising these muscles to the point of fatigue and then letting them rest completely will also help them grow stronger and more prominent.

Facial Exercise #8.4: *Freeing Up the Face*
Spend one minute contracting each of the following ten sets of muscles while performing paced breathing with a breath metronome. Hold a firm contraction until the muscles tremble, burn, or reach fatigue. After they do, focus on letting them go completely limp. As

the muscles rest, resist the tendency to resume bracing. After performing these ten exercises individually, feel free to start combining them.

1) Flare your nostrils as wide as you can while keeping the rest of your face relaxed. Many of us are afraid to flare our nostrils because it is a dominance signal. It is often used in other primates as a threat signal. Many submissive people's nostrils are completely inactive. Mine certainly were. People with very healthy nostril tone will unconsciously flare and constrict their nostrils unconsciously as they speak. Exercising them took me from having nearly zero conscious control of them to having full rhythmic control. Building subtle nostril dilation into your facial posture will lend your face more self-ownership. Because these muscles extend up into your nose, you may also find that it makes nasal breathing easier.

2) Open your jaw widely and hold it there. You might slide it from left to right or move it in a circular motion. This activates the platysma of the neck and many muscles throughout the jaw. Next, bring your jaw as far forward (underbite) and as far back (overbite) as you can and perform a chewing motion from these positions. The best default setting for your jaw is about one millimeter to one centimeter open and wholly relaxed with the lips closed.

3) Squint heavily. I have recommended not subjecting the orbicularis oculi to strain, but coactivating their firm contraction with diaphragmatic breathing will detraumatize them and help free them from passive partial contraction. So, exercise them by clamping them shut as hard as you can.

4) Raise the eyebrows as high as they will go. Hold until the frontalis muscle starts to fatigue. Repeat.

5) Furrow your eyebrows as if you were concerned or angry. Slowly alternate between letting them relax and forcing them to furrow as much as they can. Bring the procerus and corrugator *supercilii* to full fatigue. The ability to be calm while frowning fully will give your face authority.

6) Raise the chin and bottom lip by contracting the *mentalis*. This is a very powerful and dominant expression. Use it in a friendly way. It is a genteel but reserved way to greet someone. Combined with a nod, it is a strong way to provide an affirmation.

7) Pull down the sides of the mouth by contracting the depressor labii. These muscles are responsible for the down-turning of the corners of the mouth when humans make the "sad face." It constitutes what is known as the "crying face" in apes. Use this expression to play concerned or apologetic.

8) Sneer heavily. Use the levator labii superioris to raise the upper lip in an aggressive sneer. Do this with the mouth both closed and wide open. Imagine you are a ferocious monstrosity about to take a tremendous bite out of something. Making this expression will likely cause you to breathe very shallowly. Pairing it with diaphragmatic breathing will unbar this portion of the face, making you appear less fearful.

9) Crinkle the nose heavily. Crinkling the nose can be a very playful expression that demonstrates how little tension you hold in your face. Most people avoid it because whenever the muscles contract, latent trigger points here become active. Exercising it will first subdue and then purge the trigger points.

10) Contract the lips heavily. People and apes purse their lips in anger. Many of us have atrophied lip muscles because we are afraid of using this expression. If you want to improve the appearance and increase the size of your lips, exercising them will provide much more natural-looking results than cosmetic injections (injections damage muscle tissue, leading to bracing patterns that will eventually cause the lips to develop asymmetric muscle fiber contractions and become grotesque). Attractive lips are toned, not inflated. To tone yours, purse/pucker your lips hard. It can help to do this against an object such as your knuckle, the corner of your cell phone, or your wallet. Press your lips firmly into the object while extending the lips as far as they can go until they fatigue.

Aside from using these static contractions, repeated, rhythmic contraction provides other benefits. Perform each of the ten contractions above, but instead of holding a prolonged contraction for a minute, contract and release the muscle rapidly 100 times. Alternate between the firmest contraction you can muster and complete relaxation. Do this at a rate of one to three contractions per second with the goal of bringing the muscle to fatigue. This not only builds strength and optimal tone but also coordination, which can translate into interpersonal communicative skills.

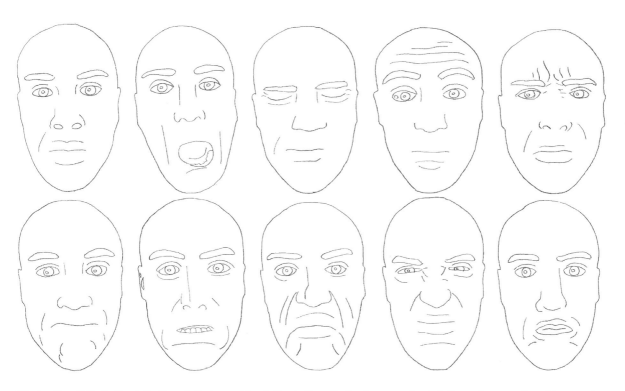

Illustration 8.3: *A. Nostrils flared; B. Jaw wide; C. Squinting; D. Eyebrows raised; E. Brow furrowed and lowered; F. Chin raised; G. Corners of mouth lowered; H. Sneering; I. Nose crinkled; J. Lips puckered.*

Chewing activates more muscle than any of the facial expressions. The muscles of mastication (including the masseter, pterygoid, and temporalis) are large and highly susceptible to strain. I had a medical doctor diagnose me with temporomandibular joint dysfunction. He said that the range of motion in my jaw was heavily encumbered and that, as a whole, my jaw was badly "closed down." Exercise 8.5 below, along with the jaw massage described in the next chapter, healed this. It ended the pain and cracking. It melted the knots away. And it resulted in the same doctor rescinding the diagnosis.

Facial Exercise #8.5: *Unstifling the Jaw*

Place a folded rag or paper towel in your mouth so that it keeps your teeth from touching when you bite down. Clench your teeth hard during your exhalations and relax the jaw during inhalations. After you carefully warm your jaw up in this way, you should be able to clench harder and harder over several days until you feel safe clenching as hard as you can. This will salvage portions of the masseter that were previously stuck in painful partial contraction and potentially contributing to headaches. Massage the masseter afterward. Combining this practice with gum chewing will cause the back of the jaw to become more muscular and toned. If you want a more strenuous jaw workout, you can cut a one-inch by two-inch strip from a cotton rag and chew it like gum. This may be painful at first, but it will feel great within a week and will improve circulation to your gums and the roots of your teeth.

Conclusion

My mother, an art historian, has cataloged and captioned many photographs of early California pioneers. She spent considerable time analyzing portraits of these hard-working, rugged people who survived on a dangerous frontier. She said many of the individuals photographed reminded her of wolves. She explained to me that they appeared wild and undomesticated. Their faces seemed less encumbered by a social mask and were emblematic of a cunning, phlegmatic, dauntless animal intent on survival. Don't wear the face of a tame, housebroken pup. Wear that of an unbroken wolf.

"There is only one inborn error, and that is the notion that we exist in order to be happy... So long as we persist in this inborn error...the world will seem to us full of contradictions. For at every step, in great things and small, we are bound to experience that the world and life are certainly not arranged for the purpose of being happy. That's why the faces of almost all elderly people are deeply etched with such disappointment." — Arthur Schopenhauer (1788-1860)

The fate described by the dismal quote above is escapable. But we have to take the reins. It is our responsibility, and not the world's, to create happiness in our lives. A great first step is to keep the etching of disappointment from happening. It is said that by old age, you manifest the face you deserve. But even some toddlers have purple creases under their eyes (usually because they are modeling their parents' expressions). The muscular contortions that lead to the disfigurement of our faces and bodies start in infancy. However, it is never too late to intervene.

Learning to embrace expressionlessness and practicing facial exercises will help keep your facial muscles from taking on additional strain as you age. However, they will not totally release your facial bracing patterns. Only soft tissue massage in the form of compression or percussion can do this. The next chapter will show you how to remove the tension from your facial muscles, making even the most expressionless face in the world look absolutely natural.

Chapter 8: **Bullet Points**

- We brace the muscles in our face throughout the day, resulting in continual wincing, grimacing, and frowning.
- Facial bracing causes the muscles to become stuck in partial contraction and develop trigger points and adaptive muscle shortening.
- The repetitive strain of facial muscle is disempowering because it anchors you to negative thoughts and emotions.
- The activation of latent trigger points in the face destroys our composure and contributes to social fatigue and introversion.
- Practicing a resting face, corpse face, or expressionlessness will stop the accumulation of strain and make your face agile and "light on its feet."
- To make expressionlessness effortless and ensure that it does not offend people, it must be combined with diaphragmatic breathing, widening of the eyes, fixed gaze practices, and positive intentions.
- Expressionlessness will reduce strain and keep latent trigger points from becoming active. However, removing the trigger points requires massage and hard contraction of the muscles involved.
- Exercising the facial muscles by contracting them beyond their normal range until they reach fatigue, and combining this with diaphragmatic breathing, will strengthen and revive them.

Chapter 8: **Endnotes**

1.   Brown, F. D., Prendergast, A., & Swalla, B. J. (2008). Man is but a worm: Chordate origins. *Genesis*, *46*(11), 605–613.

2.   Buck, R. (1980). Nonverbal behavior and the theory of emotion: The facial feedback hypothesis. *Journal of Personality and Social Psychology*, *38*(5), 813.

3.   Darwin, C. R. (1872). *The expression of the emotions in man and animals*. John Murray.

4.   Lewis, M. B. (2012). Exploring the positive and negative implications of facial feedback. *Emotion*, *12*(4), 852–859.

5.   Lewis, M. B., Bowler, P. J. (2009). Botulinum toxin cosmetic therapy correlates with a more positive mood. *Journal of Cosmetic Dermatology*, *8*(1), 24–26.

6.   Hennenlotter, A., Dresel, C., Castrop, F., Ceballos Baumann, A. O., Wohlschlager, A. M., & Haslinger, B. (2008). The link between facial feedback and neural activity within central circuitries of emotion—New insights from botulinum toxin-induced denervation of frown muscles. *Cerebral Cortex*, *19*(3), 537–542.

7.   Charlesworth, W. R., & Kreutzer, M. A. (2006). Facial expressions of infants and children. In P. Ekman (Ed.), *Darwin and facial expression: A century of research in review* (pp. 91–168). Malor Books.

8.   van Schaik, C., & MacKinnon, J. (2001). Orangutans. In D. MacDonald (Ed.), *The encyclopedia of mammals* (2nd ed.). Oxford University Press.

9.   de Waal, F. (2006). *Our inner ape: A leading primatologist explains why we are who we are*. Riverhead Books.

Chapter 9: **Massage Away Facial Tension**

Why Use Facial Massage?

The tension in our faces drives the stress response, influencing us to feel anxious and breathe shallowly. The damage it does to the muscles makes our faces appear languid, overwrought, and weak. Deep tissue massage is the only way to counteract this. Compression and percussion will reinvigorate the muscle, increase blood supply, reverse muscle shortening, remove trigger points, decrease inflammation, and permit the muscle to grow.

The results can be dramatic because the long-term strain on our muscles is the leading cause of facial aging and loss of facial composure. These two issues are probably among the biggest sources of human insecurity. Both are not only preventable but reversible. If you want your face to look healthy and feel amazing, invest some time and effort in the facial massage regimen described here.

If you press your knuckles into your brow, your cheeks, or your jaw with between 5 and 15 pounds of pressure, you will likely feel an acute aching sensation. This pain may be so intense that it makes your breathing shallow and the pit of your stomach tight. However, if you spend 10 minutes a day compressing your facial muscles while breathing diaphragmatically, the pain will be gone within three months. The sagging, puffiness, and deposits of fat will go with it. You will be washing your face, and it will feel completely different. It will feel lean, smooth, and finely contoured. You will glance at yourself in a mirror or window and won't recognize the leaner, angular, chiseled face looking back at you. You will look healthier, and that will help you feel healthier, too. Most importantly, your baseline level of stress will be significantly reduced.

Facial massage and acupressure are old arts. However, existing methods are not scientifically informed and intend to pacify the face temporarily rather than to relieve trigger points permanently. The method presented here targets the most pernicious myofascial restrictions in the face and guides you in systematically eliminating them. Once you work through these exercises, you will be able to relax facial muscles that you could not relax before, and you will have more precise control over your face's movements. Eventually, you will be tension-free and able to comfortably and gracefully transition between expressionlessness and your full, healthy range of expressions.

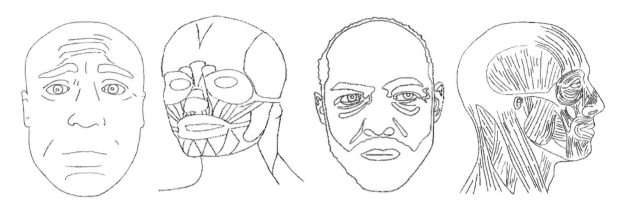

Illustration 9.1: Facial expressions.

Social Fatigue and Resting Face

When our face is continually tense, the people around us recognize it as a clear sign of self-perceived inferiority. My face was so tense that, whether someone was making a joke at my expense or complimenting me, I could not help but respond in a bashful, embarrassed way. A sheepish grimace would betray me constantly by showing others that it was easy to make me uncomfortable. By undermining my ability to stay composed and be assertive, it made me a target for mistreatment by unkind or unthinking people. Facial massage obliterates this submissiveness. If you rarely look uncomfortable, people learn quickly that they are the ones that will look bad if they try to bully you. Moreover, you will be able to keep a fantastic poker face. The person who can keep a straighter face usually controls the situation. These days I only smile when I want to, and I can even tell the punchline to a joke with a straight face. Even after a long day of gregariousness, I can easily assume a calm, expressionless demeanor.

Social fatigue occurs when prolonged social encounters become stressful, overwhelming, and cause a person to seek rest from social interaction. When you are experiencing social fatigue, people can usually see it in your face. It derives from the fatigue of facial muscles. When these muscles tire, or when their latent trigger points become active, it becomes depleting. They are draining to use, and this diminishes our ability to express and be friendly. Studies show that the amount a person smiles and makes socially engaging facial expressions are two of the best predictors of likeability. Using your face makes people want to be around you. But if your facial muscles are in perpetual fatigue, you can't emote, and you will ultimately feel dejected.

"Bitchy resting face" (or resting bitch face) is a popular term for a facial expression (or lack of expression) that unintentionally appears angry or contemptuous. When we allow our face to relax more than usual, the tense muscles that we cannot relax become readily apparent and belie our attempt to appear calm. Before I started a facial massage regimen, no one ever saw my bitchy resting face because I never allowed my face to rest, even when alone. I was so self-aware of how bad my face looked at rest that I always sported a compensatory grimace. Our goal should be to massage the face until a complete resting face is no longer bitchy. We want to shoot for a wide-eyed, peaceful resting face.

Microexpressions

All of us are constantly making microexpressions with our facial muscles. A microexpression is an involuntary expression that is evoked by emotion. They are very brief and last between 1/25th and 1/15th of a second. It is thought to be very difficult, if not impossible, to completely suppress microexpression reactions.[1] These reflexes largely dictate our genuine emotional reactions to what happens around us. Sometimes they turn out to be premature or socially unacceptable, and in these cases, we inhibit them and replace them with something else. If you find yourself compulsively thinking negative thoughts during the day, it is very likely that many of the automatic microexpressions you make are negative.

Most mammals that are not primates only wince when they experience physical pain. Primates take the innate facial reflex of wincing to physical pain and generalize it to social pain. Humans take it another step further. We wince when someone chastises us, but many of us learn to over-generalize our facial analogies, wincing even when someone congratulates us. Pained, maladaptive microexpressive habits like this are perpetuated by facial strain. Massaging the muscles using the activities below will remove the frown, the cry face, the squint, the blush, and the sneer from the involuntary microexpressions that flicker across your face.

Facial Massage Techniques and Targets

Releasing tension from your facial muscles requires the three techniques described in Chapter 6: percussion, compression, and vibration. We'll start with a simple percussion exercise, following the protocol laid out in that chapter. Use a knuckle, knuckle tool (like the Jack Knobber or Index Knobber), a coat hook, baseball, softball, or Bonger to strike the dormant, tender muscles repeatedly.

Facial Massage Exercise #9.1: *Soft Facial Percussion*
Use a knuckle or appropriate tool to gently strike all the major surfaces of your face. Find a rapid, easy-to-maintain rhythm as you go, striking your muscles 2-4 times per second. The force of each blow should be roughly what you use when clapping your hands softly. The blows that result in deep, muscular aches will succeed in reducing excessive tone as long as you are breathing deeply. Focus on your brow and cheeks, but percuss everywhere, including every inch of your nose, orbits, lips, chin, and jawline. Spend more time on areas that hurt most. The best time for this exercise is in the hours before bed so that your face can rest overnight.

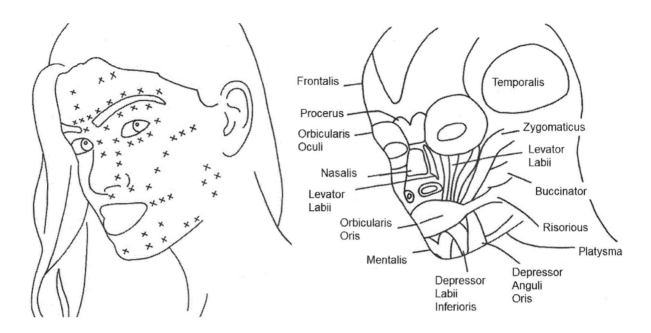

Illustration 9.2: A. Woman with major facial massage target areas marked with an "x";
B. Underlying facial anatomy

The area you massaged may feel slightly sore to the touch the next day. Even so, it should never hurt when not being touched. No part of your face should ever become chafed, swollen, bruised, or discolored; those are all signs that you are striking too hard or for too long and need to scale back. Don't skip a day just because the area is sore. Gently working through the soreness day after day will keep the hypertonia from resurfacing.

There are also a few important notes about advisability.

1) Do not massage your eyeballs, only the orbits around them.
2) If you have injected filler, or any cosmetic substances into your skin, compression may not be safe.
3) There are a wide variety of dermatological conditions that contraindicate massage, so if you have any reason to worry about your skin's sensitivity, integrity, or safety, please consult your doctor prior to attempting self-massage.

I have compressed tissues on nearly every corner of my face and have not experienced any injury whatsoever.

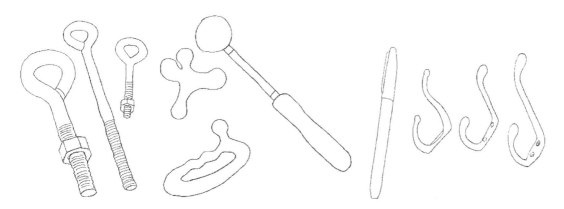

Illustration 9.3: A. These are the best tools to use on the face. Do not use the smallest coat hook (third from the right). The tip is too small and thus works too well. It will reduce muscle tone so much that it will cause healthy muscle to atrophy. Pictured from left to right: three sizes of eyebolts (1″ x 8″; .75″ x 12″; .5″ x 6″), Jacknobber Index Knobber, Bonger. The smooth end of a Sharpie marker, or coat hooks with a rounded tip can also be excellent tools.

Much of the remainder of this chapter describes how to use compression on every muscle of the face. After just six days of performing these exercises for ten minutes per day, for a total of an hour, you should attain noticeable results. The extent of the results will depend on your breathing. If you breathe five breaths per minute while performing the exercises, the results will be dramatic. If you normally breathe more than 15 breaths per minute, you may find that compressing the facial muscles is painful and that hard compression injures rather than releases them. If this is the case, you should return to Chapter 3 and spend more time rehabilitating your breathing before continuing with this regimen.

There are many layers to the tension, and it may take months or years to achieve optimal results. Your progress should be consistent and readily apparent, however, and you should expect the gains you experience to be long-lasting. Most of the exercises can be performed from a standing or seated position. The ones that use a tool (especially the eyebolt) are best performed by placing the base of the tool on the ground or a flat surface and pressing the area of the face to be compressed into the top of the tool using the weight of the head. The diagrams below illustrate how this can be done with an eyebolt seated, kneeling, or lying down.

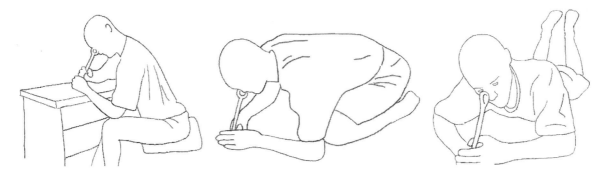

Illustration 9.4: A, B, & C. Comfortable positions for facial compression. Ensure that the tool does not slip and bump into your delicate eyeball.

For each of the facial massage exercises below, you will be using a knuckle, finger, or tool to search for and press gently against the sorest muscles. Please see the compression protocol from Chapter 6. Move slowly across the area, ensure that each press overlaps with the last. Hold each press for two to ten seconds. Once you have massaged the whole area, start over. As you practice, maintain paced breathing

Around the Eyes: Orbicularis Oculi

Most people have bags under their eyes, although the bags can vary widely in shape, size, and color. Some people have dark circles. Others have a crease that runs from the inside corner of the eye diagonally down and away from the nose. It is often darker in color and sometimes black and blue. These are all due to tension in the lower portion of the orbicularis oculi muscle caused by perpetual squinting. This tension can be the cause of frequent crying. Before compressing this area, I would often feel on the verge of crying. Since massaging them, I rarely feel tearful. You should also find that you squint much less in sunlight.

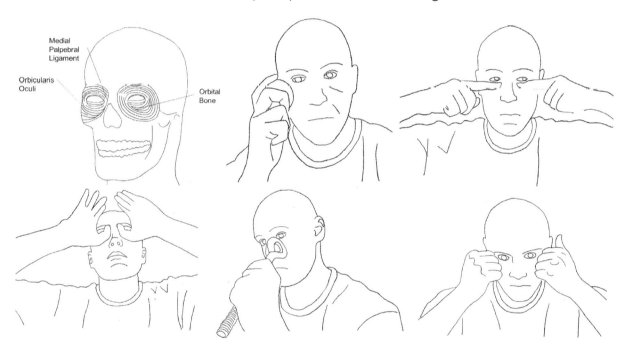

Illustration 9.5: Orbicularis oculi massage.

Facial Massage Exercise #9.2: *Outer Orbicularis Oculi*

Firmly massage your upper cheeks with a tool or knuckle. Provide moderate to hard pressure using circular strokes. Use between five and ten pounds of pressure all over the area surrounding the eye. It is okay if the affected muscles are slightly sore the next day. You might start with a squash ball until next-day soreness stops and then switch to harder implements like a baseball, knuckle, or other tool.

Facial Massage Exercise #9.3: *Inner Orbicularis Oculi*

Place the tips of your index fingers along the edge of your eyes' orbits, just under the eye (the orbit is the bony ridge that encircles the eyes). You should be able to feel hard strings of muscle. At first, I thought that these were veins, and I assumed that I should not compress them. They are merely tense muscles, and they will soften with compression. Push down on them with your fingertips and squeeze them against the orbital bone. Then, place the second knuckle of each index finger just to the side of these cords. Apply firm pressure and move slowly over them, pinning them against the orbit as you go. Finally, use your fingers, knuckles, and an eyebolt to compress the entire orbit. The portion of the orbicularis oculi nearest the nose contains the medial palpebral ligament around which there is a lot of tension. Focus on this area and the areas directly below and above it.

Facial Massage Exercise #9.4: *Lateral Orbicularis Oculi*

Compress the bony ridges of the outside (lateral) corners of your eyes. Tension here leads to the wrinkles known as crow's feet, also called periorbital lines. Your crow's feet will diminish in size and depth as the muscle becomes supple and circulation improves. Eventually, they may disappear completely. Compressing these muscles will also reduce squinting when you smile. Start by straddling the lateral orbital bone with two of your knuckles and press in to it as you stroke up and down. You may notice small painful bundles of muscle here; compress them a little more each day, and they will gradually fade away.

Facial Massage Exercise #9.5: *Eyelids*

Your eyelids contain tiny muscles that, when overly tense, can cause, swelling, itching or turn the rims of the lids bright red. To reduce excessive tone in these tiny muscles, squeeze them gently to stop them from contracting. To do so, wash your hands and then use your thumb and forefinger to pinch the outside of your eyelids. Pinch the upper lids all over from left to right especially the area near the lashes. Repeat with the lower lids. You should notice that your lids become lighter in color, less itchy, and less puffy within a week.

The Brow: Frontalis, Procerus, and Corrugator Supercilli

Most of us have very tense muscles in our foreheads and eyebrows. They become tense because we raise our eyebrows (frontalis muscle) when trying to make friends and furrow our brows (using the procerus and corrugator supercilli muscles) when we get angry. You might remember from Chapter 4 that the former are used by an animal being chased, and the latter are used by an animal chasing. Over time, these expressions can become plastered on our faces, making the brow painful by our mid-twenties.

Brow muscles can be difficult to work on. It took me three months of massaging for about 5 minutes per day before the pain faded fully. But it was worth it because it also got rid of sizeable knots and scar tissue. Previously, those knots had kept my brow in a permanently raised state, making them tremble when I was upset or nervous. Releasing your brow muscles reverses this. It will also reverse the muscle shortening letting your eyebrows descend to take on a fearless look. Your eyebrows will keep still when you talk, and only raise when you want them to.

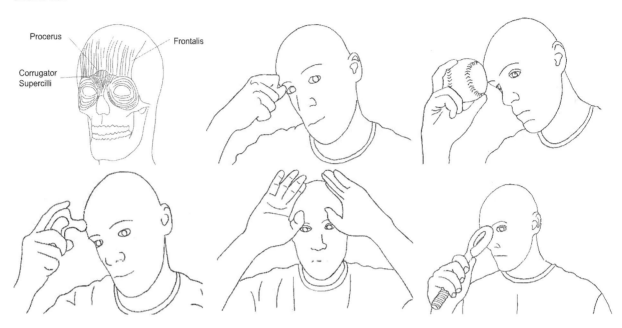

Illustration 9.6: Brow massage.

Facial Massage Exercise #9.6: *Frontalis*

Take the first knuckle of your thumb or forefinger and press it into the skin of your forehead. Be sure to cover the areas above, below, and underneath each eyebrow. You will likely find bundles of tight muscle fibers that are excruciating to compress. Begin gently and increase pressure slowly until you get the intended day-after ache. You can give your knuckle a break by pressing the full weight of your head onto a baseball, tabletop, or tool, moving the pressure all around your forehead and concentrating on areas that hurt the most.

Facial Massage Exercise #9.7: *Procerus and Corrugator Supercilli*

Press the knuckles of the thumb or an eyebolt directly between your eyebrows to compress the procerus, the corrugator supercilli, and other soft tissues in the area. I believe tension in the procerus forces us to contend with anger and that relieving this muscle is emotionally purgative. As mentioned in Chapter 6, scientists regard the corrugator supercilli as the principal muscle used in the expression of suffering. Why wouldn't we all compress these muscles until they are painless?

The Cheeks: Zygomaticus Major and Minor, Levator Anguli Oris, Levator Labii

The zygomas are the bone protrusions on either side of the human face commonly referred to as cheekbones. They are the meeting point for multiple muscles that overlap to create an intersection of tension. That tension causes inflammation and swelling. Compressing the muscles will reduce that swelling, uncovering your cheekbones and making them more visible and pronounced. It will also end chronic blushing and cheek tightness. I used to blush socially and every time I exercised. I never blush anymore.

Most smiling is nervous smiling. In fact, when we laugh or smile socially, our hearts are often beating quickly, and our breath is shallow and tense. As you know, any muscles that are routinely coactivated with distressed breathing will hold excess tension. In the case of the zygomatic muscles, that strain causes them to pull on tendons where they attach to the cheekbones, causing deep pain. The tendons become so strained that the area accumulates scar tissue and undergoes a host of degenerative cellular processes. This made my smile rotten and mangled. This was the sorest place on my entire face. Pressing a baseball into it with five pounds of pressure hurt so badly that it made me want to cry. There were tiny protuberances and what felt like sand in the area. Now it is smooth, and all the pain is gone completely.

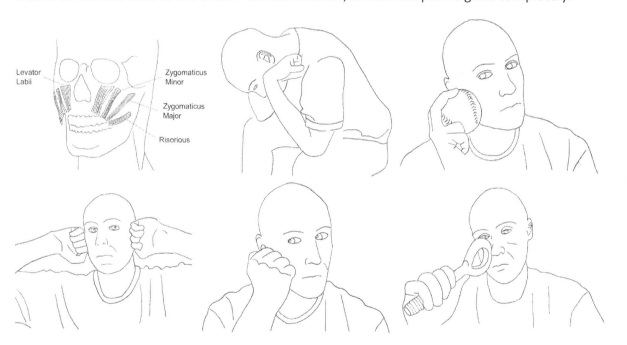

Illustration 9.7: Cheek massage.

Facial Massage Exercise #9.8: *Zygomatic Muscles*

Compress the area all around the cheekbones: above them, below them, and to the sides. You can use either a baseball, your knuckles, or the backs of your wrists. Press especially deeply into the lower, outside portion of your cheekbones where the zygomaticus (minor and major) muscles are anchored. You should be able to feel this painful point of insertion in the cheek about two inches outside (laterally) and below the corner of the eye. After a few months of compressing this, your smile will be bigger, unfaltering, and will feel full-bodied.

Facial Massage Exercise #9.9: *Zygomatic Arch*

To truly free up your eyes and your cheeks, you need to massage and compress the muscles all the way back along your cheekbones to your ears. This whole ridge (the zygomatic arch) may be painful and covered in palpably tense muscle fibers. Put this ridge between the second knuckles or your middle and ring fingers and stroke it back and forth. You should be able to ease the tension in just a few days. Additionally, try placing the ridge on a hard surface like a book and press it down at different angles. Massaging the ridge from your cheek to your ear will allow your smile to extend outward toward the ear instead of being restricted to the area around your nose.

The Nose: Levator Labii Superioris

In most mammals, the sneer occurs more conspicuously on one side of the mouth, usually the left. You may have observed this in a snarling dog. Accordingly, I had a much larger knot in my left levator labii superioris than in my right. It was probably the largest knot in my face. It was about the size of three sticks of chewed gum. Releasing this muscle was empowering for me. After releasing it, I realized that I used to walk around with a permanent sneer on my face. The sneer would grow as I became uncomfortable, making me look sour. It was stuck in partial contraction with very little range of motion. Now that the muscles are at rest, I feel less defensive and less susceptible to provocation.

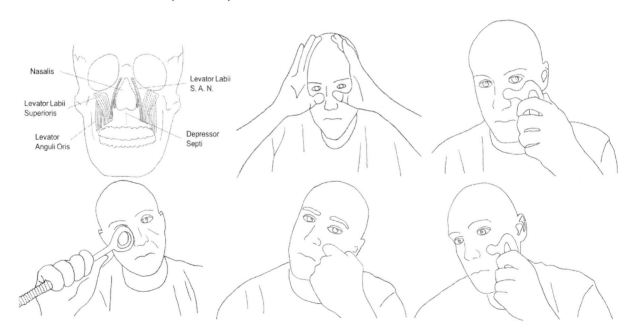

Illustration 9.8: Sneer massage.

Facial Massage Exercise #9.10: *Levator Labii*

Using a tool or the second knuckle of your forefinger, press very firmly into the space between your nose and your cheek (the upper portion of the maxilla bone). This will target the levator labii which raises the upper lip. You may be able to feel tiny pops and cracks. Very light popping is normal and indicates that the cellular adhesions holding the muscle in partial contraction are breaking down. Work your way from the top of your nose down to the corner of your mouth along your marionette lines. Use eyebolts of different sizes, pressing them into this space between your nose and cheek bone.

Releasing the muscles on the sides of your nose will make the area appear deeper and leaner, giving you a friendlier, calmer look and allowing you to smile without sneering. I felt like blood-sucking leeches had been removed from the sides of my nose. In fact, I used to wake up every morning with a dull ache on the sides of my nose. Never again.

Facial Massage Exercise #9.11: *Nasalis*

Use your knuckles to compress the bridge and the sides of your nose including the nasalis muscle, and the "levator labii S.A.N." This will provide relief to the muscles that crinkle the nose. The easiest way to do this is to lie face down on a bed, with your chest supported by pillows. Place the base of an index knobber or eyebolt on the bed and rest your head on top of the tool, with your sneering muscles as the point of contact. Move the end of the tool gently around the area, compressing deeply. The meat of the muscle lies in the bed created by the top of the nasolabial folds (marionette lines) near the nostrils. Search for and target a large knot you may find in the middle of this area.

Most people sneer heavily when they smile, and over time, this causes the nostrils to shorten and become upturned. It looks ugly. Compressing the nostrils (the alar portion of the nasalis, the dilator naris and the compressor naris) will reverse this. Also, compress the muscle under the nose (the depressor septi) with a knuckle or tool. In addition, you might put a towel down on the floor and press your nose into it, resting the weight of your head on it. Point the tip of the nose downwards, and rock back and forth to massage and compress tissues throughout the nose.

We all have a low-grade perpetual sneer burned into our facial musculature. All our lips are slightly curled due to this tension. Most people retain the coordination to relax the muscles involved but choose not to because it makes them feel uglier. I remember feeling like some kind of repulsive zombie-pig when I relaxed mine. By tensing the area, we apologize for and cover up the appearance of strained muscle. But over time, this only makes it worse. It is likely that the only time you relax these muscles is when you are exceedingly angry. Work on resting the sneer throughout the day and disregard any reservations you might have about how you look while doing this. Compressing the levator labii will remove the knots from your sneer and make it look natural to stop sneering.

People who raise dogs for dogfighting abuse them to get them to sneer. They punch, pinch, or cut the dog repeatedly until it learns to bare its teeth immediately upon provocation. They want the dog to live in a mental world where baring its teeth is the first reaction to any form of stress. This makes the dog mean. When a problem dog learns to bare its teeth at people, nipping and then biting soon follow. By relaxing and compressing your sneering muscles, you deprogram this reaction. From experience, I have come to believe that once the muscles that lift the upper lip are no longer tense, the brain's circuits for frustration and aggression are keyed down.

The Mouth and Lips: Orbicularis Oris

The right and left corners of the mouth are the point of attachment for muscles throughout the face. Muscles extending from the nose, cheeks, jaw and chin all anchor into these two corners. The bracing of our mouths and lips (orbicularis oris) is almost imperceptible. It is a subtle pouting that, over years, makes your lips thinner and your mouth appear shriveled. As you age, continuous pursing of the lips causes vertical wrinkles. Massage halts this.

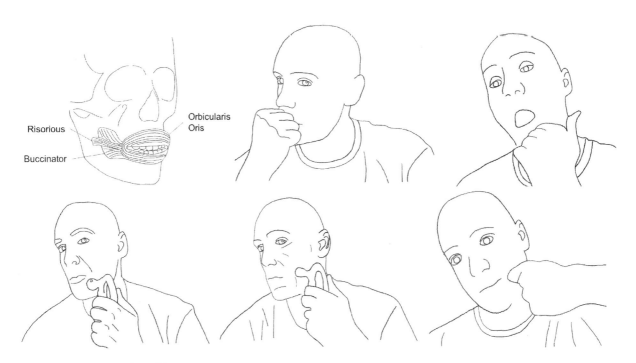

Illustration 9.9: Mouth and lip massage.

Facial Massage Compression Exercise #9.12: *Orbicularis Oris*

Press your knuckles firmly into your lips. Focus on the lips themselves and the areas above and below them. Especially focus on the corners of your mouth. You can also squeeze these areas between your thumb and forefinger, placing one on the face and the other inside the mouth. Compression and percussion here will make your lips healthier looking. Compression of the skin all around the lip area will give it a rejuvenated shape.

Facial Massage Exercise #9.13: *Risorius and Buccinator*

The risorius and buccinator are two other muscles involved in smiling. They pull the corners of the lips outward horizontally. Note the anatomical location of these muscles and compress and percuss them to make your face leaner and more muscular. Freeing these muscles up and enabling them to contract fully could help you develop prominent dimples and smile lines.

The Jaw: Masseter

The masseter muscles that allow us to control our jaws are typically very tight. That tension can cause significant pain, restrict range of motion, and prevent the muscles from growing in response to chewing. For many people, the muscles are so tense that they are slow to release—expect this exercise to yield significant results only after several months. You also need to be careful to massage relatively gently here to avoid damaging the salivary glands that lie on top of the masseter muscles. The results will be worth it, though. In addition to relieving the pain, tension, and discomfort, you'll enjoy increased jaw definition.

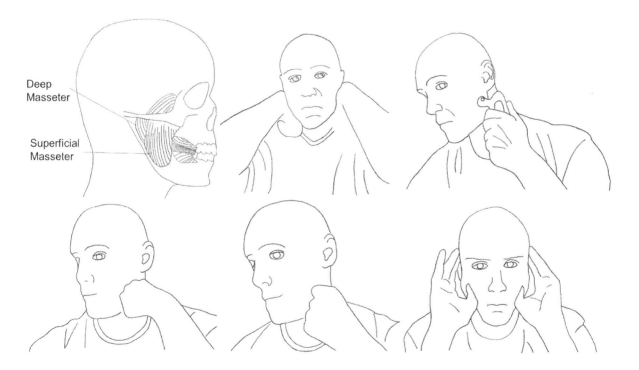

Illustration 9.10: Jaw massage.

Facial Massage Exercise #9.14: *Deep Masseter*

Start by tucking the backs of your wrists between your ear and the corners of your jaw and throat (see first image above). Allow the weight of your head to settle onto your wrists. You will likely feel substantial discomfort. Use deep diaphragmatic breathing to make the discomfort bearable and rest the head's entire weight on the back of your wrists. It took me four months of this to wipe this pain away completely.

Facial Massage Exercise #9.15: *Superficial Masseter*

Compress the entire masseter with a knuckle or tool. Also, focus on compressing the front face of the masseter by pressing your knuckles into the front facing aspect of your jawbone (last picture below). This will awaken the dormant muscle there and cause it to metabolize fat from your lower cheeks, making your face leaner.

Under the Jaw: Platysma

Poor neck posture and failing to contract the muscles under the jaw makes these muscles weak and tight. Speaking in a high, tense voice may also cause them to become taught and atrophy. As that happens, substantial deposits of fat begin to accumulate under the jaw. If you can release these muscles, your "double chin" or "jowls" will shrink or disappear, and your jawline will become much more highly defined. The result will lend an athletic and aesthetically pleasing look to your whole face. These muscles release and improve in appearance very rapidly.

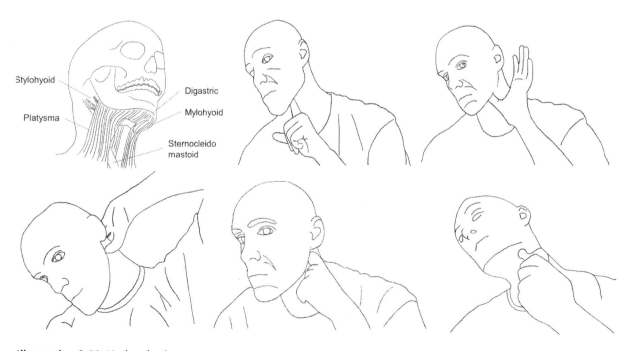

Illustration 9.11: Under-the-jaw massage.

Facial Massage Exercise #9.16: *Platysma*

Use a fingertip to press into the crease between your neck and jawline. This is the platysma. There are many other muscles in this general area under the chin that would benefit from being compressed such as the mylohyoid and digastric. To find and release them, feel around for hard and sore areas, and press into them gently.

Facial Massage Exercise #9.17: *Neck/Jaw Interface*

Behind the corner of the jaw, just under the ear, there is a very tense area implicated in neck strain and temporomandibular joint disorder. This area contains parts of a number of muscles, including the platysma, sternocleidomastoid, digastric, stylohyoid, mylohyoid and others. You should be able to find this large grouping of knots an inch directly under the ear. Press into it with your fingertips and knuckles, but be prepared to make this a long-term project.

The Chin: Mentalis, Depressor Anguli Oris, Depressor Labii Inferioris

Compressing the muscles in your chin will help it look lean and muscular. However, be advised that it may also reduce the chin's overall size as these muscles metabolize the surrounding fat. I had a painful knot of hard muscle in my depressor labii inferioris the size of a tootsie roll. Weekly compression made it smaller and smaller until it was unnoticeable. Again, this muscle is responsible for the cry-face seen in apes and humans. There is practically no scientific study on the muscular aspects of the cry-face, so I won't even speculate on what removing these painful knots has done for my psyche. However, I imagine that it is overwhelmingly positive.

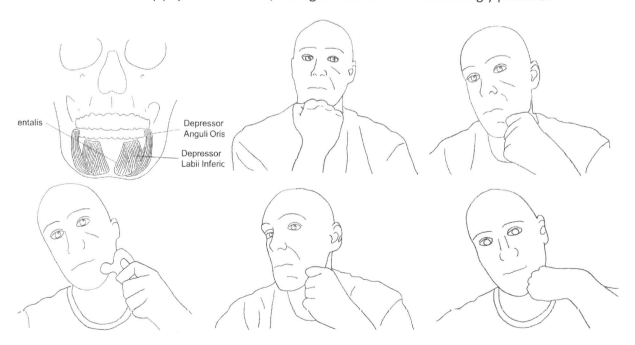

Illustration 9.12: Chin massage.

Facial Massage Exercise #9.18: *The Chin*

Compress the mentalis, the depressor anguli oris, and the depressor labii inferioris with knuckles or tools.

Keep at It

The exercises above may seem time-consuming but focus on the ones you find most interesting or potentially helpful. After a bit of practice, they'll become automatic, and you will find yourself doing them while watching TV or reading. The slower your diaphragmatic breathing is, the easier it will be to release the muscles. Given the easy, rapid results I experienced, I am amazed facial muscle release regimens are not widespread. I have concluded that without diaphragmatic breathing, tense muscles are too recalcitrant to make such a regimen feasible.

The main thing is to keep at it. Each exercise above provides suggested durations for achieving and maintaining results, but those are just guidelines. The only real standard is how you feel: how your face looks, and how your moods and thought patterns are affected. Give each exercise at least a few weeks before reaching a verdict, experimenting with different tools and small changes in pressure, angle, and rhythm. You'll soon find a method that works best for you.

Benefits to Your Skin

In addition to the myofascial release that you're expecting by now, facial self-massage has an additional benefit as well: cosmetic improvements to your skin. Skincare is a huge industry, with hundreds of millions of people trying to achieve a clear, even skin tone using tanning, moisturizers, toners, serums, lasers, masks, and surgical treatments. These can become extremely technical and remarkably expensive. They also mostly fail to address the root cause of skin problems: our skin is designed to handle a great deal of contact and use. It becomes stiff and unhealthy without physical stimulation.

When the face is not handled, tugged, or pulled for many years in a row, the system of blood vessels (or "vasculature") slowly diminishes. The result is a pale, sallow appearance that accentuates the prominence of moles, freckles, and wrinkles. The exercises presented in this chapter lightly stretch your skin, causing the creation of small blood vessels—a process known as "angiogenesis." Angiogenesis will make your skin darker, healthier, younger, and more evenly toned. The mechanical sheer forces also cause very slight damage to cutaneous and subcutaneous tissues, prompting the rebuilding and revitalization of countless dermal structures.

Benefits to the Structure of Your Face

Self-massage affects your facial muscles' shape and structure, which means it shares some similarity with treatments like cosmetic surgery and Botox injection. Botox paralyzes the muscle, decreasing tone and metabolic activity, thereby temporarily decreasing the strain muscles are under. It is popular because it makes a face appear relaxed and reduces the appearance of wrinkles. As discussed in the previous chapter it also has positive emotional effects. For instance, it can reduce negative emotions and susceptibility to crying.[2] Botox has downsides, however. The paralysis prevents muscles from contracting, which vastly reduces the flow of blood, oxygen, and nutrients to them. That, in turn, causes the muscles to atrophy and become weak. Besides these underlying problems, Botox and cosmetic surgery create an artificial look that many people can recognize. Also, Botox cannot be injected near the eyes because there is a risk it could leak into and paralyze the ocular muscles that control eye movements.

Your most beautiful face is not the one that a cosmetic surgeon can give you. They will attempt to create a face that *looks* muscular, lean, and without tension, without actually giving you any of these things. The surgeon's needles and scalpel traumatize soft tissues, reduce blood flow, and damage muscles without doing anything to reduce strain. Even the most skilled surgeon cannot come close to creating an all-natural look. This is a limitation inherent in their procedures, tools and techniques.

Compression comes with none of these risks and harms, and it costs nothing. It does take longer, and it can be uncomfortable, but it has much more dramatic, authentic, and longer-lasting effects. Furthermore, surgery and Botox crimp facial expressions, whereas compression grants you greater control over them. For example, my chin and cheeks moved sluggishly before with a reduced range of motion. Now they are surprisingly brisk and nimble. More than this, muscular release just feels good. Today, I smile wider and more frequently than I ever have, but my facial wrinkles are less pronounced. That and numerous other observations have suggested to me that wrinkles in the skin don't necessarily come from using the muscles. Rather, wrinkles are more likely to form over strained, dormant muscle. Scientists have long questioned what it is that constitutes physical beauty. The academic consensus now points to smooth skin, well-proportioned features, the appearance of youth, symmetry and being close to the population averageness.[3] More than these other criteria, I think that the absence of facial muscle strain is the primary determinate of attractiveness. In fact, the extent of facial tension can probably be seen as a marker of the status hierarchy that we wear on our faces.

Be Dominant but not Domineering

As your face become less tense, you will become more dominant. As your composure improves, people in your life, as well as people on the street, will be more respectful. Because of this, you might notice that you start to desire respect and even submissive displays from others. You will inevitably find yourself asserting your will over others in an arrogant way, whether inadvertently or not. You might find yourself holding your head high, looking above the eye line, with a perfectly calm face until another person feels compelled to look down. You might stare at a stranger on the street until they look away. This is not good or just. Keeping a stolid composure is good, but you will generate animosity if you intentionally elicit subordination displays from others.

If you combine your reprogrammed displays with rude comments and antagonizing behavior, there will be a backlash. This could result in losing a best friend, or literally being mauled in the street by strangers. This is an immensely serious point. Be humbler than you were before. If you are going to walk around without sneering or raising your eyebrows, retaining humility is imperative. The person that carries a big stick and speaks loudly must choose their words carefully.

Before, my face belonged to everyone else. They knew this, and they toyed with it. My default facial expression was what they made it. Today my face belongs to me. What will you do with your face now that you have a choice in the matter?

Conclusion

A few years ago, my cat got into an unhealthy habit of showing me with his face how hungry he was. His cries would be accompanied by pitiful facial wincing. His eyes would become tight, and his whole face would crinkle up. When I saw it, my face would empathically do the same. It pulled at my heartstrings. Here is a species, removed from humans by 85 million years of evolution, that uses remarkably similar facial signaling for distress. Of course, I started feeding him more regularly, but I also started massaging his face.

Every few weeks, I hold him in my lap and use my knuckles to gently press into his orbits, cheeks, nose, and jawline. It was uncomfortable for him at first. He found it the most uncomfortable when I used my thumbs to raise and press into his upper lips. Clearly his sneer, like mine, was strained. After four or five sessions, I could tell that it had become painless for him. He never makes those deplorable faces anymore, and people regularly comment on his poise and beauty. He showed dramatic aesthetic facial improvements even though I did not begin this routine with him until age 10.

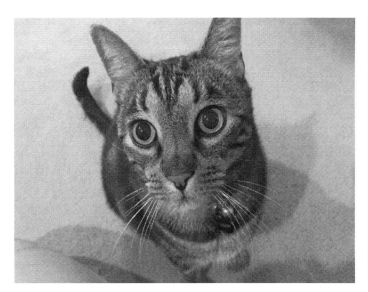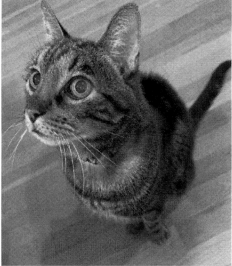

Figure 9.1: A. My cat Niko at age 11; B. Niko again at 16. Both pictures exhibit a lack of facial tension.

I recommend that people consider releasing the facial muscles, not only of their pets, but also of their spouses and children. As in the pruning of a bonsai, the sooner you can begin your manipulations, the more dramatic the effects will be. The exercises above act as a guide, but you really want to compress every square inch of your face. When you have found an area of your face or spine that is tender and sore to gentle pressure, you have uncovered a gold mine. You have discovered a location that, when rehabilitated, will allow personal and spiritual growth. You will experience decreased chronic stress, improved sleep, the release of emotional tension, and better autonomic balance. Whether you are a child, an elderly person, or anything in between, I implore you to compress all the pain out of your face.

Chapter 9: **Bullet Points**

- Deep tissue compression and percussion will reduce bracing, dormancy, and hypertonia in your facial muscles.
- Pressing firmly into any muscles that ache while breathing diaphragmatically will pull them out of partial contraction, making you more attractive and better composed.
- Massaging your face will make it so that you rarely experience social fatigue and so that your resting face is inviting and receptive.
- Your facial muscles will become more prominent and will have increased range of motion.
- Your skin and facial definition will improve. Your face will appear leaner and will have reduced pain and inflammation.
- Your neutral "resting" face will become authentic and it will be easier to be expressionless.
- Being expressionless and keeping a stolid composure is empowering. However, keep in mind that you will generate animosity if you use your composure to elicit subordination displays from others.
- Aside from the physical benefits there are emotional benefits as well because you are wiping out the low-grade wincing and frowning and the related microexpressions.

Chapter 9: **Endnotes**

1.   Eckman P. (2003). *Emotions revealed*. Henry Holt and Co.

2.   Havas, D. A., Glenberg, A. M., Gutowski, K. A., Lucarelli, M. J., & Davidson, R. J. (2010). Cosmetic use of botulinum toxin-A affects processing of emotional language. *Psychological Science*, *21*(7), 895–900.

3.   Valentine, T., Darling, S., & Donnelly, M. (2004). Why are average faces attractive? The effect of view and averageness on the attractiveness of female faces. *Psychonomic Bulletin & Review*, *11*(3), 482–487.

Chapter 10: **Strengthen and Tone Your Smile**

"There's daggers in men's smiles." — Shakespeare (1564-1616)

The quote above from *Macbeth* hints at some of the complexity and ambiguity of the smile. You might be used to thinking of the smile as something fairly simple: an expression of happiness or affection. And you're right, but it is much more than that. Smiles play a nuanced and highly variable role in social interaction. They are central to how we present ourselves, are loaded with context-dependent meaning, and are used to display our intentions and feelings— whether honestly or otherwise.

Smiles are also controlled by some of the same facial muscles that you've been working hard to free from bracing for the last two chapters. Leaving those muscles braced will make your smile frail and submissive and make it harder to connect positively with others. Relieving them from tension and then strengthening them under diaphragmatic conditions will make your smile beam. Before we dive into the exercises you can use to do that, it will help to have a look at how and why animals smile.

The Origins of the Smile

The smile has a convoluted but fascinating origin. In most mammals, drawing back the lips to reveal the teeth is done in preparation for biting. Baring the teeth keeps the animal from biting into its lips. It is also used as a flash of the fangs, warning other animals that it is angry. When accompanied by a growl, it is called a snarl. Thus, revealing the teeth is an expression of blatant aggression or the intention to take a bite.[1] In primates, the signal is more complicated.

In monkeys, lifting the top lip communicates that the displaying animal feels threatened. This often occurs when the animal is cornered, trapped, or cannot take flight. In nearly all primates, the startle reflex is accompanied by a grin (mouth corner retraction) and a shrill vocalization. This reflexive "grin-and-shriek" pattern communicates that the animal is jeopardized or intimidated.[2] As you can see, baring the teeth is tied to the neural circuits responsible for fight or flight. The flash of the teeth, especially teeth held together, is used to appease dominant group members, exclaiming, "I am stressed, but my mouth is closed and I am willing to submit." It is a self-handicapping signal and an admission of fear. As submission increases, the gaze is averted, the ears are drawn back, and the lips are retracted further, both horizontally and vertically, revealing more of the teeth and even parts of the gums. This can be contrasted with the facial response associated with anger. As anger increases, the stare widens, the ears are brought forward, and the lips are contracted, obscuring the teeth.

In short, fear is associated with displaying the teeth and dominance with concealing them. In many monkey species, if a dominant male chases a subordinate and the subordinate grins, expressing fear, the dominant animal will relent, stop chasing, and leave them alone.
If the dominant male were to grin, by contrast, the subordinate would approach and embrace him. Thus, the precise function of the signal is context-bound.

Things get even more complicated when we narrow the field to our closest relatives, the great apes. Among apes, baring the teeth can serve a range of purposes depending on the situation and what other expressions are involved. Like the human smile, an ape's grin can function to show submission, attempt appeasement, or solicit affection.[3] A quick grin is often flashed between social equals. Chimpanzees, for instance, can often be seen grinning at each other before they embrace. A silent bared-teeth expression is usually associated with assurance and affiliation. A relaxed face with an open mouth, baring the bottom teeth, is associated with play.

So, where a monkey's grin communicates either surprise or insecurity, humans and other apes have generalized and expanded the expression to convey compliance, affiliation, and play. However, because it has its origins in fear and appeasement, even the human smile is neurologically linked to distressed breathing and the sympathetic system. In other words, our smiles carry within them both the positive and negative signals that were inherited from our ape ancestors. Consequently, they do not automatically communicate goodwill. This is unfortunate because it means that fun and affection can be intrinsically tied to stress. The exercises in this chapter will teach you how to dissociate this negativity from your smile.

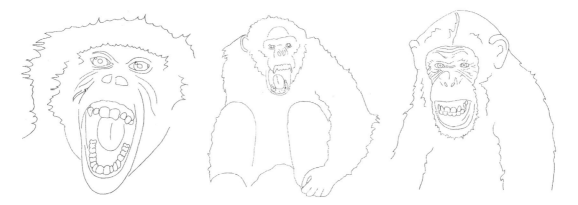

Illustration 10.1: A. Baboon baring the teeth; B. Chimpanzee making a threat display; Chimpanzee with a friendly grin.

Why Our Smiles Are Tainted

We can start by reviewing how our smiles come to be linked to negative emotions in the first place. Consider the people who have the best, most reliable smiles: models, cheerleaders, professional greeters, or front-desk staff. These are people who have been expected to keep unflinching smiles on their faces for hours at a time. At first, the experience must have been uncomfortable for many of them, causing defensive, nervous breathing. Over time, though, these professional smilers would have had no choice but to learn to breathe sustainably while smiling, leading to the gradual pairing of relaxed breathing with their grins. This is what I want for you.

Most of us don't possess that healthy link because we have never had to smile consistently for long periods. Without that kind of training, a smile typically speeds up our heart rates, makes our breathing shallow, places stress on our vocal cords, and activates trigger points in our faces. The social smiling behavior of humans is often nervous and compulsory. For instance, we smile when something awkward happens because we feel like we have to. Because most of us routinely pair smiling with distressed breathing, we have badly strained smiling muscles and offer insincere, uncomfortable smiles.

Dominant people are less likely to smile and more likely to frown. On average, bosses and managers smile less often than their employees, for instance. High-status individuals are permitted to display their negative emotions more freely and are not expected to provide appeasement displays to the people around them. On the other hand, low-status people are expected to stifle negative and competitive feelings and actively display signs of affiliation.[4] Studies have found that low-ranking children smile more when approaching high-ranking children than high rankers do when approaching low rankers. Studies also show that smiling is commonly associated with approval seeking and low social status in adults. In children, it is associated with low peer "toughness" ratings. In light of such relationships, smiling is often taken for weakness.

Several studies have found that women prefer men who don't smile. Other researchers discovered that in mixed martial arts, the fighter who smiles less during the weigh-in is more likely to win the match. However, the researchers in both cases were indiscriminate about the type of smile they looked for—they didn't distinguish between healthy, assertive smiles and sheepish, startled, submissive ones. An assertive, optimal smile is highly attractive and would likely predict victory in a fight. Smiling indicates social weakness only if the smiling muscles are strained and if smiling automatically recruits distressed breathing. Retraining your smile by pairing it with diaphragmatic breathing will make it so that your smile does not drain you but is, instead, effortless and empowering.

Smile Exercises

When I was a very young child, my grandmother told my mother that she was concerned about me because she could not perceive any joy in my smile. Some early experiences had caused me to pair smiling with shallow breathing, and my smile always appeared puny, melancholy, and forced. Chimps from the same group will show great variation in their capacity for smiling. Some smile feebly and yet other demonstrate "gingival" smiles, showing their gums. In my twenties, I started working toward that healthy smile. I decided to spend time smiling intensely to build up my smiling muscles. I would go on long walks or watch entire movies, smiling widely the whole time. Most of the time, I was also squinting and breathing shallowly, but even so, I achieved noticeable results within a few weeks. After ten cumulative hours of smiling widely, my face looked bigger and stronger, my cheeks were more muscular, and my smile was more believable.

Two close friends, on separate occasions, commented on the increased size of my smile. Then they told me to smile more widely still. When I tried, they each said: "No, smile up higher." I couldn't. They made a disappointed face and dropped the subject. They were disappointed because even though I was able to build lower sections of my smiling muscles, the section closest to the tendon that anchors into the cheekbone (the section with the biggest potential for growth) had not grown. This higher section, where the zygomatic muscle attaches to the cheek, didn't respond to the exercise because it was dormant. After diligently practicing the facial massage Exercise 9.8 from the last chapter, I was able to smile up into my cheekbones. The before and after pictures below illustrate the difference.

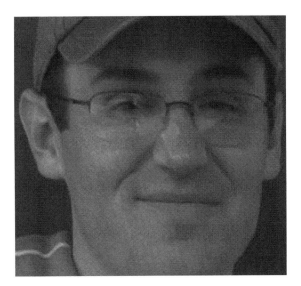 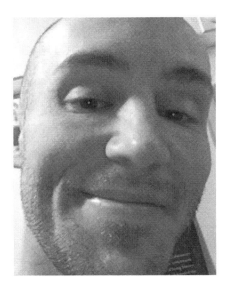

Figure 10.1: A. My smile at age 28 looks sour and unsustainable. I have rings under my eyes, thick lower eyelids, upturned nostrils, deep marionette lines, heavy sneering, and the bulk of the smile is located around my nose rather than on my cheekbones; B. By 34, each of those patterns has been reversed. The change resulted from gradually massaging away the tension and pain and strengthening the smiling muscles using firm contractions and deep breathing.

The massage of your zygomatic muscles described in Chapter 9 is complemented by the following muscle-building exercise.

Smiling Exercise #10.1: *Smiling Big with Calm Breathing*

Smile as widely as you can. Keep your face expressionless beyond the contractions involved in smiling and carefully check that you aren't squinting or raising your eyebrows. There should be no hint of apology or embarrassment in your smile. Practice paced breathing throughout the exercise, noting when the smile makes you want to breathe shallowly. You should notice that, at first, smiling big practically takes your breath away. Also, notice how, as you impose diaphragmatic breathing over the smile for several minutes, you can relax into a larger and larger smile.

You should feel your smiling muscles quiver and falter, but if you can smile through this, it will become more enduring and invariable. This will tone, enlarge, and strengthen the muscles and help them contract effortlessly without provoking your sympathetic nervous system. When your muscles reach exhaustion and start to burn, allow them to rest for at least a minute. In addition, massaging them after they reach exhaustion is a great way to stimulate regeneration, recovery, and growth.

Smiling as wide as I could stretched my lips so much that they would become chapped or even crack after doing the exercise above. Don't get discouraged by this. Gentle smiling for a few minutes a day will stretch your lips back to their optimal length over a few weeks.

Smiling Activity #10.1: *Waxing and Waning a Smile*

A genuine smile grows gradually and evenly. Sit in front of a mirror and practice growing a smile. Start with a very small smile and expand it over for five to 10 seconds until you have the biggest smile you can muster. Then, over the same period, practice letting the smile fade until your expression is neutral again. You will notice discontinuities where the expansion and relaxation jump in a jerky fashion. Focus on ironing out those irregularities in the movement, making the progression as smooth as possible. Most people find a steady, slow-growing smile captivating.

Smiling Activity #10.2: *Variants of Diaphragmatic Smiling*

Normally, every time we smile, it follows the same inflexible pattern. To vary the dynamics of your smile, practice the following:

1) Smile as widely as you can, with and without showing your teeth.
2) Smile with your teeth lightly clenched.
3) Smile with your top teeth visible and your bottom lip placed against them.
4) Smile with both sets of teeth fully revealed and your mouth slightly open.
5) Smile with both sets of teeth fully revealed and with your mouth wide open.
6) Smile while gradually squinting the eyes into a full squint, then gradually release them to wide eyes. Repeat.
7) Smile while slowly raising the eyebrows all the way, then slowly lower them until they are fully relaxed. Repeat.
8) Smile while chewing.

Smiling Exercise #10.2: *Smiling While Reading Out Loud*

Some people can smile comfortably while they talk, but most cannot. The ability to do it convincingly is so rare and so striking that it's practically a superpower. If you have not been acclimated, it is very awkward. Read a few pages of a book out loud while smiling. Practice diaphragmatic breathing, inhaling completely, and reading aloud until you are out of breath. The ability to smile while speaking is easily attained (and improved) in this way. After a total of five hours of practice, all your friends will notice the difference.

Smiling Activity #10.3: *Eye Contact with a Smile*

Sit in front of a mirror and use your reflection to model prolonged eye contact with another person. Smile. Keep your smile wide and your expression open. It will feel incredibly goofy, but only for the first few minutes.

You can also model the initiation of smiling eye contact. To do this, start by looking away, at, or above your eye line. Make the calmest face you can, and then look yourself in the eyes for a second while keeping your expression neutral. Over the next few seconds, gradually grow a heartfelt smile while continuing to make eye contact. Hold both your gaze and your smile for several seconds. Repeat. After you have practiced this exercise in a mirror, try it with a friend.

Isolate Your Smile

One of the rewards of maintaining a smile for several minutes while breathing diaphragmatically is the involuntary relaxation of muscles you don't need but that you normally tense up while smiling. Within a minute or two, you'll feel the tension in muscles all around your face, head, and neck start to ease. The process will gradually isolate your actual smile from the facial contortions that typically accompany it. That isolation has significant benefits. Usually, some 15 different muscles are involved in smiling; when you stop smiling, many of those muscles remain tense because the smile forced latent trigger points within them to become active. This is part of why smiling causes many people to lose their composure quickly, which can make them reluctant to smile at all.

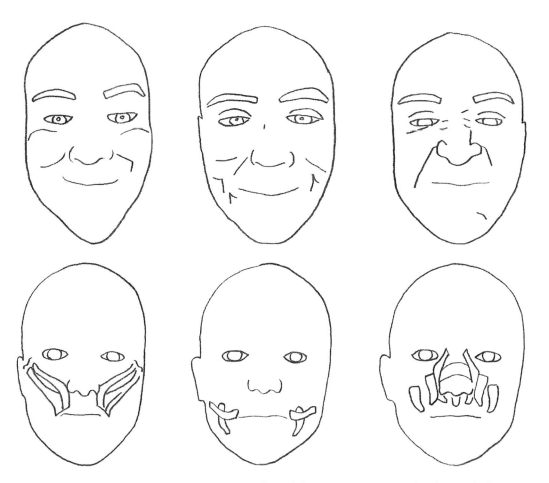

Illustration 10.2: The first column shows a zygomatic smile and the zygomaticus muscles that underlie it. The second shows the risorius and buccinator muscles and their contribution to the smile. The third shows the sneer and the muscles that contribute to it. Try to use more of the first two and less of the third in your smile.

Completely relax the sneer, the squint, and the eyebrow raise when you practice diaphragmatic smiling. You want to contract *only* the muscles needed (zygomatic, risorius, and buccinator). At first, your isolated smile will look and feel uncomfortable and you might feel like a kooky weirdo. It might also feel sarcastic or counterfeit. With time, though, this will become your preferred way of smiling. In essence, the expression you're practicing takes the expressionless face we developed in Chapter 8 and places a smile on top of it. The longer you breathe calmly while holding that isolated smile, the more natural and affable it will become.

Reduce the Extent of Squinting When You Smile

There are many kinds of smiles. Most famously, mid-19th-century French neurologist Guillaume Duchenne identified two types of smiles. The first is a fake smile, also called a "Pan Am" smile, named for the polite expressions worn by the (now defunct) airline's flight staff. Second, he described an authentic or "Duchenne" smile that employs the orbicularis oculi muscles and forms crow's feet around the eyes. Subsequent research has found that the Duchenne smile (with its associated crinkle of the eyes) is more closely associated with positive emotions.[5] That has led some scientists to assume that, to elicit happiness, smiles must include heavy squinting. I disagree.

In my experience, emotionally damaged people often squint the hardest when they smile, and emotionally healthy people squint the least. Methodically reducing the extent of your squinting will reduce eye strain without making your smile any less authentic. Work on smiling without much squinting, without raising your eyebrows, and more generally without contracting anywhere but in the smiling muscles themselves. Using the exercises from the last chapter to massage your forehead and the orbits of your eyes will help with this. It will also help you develop the ability to smile big, all the way up the sides of your cheeks, without squinting much at all. If you had been raised in an ideal, utopian environment with no threats, that's how you would smile. It might look like the smile of a deranged clown right now. But that's okay because it will become splendid once you become accustomed to doing it while breathing with your diaphragm.

Smiling Exercise #10.3: *Smile without Squinting*
Practice making the biggest smile you can muster. You might allow it to pour into your cheeks and eyes, but do so without squinting. To minimize squinting, you can monitor your eyelids in the mirror or place a finger under each eye. To do this, make a peace sign with your hand, extending the middle and forefinger. Place them just under each eye on the orbital bone. Squint a few times and become accustomed to how the muscles move under your fingertips when you squint. You will feel a mass of tissue bunch up. Continue smiling using your fingers to ensure you aren't squinting. You might want to combine this form of smiling with the upside-down TV watching exercise from Chapter 4.

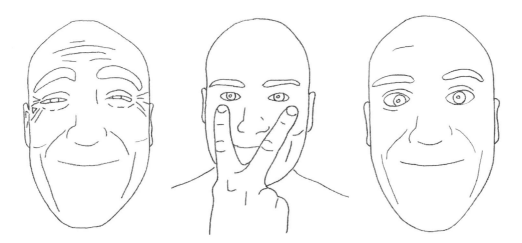

Illustration 10.3: A. Smile with heavy squinting; B. Using the fingertips to sense squinting contractions; C. Smile without squinting.

In Chapter 5, I described my efforts to remain calm while babysitting a two-year-old. That day I sat next to some blocks and pretended to play with them, lifting them, stacking them, and passing them to the little girl. I used a completely isolated, wide-eyed smile that would have looked wacky to anyone over the age of three. She saw it, she sensed that my breathing was calm, she liked the way I was sharing the blocks in a respectful way, and so she reciprocated the same smile. Within a few minutes, I lost all concern that she was judgmentally inspecting my smile. We played for hours with these silly, calm little smiles. By the time her parents came home, our smiles had gone from kooky to credible, and I have been able to utilize that same relaxed smile in the company of adults ever since.

It might help you to find a safe situation in which to practice your new smile. You might work on your "calm smile" with a stuffed animal, a pet, or even a friend you have recruited to help you. After practicing in these situations, you can start to generalize this ability to situations that feel less safe, like running errands or sitting in traffic. This is another case in which we can benefit from a "fake it until you make it" approach. If you don't create concocted social environments where you feel perfectly comfortable smiling carefree, you will never do it. Like Schopenhauer, I was cynical in my belief that life (or other people) was not creating these optimal scenarios for me. It is our responsibility to create them for ourselves and to share them with others.

Creating Dimples and Smile Lines: Contracting the Risorius and Buccinator

It is important to incorporate a full contraction of the risorius and buccinator muscles into your smile. Both pull your lips horizontally. The risorius muscles lie about an inch below your cheekbone, anchoring to the corner of your mouth on one side and the soft tissue of your cheek on the other. The nearby buccinator muscles aid in the risorius smile as well as in whistling, puckering, and chewing. I previously used my risorius and buccinator muscles very little in my smile. When I fully contracted them, they made my smile look pretentious and fraudulent. I took this as an indication that I needed to use them more. The muscles were very tense, and if I pressed my knuckle into them, it was painful. I have since rehabilitated them with compression and contraction, making them much stronger, leaner, and painless.

I never had dimples or smile lines in the past as the first photo at the beginning of this chapter evinces. Genetic testing revealed that I do not have the genetic markers associated with dimples. But exercising the risorius and buccinator muscles has given me somewhat pronounced smile lines/dimples. This surprised me. It even surprised my mom. I was 35, and I was spending time with her for the first time in months when she said, "Oh my, you have dimples now. Is that from a specific Program Peace exercise?" My experience suggests to me that everyone can develop them. At first, your dimple beds (the pockets between the contracted risorius muscles and the jaw muscles) may be completely covered by the fatty tissue in your cheeks. Contract the risorius and then use your fingers to search for this pocket. It may be filled in with fat now, but as your smiling muscles grow, it will slowly come to form a depression—a dimple.

Smiling Exercise #10.4: *Risorius Smiling*

Smile in the following ways:

1) Smile with only the risorius muscle. To do this, your smile should not be drawn upward toward the cheekbone at all. Only draw it horizontally. Try to contract the muscle fully and to exhaustion. That contraction will turn into a friendly, polite smile that you can use all the time. You can offer a solemn but polite greeting by accompanying this smile with a slightly lifted chin (created by contracting the mentalis).

(2) Incorporate the buccinators into your risorius smile. To do this, squeeze the risorius smile as hard as you can, forcing the buccinators to contract. You'll know you're succeeding when you feel the inside of your cheeks pressing against your teeth. The more you exercise these muscles, the leaner your cheeks will become and the more pronounced your smile lines or dimples will be.

Creating a Muscular Smile: Contracting the Zygomatic Muscle

The most important smiling muscle is the zygomaticus major. It connects the corners of your mouth to your cheekbones. The muscle is likely to be feeble and feel uncomfortable when isolated at first. However, contracting it firmly will gradually create noticeable lumps of muscle under your cheekbones that appear when you smile. Many famous actors have well-developed zygomatic muscles, and in women, they tend to be much larger. Conditioning the zygomatic muscles will make your smile unambiguous and make your face leaner and friendlier.

Smiling Exercise #10.5: *Zygomatic Smiling*

Smile with only the zygomatic muscle (leaving the risorius and buccinators relaxed). To do this, pull the corners of your mouth diagonally upward toward your cheekbones (a sneer pulls the lips up vertically, the risorius pulls them out horizontally). I believe the zygomatic smile is more draining than the risorius smile because it is more closely tied to the stress system. The more you pair it with diaphragmatic breathing, the less effortful it will be to use.

Repeated rhythmic contractions as in Exercise 8.4 can also help build muscle, tone, and coordination. Instead of holding a prolonged contraction, you may consider performing 100 rapid zygomatic and risorius contractions.

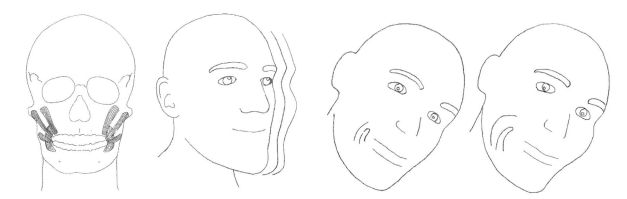

Illustration 10.4: A. Each of the muscles involved in smiling is anchored at the corners of the mouth. The two zygomatic muscles stretch up to the cheekbone, the risorius extends laterally toward the side of the face, and the buccinator is the large muscle underneath the others; B. Zygomatic exercises will help strengthen the muscles centered around the cheekbone. C. & D. Risorius and buccinator exercises will increase the prominence and size of smile lines and/or dimples.

As you practice the exercises in this chapter, your entire cheek will become much leaner and more muscular, giving the impression of a long history of relaxed, confident smiling. People will see this and implicitly assume that you are a happy person who has been smiling healthfully all their life. When you exercise the smiling muscles, you may notice other facial muscles reaching fatigue before your smiling muscles due to their relative lack of exercise. This is most likely to be a problem with the heavily strained sneering muscles. Luckily, the issue is fairly simple to address.

Refrain from Sneering

In my twenties, a friend told me that I smile like the Grinch. It hurt to hear, but he was right. My sickening smile was perverted from the repetitive strain of muscles around my nose. These included the three pairs of levator labii muscles which run along the sides of the nose from the height of the eyes down to the lip. They work in tandem to lift the upper lip and reveal the canines.

As you know, revealing the upper teeth is a threat display in most primates. Chimps bare their top teeth in a grin when they are frightened, uncertain, or uncomfortable. It often means they are ready to fight. Interestingly, baring the teeth *during* a fight is a sign of uncertainly and fear. High-ranking chimps seldom show their top teeth[6] while low-ranking animals frequently do it. All of this indicates to me that the muscles that lift the top lip are the smiling muscles most closely associated with stress and submission. Check the action of these muscles in the mirror. What do you think?

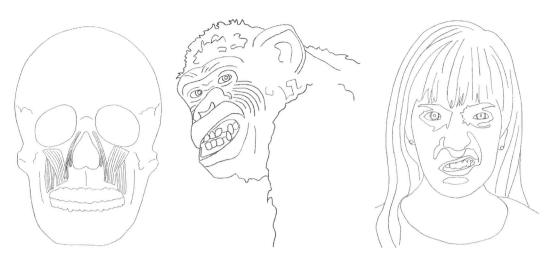

Illustration 10.5: A. Muscles involved in sneering; B. Chimpanzee sneering; C. Girl sneering.

Sneering is common in human infants. For example, all infants sneer in fear when they are momentarily left alone by their mothers (using the logic presented in Chapter 7, this suggests a link with grief). Scientists believe older humans learn to inhibit the sneering reflex because sneering is not accepted in polite society. Most adults only knowingly sneer to communicate disgust or disdain. Much more accepted is an unconscious partial sneer, bracing the sneering muscles just slightly. We see this in people who curl their lip for minutes at a time. By doing that, they subject their muscles to repetitive strain. Over time, that leaves the muscles in a state of partial contraction.

The use of the sneering muscles amounts to a fascinating psychological complex. When trigger points within the sneer change from latent to active, you become committed to a negative emotion because it is now advertised on your face. Once you know someone else has seen your sneering muscles become tense, it forces your hand. You implicitly decide you must either act scared or aggressive. The activation of latent trigger points within the sneering muscles is the incendiary event in many negative confrontations. Since using massage to obliterate the trigger points in my sneering and frowning muscles, I have been virtually free of heated reactions. I previously thought my anger was unjustly provoked by others, but now I realize I was allowing others to activate latent trigger points in my sneering muscles, and it was this that compelled me to react prematurely and discourteously.

If you can release the tension in your levator labii, it will make your resting face appear less guarded. Some people will not be able to tell whether you look unguarded because you are friendly or because you are angry. This is because dominant people often completely release the levator labii when provoked. Thus, when you let this muscle relax, you will either appear calm and angelic or calm and dangerous. Your other postures and actions will determine which. The first step in making your sneerless expression noncombative is becoming more aware of the tension in your sneering muscles, which you can do using the activity below.

Smiling Activity #10.4: *Sneer Awareness*

Sit, stand, or kneel in front of a mirror. It is best to have a light overhead that casts a shadow over your marionette lines (nasolabial folds) so that you can see them move. Play around with the sneering muscles that lift and curl your upper lip. Practice making the smallest sneer and the largest sneer that you can. Transition gradually between them. Become aware of the sensation of sneering slightly and how that differs from not sneering at all. Pretend to say something rude to an acquaintance and notice how you maintain a light sneer afterward. Just as you want to stop squinting and raising the eyebrows chronically, you want to end your chronic sneer.

When people see that your sneering muscle is relaxed, they will try to imitate this. Unless they have practiced it and massaged the muscles, they will likely not be able to do it comfortably for long. This is because once the sneer is relaxed, even a slight emotional aggravation can make this tense muscle snap back to full contraction reflexively. Thus, you may find that people flash sneers at you inadvertently. Just ignore this, keep your sneering muscles calm, and continue being kind.

Be particularly aware of the presence of the sneer in your smile. Strained sneering muscles cause us to smile when we are nervous—we use the smile to cover up the sneer. In fact, a strained sneer tarnishes our every smile. Our smile has become conflated with our sneer, and often, even we don't know whether we are sneering or smiling (see the first picture of me above). The exercise below will help guide you to use the risorius and zygomatic muscles without using the levator labii to create a sneerless smile.

Smiling Activity #10.5: *A Sneerless Smile*

Sit, stand, or kneel in front of a mirror. Look carefully at your lips. Raise the corners of your mouth while the center of your top lip stays still. This involves using your risorius muscle to draw the corners of your lips outward horizontally and using the zygomatic muscle to raise them diagonally. Do this without squinting or sneering. Ensure that you are not sneering by keeping the center of your top lip (cupid's bow) neutral.

You can also monitor your sneer with your fingers. To do this, make a peace sign with your hand, extending the middle and forefingers. Place them just to the side of each nostril. Sneer a few times and become accustomed to how the muscles move under your fingertips. You will feel the skin rise. Return to smiling without sneering, using your fingers to track your success.

The sneer-free smile will look ridiculous at first, but the more you pair it with diaphragmatic breathing, the more sincere it will feel to you and the more genuine it will appear to others.

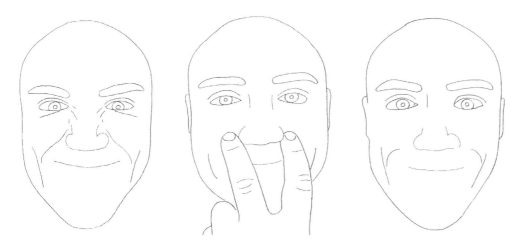

Illustration 10.6: A. Smile with heavy sneering; B. Using the fingertips to sense sneering contractions; C. Smile without sneering.

Smiling Exercise #10.6: *A Sneering Smile*

You don't want to stop using your sneering muscles entirely. In this exercise, practice making the most intense sneer you can. This time, do not smile. Ensure that your top lip is maximally curled and that you are showing as much of your top and bottom teeth as possible. It will continue to feel like you are performing a barbaric threat display until you can breathe diaphragmatically while doing it. This exercise will allow you to pull your upper lip higher and do so with more force. It will also help strengthen your sneering muscle and clear out the trigger points, giving you greater control and separating your sneer from the activation of your stress system.

Smiling Activity #10.6: *Crinkling the Nose*

Crinkling the nose adds a momentary sneer into your smile, but that can be a good thing. Crinkling for about half of a second adds affection and dynamism to the expression. Spend a few minutes smiling in front of the mirror while intermittently crinkling your nose. Try looking yourself in the eyes in the mirror and say, "It's gonna be fun." When you do this, briefly crinkle your nose while you say the "f" sound in the word "fun." Let it be playful and relaxed.

Smile Dominantly

According to body language experts, smiling with the brow lowered is extremely dominant. There is solid research indicating that leaders and people judged by others to have high leadership aptitude are capable of smiling with a lowered brow.[7] This combination of a frown and a smile has been called "the Bill Clinton effect." Experiments find that people rate those who use it as particularly dominant and are more likely to vote for them for leadership positions.[8] Most people have never actually tried it. It takes a lot of time and confidence to develop this socially. Or, you can just practice it by yourself for several minutes until it is intrepid.

Smiling Exercise #10.7: *A Frowning Smile*

Smile big without sneering or squinting. Next, frown by pulling the eyebrows together and down toward the eyes. Try to keep your eyes wide and hold this expression. You might start in front of a mirror and then practice in front of a TV. You can use this expression to exclaim things like "isn't that ironic," "what a coincidence," or "that's really amusing."

We are all hesitant to smile optimally because we don't want to come across as inauthentic or psychopathic. We remember being afraid to smile around our parents, grade school teachers, or bullies, thinking they might misinterpret our expression as flippant or impudent. The good news is that this feeling will fade. Smiling large, carefree smiles made me feel like a sinister demon or a sarcastic jester when I first started. Now, it just makes me feel happy.

Smiling Activity #10.7: *Smile with Impunity*

Spend a few minutes smiling just for yourself. Notice your inclination to inhibit your smile and recognize that the instinct comes from a petrifying fear that other people will misperceive or misunderstand you. Notice how you perceive your smile to be facetious or vindictive. Now, let those misgivings go. Perform the smiling exercises in this chapter staunchly with full confidence that your smile is positive, coming from a good place, and will be perceived as such by others.

Conclusion

"Buddha's contemporaries described him as 'ever-smiling' and portrayals of Buddha almost always depict him with a smile on his face. But rather than the smile of a self-satisfied, materially-rich or celebrated man, Buddha's smile comes from a deep equanimity from within." — Mark K. Setton (1952)

Genuine smiling induces the release of feel-good neurotransmitters like dopamine, endorphins, and serotonin. That's part of why the intensity of our smiles in childhood photographs predicts life satisfaction, marriage stability, and a longer lifespan.[9] Studies have found that even faked or forced smiling can increase happiness and decrease depressive states.[10] Those studies don't distinguish between genuine, healthy smiles and forced, strained ones. Imagine how much more dramatic the results would be if they had! The lesson here is straightforward: smiling more and properly increases your standard of living.

I believe the best default facial posture is to have the entire face at rest except for a small smile involving only the zygomatic, risorius, and buccinator muscles. If you can direct this toward others, it will cause them to unconsciously imitate your smile.[11] This will lift their mood and make them want to be around you. Since performing these exercises, I regularly notice strangers smiling at me—something that was unusual before. Every time this happens, I wonder why they smiled at me, and then I realize it was because I was smiling. It can become so effortless that you don't realize you are doing it.

Smiling Exercise #10.8: *The Miniscule Smile*

Practice holding the smallest smile you can. With time, this will create a new mode of operation for you where you find yourself smiling for prolonged periods with very little effort. It will look and feel preposterous at first but coupling it with paced breathing will make it both renewable and pleasurable. After a few hours of training, you will find that this smile arises on its own and slowly turns you into a more optimistic and idealistic person.

Fully contracting the muscles helps them grow but contracting them lightly and continuously builds tone and comfort. Do you sit in front of a computer during the day? Turn on your paced breathing app and smile. Just make sure that you do not subject the muscles to repetitive strain and don't forget to massage your face after long sessions of smiling. Allow the muscles intermittent rests, especially once they reach fatigue. Spend time smiling as you lie down or fall asleep. A "resting smile" may sound like an oxymoron, but it shouldn't.

Chapter 10: **Bullet Points**

- In monkeys, baring the teeth is a threat and subordination display, so the smile is intrinsically tied to the stress system.
- Our smiles have become tainted by repetitive strain, and the smiling muscles are stuck in partial contraction, full of trigger points, and painful. Our tight, braced smiles aren't happy—they're just submissive and tense.
- Contracting the smiling muscles completely while breathing diaphragmatically (and then compressing the muscles afterward) will reverse the bracing.
- Isolating and fully contracting the zygomatic, risorius, and buccinator muscles will improve your smile.
- Careful practice will enable you to remove the squint, eyebrow raise, and sneer from your smile, freeing it to be a purely positive expression.
- Practicing a smile while making eye contact with yourself in front of a mirror will help you smile while making eye contact with others.
- Practicing smiling while reading out loud will help you smile while speaking to others.
- As often as possible, practice wearing either the biggest or the tiniest smile that you can.

Chapter 10: **Endnotes**

1.   Pennisi, E. (2000). The snarls and sneers that keep violence at bay. *Science, 289*(5479), 576–577.

2.   Fridlund, A. J. (1994). *Human facial expression: An evolutionary view*. Academic Press.

3.   Chevalier-Skolnikoff, S. (2006). Facial expression of emotion in nonhuman primates. In P. Ekman (Ed.), *Darwin and facial expression: A century of research in review* (pp. 11–90). Malor Books.

4.   LaFrance, M., & Hect, M. A. (1999). Option or obligation to smile: The effects of power and gender on facial expression. In P. Phillipot, R. S. Feldman, & E. J. Coars (Eds.), *The social context of nonverbal behavior* (pp. 45–70). Cambridge University Press.

5.   Messinger, D. S., Fogel, A., & Dickson, K. (2001). All smiles are positive, but some smiles are more positive than others. *Developmental Psychology, 37*(5), 642–653.

6.   Petersen, R. M., Dubuc, C., & Higham, J. P. (2018). Facial displays of dominance in non-human primates. In Senior C. (Ed.) *The facial displays of leaders* (pp. 123–143). Palgrave Macmillan.

7.   Senior, C. (2018). The facial displays of leadership: A systematic review of the literature. In C. Senior (Ed.), *The facial displays of leaders* (pp. 1–25). Palgrave MacMillan.

8.   Campbell, R., Benson, P. J., Wallace, S. B., Doesbergh, S., & Coleman, M. (1999). More about brows: How poses that change brow position affect perceptions of gender. *Perception, 28*(4), 489–504.

9.   Abel, E. & Kruger, M. (2010). Smile intensity in photographs predicts longevity. *Psychological Science, 21*, 542–544.

10. Freitas-Magalhães, A., & Castro, E. (2009). Facial expression: The effect of the smile in the treatment of depression. Empirical study with Portuguese subjects. In A. Freitas-Magalhães (Ed.), *Emotional expression: The brain and the face* (pp. 127–140). University Fernando Pessoa Press.

11. Hatfield, E., Cacioppo, J. T., & Rapson, R. L. C. (1992). Primitive emotional contagion. In M. S. Clark (Ed.), *Emotional and social behavior* (pp. 151–177). Sage Publications.

Chapter 11: **Breathe Less, Nasally, and without Pharyngeal Tension**

"The yogi's life is not measured by the number of his days, but by the number of his breaths."
— B.K.S. Iyengar (1918-2014)

In Chapter 3, we established the first four tenets of diaphragmatic breathing: 1) extend the breath over longer intervals, 2) breathe deeper to increase the tidal range, 3) breathe at a steady, smooth rate, and 4) breathe assertively regardless of social pressure. We also talked about how, if you are doing these things properly, your inhalations should be recruiting your diaphragm, thereby pushing your belly out. In Chapter 5, we added the passive exhalation, pointing out that you can let your breathing muscles go limp on the outbreath to provide them with a microbreak.

Hopefully, by now, you have practiced these using a breath metronome and have learned what paced diaphragmatic breathing feels like and how to sustain it. You should feel comfortable breathing for several minutes at a rate of around five-second inhalations and seven-second exhalations. Perhaps you have advanced closer to eight and 12. This chapter will return to the topic of breathing, offering further background and more breathing techniques to complement what you have already learned.

Stop Hyperventilating

I remember being pulled around by the pressures and concerns of life. Everything felt rapid, loud, and urgent, and I would breathe fast and hard in an attempt to keep up with it all. Then, when things slowed down, and I found myself in a quiet room with others, my over-breathing stuck out like a sore thumb. They could hear me heaving, taking two or three breaths for every breath they took. I found it embarrassing, but because my body had adapted to hyperventilating, there was little I could do about it in the moment.

Today, many self-help breathing gurus tell their followers they are not inhaling enough air and, consequently, are not getting enough oxygen. The people giving this advice are mostly confused. It is over-breathing that is unhealthy, and it is the rapid cycles of heavy inhaling and exhaling that we want to stop. This excessive breathing is called hyperventilation and results in abnormally high oxygen levels and low levels of carbon dioxide. This is why medical personnel give people who are hyperventilating a paper bag to breathe into; it depletes them of oxygen. Rebreathing exhaled carbon dioxide trapped in the paper bag helps them reduce over-oxygenation and quell their panic. Inordinate oxygen intake can be just as bad as insufficient oxygen intake.[1] Like overeating, over-breathing amounts to too much of a good thing.

During stress, thoracic breathing is accentuated to meet the anticipated increases in oxygen demands. If the anticipated event never arrives, there is no increase in physical activity and the extra oxygen is never used. This is why hyperventilation leads to problems. During hyperventilation, oxygen levels become so high that, paradoxically, many body tissues are deprived of oxygen. This is especially true in the brain, leading to reduced neural and mental function.[2]

A common criterion for hyperventilation is 30 liters of air per minute, and many people breathe normally in this range. Conventional medicine deems five to six liters of air per minute (at around 500 milliliters of air per breath) normal.[3] This would be about as much air in three empty two-liter soft drink bottles. It is likely that you, like most people, inhale significantly more than this.

I was a chronic hyperventilator, and I was well acquainted with the symptoms: dizziness, poor concentration, muscle tension, cramps, irregular and rapid heartbeat (tachycardia), heart pounding (palpitations), and gastrointestinal upset. It is also strongly associated with nasal congestion, tightening of the airways, fatigue, tremor, shakiness, tight muscles, stiffness, muscle pain, weakness, constriction of blood vessels, asthma, rhinitis, and snoring.[4] Because over-breathing is hard work, it leads to exhaustion, chest tightness, and pain around the ribs. Hyperventilation also leads to feelings of breathlessness, choking, and smothering.

Hyperventilation is thought to be a significant factor in medical conditions caused or aggravated by mental stress (psychosomatic diseases). These include headaches, backaches, nausea, dry mouth, sweaty palms, insomnia, ulcers, and many others. This may be partly accounted for by the fact that hyperventilation increases the concentration of stress hormones in the blood. In one study, a few minutes of hyperventilation increased adrenaline levels in subjects by 360 percent.[5] The diaphragmatic breathing retraining regimen outlined in this chapter will reduce the amount you hyperventilate and potentially provide you with relief from symptoms you didn't even realize you had.

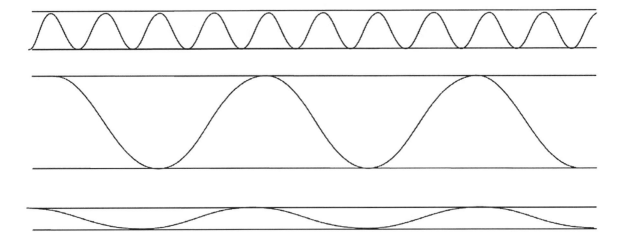

Figure 11.1: A. The first sine wave depicts shallow rapid breathing characteristic of anxiety; B. The second wave depicts calmer, deeper breathing at longer intervals; C. The third depicts a form of breathing that involves the movement of a much smaller total volume of air. Breathing less than usual in this way as an exercise can reduce the tendency to hyperventilate. Again, the x-axis represents time and the y-axis represents the volume of air in the lungs.

The benefits of breathing less have been appreciated for a long time. In the 1950s, Russian physiologist Konstantin Buteyko developed a now popular breathing program to counteract hyperventilation. He observed that the closer his patients were to death, the faster and shallower was their breathing. Today, his program is called the Buteyko method and is used for asthma, anxiety, and to increase pulmonary function in athletes. Reviews of the medical literature have come to different conclusions about the strength of the evidence supporting the Buteyko method,[6] but it has a large number of steadfast adherents, and I think in principle it is credible and compelling.

The Buteyko method uses breath holding, resistance breathing, and breath restriction exercises to counteract over-breathing. The practice focuses on reducing breathing movements until you feel a tolerable air shortage and hunger for air. I do not recommend reducing breathing to the point of air hunger per se, but I do recommend the bread and butter of the Buteyko system: 1) resistance breathing, 2) breathing through the nose, and 3) breathing "slower and less." These are legitimate methods to counteract hyperventilation. Allow me to explain why.

Resistance Breathing

Resistance breathing is any kind of breathing that creates resistance to the flow of air. You can create resistance by breathing through clenched teeth, pursed lips, or a straw. Resistance breathing forces the breathing musculature to work harder, thus strengthening it substantially over time. Because it proceeds slower and disallows air gulping, it forces the diaphragm to do the work.

Many people use "elevation training masks" during exercise to create intense pulmonary resistance to strengthen the muscles of respiration. These masks are meant to simulate the benefits of training at high altitudes. Studies show that the masks are useful, and I imagine the masks might be very helpful when used with diaphragmatic breathing. However, simply breathing through the nose is a free and easy alternative to train resistance breathing.

Why Nasal Breathing is Healthier Than Mouth Breathing

Because the nasal passages are narrower than the oral one, taking a full breath through the nose takes significantly more time and effort. It takes 50% more work to breathe exclusively through the nose compared to breathing through the mouth. It is hard work for the diaphragm and will make it stronger fast. Also, it forces you to breathe more slowly, at an even pace. You'll notice that you cannot gasp through the nose, and several researchers agree that "one cannot easily hyperventilate when breathing through the nose."[7] I consider nasal breathing the sixth tenet of optimal breathing.

Most mammals breathe exclusively through their noses with their mouths closed, but there are a few exceptions. Some mammals will breathe through the mouth when engaging in intense cardiovascular activity. Others use mouth breathing for evaporative cooling, like a dog panting on a hot day. Some mammals will breathe through their mouth during an aggressive confrontation. Usually, the dominant animal will breathe exclusively through the nose and the subordinate one will open the mouth and pant non-diaphragmatically. Many dog trainers interpret nose breathing as defiant and mouth breathing as acquiescent. The dog that pants rapidly with an open mouth is usually seen as the most obedient. Chronic mouth breathing, like hyperventilation, is a submissive, handicapping signal. Otherwise, mammals breathe almost exclusively through their noses. Whenever a veterinarian sees a mammal at rest breathing through its mouth, it is taken as a sign of sickness or serious injury.

In humans, mouth breathing is thought by many experts to increase the stress response.[8] It has been shown to lead to high blood pressure, poor posture, cognitive disturbances, and heart problems.[9] In newborns, it is a sign of failure to thrive. However, there is no medical consensus merely because not enough studies have been performed. Neither is there any rubric in medical science helping people to stop breathing through their mouths. This is a serious oversight.

Shut Your Mouth and Save Your Life

In 1862, George Catlin wrote the book *Shut Your Mouth and Save Your Life*, in which he extolled the virtues of nose breathing. He was an American adventurer who specialized in painting portraits of Native Americans in the Old West. He observed a large proportion of Native Americans breathing exclusively through the nose, even during sleep. He attributed their good health and serene countenance to this habit. He even saw mothers encouraging their infants and children to breathe through their noses. If a baby opened its mouth to breathe, the mother would gently push the baby's lips together to ensure nasal breathing. He compared this to Europe, where it seemed to him everyone breathed with their mouths.

He claimed the American Indians referred to the white men not only as "pale-faces" but as "black-mouths" due to their penchant for breathing through their mouths. He said that breathing through the mouth leads to a derangement of the "whole face, which is not natural; carrying the proof of a long practice of the baneful habit, with its lasting consequences; and producing that unfortunate and pitiable, and oftentimes disgusting expression which none but 'civilized' communities can present." He called mouth breathing "the most abominable and destructive habit that ever attached itself to the human race."

The following are two drawings by Catlin from the book. They illustrate what he saw as the difference between English mouth breathers and Native American nasal breathers.

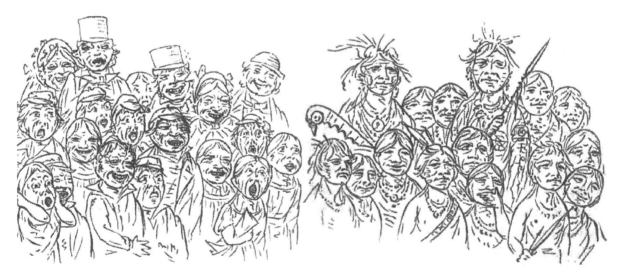

Illustration 11.1: George Catlin's 1862 sketch comparing mouth-breathing Londoners to nose-breathing American Indians.

Catlin wrote that no "excitements" could cause the Indians to part their lips. He said their mouths remained closed unless they were eating or speaking and that they even smiled with their mouths closed. He recounted a story in which a quarrel arose between a white fur trader and a Sioux brave. The men decided to settle the dispute naked, in a prairie, with knives.

Minutes before the fight, Catlin intervened and convinced the men to reconcile and shake hands. Afterward, he asked the brave whether he was afraid of the other man, who was both bigger and stronger. The Indian replied: "No, not in the least; I never fear harm from a man who can't shut his mouth." He wrote that both Indian mothers and medicine men told him that Native Americans breathe through their noses to ensure strength, confidence, athleticism, and long, peaceful lives.

If I were asked to name a single habit that could be corrected to increase longevity and quality of life, it would be mouth breathing. So, the question arises: "What is the best way to ensure nasal breathing?" Well, at first take, it's not easy. There are two main hindrances to nasal breathing: 1) it is easy to forget to breathe nasally, and 2) we transition from nasal to mouth breathing unconsciously when we become stressed. However, spending time with the mouth taped can help you to overcome each of these issues.

Taping the Mouth to Ensure Nasal Breathing

You may think you breathe through your nose but you likely often switch to mouth breathing. Many people switch from nose to mouth breathing when they feel nervous or when they are socializing. You may have never noticed it, but you probably make this switch repeatedly as your stress levels fluctuate throughout the day. In many cases, the diaphragm is not strong enough to support nasal breathing under stressful conditions. Breathing through the nose is unnerving for many people in social situations.

I was very uncomfortable nose breathing in my twenties, partly because it made me look expressionless. I was afraid people would think I looked "bold-faced" or insolent. But my face looked "disrespectful" while nose breathing only because I was uncomfortable doing it. Once you become complacent breathing through the nose, with mouth closed, you can get away with sporting a highly expressionless face. In other words, nasal breathing builds composure. Spend time breathing with your mouth shut more often. Practice it in public and with social contacts. Notice how difficult it can be in certain situations and how you have the repeated impulse to switch to mouth breathing. If you allow yourself to transition to mouth breathing when you feel stressed or excitable, you will resort to hyperventilation.

To address this, I strongly recommend taping the mouth shut as often as possible. It stops you from taking intermittent gasps and sighs through your mouth. The gasping and sighing compensate for the air hunger created when stress rises and nasal breathing becomes nonassertive and weak. Even when you are making a concerted effort to breathe through the nose, you will probably only do it halfheartedly because you know in the back of your mind that you can always switch to mouth breathing if you need to.

Taping your mouth will teach you to breathe through your nose without recourse to the mouth. Nasal breathing will be your only option, so you will unconsciously lean into it more. This will train your diaphragm to be self-sufficient and uncompromising. I recommend using a bandage or surgical tape, which can be found in drug stores as it is made for contact with skin and won't chafe your lips or strip them of their natural oils. When I started taping my mouth, my nasal passages stung from the heavy increase in airflow. Each breath felt cold and dry, but this only lasted a few days. I urge you to tape your mouth as often as you can for a few months until you are nasal breathing by force of habit.

Breathing Exercise #11.1: *Taping Your Mouth Shut*

Put a piece of tape over your mouth for an hour. Place it horizontally across the mouth so that it makes contact with both the upper and lower lips. Concentrate on the work involved in breathing through the nose. Notice that you will breathe too shallowly, get too little oxygen, and will panic, wanting to switch back to mouth breathing. You can overcome this by making your breaths longer, deeper, and steadier. Next, try it while walking, reading, watching television, working, and exercising. Tape your mouth often to train exclusive nasal breathing in all situations. You should find that flaring the nostrils (a dominance signal) may help to gradually open your nasal passages.

While your mouth is taped, you will inevitably find some mundane stressor to get worked up about. Let's say, for instance, that your doorbell rings and you aren't expecting anyone. Your respiratory rate will increase ahead of the anticipated social demands, and you will feel air hunger. However, you won't be able to sustain an increased breathing rate because you cannot gasp through your mouth. As you are forced to continue to breathe through your nose, the worries about the doorbell fade. This will ensure that the person who answers the door is courageous rather than fretful. Every minute your mouth is taped, you have small victories like this one that will take the reins over your diaphragm from the environment and place them in your own hands.

After 20 cumulative hours of taping my mouth in the first month, I could feel I was breathing far less and had conquered the restlessness in my chest. After three months, I realized that, for the first time in my adult life, I was holding eye contact with others while breathing calmly through the nose. I also found that when I was having a conversation with someone, I would close my mouth as soon as I stopped talking. This shifted my entire style of communication from overexcited and frivolous to levelheaded and measured.

Everyone should be breathing exclusively through their nose even while sleeping. Many nose-breathing adherents recommend taping the mouth shut before going to sleep to strengthen nocturnal nasal breathing.[10] They claim, and I agree, that it helps you fall asleep more quickly, stay asleep longer, and wake feeling energized. It also limits snoring, stops drooling, keeps the mouth and throat from getting dry, reduces bad breath, and keeps you in the diaphragmatic sweet spot throughout the night. For all these reasons, I strongly recommend you tape your mouth before bed. However, it is a sharp right turn into hard diaphragmatic demand. You might need to work your way up to it using other Program Peace breathing exercises (including taping your mouth during the day) before you can start to tape your mouth at bedtime.

Breathing Exercise #11.2: *Taping Your Mouth During Sleep*

Put a piece of tape over your lips before your head hits the pillow. When most people start, they wake up with discomfort in their chest. This happens because their chest was kept from heaving throughout the night. If you feel this way, it means that you must do more remedial diaphragmatic breathing first. The soreness in your chest upon waking is a measure of how non-diaphragmatic your breathing is and how much your habitual breathing pattern fights against calm, restorative breathing.

Some people claim that they cannot breathe through their nose due to nasal obstruction or congestion. If this is true for you, know that your nasal passages will clear from nasal breathing practice. Mine certainly did. Before taping my mouth, I was lucky to have one nostril clear of congestion. However, you should find that after you start taping your mouth, the congestion clears on its own. Just like you don't let dry eyes keep you from widening your eyes or dry lips keep you from smiling, don't let a stuffy nasal cavity keep you from breathing through your nose. You might want to try nasal irrigation (i.e., a neti pot, Nasaline, or nasal relief spray), a personal hygiene practice used for flushing excess mucus and debris from the nasal cavity and sinuses.

Also, make an effort to breathe through the nose while chewing. Because I breathe through my nose now, I can close my mouth while I chew. Thus, much to the pleasant surprise of my friends and family, I no longer smack my lips.

The "alternate nostril breathing" technique is common in yoga and stress reduction circles. In this exercise, the index finger is used to close one nostril at a time. Many hypotheses have been advanced regarding why breathing through only one nostril seems to have a calming effect on people. Some scientists think you can activate different hemispheres of the brain this way. I think blocking one nostril works because it narrows the breathing bottleneck even further, increasing the resistance and necessitating that each breath is even slower and smoother. Try it. There are many guided alternate nostril breathing exercises online.

Modern-day hunter-gatherers are known to be nose breathers, and even the persistence running they do during prolonged hunts is accomplished with the mouth closed. As you get better at nose breathing, force yourself to breathe exclusively through the nose during exercise. Keep tissues with you if you need to. Blow your nose frequently, and train as often as you can with your mouth closed.

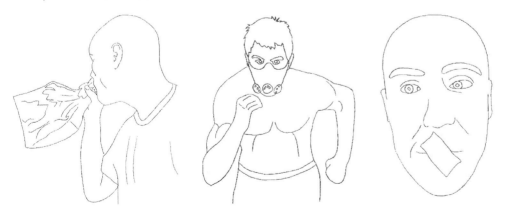

Illustration 11.2: Hyperventilating man breathing into a paper bag; B. Man running with an elevation training mask; C. Man with tape over the mouth to ensure nose breathing.

Months of paced breathing helped, but breathing exclusively through the nose was still a challenge for me when I started. Inspired by the writings of Konstantin Buteyko and George Catlin, I forced myself to do it. You haven't accomplished it until every time you think to notice, you find yourself breathing through the nose. Don't try to accomplish exclusive nasal breathing in a matter of weeks. Give yourself at least a few months to make a comfortable transition to exclusive nose breathing. Teaching myself to breathe through my nose made diaphragmatic breathing much more accessible and gave me a whole new level of composure and poise. Breathe through the nose as much as possible. It calms your mind and turns your breathing musculature into a powerful, relentless, irrepressible bellows.

The Slowest, Smallest Breath

When you breathe with a smooth flow rate, you should feel that your breath proceeds at an even tack. You should hear and feel a constant stream of breath that doesn't vary in speed. I think the best way to perfect a smooth flow rate is to inhale as little and as slowly as possible. When you do this, the tumultuous discontinuities (apneic disturbances) discussed in Chapter 3 become magnified. This enables you to perceive them and work to "iron them out."

Breathing Exercise #11.3: *The Slowest, Smallest Breath*

After a couple of deep breaths, take a single inhalation that is a tiny continuous sip of air. It should be long in duration (from 10 seconds to a minute) and deep (from the bottom of your expiratory reserve to the top of your inspiratory reserve). Take in as little air as possible, as slowly as possible, without pausing. After you finish inhaling, breathe normally for a few breaths, then repeat. Steady your breath so that you override the shudders and shivers in the flow of air. It should feel like a long, drawn-out note on a saxophone, a rocket ship sailing smoothly out of the atmosphere, or a slow ride down a gently sloped slide made from warm butter. Sometimes it helps me to visualize the slow but steady propulsion made possible by hundreds of millipede legs working in unison. Continue to practice this, making your goal to breathe slowly and evenly all the time.

Breathing slowly like this feels dangerous—either like you are not getting enough air or like it is too much work. Some of the most archaic brain areas ring their alarm bells when they can tell that the conscious system is imposing a slow diaphragmatic breath. Deep down, our unconscious mind is afraid that the diaphragm will be overexerted and that this will lead to death by some form of cardiorespiratory fatigue. It is afraid that we will ignore the pain signals from our weary breathing musculature and succumb to diaphragmatic failure. And it is true that if a person who is a heavy hyperventilator that takes in 20 breaths per minute was forced to switch to four breaths per minute without any deviation, the abrupt change in demand could lead to respiratory shutdown after many hours. However, a few minutes of diaphragmatic fatigue is not going to kill you. You don't want to push it too hard for hours at a time, but you must get past this instinctual dread of exerting the diaphragm.

To do this, embrace the feeling of "suffocating" yourself with the slowest, smallest breath exercise. These breaths should feel like prolonged, streamlined sighs that "ooze" in and out of your body. Taking extremely slow inhalations will strengthen your diaphragm and teach your mind to control it on a very precise and fine-grained scale, putting an end to hyperventilation.

When you perform exercise 11.3 above, imagine that you are training to be the best in the world. Pretend that the national pastime consists of stepping up to home plate, pressing your nostril against a microphone, and taking the smoothest inhalation and the smoothest exhalation you possibly can. You want to inspire the entire stadium, as well as the folks watching at home, with how constant and unperturbed your breath is. Of course, we will never get the opportunity to show off in this way. However, if you breathe as if you are training for it, the results will significantly affect your every word, thought, and action. It will also make your breath extremely quiet.

Several Eastern arts, such as tai chi, yoga, and qi gong, recognize the importance of quiet, gentle breathing. Japanese legend holds that samurai would be tested by placing a feather under their nose. If the feather wavered, then they were not ready to progress. Qi gong master Chris Pei explains, "Generally speaking, there are three levels of breathing. The first one is to breathe softly so that a person standing next to you does not hear you breathing. The second level is to breathe softly so that you do not hear yourself breathing. And the third level is to breathe softly so that you do not feel yourself breathing." The Chinese practice of Taoism defines ideal breathing as "so smooth that the fine hairs within the nostrils remain motionless." In the 6th-century B.C. Chinese philosopher Lao Tzu said, "The perfect man breathes as if he is not breathing."

I find these quotes inspiring, and I do believe that quiet breathing is an indicator of diaphragmatic health and precludes hyperventilation. However, the breath cannot always be inaudible. When you first transition to nasal breathing, it is often loud. Don't necessarily suppress your breath to make it quiet and don't be embarrassed by the sound of your breathing. Instead, be proud that others will hear how smooth and deep it is.

Calming Your Gasping Reflex

As discussed in Chapter 3, your default tidal range can be expanded by taking longer, deeper breaths. But your tidal range can also be reduced by teaching your body that it is safe to take more shallow breaths. When you first try to take several shallow breaths in a row, your diaphragm and other breathing muscles will stubbornly resist the process. Again, your nervous system will be afraid to let them relax. This is why breathing less feels uncomfortable and can be downright scary. It brings you face to face with your gasping mechanism.

It is difficult to breathe in a tidal range that is shallower than usual (as in diagram C in Figure 11.1 above) because it exposes a reflexive gasp that powers your every inhalation. Once you are breathing more shallowly than usual, you can feel the jerk from this gasp in your chest. It initiates each inhalation and is essentially a violent convulsion and another manifestation of trauma keeping you in fight or flight. The more time you spend breathing less, the more you experience it and the more you calm it. Calming it will tremendously reduce your tendency to hyperventilate. You can use the following exercise to do this.

Breathing Exercise #11.4: *Depowering the Heaving Gasp*

For one or two minutes, take breaths that are vastly shallower than you are accustomed to. Imagine merely taking in a few teaspoons of air. Spend about between one and three seconds on each inhalation and exhalation (.5x.5 to 1.5x1.5). When executing this pattern, the breathing muscles should be about as close to resting as they can be, moving very little. You are hypoventilating.

By the fifth to tenth breath, you should feel a sense of air hunger. This sensation of suffocation or smothering is too soon to be a legitimate need for oxygen. Instead, it is the feeling of your hyperactive breathing musculature fighting against your decision to breathe less. The discomfort should be centered around the beginning of the inhalation. Your chest is trying to involuntarily kickstart a gasp, but you are not letting it. It should feel a bit like a hiccup coming on. This should create the feeling that you need a deep inhalation and are having trouble catching your breath.

Become immersed in the sensations surrounding your gasp reflex and try to calm it for the remaining breaths. Once you have been breathing like this for twenty seconds to a minute and the feeling of air hunger starts to kick in, allow yourself to take a few normal, deeper breaths to reoxygenate and then try again. Use this exercise to learn to feel comfortable breathing much less and transform the violent, spastic contraction that initiates your inhalation into a gentle, gradual one.

I think the exercise above brings you into contact with the cramp in your diaphragm. It is the portion of the diaphragm that is always heaving in an effort carry on with hyperventilation. It is trying to overpower your current rate. It is doing this because your body is afraid that you are not going to get enough oxygen to deal with the environment that it assumes is adverse. By ignoring the gasp and feeling the air hunger you get a panicky sensation. By attenuating your breath, you ignore the panic. You should get this feeling sometimes as you come down from exercising. Treat it as if that is all it is. Even though you are not exercising, feel comfortable coming down a whole level. It is the ultimate form of underreacting and it sends a message to the body that says, "There is no way we need that much oxygen right now."

You may have to be experiencing anxiety for this to happen, but when performing the exercise above, people often breathe like an actor in a scary movie and it may feel "horrific." That gasp reflex is trying to break through. We normally try to avoid this sensation at all costs. It is like a big wave hitting the body. The idea is to let the waves hit and prove to your body that it doesn't hurt and breathing less is not the end of the world. Not startling in response to it is detraumatizing. I think this is what Buteyko was trying to lead people to do, but he didn't articulate it this way.

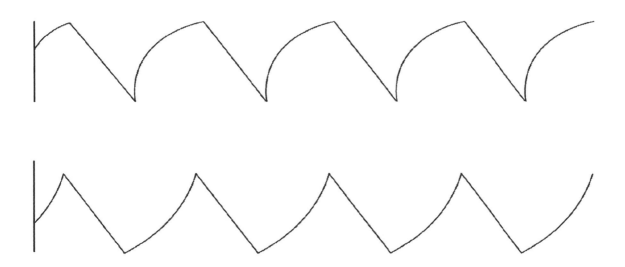

Figure 11.2: The first sine wave depicts a gasping form of inhalation. The slope starts steeply, indicating an abrupt force at the beginning. This is a violent and exhausting way to breathe that perpetuates hyperventilation and stress. The second wave depicts a relaxed form of inhalation that is not powered by an initial jerk of the breathing musculature. In both waves, the exhalation is shown as a straight line to simplify.

Breath Holding

Many breathing exercises utilize breath holding. They come with names like breath restriction, hypoventilation training, and hypoxic therapy. There are even paced breathing routines that ask you to hold your breath between each inhalation and exhalation. The popular 4-4-6-2 exercise asks you to inhale for four seconds, hold your breath for four, exhale for six, hold the breath for two, and then repeat. Try it. The 4-7-8-0 technique is also very popular. The 5-5-5-5 version is a drill. Sometimes called "box breathing," it is utilized by the military to calm and rehabilitate warfighters with PTSD. I think breath-holding exercises like these can be helpful, but I do not recommend holding the breath during paced breathing because practicing so many pauses may influence you to hold your breath habitually without realizing it. Due to the strong association between breath holding and anxiety, I think this is counterproductive. Still, doing it for as long as you can a few times per week might be beneficial. Holding the breath causes panic. By desensitizing yourself to this panic, you may harden yourself against trauma.

Breathing Exercise #11.5: *Breath Hold*

Start by taking a deep inhalation while lying down and then exhale most of it. Next, close your mouth and time yourself (using the stopwatch on your smartphone) to see how long it takes you to experience air hunger. Hold your breath as long as you can. Try to work up to holding your breath in this way for 20 seconds, then 30. After a few weeks, you should be able to get near a full minute.

You should feel strong discomfort in your chest and an unrestrainable desire to resume breathing. Calmly expose yourself to this unpleasant feeling for a least a few seconds. Your body will feel restless, and you should feel a pulsating sensation in your chest. Focus on bringing absolute peace to this reaction, as if you were ignoring the siren of a passing ambulance. As soon as you stop and take that first gasp, go right back to diaphragmatic breathing. This will teach your body not to fear the pain of suffocation and not to perceive it as a lethal state.

The first sincere desire for air will occur with an involuntary contraction of the diaphragm. The diaphragm starts to push and pull involuntarily to get breathing going again. The amount of time it takes for you to feel this sensation is a good measure of general breathing health. Many people will experience diaphragmatic contractions between 10 and 20 seconds. Breath holding practitioners maintain that a person who breathes optimally will not experience this until 30-40 seconds.

The more you practice the exercise above, the longer you will be able to hold your breath before you feel your diaphragm attempt to kickstart the breath. Buteyko adherents call the practice of breath holding the "control pause." It is also known as the "blood oxygen level test" (BOLT), and using the four rules will help improve this score. Breath holding is thought to improve your blood's oxygen-carrying capacity and increase the maximum volume of oxygen that you can use in exhaustive exercise. This metric is known by athletes as VO_2 max and is highly coveted.[11]

Stressful situations (such as a tense conversation that involves gasping and breath-holding) often lead to feelings of air hunger. Intermittent air hunger contributes to anxiety. So, once you have spent a few days desensitizing yourself to the sensations involved in breath-holding, you will notice that you feel calmer in general. You will realize that a fear of suffocation regularly intruded into your everyday life but that it does this no more.

Rapid, Shallow Breathing

Earlier in this chapter, we discussed how constant hyperventilation is extremely unhealthy. Deliberate hyperventilation on the order of a few seconds, however, may be health-promoting. Many forms of breathwork induce hyperventilation. Tummo breathing is an ancient Tibetan example. Similar forms such as holotropic breathing and the Wim Hof method have recently become popular. Each of these involves taking very rapid, full breaths for minutes at a time, often followed by breath holds. This voluntary hyperventilation leads to high levels of oxygen, low levels of carbon dioxide, the feeling of pins and needles, and even panic. But if you can expose yourself to these sensations without panicking, you can further desensitize yourself to stress. I recommend voluntary acute hyperventilation (try the Wim Hof guided breathing session on YouTube) because I think numbing yourself to it is another experience that will strengthen you as a person.

Insufficient skill in coordinating the transition between rapid inhalations and exhalations is a manifestation of trauma. For example, it keeps you from being able to project your voice strongly and decisively during times of tension. Building better coordination over the switch between breaths may make you a less hesitant, more confident breather. One reason I believe this is that chimpanzees perform rapid, loud panting displays daily. These are called ventilating displays or pant-hoots and are used to indicate dominance. They are more intense and more frequent in highly ranked individuals. The higher a chimp's dominance rank within its party, the more intensely it pant-hoots.[12] Pant-hoots are most common in the presence of high-quality food or females in estrus, indicating that it is used during social competition to designate status and priority. These vocalizations are set to almost violently fast breathing and are used to prove to others that the vocal and respiratory systems are robust.

The pant-hoot is a series of deep yells that take place while rapidly switching between inhalations and exhalations. Each cycle lasts between a half and a quarter of a second. Perform a video search on the internet for the term "pant-hoot," listen to the sound, and try to recreate it yourself. You might also search for an episode of the Arsenio Hall talk show from the 1990s. The pant-hoot was used by the audience in a collegial, energetic way to show support for the host or his guests. The crowd would often swing their arms above their head and hoot uncompromisingly. You will find that hooting is very strenuous at first yet becomes facile over just a few days. This may seem like another bizarre exercise, but remember, Program Peace is all about finding weaknesses in the body and rehabilitating them to find new strength, especially when this strength is associated with dominance in closely related animals.

Breathing Exercise #11.6: *Pant-Hooting*

Practice breathing in and out at very short intervals while vocalizing loudly. You should be imitating a chimpanzee pant-hoot that you listened to online. Alternate between inhalation and exhalation around two to five times per second. Do it rhythmically and with control. During each exhalation, yell "hoo" loudly and deeply. It should be like a bark. Time yourself using your phone's stopwatch. At first, try to reach 30 seconds of intense hooting. Over several weeks, you should be able to do it for more than a minute. Once you reach proficiency, you can try doing what the chimps do, and vocalize not just on the exhalations but the inhalations as well.

As you do this, you will notice that every few times you switch, your breathing will falter. Your timing will be off because you don't have fine enough control over the transitions between inhalations and exhalations. This kind of poor respiratory coordination may be a contributor to autonomic dysregulation. Use this exercise to iron through these irregularities and unbrace and strengthen the muscles involved. After a minute of pant-hooting intensely, your chest and voice will feel agitated. However, if you concentrate on letting the muscles go limp afterward, they will relax deeply. You will feel calmer and notice that your voice is stronger and deeper for up to a day.

I believe that humans and chimps add tension to the aspect of the diaphragm responsible for the pant-hoot as a function of their social standing. They do this as part of a submissive display that self-handicaps the bark and roar, both of which are powered by the diaphragm. This is why only the most dominant chimps are capable of performing an optimal pant-hoot. Pant-hooting loudly and forcefully will drive this underused aspect of your diaphragm into full fatigue, allowing it to recover from the tension you have imposed on it for years. I strongly believe that after just a handful of sessions, you will realize that the pant-hoot achieves a diaphragmatic detox, reaching into and purging the nucleus of your anxiety.

Completely avoiding breathing at short intervals is like being an endurance runner who never sprints. I think it is important to spend time every day not trying to lengthen or even control the breath. Let it get as shallow as it wants and breathe through your mouth if it feels right. Forget about the rules of diaphragmatic breathing sometimes and let the unconscious breath regulation modules do what they will. Stated simply, allow yourself to breathe shallowly once in a while as a form of cross-training.

Stretch and Flex the Diaphragm

The next exercise provides a great maneuver to stretch and contract your stale, stiff diaphragm. This stretch will bring it blood and help make it stronger and better at its job. Think back to the hiccup activity from Chapter 3. When simulating a hiccup, you sealed off your glottis (the vocal opening in the throat) and contracted your diaphragm. Using the following maneuver, you will similarly close the glottis so no air can enter the lungs and contract the diaphragm as if you were inhaling, creating a brief vacuum.

By restricting the flow of air, closure of the glottis isolates the diaphragm in a fixed position, allowing it to contract isometrically. To contract it, you only have to try to breathe in. With the glottis closed, you won't be able to, but trying will pull the central tendon of the diaphragm down toward the abdominal cavity, stretching the entire diaphragm as well as the organs near it. Again, I thought I originated this exercise, but after entering a description into a search engine, I found that it is a variant of an age-old yoga pose called uddiyana bandha, or "flying abdominal lock."

Breathing Exercise #11.7: *Isometric Contraction of the Diaphragm*

Lie down and breathe out completely, blowing on your fingertip until you cannot blow out anymore. Then, close and seal your glottis. This makes it impossible to breathe. From here, you can fully engage the diaphragm by trying to either breathe in or out.

1) Attempt to breathe in. You will not be able to, and the harder you try, the better stretch you will get. Try to extend this contraction up into your rib cage and hold it for at least five seconds. This may make you cough, which is fine. While contracting the diaphragm, alter the position of your trunk and thoracic spine. This will allow you to flex hard into your diaphragm at different angles. This may lead to a satisfying crack.

2) Attempt to breathe out forcefully, pressing the stomach outward at the same time. Again, the harder you press, the better the stretch. Try to hold this for at least five seconds.

From either of these two positions, you should be able to find a very achy contraction. This is the cramp in the diaphragm that has formed as a consequence of bracing and chronic hyperventilation. Now that you have isolated it, you can gradually work through it.

There are other ways to isolate and contract the diaphragm isometrically. Breathing deeply from some yoga positions offers challenging opportunities for diaphragmatic stimulation. I want to strongly encourage you to try a full inhalation from either a forward fold or plow pose because these yoga positions decrease the volume of the abdominal cavity, forcing the diaphragm to work harder than it normally does. Full breaths from these positions are hard work with a big payoff.

Intraoral Myofascial Release for the Nasopharynx

You have an extensive muscular knot behind your face that comes from constricting the nasopharynx. The nasopharynx is an opening in the back of the throat, just behind the uvula. My nasopharyngeal sphincter was highly tense and painful. Contraction of the nasopharynx is a natural reflex that occurs during swallowing to prevent food or liquid from going up into the nose, but bracing it is another manifestation of trauma. People brace it out of fear of appearing "too calm." This knot becomes tighter every time you feel stressed. It contributes to wincing and grimacing and it gets worse every day because it is never massaged or even touched. I advocate that you perform compression and self-massage specifically for your nasopharynx. It is very uncomfortable at first, but it gets easier every time, and it only takes a few weeks to get rid of the pain completely.

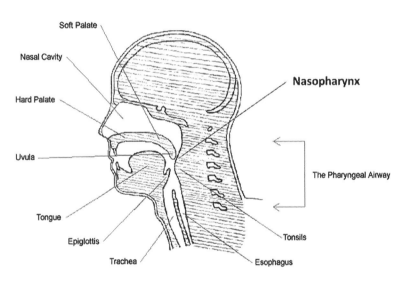

Illustration 11.3: The nasopharynx is a small opening just behind the uvula that connects the oral cavity with the nasal cavity.

You can provide compression to your nasopharynx by donning a plastic glove, putting your thumb into your mouth and up into your nasopharyngeal opening. This opening is where your nasal passage connects with your throat. To do this, insert your thumb into your mouth as if you were sucking on your thumb. To find the opening, you must feel around the roof of your mouth, traveling away from the teeth and toward the area where the hard roof of the mouth (hard palate) turns soft (soft palate). An inch behind (posterior to) this border is the uvula, a fleshy hanging structure. Just behind the uvula is the opening of the nasopharynx. The nasopharynx is an invagination that you want to explore and massage using one of your thumbs. The opening will feel tight and painful, and pressing against it will initiate a gag reflex. The best way to bypass the gagging is to breathe diaphragmatically, preferably to a breath metronome. Within the first week, you will notice that it is less painful to probe, that your face feels and looks calmer, and that mucus clearance is easier.

Breathing Exercise #11.8: *Massaging the Nasopharynx*

Put on a plastic glove. With your thumb inside your nasopharynx, you can place strong pressure on many muscles and soft tissues in the nasopharynx and nasal cavity. When you start, simply insert the thumb past the first knuckle and keep it still. It will feel sore, itchy, and scratchy, like a sore throat. Next, try to swallow a few times and feel the nasopharyngeal sphincter tighten and loosen around your thumb. The first few times, this may be very uncomfortable, but it should be painless within a few weeks.

Next, you want to gently press your thumb into different areas, massaging the soft tissues, stimulating the nerves, reducing tension in the accompanying muscles, and bringing needed blood to the area. You want to press against each of the walls and folds of the nasopharynx and even up into the nasopharyngeal ceiling. The padded side of your thumb (opposite the side with the fingernail) will come into contact with the anterior portion of this muscle (closest to the face). You want to press into it firmly while contracting it intermittently to exercise it and gain a conscious ability to coordinate its movement. As usual, learning how to control it will teach you how to relax it.

It is essential to employ paced breathing and focus concertedly on remaining calm before, during, and after this exercise. Influencing how your brain interprets intense forms of stimulation is incredibly decisive in how your body copes with them. I also recommend doing this while relaxing at home before sleep. While you have the rubber glove on, I recommend that you use the thumb to press into muscular areas all over the soft palate.

You can massage the tongue as well. This can be done in two ways: (1) squeeze your tongue between your thumb and forefinger, or (2) use your middle finger to gently compress the length of your tongue down toward the floor of your mouth. Allow your tongue to go limp and drop down to a lower point in your throat. Unbracing your tongue and allowing it to become flat and broad at its base will help relax your voice, the topic of the next chapter.

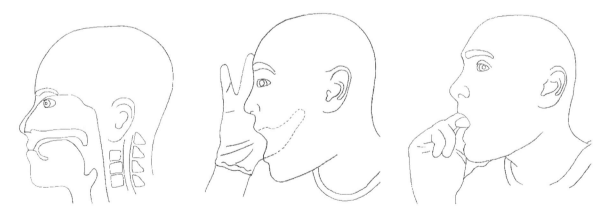

Illustration 11.4: A. Nasal cavity and nasopharynx; B. Man inserting thumb into nasopharynx; C. Man squeezing tongue.

Have you ever heard of mewing? It is a popular do-it-yourself facial restructuring technique developed by Dr. Mike Mew, a British orthodontist. Mewing involves flattening out the tongue against the roof of the mouth (the hard palate). The tip of the tongue is placed on or near the top front teeth and the body of the tongue is placed on the roof of the mouth. Proponents claim that learning to rest the tongue here habitually will define the jawline and change the shape of the face for the better. Like many similar techniques (including most of the exercises in this book), there is not enough scientific evidence yet to support the practice. However, it is interesting to point out that resting the tongue against the roof of the mouth seems prevalent in most mammals and human infants. This indicates to me that resting the tongue on the floor of the mouth (not mewing) may be a traumatized posture associated with mouth breathing and a widened airway diameter facilitating hyperventilation (discussed in the next chapter). I think it is possible that mewing could aid in nose breathing, expressionlessness, reducing oral and pharyngeal bracing, decreasing vocal tension, and reinforcing ujjayi breath (also discussed in the next chapter).

Pair Diaphragmatic Breathing with Anything and Everything

I hope you feel you now have more tools to ensure that your diaphragm is working properly. When it is working, it pacifies your interpretation of and responses to any experiences you have. It helped turn my nasopharynx from a "pit of pain" to a painless, normally functioning part of my body. I believe that this diaphragmatic generalization can similarly enhance the positive externalities from many forms of traditional and alternative therapy. Existing forms of therapy that may be vastly augmented by proper breathing may include:

Mainstream Therapies: yoga, psychotherapy, relaxation techniques, muscle and joint rehabilitation, mindfulness-based stress reduction, chiropractic, acupuncture, osteopathy, cognitive behavioral therapy, medical massage, neurotherapy, biofeedback, positive affirmation, somatic therapy, etc.

Exercise and Movement Based Therapies: personal training, physical therapy, Pilates, tai chi, qigong, martial arts, acroyoga, dance, the Gyrotonic Method, Gyrokinesis, the Franklin Method, the Alexander Technique, Feldenkrais, Nia, ChiWalking, ballistic stretching, proprioceptive neuromuscular facilitation, gymnastics, Laban Movement Analysis, somatics, etc.

Complementary, Holistic, and Alternative Therapies: meditation, prayer, cold showering, electronic pulse massage, abdominal or visceral massage, kneading, petrissage, craniofacial manipulation, gua sha and Mei Zen acupuncture, muscle stripping, guided therapeutic imagery, active release technique, Rolfing, craniosacral therapy, tantric sex, eye movement desensitization and reprocessing, visceral massage, colonic irrigation, reiki, autogenic training, hypnosis, mewing, ASMR, forest bathing, art therapy, animal therapy, etc.

Conclusion

After you perform the breathing exercises from this chapter and Chapter 3 for 12 weeks, you will notice that many of the people you know breathe two to three breaths for every breath you take. Relative to the new you, everyone else will be hyperventilating.

Chapter 11: **Bullet Points**

- Distress causes over-breathing, also known as hyperventilation, which is strongly associated with anxiety and has many negative symptoms and repercussions.
- Taking exaggeratedly slow breaths will put you on an "air diet," reducing distressed breathing and hyperventilation.
- You want your diaphragm to approximate a large piston moving in slow motion.
- Because nasal breathing forces you to breathe more slowly, it will strengthen the diaphragm and greatly reduce distressed breathing. Taping the mouth helps with this.
- Breathing in for as long as you can will force the diaphragm to contract completely, expanding its range, pushing it to fatigue, and allowing it to rest afterward.
- Stretching the diaphragm and contracting it isometrically will make it stronger and increase its range of motion.
- Breath holding, mewing, and pant-hooting may help rehabilitate your breathing habits.
- Providing compression to the nasopharynx, soft palate, and tongue will remove trauma in these areas.

Program Peace: *Breathing Exercise Progress Tracker*

Use the boxes below to tally your number of hours of nasal breathing as in Exercise 11.1.

Hours Nasal Breathing								

Use a stopwatch to see how long you can prolong an inhalation and an exhalation as in Exercise 11.3. Use the table below to keep track of your best times.

Longest Inhalation								
Longest Exhalation								

Use a stopwatch to see how long you can hypoventilate as in Exercise 11.4. Use the table below to keep track of your best times.

Longest Hypovent.								

Use a stopwatch to see how long you can hold your breath as in Exercise 11.5. Use the table below to keep track of your best times.

Longest Breath Hold								

Use a stopwatch to see how long you can pant-hoot as in Exercise 11.6. Use the table below to keep track of your best times.

Longest Pant-hoot								

Use a stopwatch to see how long you can hold an isometric contraction of the diaphragm as in Exercise 11.7. Use the table below to keep track of your best times.

Longest Dia. Contraction								

Chapter 11: **Endnotes**

1.   Sauty, A., & Prosper, M. (2008). The hyperventilation syndrome. *Revue medicale suisse*, *4*(180), 2502–2505.

2.   Sauty & Prosper, 2008, The hyperventilation syndrome.

3.   Naifeh, K. H. (1994). Basic anatomy and physiology of the respiratory system and the autonomic nervous system. In B. H. Timmons R. Ley (Eds.), *Behavioral and psychological approaches to breathing disorders*, (pp. 17–47). Springer.

4.   McKeown, P. (2015). *The Oxygen advantage: The simple, scientifically proven breathing technique that will revolutionize your health and fitness*. Harper Collins.

5.   Staubli, M., Vogel, F., Bärtsch, P., Flückiger, G., & Ziegler, W. H. (1994). Hyperventilation-induced changes of blood cell counts depend on hypocapnia. *European Journal of Applied Physiology and Occupational Physiology*, *69*(5), 402–407.

6.   Rosalba, C. (2008). Strengths, weaknesses, and possibilities of the Buteyko Breathing Method. *Biofeedback*, *36*(2), 59–63.

7.   Fried, R. (2013). *The psychology and physiology of breathing: In behavioral medicine, clinical psychology, and psychiatry*. Springer Science.

8.   Park, Y. S. (2012). *Sleep, interrupted: A physician reveals the # 1 reason why so many of us are sick and tired*. Jodev Press.

9.   Park et al., 2012, *Sleep, interrupted*; Morais-Almeida, M., Wandalsen, G. F., & Sole, D. (2019). Growth and mouth breathers. *Jornal de Pediatria*, *95*(1), 66–71; Masahiro, S., Sano, S., & Kato, T. (2013). Increased oxygen load in the prefrontal cortex: A vector-based near-infrared spectroscopy study. *Neuroreport*, *24*(17), 935–940.

10. Nestor, J. (2020). *Breath: The new science of a lost art*. Penguin.

11. McKeown, P. (2015). *The Oxygen advantage: The simple, scientifically proven breathing technique that will revolutionize your health and fitness*. Harper Collins.

12. Fedurek, P., Donnellan, E., & Slocombe, K. E. (2014). Social and ecological correlates of long-distance pant hoot calls in male chimpanzees. *Behavioral Ecology and Sociobiology*, *68*(8), 1345–1355.

Chapter 12: **Release Vocal Tension**

"A determined man, by his very attitude and the tone of his voice, puts a stop to defeat, and begins to conquer." — *Ralph Waldo Emerson (1803-1882)*

There is an intimate connection between the voice and well-being. Our voices are right at the center of how we feel about ourselves and how we interact with the people around us. For most of us, however, interpersonal pressures and internal discomforts gradually put stress on our vocal cords. This chapter deals with the causes of this critical source of bodily dysfunction, then gives you a detailed and accessible guide to undoing it, building on the work you've done in previous chapters. It will cover healthier vocalization, clear articulation, coughing, yawning, muscle strengthening, and how to find relief from your internal monologue. First, let's touch on the basic facts.

The vocal cords are two membranes in the throat that are spread apart when breathing and pulled together for speech. When they are touching, and air from an exhalation is forced through them, they vibrate against each other, giving rise to the voice. Sound is generated as a steady flow of air is chopped up by the cords into little puffs of sound waves. More than a dozen different muscles manipulate the vocal cords within the voice box (larynx). We modulate our speech sounds by contracting these muscles along with muscles of the tongue, mouth, lips, and an entire wall of muscles extending from the voice box to the last molar. All of these muscles take on trigger points and partial contraction from intermittent bracing.

That brings us to the link between voice and emotion. Behavioral ecologists have long noted that dominance displays in mammals feature low-pitched vocalizations while subordination displays feature high-pitched squeals and whimpers. In primates, high-pitched noises are common during juvenile play, submissive threats, appeasement, and begging for food. Human voices similarly rise in pitch as a result of insecurity, stress, and social submission. Higher pitch is caused by vocal cord tension: the tauter the cords are, the faster they vibrate back and forth, and the higher the frequency of the sound they produce.

Voice pitch rises when we ask for a favor, apologize, whine, or attempt to show affection or goodwill. Negative emotion, in general, increases the pitch of the voice. When you are nervous or scared, for instance, the muscles around the larynx automatically tighten up, involuntarily creating a higher-pitched sound. In Chapter 7, we saw how the brain's grief system elicits reflexive distress vocalizations in mammals and birds. It ensures that lost babies call out for their mothers. Our grievances activate this ancient neural pathway, intensifying vocal bracing. When we are anxious, we are, in essence (even in silence), calling out for our mothers.

Dominant voices maintain or lower in pitch when finishing a sentence. Lowering intonation midsentence conveys unshaken confidence. Submissive voices do the opposite, rising in pitch as if asking a question. This is commonly known as upward inflection. When you speak at an artificially high pitch, you can strain your larynx in as little as a few minutes. Accumulated over months and years, that strain changes the resonance of your voice, making it softer and higher. This effect—when tension in the vocal muscles affects the voice—is called *muscle tension dysphonia*. When this condition leads to pain and inflammation in the larynx, it is called *globus pharyngis*, or *laryngitis* when truly acute.[1] Few of us are formally diagnosed with these ailments, but we all have hoarseness and diminished voices from the self-imposed repetitive strain on our vocal muscles.

Have you ever found that when you are in a calm state (i.e., after a massage or upon waking), your voice is very deep, loud, and full? Your voice sounded like that because you gave it a rest from bracing. That is your true voice and should be your voice all the time. To reclaim it, all you need to do is learn to stop tensing it.

I used to talk in an artificially high voice all the time, and there were many friends with whom I would never speak in my normal voice for fear of offending them. By age 25, this led to my normal voice being completely unavailable, and it continued to get weaker every year. The sustained high-pitch mangled my voice. It wrenched my larynx, took all the bass out of my speech, and ruined my singing ability. By the time I turned 30, even my ability to modulate and inflect was greatly reduced. The weakness in my voice led me to talk and socialize less. My laryngeal posture became so compromised that I developed a persistent lump in my throat.

The constriction in my gullet affected my swallowing, too, and I developed dysphagia. The airway around my voice box was so tight that I would choke at almost every meal. The following exercises and techniques completely resolved this problem. The lump in my throat is gone, and the improvement in my voice has been profound. Use the exercises in this chapter to get the frog out of your throat and turn your croaking into crooning. We will start, once again, by applying deep breathing to the situation.

Diaphragmatic Vocalization

Enter the terms "vocal cord endoscopy" into a video search engine to see the vocal cords in action. When you watch this medical exam, you can hear the doctor giving the patient instructions about when to vocalize and when to be silent. You will see multiple muscles in the throat contracting to modulate the patient's voice. If you watch carefully, you should notice the patient contract the muscles that pull the vocal cords together in preparation for speech before any vocalization begins. You are most likely to spot it if the doctor interrupts the patient before they start speaking, at which point you can see the musculature either stay tense or return to rest. Seeing this will make you question how often you unknowingly tense the muscles of your vocal apparatus in anticipation of speech, even when you are not speaking. In reality, we are constantly bracing our vocal musculature in neurotic preparation for high-pitched speech.

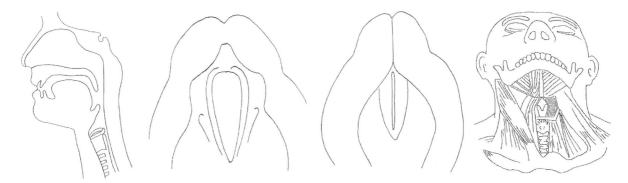

Illustration 12.1: A. Side view of vocal cords; B. Vocal cords open from above; C. Vocal cords closed; D. Exterior throat anatomy with the voice box in the center

When you go to a loud party or concert and your voice is frazzled the following day, it is not because you were yelling too loudly. Rather, it is because you yelled with strained vocal cords and then braced them for the remainder of the evening while breathing thoracically. Our vocal apparatus was designed for shouting, but not for shouting combined with shallow breathing. That is a very different type of muscular stress and one we are not well equipped to endure.

Most people hyperventilate when they speak, often needlessly doubling their intake of air. The discomfort of hyperventilation is a major contributor to the widespread fear of public speaking. This tendency causes us to speak in an even shallower tidal range than the one we breathe in. The breathing exercises from Chapters 3 and 11 will expand this range, allowing you to continue speaking when your lungs are nearly empty. That greater range adds depth to your voice. Any speech expert (or "vocologist") will tell you that practicing diaphragmatic breathing is one of the best ways to achieve a better-sounding voice. As you will see in the next exercise, breathing diaphragmatically while vocalizing is even better.

Vocal Exercise #12.1: *Sing Loudly without Gasping*

Sing from memory or along to a song. Don't let yourself gasp. When it comes time to inhale, do so completely without singing, even if the vocalist in the song you are listening to is singing. Once you have taken in a full breath, resume singing until you have no more air left to exhale. You might do this in the car or with headphones on.

Select songs that make you feel powerful. Pull up the lyrics online and read along if it helps. Sing your heart out. Singing loudly will make your voice stronger very quickly, and doing it with passion will produce endorphins and confidence. Bring your voice to a healthy state of fatigue over and over, taking breaks between songs to let it go completely limp. The more you do this exercise, the closer your standard social voice will come to that audacious singing voice.

The next exercise will ask you to make several types of vocalizations, including yelling, while breathing diaphragmatically. Coupled with distressed breathing, these exercises would wear out your voice or even damage it. But diaphragmatic breathing protects it by disallowing vocal bracing and the activation of the sympathetic nervous system. After several minutes of practice, this will allow you to start vocalizing with, and rehabbing, muscles that were previously stuck in partial contraction. These exercises will also train your vocal muscles to coordinate more efficiently, resulting in more sound production with less energy expenditure.

Vocal Exercise #12.2: *Diaphragmatic Vocalization*

Perform the following vocalizations after taking a deep, smooth inhalation. Once your lungs are full, vocalize until you are almost out of breath. Repeat. Choose a location like a closet or a car—somewhere you won't be apprehensive about being overheard. Let loose. The real work of these exercises involves paying attention to the wavering and instability in your voice and using repetition to smooth out such weaknesses. Full-range vocalization repeated over and over will tune up the voice by teaching your diaphragm to provide your vocal cords with constant, unfaltering air pressure.

1) Take a deep breath and sing a single note (or a scale) until you are out of air. Do this loudly. Bellow. Keep singing/exhaling until you have absolutely no air left. The last few seconds will be uncomfortable, but it will start to feel good after completing the exercise a few times over the course of a week. Focus on making your voice ring like a bell, pure and unflinching, and it will become one. If you prefer, you can also perform this exercise with humming or vocal sighs.

2) Yell loudly without straining, projecting as much as you can comfortably. Alternate between a roar, a howl, and a bark. Try yelling at different registers and frequencies. You can yell the vowels A, E, I, O, and U one at a time. Keep it up until you have emptied your lungs of air. Repeat this over and over in an effort to increase your volume at the end of your expiratory reserve.

3) Sing using vibrato. Vibrato is a vocal technique that involves shifting the voice quickly between two pitches. An example of vibrato would be wavering back and forth between C and C# with regular pulses around six times per second. To hear a good example, listen to Johnny Mathis sing "Chances Are." It is commonly used by professional singers but is very difficult to achieve unless the vocal cords are relaxed. Start by switching between two notes that are very close together. Go back and forth slowly and easily and then gradually speed this up to achieve vibrato. Practicing vibrato will improve your voice's melody and prosody while building vocal relaxation and agility.

4) Practice vocal fry. The vocal fry register is the lowest range of tones available to the human voice. It involves a rough, creaky sound and is produced by loose glottal closure which permits air to bubble through slowly, creating a rattling effect at a very low frequency. If you are not familiar with creating vocal fry, use an internet search to listen to some examples. Once you get the hang of it, practice producing vocal fry that is as loud and smooth as possible. Find the tone that feels the itchiest and scratchiest and concentrate your efforts there. Rehabbing it will renovate the substructure of your voice.

After completing the exercises, lie down and focus on the sensations in your vocal tract. You will be bracing it. Find the throat posture that allows the tension you created to subside. This is your most relaxed vocal posture, and the one you want to hold all the time.

If you are nervous before an important meeting, a big presentation, or a hot date, chances are much of the nervous energy will be concentrated in your vocal muscles. Much of your anxiety stems from knowing that the tension leakage will be audible the moment you open your mouth. However, if you sing along loudly and deeply to a few songs you know by heart during the drive there, you will push your vocal muscles through a full contraction. This will wring out the stiffness from those muscles and prime them for use. Also, singing loudly with energy is one of the best ways to improve your mood because it causes the release of endorphins.

If, after singing, you then spend the second half of the drive breathing to a breath metronome, those same muscles will get a full chance to relax and regenerate, ensuring that the exercise they got didn't push them into spasm and activate latent trigger points. You will arrive at the event with the most powerful version of your voice.

To acquire a more fully faceted voice and "deep resonance," you must reestablish the muscles responsible for growling. The need for this kind of rehabilitation comes from a lifetime of disuse. We suppress any hint of a growl, concerned that others will interpret it as adversarial. But by avoiding even minor tonal suggestions of anger, we repress the vocal muscles needed for dominant vocalizations. Whole sections of our vocal tracts are cramped and dormant as a result. The next exercise addresses this.

Vocal Exercise #12.3: *Activate Your Aryepiglottic Folds*

Vocalize using the breathing method in Vocal Exercise 12.2 above, but this time growl loudly. Create the guttural vocalization of a husky character with a gruff voice. This will force unused portions of the vocal cords, including the aryepiglottic folds, to get involved in producing sound. Almost everyone stifles the aryepiglottic folds, leaving them underdeveloped in all but a meager portion of the population. You may have never used yours, but they have always been available to you. By practicing the growl, you will un-stifle your aryepiglottic folds.

If you don't know what the use of aryepiglottic folds sounds like, listen to Louis Armstrong sing "What a Wonderful World." Also, channel Cookie Monster, Barry White, Marge Simpson, and Batman. Hold a deep note in a low, loud growl throughout your exhalation. After you've practiced the growl alone, try singing with a growl. After two to five hours of cumulative practice, you should be able to unleash your inner monster, permitting you to overlap a growl with your normal speech any time you choose.

Using portions of your throat to which you are unaccustomed in the exercises above will make you choke and cough. Especially using the aryepiglottic folds will feel sensitive, scratchy, and achy (as in a sore throat). Utilizing these achy sections of the vocal tract will rehab them. The soreness will dissipate, and accumulated phlegm will clear. Whole sections of your vocal apparatus only vibrate when you cough or scream, but you can use diaphragmatic rehabbing to coax them to flutter with every word you speak. Try using noise-reducing earmuffs with these exercises so that you are not focused on the timbre of your voice but rather the rattling sensations in your throat.

Feel good about vocalizing forcefully. Don't equate vocal power with discourtesy, and don't inhibit it to be polite. Model your favorite radio personality or disc jockey, emulating how they can speak richly and deeply yet also congenially on the air.

Chin Lock

Tucking your chin back into your throat firmly allows you to contract many muscles in the throat and vocal tract. It is a great way to find and activate lengths of muscle that have gone dormant. In yoga, this position is known as a chin lock (jalandhara bandha). The muscles it strengthens include the underused longus colli and longus capitus, both in the front of the neck, alongside many others. As you explore the chin lock over several weeks, you will discover there are many layers to the dormancy in your laryngeal muscles. As you gain the ability to contract and relax new portions of these muscles, in addition to recovering your voice, your neck will become straighter and your throat and jawline will become leaner.

When trigger points in dormant laryngeal muscles become active, we feel "choked up." Most of us are familiar with the acute version of this sensation that accompanies crying, but it can easily become a chronic problem. The feeling of being strangled by the tension in my own throat was a daily occurrence. After only a slight provocation, my voice would waver as if I had just been in a fight. People around me could hear the strain in my voice and recognized it as an impairment and a clear indicator of uncertainty. I recovered, slowly and with work, through a gradual process of strengthening these strained, weakened muscles.

You will find sections of muscles that ache intensely when contracted in a chin lock. Stimulating them daily with contraction will reanimate the dormant muscle fibers, clear up the trigger points, increase circulation, remove the achy feeling, and—eventually—make this chakra-like module steadfast and unfaltering. Once this has been done, it will be impossible for you to feel choked up.

Another technique to "reach" inaccessible dormant muscles is to swallow while holding a chin lock. This will ensure that you are not unnecessarily engaging the swallowing muscles in a state of fear, as many people do. You have probably seen cartoons where the protagonist gulps after they are threatened by a bully. Remove this tendency by using the exercise below.

Vocal Exercise #12.4: *Speaking and Swallowing Through a Chin Lock*

Bring your chin back to your Adam's apple, then toward your chest. Visualize the tip of your chin reaching for your collar bones. From that position, flex the muscles in your throat as deeply as possible. Search for sore muscles and contract them firmly for up to 15 seconds to bring them to fatigue. While you are holding this chin lock, perform the following exercises:

1) To intensify the chin lock, open your mouth wide. Place your fingertips on your bottom teeth and pull your lower jaw down to flex your throat muscles more deeply.
2) Swallow while holding a chin lock. This may be difficult or painful at first, so do it gently and carefully.
3) Freeze your swallowing musculature halfway through the swallow action. (You may need to hold your breath.) This position will allow you to gently contract an array of laryngeal muscles.
4) Chew and swallow food, maintaining a chin lock throughout an entire meal.
5) Speak or sing through the chin lock. Does your voice sound foreign or strange? At first, it should sound deep and bold but muffled. What you are hearing is your optimal vocal tone. Your end goal should be to speak in this register all the time.

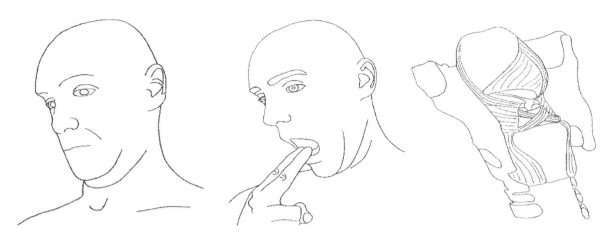

Illustration 12.2: A. Man performing chin lock; B. Man using fingers to accentuate chin lock; C. View of the muscles of the larynx from the back.

I cannot emphasize enough that many of these exercises, such as the chin lock and the isometric contraction of the diaphragm (Exercise 11.7), require months of explorative work but result in gradual progress that makes real and lasting changes to your quality of life. It took me two years of practicing a couple of minutes a month, but I eventually used the chin lock to push into and break up the partially contracted lump in my throat. Using the chin lock to reanimate dormant muscles in the larynx will instate your fullest, most optimal voice and enable you to speak in deep, rich tones.

Ujjayi Breath: Fogging Up a Glass

I have spent numerous hours searching for an optimally relaxed throat/vocal posture. After trying countless configurations, I concluded that the age-old "ujjayi breath" pose is the best among them. Ujjayi (Sanskrit for "one who is victorious") breath is a common Taoist and yoga breathing technique, which instructors usually describe as "breathing while constricting the back of the throat." This "constriction" is accomplished by complete relaxation, and you can find the ujjayi posture by allowing your vocal cords to go completely limp. Ujjayi breathing makes a hoarse, throaty sound because when completely relaxed, the vocal cords sit very close together and vibrate softly as air moves in and out.

When at rest, the vocal cords should be separated by about eight millimeters of space. During cardiovascular exercise, that distance doubles to allow unimpeded breathing. The space between your vocal cords also expands when you are under intense stress. This response happens because your body assumes you are going to be breathing heavily. For that reason, a permanently widened vocal opening is a sign of chronic stress. If you stop bracing those muscles, though, the opening will go back to its normal eight millimeters. But how are we supposed to learn to relax a structure we can't see or feel? Luckily, the answer is easy. Everyone knows how to do it. To perform ujjayi breath, simply breathe as if you were trying to fog up a glass.

Vocal Exercise #12.5: *Fogging Up a Glass*

Breathe as if you are trying to fog up a window or mirror. Concentrate on relaxing your throat and the entire vocal apparatus. Imagine all the tension in your voice box evaporating. Even though you cannot fog up a glass by inhaling, maintain this vocal posture even during the inhalation.

As long as your breath can fog up glass, the deep sound-producing muscles should be completely relaxed. You should find that after performing vocal exercise 12.2, your fatigued vocal cords can be coaxed into this resting posture more readily. This is because it is easier to make muscles go limp after exercise, as long as you focus on the process.

When a trauma-naïve kitten or puppy jumps down to the ground, they belt out a soft "hmm" sound as their paws make contact. This is because ujjayi breath is their default, and their vocal cords always sit right next to one another. Every breath for them is the softest cooing hum. As you practice, try to emulate that pure and innocent vocal relaxation.

You are performing ujjayi breathing properly if you are mere millimeters from a hum. You should hear a breathy, wheezing sound as you take each breath, a sort of white noise. White noise contains many frequencies with equal intensities. Examples include radio static, applause, or the sound of surf. It is not a coincidence that ujjayi breath is also known as "ocean's breath." The sound is created by air resistance when the vocal opening is the bottleneck of the breathing tract.

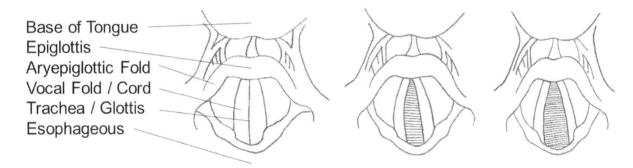

Base of Tongue
Epiglottis
Aryepiglottic Fold
Vocal Fold / Cord
Trachea / Glottis
Esophageous

Illustration 12.3: A. Vocal cord closure; B. Vocal cords at rest; C. Vocal cords braced open.

Once you develop proficiency breathing with your throat in this configuration, try speaking while retaining it. Speak like you are trying to fog up a glass. I think of this as "ujjayi voice." It may sound weak now, but it is the optimal way to speak. In fact, I want to encourage you to perform the vocalization exercises above using ujjayi voice. You might also consider the "ujjayi smile," pairing your smiling with relaxed breathing. Most humans separate the vocal cords widely when they smile, the same way that an eager dog pants as it wags its tail. Your every smile should be accompanied by ujjayi breath.

When you relax the throat and breathe as if you were fogging up a glass, it becomes a little harder to breathe. Your airway diameter narrows even further. Remember from the last chapter that this is a good thing. Ujjayi is an advanced form of resistance breathing. Once you have mastered nose breathing, add ujjayi on top of it to increase the resistance even further.

Breathe this way all the time to develop a more powerful voice and a stronger diaphragm. I consider ujjayi breath as the seventh tenet of optimal breathing.

Hot chicken soup can help you stop bracing vocal muscles. The delicious taste combined with the warming liquid reduces bracing, allowing you to hold the muscles in your throat under the trigger point activation threshold. I believe this is why warm broth or hot tea with honey is commonly thought to help in healing respiratory infections. They encourage the restive ujjayi posture. Take advantage of this effect and have a hot soup or drink after practicing the exercises above.

Rehabilitate and Detraumatize Your Cough

A cough is a protective reflex that clears the large breathing passages of foreign particles, microbes, phlegm, saliva, and other fluids. It involves a forced exhalation of air against a closed glottis. The diaphragm creates pressure, and when this pressure reaches a certain level, the glottis and vocal cords open suddenly, resulting in a violent release of air. It is essentially a hiccup in reverse. I believe that it may also be a mechanism for delivering blood to sensitive respiratory tissues and, thus, could play a vital function in overall health.

A healthy and effective cough depends on hardy and active respiratory muscles, so it is negatively affected by a lifetime of tension. By the time they are old, most people have weak, strained coughs that probably no longer perform their health-promoting functions. For many people on their deathbed, debilitated coughing appears to be their weakest link and a factor that contributes to disease progression. For these reasons, this short section will guide you in rehabilitating your cough.

Most people cough too hard and strain the muscles involved by doing it haphazardly. This leads to coughing that pits different muscles against each other, damaging some and wearing others down. Most people cough violently or not at all. This may be because we are accustomed to thinking of coughing as a negative reaction associated with disease and death. Of course, that is far from true—instead, think of coughing as health promoting and learn to do it gently but vigorously. Since performing the exercise below twenty times (equating to around 1,000 coughs) my coughs have been crisp, lively, and completely pain-free.

Vocal Exercise #12.6: *Detraumatize Your Cough*
Cough 60 times in three minutes. Start softly and find a safe, sustainable cough. Build up to a more forceful cough while ensuring that there is zero associated pain or strain. As you go, breathe in cycles, inhaling slowly and deeply, then coughing until you have no air left, and repeating. You should be coughing five to ten times in a row in between inhalations. You may find that your body instinctively takes over this process, so allow these involuntary action patterns to do their work. It should feel good. Focus on coughing in different ways, at different depths, and with different intensities and pitches. Stick out your tongue. Experiment with a barking cough, a whooping cough, and a staccato cough. Try to extend a cough by creating a prolonged raspy sound over several seconds. Think of this as a search for frailty and seek out dormant muscles that you can activate. Afterward, pay attention to any tension or bracing that may have been caused by the exercise and gently quell it.

Strengthen Your Yawn

Your yawn may be another subroutine that you can benefit from rehabilitating. Yawning is a mammalian reflex consisting of inhaling while stretching the face, throat, jaw, tongue, pharynx, and eardrums. Yawns are largely diaphragmatic and are the longest, smoothest breaths that many mammals take all day. Dozens of explanations for yawning's adaptive value have been proposed by scholars, but there is still little agreement about its purpose.[2] It has even been called "the least understood human behavior."

When mammals yawn, they often stretch their spines in some way, and the pairing of these two actions is called pandiculation.[3] When your cat or dog yawns while standing, they usually perform a deep backbend or some other stretch at the same time. One likely possibility is that pandiculation is nature's way of pairing a diaphragmatic breath with stretching and isometric contraction (the topic of the next few chapters). If this is the case, the sheer normalcy of pandiculation in the animal kingdom suggests that this pairing is something we should emulate.

From the perspective of muscular rehabilitation, yawning is not so different from coughing. It is a valuable opportunity to stretch and contract a large number of muscles throughout the head and neck. And like coughing, in most people, yawning becomes weak and regressive over the course of their lives. This is probably because to yawn substantially and resolutely, you must put your social guard down. An unrestrained yawn is a great way to prove to your body and others that you are relaxed. I recommend yawning as heartily as you can to explore and strengthen it. Practice it before bed because its link with drowsiness may help you fall asleep.

Vocal Exercise #12.7: *Strengthen Your Yawn*

Yawn twenty times during the next three minutes. Practice extending a yawn for at least five full seconds or as long as you can. Take a broad diaphragmatic inhalation while stretching your throat, jaw, and tongue. Open your mouth wide and clear your Eustachian tube by firmly popping your ears. There is also an underused suite of muscles involved in swallowing and voice production that your yawn should hit. This suite may ache but you can rehab it in only a few sessions. If you watch your yawn in the mirror with your mouth open, you can contract this group by maximizing the distance between your uvula and your tongue. Hold the entire set of various contractions in an unfathomably deep, silent roar. Yawn like a lion without worrying who sees it.

Compression for the Throat and Larynx

The vocal folds are shielded by cartilage, so, unfortunately, we cannot press our fingers against the neck to massage or compress them. However, you can give them some relief by compressing the tissues around them.

Vocal Exercise #12.8: *Compression of the Front of the Neck*

Use your thumbs and fingertips to press firmly but gently into your throat. Press all over and from all angles. Apply pressure from the jawline all the way to the collar bones and sternum. Another way to find relief is to lean onto the side of a bed while pressing your upper chest and throat into a basketball. Use the basketball to compress the sternum and clavicle. This also results in reducing clavicular and thoracic breathing. The sensation may make you cough or gag, but it is highly beneficial because it moves and stimulates muscles and tissues that are usually completely still. Be very gentle with this exercise, taking it easy and focusing on dissipating the tension in your throat over a span of several weeks.

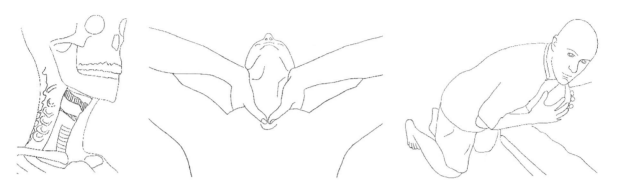

Illustration 12.4: A. Larynx; B. Compression of tissues surrounding the larynx; C. Compression of the throat and chest with the use of a basketball.

Rushed Speech, Enunciation, and Clarity

There are many verbal indicators of dominance that are recognized in psychology. More dominant people have more vocal control, are louder, speak at a lower average pitch, talk more, and are more comfortable speaking at a variety of speeds. They exhibit more prosodic variety with increased use of rhythm, intonation, and melody. They also speak with fewer disfluencies (false starts, stammering, repeated words, mispronunciations, fillers, repaired utterances, etc.). They are less hesitant to interrupt others, are less tolerant of being interrupted, and overlap their speech with that of others more often.[4]

People who have been heavily subordinated, on the other hand, hardly move or open their mouths when they speak. They usually sound uncertain and defensive. They also ramble, murmur, and stammer to create space for a more charismatic person to interrupt them. I speak from experience here. In my twenties, I acted like I was about to be interrupted every time I spoke. I tried so hard to downplay my strengths in front of my friends that I enunciated and articulated poorly, choosing not to use descriptive terminology when speaking. Over several years, this rendered my speech indistinct and reduced my once-hefty working vocabulary into a limited one.

Instead, when you are speaking, act as if you have the floor. That will build credibility, suspense, and engagement with your listeners. Perhaps most importantly, take your time. Hurried speech and quick responses to other people's questions are submissive and will quickly cause you to become tongue-tied. Do not rush to respond.

Employ dramatic pauses. For instance, pause for two seconds before you speak. Pause for a second or so between some sentences. Doing so conveys that you are so assured of your own power that you trust others won't interrupt. The more slowly you speak when talking about something important, the more thoughtful and deliberate you will appear.

Act like whatever you said is helpful, interesting, and stands alone without feeling forced to elaborate on it. People will commonly under-react to your points and good ideas. This will influence you to flounder in an attempt to better explain yourself breathlessly and unnecessarily. Instead, say what you want to say in definitive terms and conclude with confidence and finality. Don't feel like you have to repeat, reiterate, or reexplain yourself. Chances are your listeners got it the first time, even if they act like they didn't.

Don't let silence during a conversation worry you. In professional negotiations, often the person who is less comfortable with silence loses. This is partly because silence makes most people breathe shallowly. Breathe comfortably with all nonverbal aspects of your conversations, and you will become the proverbial 500-pound gorilla in the room.

Monitor your breathing carefully during conversations; don't let it become shallow. Take deep breaths when the other person talks. Pause and breathe in slowly and completely after every few sentences. Don't feel apologetic for making people wait for you to finish your inhalation. Do not jump back into the conversation quickly using a gasp. Finish the breath you were on. Your breath comes first.

Speaking clearly, articulately, and with charisma is not showing off. Start now. Enunciate as properly as you can, and within a few months, your utterances will be crystal clear and will sound more intelligent and persuasive. Don't forget to practice these new habits as you speak to yourself.

Relieve Subvocal Tension in the Vocal Cords by Muting the Internal Monologue

An especially useful form of meditation focuses on subduing the restless subvocalizations within both your head and your larynx. The part of your brain responsible for generating speech, called Broca's area, is always active, producing speech patterns. Because of its incessant activity, language often proceeds through our minds, whether it is involved in planning the day, singing the words to a song, or defending ourselves in a hypothetical argument.

Sometimes, of course, the activity in Broca's area and other language regions is not broadcast to the brain's conscious areas, and so we are not aware of it. When this happens, we gain a brief respite from our internal monologues. Usually, however, not only is it broadcasting its speech to much of the cortex, but it is broadcasting instructions for speech to the cortical motor areas responsible for moving the vocal cords. That input causes us to constantly tense our throats, silently going through the motions of speech even as our mouths stay shut. Sometimes, the lips and tongue move along with these silent words, sometimes they do not, but the voice box almost always follows along. Giving ourselves a reprieve from this interminable activity gives those muscles a rare chance to relax, removing some of the strain they usually feel. Try to become aware of your own pressured, subvocal speech. Using ujjayi breath can help because vocal bracing is vastly reduced if you breathe as if fogging up a glass.

Also, notice how your vocal posture becomes more relaxed in the following situations: when you are around other people with low, relaxed voices; when you wake up in the morning; when you drink a hot beverage; after drinking alcohol; after taking a cough suppressant; and when reclining in complete safety. You might also experiment with the corpse activity from earlier chapters, taking on the limp vocal configuration of a deceased person. Spend some time trying to find your most relaxed vocal posture with the intention of being able to reproduce it on command.

Conclusion

Predatory mammals are less likely to attack those who have a deeper voice. After reading that last sentence, notice how your vocal posture altered. You probably felt tissue in the back of your throat drop to a more secure configuration. However, keeping this posture for more than a few seconds is uncomfortable because it feels so "unguarded." But this is what you want to pursue. Doing it habitually will make your voice unshakable.

Speak to your pets in a deep voice rather than a high squeaky one. Do the same with your children. Addressing them in a full voice is not only beneficial for you but will also encourage them to develop strong voices of their own. A higher-than-natural voice results in braced and dormant laryngeal musculature. The most powerful version of your voice results from the least expenditure of energy. Sonic dominance is one thing: vocal efficiency and efficiency derives from calm practice.

The people with the most beautiful, stentorian voices are those who were able to pair tranquil diaphragmatic breathing with forceful vocal projection while growing up. Even if you didn't have this luxury in childhood, you can create it by employing the exercises in this chapter. Hence the final exercise, which incorporates several of this chapter's key principles.

Vocal Exercise #12.9: *Reading Out Loud*

Read several pages from a book out loud, as in exercise 3.7. Speak in a calm, kind, full voice. Take slow, full inhalations and read aloud until you have no air left to exhale. Focus on articulating loudly and deeply and allow the vocal tract to fully relax during each inhalation. Read slowly and fluently, enunciating as clearly as you can. Maintain a subtle ujjayi throat posture and chin lock. Throughout, preserve a healthy posture in the rest of your body with wide eyes and a calm face. You might gesticulate with your free hand as you talk or make eye contact with yourself in a mirror between sentences. You might perform a zygomatic smile while you speak. Read to your pets, a friend, or the following imaginary audiences:

1) A battalion of soldiers hanging on your every word
2) A huge auditorium or amphitheater filled to capacity
3) A group of third-graders in a library captivated by your story
4) A congregation listening to your sermon
5) The listeners of a major broadcasting station
6) A being with a weak heart who could use a loving voice

Chapter 12: **Bullet Points**

- Stressed and submissive mammals vocalize in an artificially high range. This is also true of humans.
- Over time, persistent high pitch strains the voice box, leads to the degradation of the voice, and creates a stubborn lump in the throat.
- Speak deeper, louder, and more assertively. Start using your outside voice indoors and your distance voice in close quarters.
- Never whine. Stop yourself whenever you notice that you are speaking in a voice that it higher than natural.
- Tense throat muscles can be rehabilitated in several ways, including exercising the muscles involved by holding a chin lock, therapeutic coughing, massaging the throat muscles externally, muting your internal monologue, developing a relaxed default vocal posture, and engaging in diaphragmatic vocalization.
- Diaphragmatic vocalization will pull your vocal muscles out of dormancy. To do this, you take a deep inhalation and then vocalize until you have no air left. You can hum, sing, speak, growl, cough, or yell. Repeating this over and over with the voice deep and relaxed will rehabilitate your vocal tract. Afterward, it is essential to let these exercised areas rest completely.
- The optimal resting vocal posture includes limp vocal cords, a relaxed glottis, and breathing as if you are fogging up a glass.

Chapter 12: **Endnotes**

1.   Morrison, M. D., & Ramage, L. A. (1993). Muscle misuse disorders: Description and classification. *Acta oto-laryngologia*, *113*(3), 428–434.

2.   Morrison, M. D., & Ramage, L. A. (1993). Muscle misuse disorders: Description and classification. *Acta oto-laryngologia*, *113*(3), 428–434.

3.   Anderson, J. R., & Meno, P. (2003). Psychological influences on yawning in children. *Current Psychology Letters*, *2*(11).

4.   Gupta, S., & Mittal, S. (2013). Yawning and its physiological significance. *International Journal of Applied and Basic Medical Research*, *3*(1), 11–15.

5.   Dunbar, N. E., & Burgoon, J. K., (2005). Perceptions of power and interactional dominance in interpersonal relationships. *Journal of Social and Personal Relationships*, *22*(2), 207–233.

Chapter 13: **Reprogram Your Posture for Power**

"By adopting a certain physical posture, a resonant chord is struck in spirit." — Bruce Lee (1940-1973)

Ideal Posture, Spinal Health, and Psychological Well-Being

Poor posture uses tension to hold you upright. Because poor posture is less biomechanically efficient than proper posture, it takes much more effort to maintain. This inefficiency makes it so that muscles are used even when not needed and so do not get a chance to rest. This places muscles throughout the spine in a state of perpetual fatigue. Over time, the lack of rest pushes these muscles into dormancy, which in turn bends the spine out of shape.

As age advances, the extent of degeneration increases and posture generally worsens. The spine curves into a C-shaped orientation, and spinal mobility declines. Between young adulthood and older age, there is a 20-45% reduction in all planes of neck movement. There is about a 30% reduction in all planes of lower back movement.[5] But this is not an inevitable consequence of aging. Implementing some additional key postural correctives will ensure that you retain excellent posture. It will also enhance your ability to perform activities of daily living for the rest of your life.

The present chapter provides you with the central principles of proper posture, communicating exactly how to hold your body in space. As with the diaphragm, however, knowing the tenets of proper placement is only half the battle. Like the diaphragm, your postural muscles are stuck in partial contraction, and the only way to release them is to push them through their full range of motion, over and over again. Releasing the muscles from dormancy in this way is the other half of the battle and the focus of the next four chapters.

Proper Posture:

- Ensures bones and joints are in alignment and working efficiently
- Prevents the spine from being set in destructive abnormal positions
- Prevents fatigue, strain, and overuse
- Decreases wearing of joint surfaces that can result in arthritis
- Increases the ability to generate appropriate levels of force at desired joints
- Stabilizes the body against reactive forces and gravity
- Makes you come across as a predator rather than as prey

Poor Posture is Caused by Chronic Subordination

We are all born with perfect posture, and many of us maintain it as far as early childhood. It breaks down due to inattention. Postural neglect, or a lack of body awareness, blinds us to our protruding head, rounded back, and uneven hips. Most people are similarly unaware of the soft tissue adaptations that reinforce these bad habits. When poor posture begins to feel normal, the muscle memory for good posture becomes inaccessible. We permit countless blind spots of overuse and underuse that crumple our bodies. These cause incoordination, hinder proprioceptive messages sent to the brain, and speed up the formation of trigger points.

Where does poor posture start? We ignore our stooping and make little attempt to correct it because we tacitly assume that any effort to enhance our posture will offend people.

Bad posture is a social signal that communicates defeat. Slouching with head bowed and shoulders forward signifies inferiority in many mammals (especially monkeys and apes). This posture constitutes a mode of operation for looking downward under the eye line of more eminent individuals. It also declares a defective spine and a reluctance to challenge. Primates commonly use poor posture to avoid being attacked.[6] They are sending a signal that they are already defeated, despondent, and willing to submit to the wills of others. But by impoverishing their posture, nondominant mammals promote the formation of dormant muscles in the spine. This makes them likely to become hunched, distorted, and weak as they grow older.

It is much the same with humans. Most people hold themselves as if a lion is about to attack them. Our slouching is heavily braced. We do this either to appease others or to put them at ease.[7] We try not to appear like our motions are effortless by attenuating them. We try not to stand to tall by making ourselves look stymied and compacted. This is so commonplace that submissive posturing has become a conventional standard of modern behavior.

Poor Posture Creates Pain, Stress, and Depressive Thinking

Social conflict pressures us to adopt bad posture, which unfortunately leads back to more stress. Trigger points and muscle shortening cause pain, so the more deviated you are from your most biomechanically efficient posture, the more pain messages besiege your brain. Also, because we know that dormant muscles are weak points that will buckle and collapse if loaded improperly, they cause us to move with unease and apprehension. This restricted dynamism makes us feel defenseless and semi-disabled, turning our personality into that of a cornered animal.

There are many methods for increasing stress in lab rats. One of the most effective is to restrain them by shackling their feet. This is known as "restraint stress." Their stress hormones go through the roof, even when detained for only a few seconds. Looking back, I know that the curved postural restrictions in my spine were equivalent to shackles and were a source of restraint stress for me. As when our face holds a grimace, a stiff, stooped spine affects our unconscious appraisals of the environment.[8]

Slumping impedes the lungs' ability to fully inflate. Adopting a stooping stance causes experimental subjects to breathe more shallowly because the diaphragm has less room to descend. This accounts for why those same subjects find it much more challenging to learn how to breathe with the diaphragm when their posture is collapsed instead of erect.[9] By suppressing the diaphragm, poor posture also mobilizes the sympathetic nervous system.

As you might have perceived, slumping is common in depression.[10] Studies show that slouching tends to increase access to helpless, hopeless, and depressive thoughts.[11] Contrastingly, assuming an upright posture results in faster recall of positive memories,[12] increased energy levels,[13] better body image,[14] and improved affect.[15] This is what we want. So, next, let's look at the specifics of how to position your body dominantly and optimally.

Self-Assess and Recalibrate Your Posture

Before we discuss the characteristics of optimal posture, take a baseline look at your current posture.

Postural Activity #13.1: *Assume What You Think Is Good Posture*

Take photographs of yourself without a shirt, standing as you usually do. Take at least one from the front and one from the side. Next, take two more pictures standing in the way you believe constitutes good posture. Pay careful attention to your positional choices so you can compare them to the postural principles later in this section. Six months from now, repeat this exercise to see how your posture has changed.

Ideal posture occurs when you use the least amount of energy to balance your body weight. You have three major weights in your body: your head, chest, and pelvis. Whether you are sitting or standing, you want to use the curves in your spine to ensure these three weights are neatly stacked atop one another. You can do this by ensuring that your earlobes are in line with your shoulders, which, in turn, are aligned with your hips.[16] If they are not aligned, you will be out of balance and on a path toward pain. You can tell whether they are aligned by examining the pictures you took above, or by placing your back against a wall.

Postural Activity #13.2: *Use a Wall to Improve Your Posture*

Stand in a neutral position against a wall. Your buttocks should be touching the wall and your heels should be about two to three inches away from it. How much space is there between your lower back and the wall? Make it so that there is only enough to insert your hand. Now pull your head and shoulder blades back to touch the wall. Unless your posture is excellent, you will find that you must use tension to keep them back. Try walking away from the wall while maintaining this alignment. This is your optimal posture.

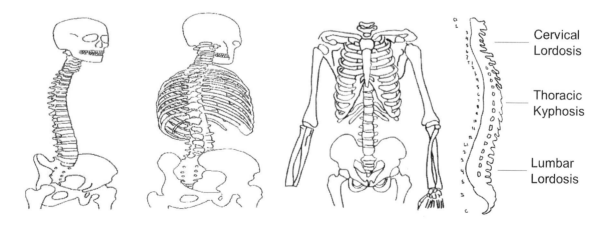

Illustration 13.1: A. Spine from the front, B. Spine and ribs from the back; C. Upper skeleton from the front; D. Spine from the side (facing left) exhibiting the three spinal curves: cervical (neck), thoracic (middle back), and lumbar (lower back).

A "neutral" or properly aligned spine exhibits three curves from the profile (pictured above). These natural curves can be excessively pronounced or not pronounced enough. For most people, they are overly pronounced.[17] The curves are: 1) a backward curve in the neck region known as "cervical lordosis," 2) a forward curve in the upper back called "thoracic kyphosis," and 3) a backward curve in the lower back called "lumbar lordosis." You had to alter these curves for your head, butt, and shoulder blades to meet the wall in the activity above. To repair these natural curves and ensure that they are not under- or over-pronounced, use the following optimal posture protocol.

Optimal Posture Protocol:
These are the five principles of proper standing posture:

1) Keep your feet shoulder-width apart, pointing straight forward. Don't lock your knees; keep them bent slightly.
2) Tilt your hips backward by contracting your gluteus muscles. You don't want your hips tilted forward, your lower back arched, or your butt sticking out.
3) Tighten the abdominals and pull your abdomen in slightly.
4) Let your arms hang down by your sides. Pull your shoulders back and down, spreading your chest. Lean your midback backward. The goal is to avoid slumping forward in the C-shape while rounding and shrugging your shoulders.
5) Pull your head backward. Pull your chin toward your throat. You do not want your head hanging forward or your jaw jutting out.

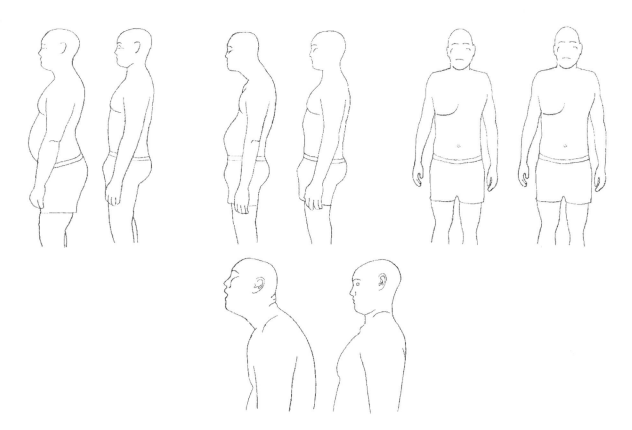

Illustration 13.2: Four of the five postural fixes: A. Contract the gluteus muscles and allow this action to roll the hips backward and reduce the arch in the lower back; B. Flex the abs and pull the belly button toward the spine; C. Lean the torso back, pulling the shoulders back and down; D. Lean the head backward with the chin tucked in toward the throat. A counteracts excessive lumbar lordosis, B and C counteract excessive thoracic kyphosis, and D counteracts excessive cervical lordosis.

Try to use these postural tenets at least half the time you are standing up. They will feel oppressive and phony at first, but pairing them with full breaths using the upcoming exercises will make them your new set point.

Anti-laxity: Temporarily Bracing Optimal Posture Will Strengthen It

The exercises in this section involve lightly bracing postures that are integral to postural strength. Up to this point, I have vilified bracing. However, the form of bracing used in this section is deliberate, temporary, and not destructive because you will be taking breaks and pairing it with proper breathing.

Unfamiliar muscular contractions increase the stress response. Previously, we discussed that widening the eyes, smiling, and looking up cause sympathetic activity to spike. Standing up straight does this too. It is the same with flexing the buttocks, the abdominals, and even the biceps. This link between firm contraction and stress keeps our muscles from having ideal tone at the joint. This reduction in tone is known as muscle laxity. Forceful contractions make us feel like we are showing off or like we are doing something unnatural. This, in turn, makes us breathe shallowly. This results in countless muscles going lax, and a reluctance to engage physically with the environment. We can reverse it with diaphragmatic breathing.

In general, people who breathe shallowly in response to unfamiliar contractions have the lowest tone and the smallest muscles. On the other hand, people who breathe comfortably, even under heavy loads, tend to be muscular. These tendencies form in childhood, but you can still influence them now. The following exercises will ask you to pair paced breathing with different forms of muscular bracing and loading. When you breathe calmly through the discomfort this causes, you are utilizing the Program Peace "anti-laxity" method.

When performing anti-laxity, you are looking for any unfamiliar loading patterns that cause you to tremble, require great concentration to maintain, or take your breath away. During episodes of anxiety or submission some muscles go lax more than others and feel uncomfortable to contract. These are the muscles you are targeting. An example of this is performing a plank. Most people quiver and experience discomfort when planking. You want to spend time in these kinds of configurations, teaching your body that they are safe, and learning to breathe easily within them, even for several seconds at a time. After 10 cumulative minutes of exerting yourself at a moderate intensity in these loading configurations, they will become familiar, stable, and sound. The chin lock, facial exercises, and eye-widening from previous chapters are all examples of anti-laxity exercises.

Anti-laxity Protocol

1) Find a group of muscles you have neglected because you feel uncomfortable or self-conscious contracting them.

2) Hold a firm contraction in these muscles for five to 30 seconds until they start to fatigue. Let them rest for twenty seconds and repeat. These contractions are generally meant to be isometric, meaning that they do not involve motion. Without risking strain or injury, alternate between clenching them softly and then very tightly (between 10 and 90% of their maximum).

3) These contractions may make you startle or tremble, may require concentration, or may make you breathe shallowly. If it feels shaky, feeble, or wobbly, you know it needs anti-laxity.

In Chapter 5, I said that we lightly brace our hands all day in the form of a claw. However, we are afraid to ball our hands into tight fists because other people may notice and think we are preparing to fight. This is why simply clenching our hands into fists raises our heart and breathing rates. The exercise below will use anti-laxity to heal this, priming your fingers and forearms for building strength. The exercises that follow do the same for other postural systems. Perform each with your breath metronome.

Postural Exercise #13.2: *Making a Fist*

Clench your fists into tight balls. Feel the contractions in each knuckle. Alternate between clenching softly and then as tightly as you can. Start with your wrists straight. Spend time rolling your wrists in wide circles while the fists are clenched. Become comfortable with the sensations you feel throughout your hands and forearms.

Postural Exercise #13.3: *Clench the Elbow*

Clench your elbows by contracting your biceps, triceps, and forearm muscles. Do this with the arms bent at different angles from 10 to 170 degrees. Do it with the wrists rotated to different extents. Pose like an action movie star, your arms crossed in front of you with all the muscles flexing. Try it with the arms behind the back. Over a matter of days, this will go from feeling enfeebled to electrifying.

Postural Exercise #13.4: *Clenching the Buttocks*

While standing, clench your gluteus muscles into tight balls. Do this while placing your legs and lower back in different positions. If you do this while lying on your back, each gluteal contraction should lift you slightly off the ground.

Postural Exercise #13.5: *Clenching the Abdominals*

Flex your abdominal muscles. While you do this, suck your gut all the way in. You should be able to absorb a light punch to the stomach without the punch hitting your internal organs. Take a knuckle or a tool and lightly strike the abs in different regions from the ribs to the pubic bone to ensure that the abs are taut in all areas.

Within a minute of performing the abdominal exercise above, you should notice your back round forward and your chest cave in toward your stomach. You don't want to reinforce this. Continue to perform the exercise but with your back extended and your chest puffed out (optimal posture tenet four). This will overhaul your tendency to collapse the middle of your back when your abdominal muscles contract. Combining this with a contraction in your glutes will align your ribcage with your pelvis. Combining it with the next two exercise will align these with your neck.

Postural Exercise #13.6: *Shoulders Down While Supine*

Lie down on the floor on your back and slightly tuck your shoulder blades underneath you. Put your arms at your sides and raise your hands off the floor to the level of your hips. Next, push your arms down as if you were reaching for your knees. This will prime your shoulders to remain down and back.

Postural Exercise #13.7: *Bringing the Chin Toward the Chest*

While standing, gently lean your head back until it aligns with the rest of your spine rather than in front of it. Next, bring your chin in toward your neck. This firm contraction in the front of your neck is a chin lock, previously described in Chapter 12. Feel how this resituates the neck.

You may want to start out performing exercises 13.4-7 on your back on the floor. This remedial position will help you isolate, relax, and focus. When that feels comfortable, try using all of them simultaneously while standing up as in the next exercise.

Postural Exercise #13.8: *Optimal Posture While Standing*

Stand up straight and perform exercises 13.2-7 simultaneously. Contract your glutes and abdominal muscles as you tuck your shoulder blades behind you. Puff out your chest and press your arms toward the floor as you straighten the back of your neck. Using anti-laxity, stand tall, strong, and resolute.

While you may feel apprehensive about how others will perceive you in this stance initially, don't let this undermine your posture. Stand as if 100 people staring at you wouldn't reduce your resolve. Stand as if a 45-caliber handgun discharge wouldn't make you flinch. Stand as if you wouldn't surrender even one iota of your optimal form even if you were being tased. Steel yourself against any startling or trembling.

Shift your weight and the distribution of contractions to explore this configuration. Even just 20 cumulative minutes over several days will appreciably desensitize you to the discomfort involved in sustaining this position. After a total of an hour, it should become credible to others and dependable for you.

Most programs aimed at improving posture tell us not to stand unnaturally erect like a soldier. While they are correct in claiming that this can create more tension, they are wrong to think that it should never be done. Tensing and bracing hard within the four postural tenets (Exercises 13.4-7) is the best way to augment posture as long as you limit it to under a minute at a time, allow for ample regenerative breaks, and breathe properly. If you use anti-laxity to repeatedly fatigue your deep postural muscles, and then give them the rest they need, they will gain the strength and endurance to buttress your optimal posture. The following illustrations provide some examples of positions and poses you can perform anti-laxity within.

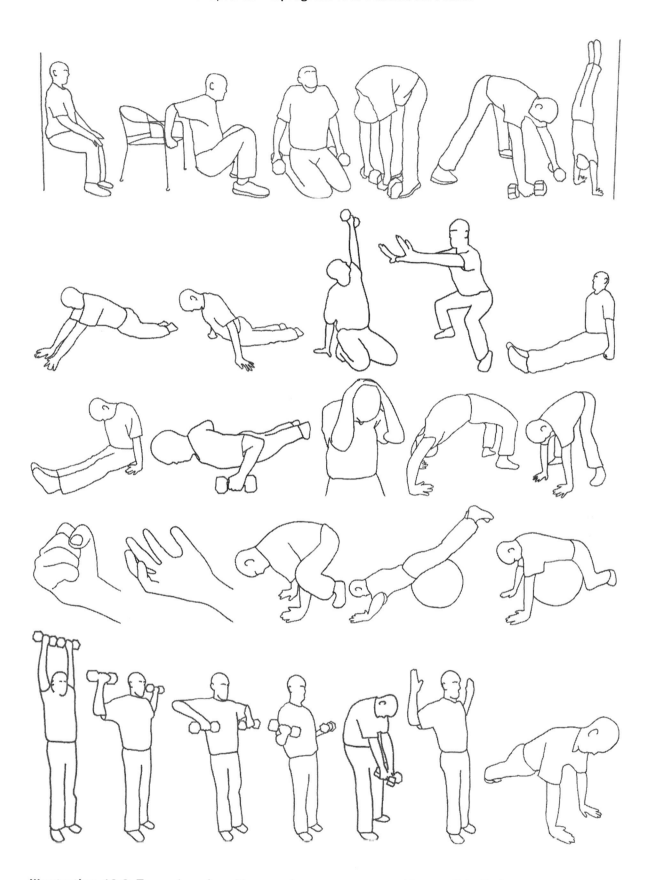

Illustration 13.3: Examples of positions and poses you can achieve anti-laxity from.

Good Posture Requires Healthy, Active Spinal Muscles

The spine, also known as the backbone or vertebral column, is a stacked set of bone disks. It gives the trunk stability and protects the spinal cord. The human spine comprises a complex chain of ligaments, fascia, bone, and intervertebral discs, and their health is dependent on the tone of the surrounding spinal muscles. When the tone is either too high or too low, dormancy and damage ensues.

When I think of the spine, I envision an inner worm that wants to stretch out and squirm in all directions. Dormant spinal muscle is like an oppressively tightened straitjacket that warps and restricts the worm's movement. Large sections of the back, neck, and hips are not just braced in most people; they are splinted, as in a body cast. Due to the discomfort involved, we try to keep these joint configurations as still as possible. We move the rest of the body around these rigid, wounded areas. When we accidentally use them, they force us to startle and take our breath away. Thus, I see the entire spine as a kind of chakra of its own; one capable of holding massive amounts of trauma in the form of painful muscle shortening.

The muscles that encase your spinal column constitute your true "core" and, as a unit, are the ultimate module to rehabilitate. These muscles run up and down your spine, interdigitating between your vertebrae and connecting them to various other body parts. By pushing and pulling against the vertebral bones, spinal muscles help your core bend, twist, and turn. It is difficult to move athletically without a mobile spine because the neck, shoulders, and hips are anchored in the spine, where they provide a base for the head, arms, and legs. Joseph Pilates referred to the neck, shoulders, and hips as the "powerhouse" of the body and insisted that they provide the foundation for all movement. For this reason, spinal dormancy is a primary limiting factor for people trying to build strength in their arms and legs. Are you having trouble putting on muscle or losing fat? You need to rehab your spine first if you want to reap the benefits of exercise.

You want all the minor muscle groups in and around your spine to be capable of contracting entirely, have full range of motion, and articulate effortlessly during everything you do. When the muscles lining your vertebrae are active from top to bottom (atlas to coccyx), you can't help but move nimbly, hold yourself gracefully, and think confidently. In the previous section we started to train them to hold a specific configuration. In the next section, we will wake them up.

Backward Spinal Stretches Will Straighten You Out

Social apprehension causes us to bend our spine forward (flexion) but rarely backward (extension). This results in difficulty and pain in any motions that require backward bending. Habitual stooping shortens the joint structures in the front of the spine and lengthens those in the back. This creates the characteristic "C" shape.

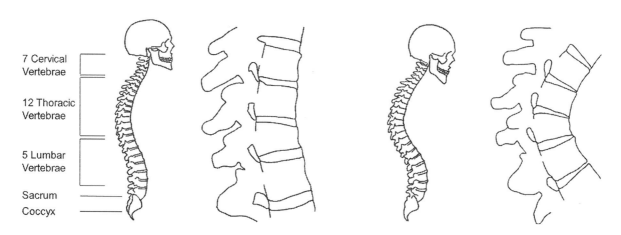

7 Cervical
Vertebrae

12 Thoracic
Vertebrae

5 Lumbar
Vertebrae

Sacrum

Coccyx

Illustration 13.4: A. Healthy spine with natural curvature; B. Collapsed unhealthy spine with excessive curvature and exaggerated C-shape.

The best way to override the C-shaped spine is to regularly bend in the opposite direction, creating a backward "C." There are many poses introduced in upcoming chapters to help with this, but the best way to start is to lie back onto a ball. Start with a large, inflatable stability ball. Spending time lying on your back on top of a stability ball will stretch the compressed muscles in the front of the spine and contract the atrophied muscles in the back. After a few weeks or months, try this with a foam roller. Lie on your back on the carpet and place the foam roller in different places under your spine. Very carefully move the foam roller to different areas, relaxing and breathing into the stretches. You are spot-treating your backward arch. Once you are accustomed to this, try rolling down the length of your back on the foam roller. Please be careful. The probability of a person with a bad back hurting themselves in this way is so high that foam rollers are rarely advertised for this purpose. You can gravely injure yourself by doing this too aggressively without listening to your body. It should never hurt. Rolling down the length of your spine on top of a basketball is even more ambitious. However, after working up to it, anyone would benefit from performing this daily as in the exercise below.

Postural Exercise #13.9: *Backward Extension on a Ball*

Lie on your back and place a basketball underneath your neck, between your shoulder blades. Beginners should use a deflated basketball and work up to using a fully inflated ball. Carefully roll from the top of your spine to the bottom three times. Stop at the kinked portions and stretch into the position from all angles. This will help you achieve spinal contractions in the weakest of muscles that you could never ordinarily reach while standing or sitting. If you use the anti-laxity protocol while doing this, the contractions will make your back strong and straight. Make sure you are relaxed and breathing deeply. Without paced breathing, you will resist the ball's curvature. With paced breathing, you will melt into it. This will literally straighten you out.

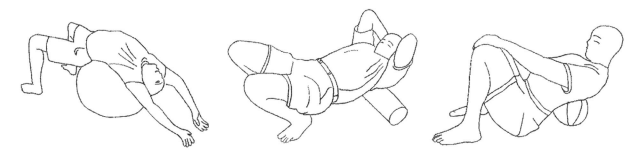

Illustration 13.5: A. Backward bend on a stability ball; B. Achieving a full backward bend at different spinal segments using a foam roller; C. Rolling down the length of the spine on a basketball.

Maintain Good Posture in Bed and When Waking

We have talked about optimal posture while standing. In this section we will discuss it during sleep, and in the next section during sitting. The best sleeping posture is limp and linear. You want to sleep with a straight back and neck. Avoid curling up into the fetal position, which usually involves bracing and reinforces the C-shaped spinal configuration. Attaining proper support can help. When sleeping on your back, try placing a pillow under the knees. When sleeping on the side, place a pillow between the knees. If you sleep predominantly on your side, buy a body pillow and hug it, straddling it with your arms and legs. You also want a firm mattress that does not sag or contour your existing posture. An extra-firm mattress may take weeks to get used to, but it will straighten your spine as you slowly learn not to brace against a flat surface.

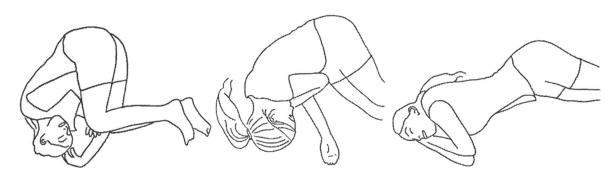

Illustration 13.6: A. Woman curled into a C-shape while sleeping; B. Slightly improved sleeping position; C. Much-improved straight sleeping position.

Postural Exercise #13.10: *Stretches to Do in Bed*

When your alarm clock goes off in the morning, hit the snooze button once and buy yourself five minutes to perform three fundamental stretches. Employ anti-laxity while doing the following:

1) Lay on your stomach. Lie there with your head turned to each side for a few minutes to get a good stretch in your neck. If laying on your stomach puts a strain on your lower back, bend one knee and bring it toward your chest.

2) Lay in the yoga "L" shape pictured below and slowly rock your feet in different directions to get a good stretch through your hips.
3) Lay on your back and place a pillow or two under your thoracic spine. Spend time lying motionless, then try stretching your chest, neck, and back from this position.

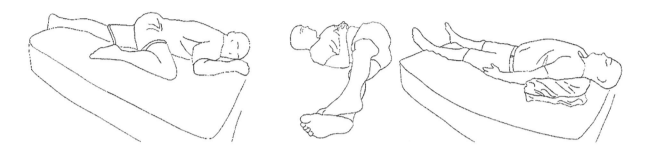

Illustration 13.7: A. Laying stomach, head to the side; B. L-shaped stretch for the hips; C. Pillow under the thoracic spine.

Postural Exercise #13.11: *Stretches to Do Out of Bed*

After you get out of bed, set your breath metronome for five minutes and perform the following anti-laxity exercises to wake up your spine. You can combine these stretches with Exercise 4.10 by performing them while looking into your own wide eyes in a mirror.

1) Start with knees, shins, backs of the feet, and hands on the floor. For the first minute, press away from the ground while shrugging the shoulders. Do this while warming into the forward curves (kyphosis) in your neck, middle back, and lower back.
2) For the next two minutes, warm up the backward curves (lordosis) in your neck, middle back, and lower back.
3) For the final two minutes, sit on the floor with the back of your legs flat against the ground. Let your head hang and sink your head and neck toward your knees.

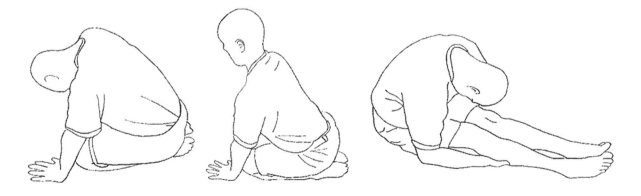

Illustration 13.8: A. Kneeling shoulder shrug with full kyphosis in the neck and lower back; B. Kneeling backward stretch with full lordosis in the neck and lower back; C. Sitting forward stretch with full kyphosis in the middle back.

Sitting with Poor Posture Is Extremely Unhealthy

Most of us sit far too much. Many of us are forced to sit just to earn a living. It is estimated that 90 percent of office workers use computers, with 40 percent reporting usage of at least four hours per day. Unfortunately, using a computer for four or more hours per day greatly increases the risk of musculoskeletal disorders.[18] This is one of the reasons office workers who sit in chairs garner more musculoskeletal injuries than any other industry and have the highest risk of heart disease, diabetes, metabolic syndrome, cancer, and back and neck pain.[19] Even people who do not work in an office setting develop misalignments from sitting. This happens at school, in the car, and in front of the television.

Sitting intensifies the rounding of our spines into the C-shape. When the spine is rounded, the weight distribution changes, creating perpendicular shear forces. This "resting tension" compresses the spine and weakens crucial muscles, robbing you of the mobility and strength you need to sit, stand, and walk properly. Worse yet, because your body adapts to the position you assume throughout the day, the more you sit, the more you want to sit.

In his book, *Deskbound*, physical therapist Kelly Starrett[20] calls sitting a "toxic position that feasts on athletic potential." It truly is. The best recourse is to vary your posture often to get blood to stagnant, poorly perfused muscles. You should shift positions every two minutes from one neutral position to another. Every 20 minutes, straighten your legs, squeeze your thighs together, and flex your glutes. Grab the back of the chair behind you and use it to twist. It is also important to take five-minute breaks during which you walk away from your chair every hour. Don't be afraid to lie down, take a walk, or stretch during your breaks.

The postural misalignments due to sitting are made worse by shallow breathing. Studies show that people automatically engage in shallow breathing when working at a desk, especially if they are behind a keyboard.[21] In some studies, every participant who placed their hands on a keyboard demonstrated an increased respiration rate[22] and reduced motion of the diaphragm. This happens because sitting positionally inhibits the diaphragm. As mentioned earlier, slumping encroaches on the diaphragm's natural range of motion, forcing shallow breathing, which in turn causes the release of stress hormones.

Sitting up straight in your chair deepens your breath, as does breathing through your nose. So, you might want to think about taping your mouth at your desk to ensure nasal breathing. I also strongly suggest using a breath metronome at your desk. Remember how hard it was back in Chapter 3 to eat a meal while following a breath metronome for the first time? Trying to do office work while engaged in paced breathing is even more difficult to coordinate at first. It will initially interfere with your concentration.

Most people hold their breath intermittently when trying to focus their attention in what has been called "concentration apnea."[23] As you read in Chapter 7, shallow, distressed breathing helps us focus in the short term due to its association with adrenaline and alertness. However, after using a breath metronome at your desk for a week or two, you can override your tendency toward concentration apnea and develop the ability to focus concertedly while breathing diaphragmatically. Place your phone with the breathing app software running next to your computer monitor and follow it out of the corner of your eye. Don't be surprised if pairing paced breathing with desk work helps you change your whole attitude about your job while increasing your productivity and work ethic in general. It is much like "whistling while you work."

The Ideal Sitting Posture

To sit optimally, you must maintain the natural lordosis in your neck and lower back that is present while standing. To do this, sit up in your chair with your back straight. Shoulders should hang straight down. Elbows should not be in front of the torso, and hands should be below the level of the elbows. Place your keyboard accordingly.

When it comes to your lower back and hips, it is essential to distribute your weight equally. Remove anything from your back pockets such as a wallet or phone to assist with this. When sitting, keep your knees a few inches wider than your hips, as this will stabilize your pelvis. Your knees should also be level with or slightly below the hips but not above them. Keep the toes pointed forward, with the feet flat on the floor. If your back is leaning against the chair, press your buttocks against the chair back, too. If not, sit at the edge of the seat placing about 40 percent of your weight is on your feet.

It is obligatory to sit with most of your weight transferred to the chair through your sitz bones (ischial tuberosities). The sitz bones are two protuberances at the lowest point of the hip bone (pictured below). The cushion on many chairs makes it challenging to find your sitz bones. However, when sitting on a hard surface, you should be able to find them easily. If you cannot feel two hard contact points, one under each gluteus, then you are not sitting on your sitz bones and your spine is likely curved. Curved pillars have little structural integrity. Rock back and forth on your sitz bones to find a sturdy upright posture. This is active sitting. You are more likely to stay seated on your sitz bones when you sit on the edge of the chair, sit on a hard wooden or metal chair, or place a hard object like a book underneath you.

Most people actively avoid sitting on the sitz bones, sitting instead on their tail bone, and tucking the pelvis like a shrimp. This is a form of lumbar kyphosis, also known as "posterior pelvic tilt." A tucked pelvis inactivates our hip flexors, putting all the strain of sitting on the lower back. Avoid this by pretending you have a vestigial tail extending from the base of your spine. Don't sit on the base of your tail. Instead, sit below it (on the sitz bones), allowing your imaginary tail to emerge just above the place of contact with your chair.

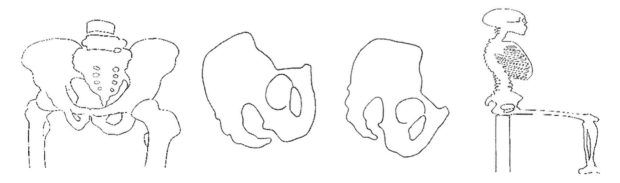

Illustration 13.9: A. Pelvis with sitz bones at the bottom; B. Pelvis seen from the side, resting on tail bone; C. Pelvis resting on sitz bones; D. Skeleton sitting on sitz bones.

It can be tiring to sit on your sitz bones all day. Therefore, do what postural experts advise against and sink down in your chair, sitting on your tailbone for at least two to five minutes every hour. You can use this position as a brief counterpose. When you do so, stretch lordotically and kyphotically and swivel the hips. Standing is good, too. Many people use standing desks. You might consider placing your laptop on a bookshelf around waist height for a few hours at a time to create your own standing desk.

The design of most chairs conforms to the average person's poor posture. However, you can avoid this trap by buying an ergonomic, posture-conscious desk chair. You might consider buying a lumbar pillow specially designed to support your lower back. You can also place a roll vertically down your spine, helping you to push your shoulders back. Change the settings on both your chair and car seat frequently to expose your sitting posture to different loading profiles. If your seat reclines, spend a portion of your sitting time leaning back at an angle. The more positions you can use, the better.

Cross and spread your legs more often. Being comfortable sitting with the legs spread is one of the most telling signs of dominance. We must remove the stigma against men crossing their legs and women spreading their legs. Similarly, many people inhibit pronounced flexion and extension of the lower back because they fear others will see it as sexual. We need to feel comfortable assuming these postures in public because they allow us to refresh our hips, groin, and lumbar spine, leading to more postural variation and stronger, more mobile backs.

Daily sitting time is a major risk factor for diabetes and cardiovascular disease.[24] This is the case even in people who exercise regularly. Studies have shown that even daily exercise cannot counteract the effects of sitting and sedentariness. However, I think that diaphragmatic breathing, postural variation, anti-laxity and anti-rigidity (discussed in the next chapter) may. Remaining in a static sitting position for years on end dramatically reduces circulation and mobility. We can avoid this by using other postures that serve as alternatives to traditional ways of sitting. The figures below offer some for your consideration.

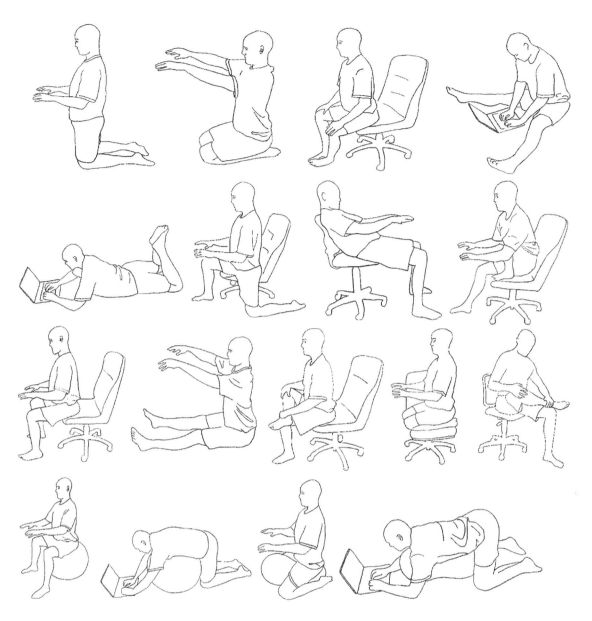

Illustration 13.10: Several different positions for working or reading that are good alternatives to conventional sitting. The oblong ball pictured in the last two illustrations is an "inflatable peanut."

　　Our ancestors rarely sat on a raised surface like a chair. Rather, they sat on the ground, knelt, or squatted. In other words, chair sitting is unnatural for humans. Yet Americans sit in chairs or sofas for an average of 13 hours a day.[25] Many experts believe that musculoskeletal integrity is much better in countries where people sleep on the floor, use squat toilets, and do not use chairs. This is because they must crouch, kneel, and bend over several times per day.[26] Many Americans do not crouch, kneel, or bend over at all.

　　The main reason older people are placed into nursing homes is that they cannot get off the ground on their own. Indeed, the ability to get up from and down to the floor is a good predictor of overall mortality.[27] This should motivate you, whether reading, watching TV, or relaxing, to spend as much time on the ground in as many different positions as possible.

Don't watch TV from the couch. Watch it from a million different positions on the floor. You might start with some of the following:

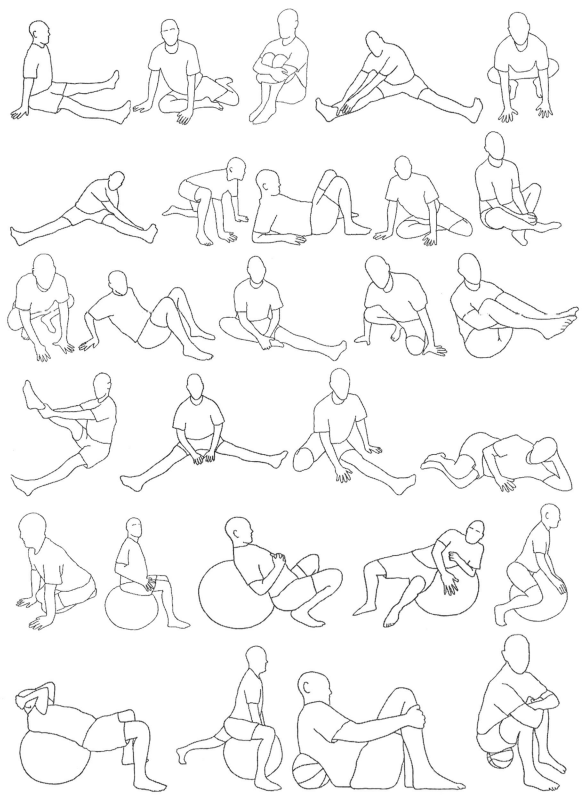

Illustration 13.11: Several positions for lounging or watching TV.

Conclusion

I believe that in the workplace, in classrooms, and even within families, we are constantly sending each other nonverbal feedback, practically bullying each other into slouching. When someone else stands straight, we have a natural inclination to be offended. Our instinct is to try to pull them back down. What we should do is applaud them while being reminded to better monitor our own posture. If you notice people trying to coerce you back into slouching, just ignore it, and reassure yourself that they are in the wrong.

This chapter guided you to brace within the five tenets of optimal posture and pair this bracing with diaphragmatic breathing. While doing so, you should have noticed that some points within each posture were marked by weakness and pain. Holding your back, neck, and shoulders in firmly upright positions probably feels tight and somewhat intense. It is a brittle, aching pain, almost as if the muscles are asking you to leave them alone—warning you that excessive use will lead to injury. This aching is the signature of dormant muscle and to treat it we need an entirely different technique. The next chapter will show you how to rehab it by contracting into it and breathing through the discomfort using a method I call "anti-rigidity."

Chapter 13: **Bullet Points**

- Mammals signal submission with their body posture. They collapse the spine, which, over time, strains it and causes pain.
- Postural concessions lead the muscles that support confident posture and dominance poses to become frail, shortened, and stuck in partial contraction.
- Stooping to look non-threatening will bend your spine into a forward C-shape over time.
- Backbends repair this forward C-shape by strengthening your backward C.
- Laying backward over an inflatable stability ball, foam roller, or basketball will straighten your spine.
- The five tenets of optimal posture are:

  1) Space your feet shoulder-width apart with toes pointing forward.
  2) Roll your hips forward and contract your gluteus muscles.
  3) Tense your abdomen taut and gently pull your belly button toward the spine.
  4) Pull your shoulders back and down.
  5) Tilt your head back and pull your chin toward your throat.

- Building postural muscles can be accomplished by pairing paced breathing with firm contractions in the muscles that support the five tenets above.
- Combining very firm contractions of muscles that are not used to contracting firmly (and may tremble under load), and combining this with paced breathing is a therapeutic method called anti-laxity.
- Vary your position often, whether sitting, standing, or lying down.
- Postural inattention is a major contributor to poor posture, so be mindful of your posture during everyday activities.
- Sitting tense, motionlessly, while shallow breathing is highly detrimental to posture and health in general.
- Sitting directly on the sitz bones rather than the tailbone will support your lower back and keep it strong.
- It is much healthier to sit on the floor in various positions than to sit in a chair or a couch.

Chapter 13: **Endnotes**

1. Satariano, W., Guralnik, J. M., Jackson, R. J., Marottoli, R. A., Phelan, E. A., & Prohaska, T. R. (2012). Mobility and aging: New directions for public health action. *American Journal of Public Health, 102*(8), 1508–1515.

2. de Waal, F. (2013). *The bonobo and the atheist: In search of humanism among the primates.* WW Norton & Company.

3. Collins, A. (2003). *Gestures, body language and behavior.* DKC.

4. Dael, N., Mortillaro, M., & Scherer, K. R. (2011). Emotion expression in body action and posture. *Emotion, 12*(5), 1085–1101.

5. Mason, L., Joy, M., Peper, E., & Harvey, R. A. (2017, March). *Posture matters* [Poster presentation]. 48th Annual Meeting of the Association for Applied Psychophysiology and Biofeedback, Chicago, IL.

6. Michalak, J., Troje, N. F., Fischer, J., Vollmar, P., Heidenreich, T., & Schulte, D. (2009). Embodiment of sadness and depression: Gait patterns associated with dysphoric mood. *Psychosomatic Medicine, 71*(5), 580–587.

7. Peper, E., Booiman, A., Lin, I. M., & Harvey, R. (2016). Increase strength and mood with posture. *Biofeedback, 44*(2), 66–72.

8. Peper, E., Lin, I-M., Harvey, R., & Perez, J. (2017). How posture affects memory recall and mood. *Biofeedback, 45*(2), 36–41.

9. Peper, E., & Lin, I-M. (2012). Increase or decrease depression: How body postures influence your energy level. *Biofeedback, 40*(3), 126–130.

10. Canales, J. Z., Cordas, T. A., Fiquer, J. T., Cavalcante, A. F., & Moreno, R. A. (2010). Posture and body image in individuals with major depressive disorder: A controlled study. *Revista Brasileira de Psiquiatria, 32*(4), 375–380.

11. Wilkes, C., Kydd, R., Sagar, M., & Broadbent, E. (2017). Upright posture improves affect and fatigue in people with depressive symptoms. *Journal of Behavior Therapy and Experimental Psychiatry, 54*, 143–149.

12. Pavilack, L., & Alstedter, N. (2016). *Pain-free posture handbook.* Althea Press.

13. Bond, M. (2007). *The new rules of posture: How to sit, stand and move in the modern world*. Healing Arts Press.

14. Sjogaard, G., Lundberg, U., & Kadefors, R. (2000) The role of muscle activity and mental load in the development of pain and degenerative processes at the muscle cell level during computer work. *European Journal of Applied Physiology, 83*(2-3), 99–105.

15. Starrett, K., & Cordoza, G. (2013). *Becoming a supple leopard: The ultimate guide to resolving pain, preventing injury, and optimizing athletic performance*. Victory Belt Publishing.

16. Starrett, K., Starrett, J., & Cordoza, G. (2016). *Deskbound: Standing up to a sitting world*. Victory Belt Publishing.

17. Peper, E., Harvey, R., & Tylova, H. (2006). Stress protocol for assessing computer related disorders. *Biofeedback, 34*(2), 57–62.

18. Peper, E., Burke, A. & Peper, E. J. (2001). Captured by the computer: A psychophysiological profile of boys playing computer games. *Proceedings of the Thirty Second Annual Meeting of the Association for Applied Psychophysiology and Biofeedback*. Wheat Ridge, CO: AAPB.

19. Olsson, A. (2014). *The power of your breath. The secret key to reshaping your looks, your body, your health, and your weight*. Anders Olsson.

20. Bailey, D. P., Hewson, D. J., Champion, R. B., & Sayegh, S. M. (2019). Sitting time and risk of cardiovascular disease and diabetes: A systematic review and meta-analysis. *American Journal of Preventative Medicine. 57*(3), 408–416.

21. Levine, J. (2014). *Get up! Why your chair is killing you and what you can do about it*. St Martins Press.

22. Starrett, K., Starrett, J., & Cordoza, G. (2016). *Deskbound: Standing up to a sitting world*. Victory Belt Publishing.

23. Brito, L. B., Ricardo, D. R., Araújo, D. S., Ramos, P. S., Myers, J., & Araújo, C. G. (2014). Ability to sit and rise from the floor as a predictor of all-cause mortality. *European Journal of Preventive Cardiology, 21*(7), 892–898.

Chapter 14: Anti-rigidity Therapy: Bring Dormant Muscle to Fatigue

The last chapter explained that to have optimal posture, you must free your postural muscles from partial contraction. This chapter emphasizes that to do this, you must search your body for these segments of dormant muscle and push them through their full range of motion. These full, firm contractions should be held long enough to push the muscle to fatigue. As soon as fatigue is reached, it should be followed by full relaxation. This chapter will describe how to use this new technique that I call "anti-rigidity" therapy to reinstate motion diversity in your life. I created this technique by experimenting on myself and developed it further while using it with my clients. It will work for you, but only if you are breathing diaphragmatically.

Using Dormant Muscles Wakens Them from Dormancy

The lives of our nomadic hunter-gatherer ancestors featured endless variation in movement. They spent their time foraging, hunting, scouting, ranging, and setting up and breaking down camps. They dug for vegetables, picked fruit, made weapons, cleaned animal hides, prepared food, and carried wood, water, and children. On the other hand, the modern human habitat is one of urban dwelling, sedentary technology use, and cultures of convenience. Most people go months without extending their muscles beyond the requirements for mere walking. Compared to our ancestors, the geometric diversity of our daily motions is impoverished.

We are essentially animals in captivity, imprisoned by the incredibly low variation of our movement patterns. By moving in the same limited ways, we deny our bodies the nutritious movement they are starving for. We self-limit our ranges of motion because of bracing, postural inattention, intimidation, sitting, restraining working positions, laziness, surgery, injury, and load-bearing (including things like pregnancy, heavy backpacks, breast augmentation, and obesity). The tension from these activities results in shortened, hypertonic, dormant muscle.

Medical experts have documented that dormant segments of the spine exhibit many of the same physiological properties as cadaver spine. They get so little blood that they might as well be zombie flesh. Because their oxygen and nutrient supply has been strangled off, these beef jerky-like muscles in your back hurt. Pushing them into contraction outside of their customarily restricted range causes pain. Accidentally forcing them into rapid full contraction (e.g., during a fall) can be excruciating. This pain, and fear of it, can influence us to avoid using dormant muscle entirely.

We engineer the use of dormant muscles out of our lives and find ways to get around having to use them, which leads to a poorly balanced and ungainly physique. This compensation leads us to use other muscles that are biomechanically less efficient at completing the task. Then these muscles also take on strain. To correct this problem, we must reteach ourselves to use the dormant, partially contracted muscle by flexing through the untapped phases of its contractile range.

Anti-rigidity Training: The "Aching/Cracking Method"

The anti-rigidity technique involves finding the most dormant parts of the body and subjecting them to a full-range stretch and full-range contraction. The first step is to find a dormant joint. To do this, you must search for two sensations that are usually found together: 1) cracking or popping of the joint, and 2) sore, achy muscle. You should notice that as you bring a joint into the range where it cracks, it will feel sore if held in that position. These areas feel brittle because they are frail from disuse. Once you have found a position like this, you want to gently contract the muscles involved while engaging in paced breathing.

At first, it feels unnatural to hold a posture that cracks for a prolonged period. Your impulse will be to achieve the crack and allow the muscles to relax immediately thereafter. Avoid this inclination. Whether the joint cracks is not important. What is important is that you take your time stretching and flexing into the joint configurations susceptible to cracking. Cracking provides temporary relief from joint pain through the release of endorphins but does not heal tension. You want permanent relief that is provided only by strengthening the joint and the muscles surrounding it.

Anti-rigidity Protocol

1) Find a contraction or active stretch that feels stiff and achy when held. This often involves an unfamiliar position or posture and leads to cracking at the joint. The point where this configuration cracks is the most in need of rehab. Engage, stabilize, and hold the position until it fatigues. This usually takes between five and 30 seconds.

2) Hold the general parameters of the posture while varying others. Move the joint dynamically, utilizing its range of motion in every possible vector, flexing into the ones that seem the stiffest or sorest. If you can continually reposition, you can approach the problem from different angles. Anti-rigidity can be done with concentric contractions (in which the muscle shortens), eccentric contractions (in which the muscle lengthens), or isometric contractions (in which the muscle does not change length).

3) Allow the area at least 15 seconds of complete rest before you try again. Use this respite to recognize what the muscle feels like when it is completely resting.

4) Stimulate dormant muscles throughout the body in this way while breathing correctly. As long as you are breathing diaphragmatically, you should feel the ache diminish in a matter of seconds. At first, the ache may be so intense that it makes paced breathing difficult. In that case, just ensure that you are taking long, passive exhalations. You can facilitate this by taking deep inhalations through the mouth and then puckering your lips and blowing out for as long as possible to reinforce the relaxation response.

5) After your anti-rigidity training session, it is essential to allow these muscles to relax completely, so lie down (employing the corpse pose, body scan, or progressive muscle relaxation from Chapter 5) and let the contractions subside.

Start by targeting raw and achy areas in your shoulders, neck, back, and hips. This achiness is the deep somatic pain and myalgia that we discussed in Chapter 5. Search for this discomfort within your unexplored end ranges of motion. It helps to position yourself in ways that are out of the ordinary. Wiggle and writhe in these positions as you hunt for tissue to restore.

Gently jostle the muscles to get them moving. Start with what you can find and then spend the most time in the configurations you would like to heal. You are hunting for that crick in the neck, tweak in the shoulder, and twinge in the lower back. By the time you have used anti-rigidity to dispel all the achiness from your body, your posture will be statuesque.

Anti-rigidity Activity #14.1: *Sense the Tightness in Your Shoulders*

Stand or sit with your hands on your hips. Keep your hands there and press your elbows out in front of you. You should feel a tight, stiff sensation in your upper back, shoulders, and arms. This is the aching sensation that I am asking you to locate throughout your body. Play with the posture, gently shrugging, bending your elbows, and flapping the arms. Use the anti-rigidity protocol above to find sore muscles while stretching and contracting within this pose.

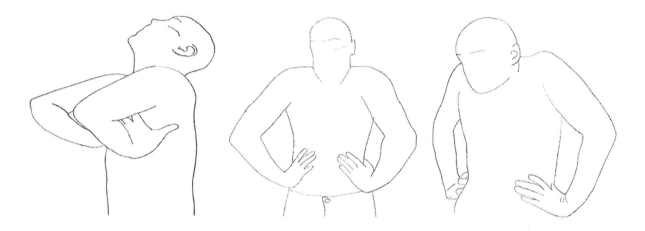

Illustration 14.1: Anti-rigidity for the shoulders.

Anti-rigidity Activity #14.2: *Contract Dormant Muscle in the Neck*

Locate the achy muscles in your neck. There should be many uncomfortable positions that feel sore and crack. Try looking up as far as you can while rotating your head to both sides. Try looking down as far as you can and then to both sides. Try touching your chin to your chest and then tilting your head to each side. Try touching your chin to each shoulder repeatedly. When you find an uncomfortable position, hold it for several seconds while maintaining paced breathing.

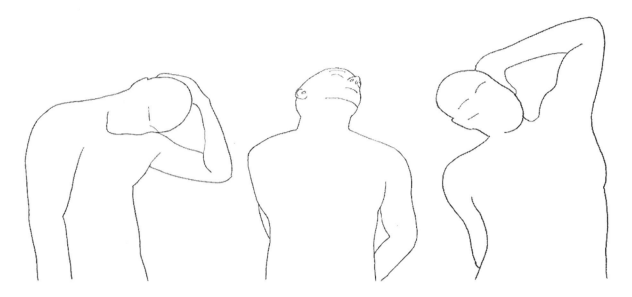

Illustration 14.2: Anti-rigidity for the neck.

As you work through these tender areas, integral sections of your body will start to open up. You might ask yourself: "Is this whole region going to become unlocked and available to me?" Yes, it will. If you keep practicing, eventually it will all come unglued. Below are illustrations of some anti-rigidity poses that will help you to expose and recondition frailty. As you practice these, you will inevitably come up with poses of your own that are better suited for your particular strain pattern.

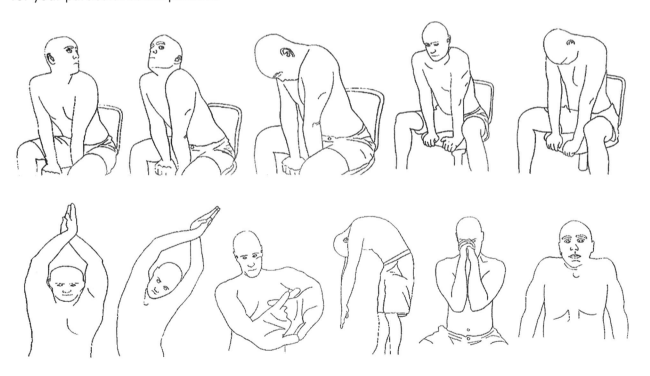

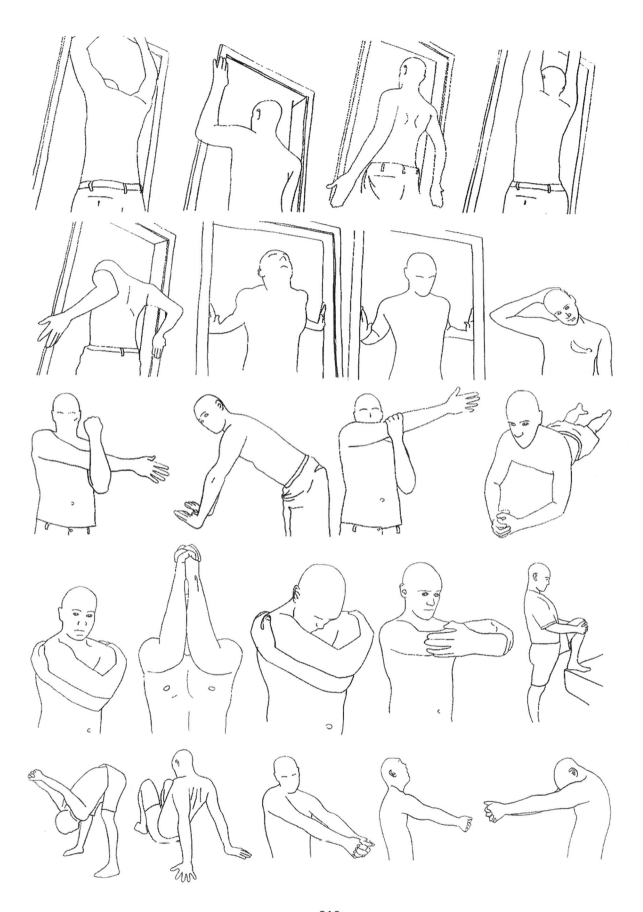

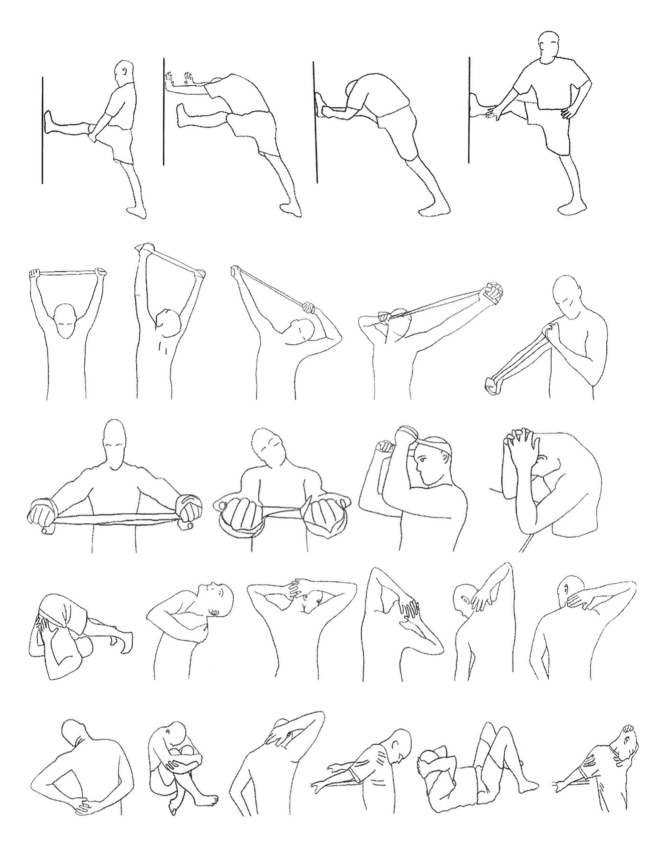

Illustration 14.3: Various anti-rigidity positions and techniques.

At first, anti-rigidity work feels unnatural, but after a while, your muscles will thirst for it, and you will find yourself doing it without realizing it. Relish the alleviation of the ache. Bask in the sensation of sending fresh blood through dormant tissue. Memorize the sensorial signature of tensity. It feels a little like the gnawing burn that accompanies lactic acid buildup. It is also similar to the soreness you feel when massaged. Anti-rigidity will help you locate the best candidates for compression and percussion. If, for example, you used anti-rigidity to identify the precise location of tightness to the right of your lower cervical spine, you should then try to compress it. Using massage to release muscles after anti-rigidity training will allow them to fully relax so they can heal.

After anti-rigidity, the muscle you treated will have increased blood flow for several hours. This means that any other activity or exercise you perform during this time will recruit that muscle and condition it to be more easily recruited in the future. However, within just a few hours of disuse, the muscles will stagnate again. The more frequently you refresh dormant muscles with anti-rigidity, the faster they will come out of dormancy. I recommend using it before and after long periods of sitting, upon waking, before bed, and after your usual exercise routine.

Using anti-rigidity, you teach your brain to control muscle that it has come to ignore through learned disuse. You are actively relearning how to incorporate these neglected muscles into your daily routines and overall posture. This will develop your proprioceptive awareness (knowledge about where your muscles are in space) and kinesthetic awareness (ability to coordinate muscles cohesively) while enhancing neuromuscular coordination and agility. Anti-rigidity will also reduce the fidgeting and restlessness that painful dormant muscle causes. It might look strange to others, but don't worry about that. Feel comfortable performing anti-rigidity training wherever you go, whether in front of friends or in public. I believe that anti-rigidity therapy is one of the most beneficial "somatic self-healing" techniques available.

How Anti-rigidity Works

Anti-rigidity causes mechanical deformations in muscle that result in cascades of beneficial biochemical processes. For instance, it is known that contracting dormant muscle compresses embedded arterioles and other blood vessels, causing their walls to relax and spread open (vasodilation). The walls open wide, drawing blood into the surrounding capillaries. This pulls oxygen into the area and allows the clearance of waste products built up from sustained contraction. Over time, it enhances the resilience and pliability of not just muscles but also tendons, ligaments, and fascia.

Some of your muscles get this perfusion and clearance every day, but the dormant ones are deprived of it. Even during a full-body workout, dormant muscles often receive only minimal contraction. Exercise only improves the distribution of oxygen and nutrients to the muscles used in that particular exercise. In other words, the benefits of exercise are not systemic. This is why pursuing varied movement is so important. Missing out on essential loads is like missing out on essential vitamins.

In physical rehabilitation and sports training, there is a popular principle called SAID (specific adaptation to imposed demand). This states that your muscles will gradually get better at the demands you place on it. If you contract seldom-used muscles, they will adapt, and with time be able to contract fully. The best way to take advantage of the SAID principle is to make small demands on the body and to gradually increase the intensity as the body adapts.

Anti-rigidity gently forces trigger points to contract causes them to unravel and burn out. This lengthens the muscle, quells muscle spasms, extinguishes ongoing inflammation, and unfurls myofascial restrictions. As you do this, you are weeding the trauma out of your spine, scaling down your chronic pain, and diminishing its emotional burden. By providing the muscle the exercise it has been deprived of, full contraction affords it the ability to rest and recover. In essence, by pushing muscles with minimal capability for endurance to full fatigue, anti-rigidity builds their endurance. Because much of your dormant muscle is postural, converting it into muscle capable of enduring body weight will resurrect your body's foundation.

For clarity, the following table summarizes some of the important distinctions between anti-laxity and anti-rigidity. It is important to note that the two do overlap to an extent and that they also complement each other in practice.

	Action	Target	Consequence	Sensations Involved	Goal
Anti-laxity	Firm isometric contraction	Hypotonic, atrophied muscle	Reinforcing postures of strength	Weakness and trembling	Increasing strength and tone
Anti-rigidity	Stretch combined with firm contraction	Hypertonic, dormant muscle	Rehabilitating muscles stuck in partial contraction	Aching, soreness, and cracking	Decreasing weakness and excessive tone

Table 14.1: Comparing Anti-laxity with Anti-rigidity

Anti-rigidity Fills in Missing Corners

Dormant muscles are responsible for the "missing corners" in your range of motion. Because the muscle is stuck in partial contraction, it is incapable of moving pliantly. People of Eastern philosophical persuasions call these "energy blocks." While prior chapters have examined the effect this has on the diaphragm, eyes, face, and vocal apparatus, this chapter focuses specifically on the spine, core, and postural muscles. There are numerous muscles throughout your spine that you only contract within 25 percent of their full range of motion. Find them and rescue them by pushing them toward 100.

As you rehab missing corners, you will expose other missing corners beneath them. There are hierarchies of missing corners to reestablish. When one spinal segment is curled up and inoperative, it undermines those nearby it, rendering them inaccessible. Correcting one provides leverage for correcting others. Using the anti-rigidity method regularly, you will continue to discover repositories of strength you never knew you had.

You may come to recognize that many of your most dormant muscles derive from previous injuries. Using anti-rigidity, I encountered many previous strains and sprains from adolescence and young adulthood that I had forgotten about. The process is like unearthing fossils. If you drive, then you probably have dormant muscle in your right ankle, knee, and hip from working the gas and the brake. Likewise, if you work on a computer, you probably have strain in your right shoulder that runs up your neck from bracing while holding the mouse. I had pronounced lumbar knots from decades of bending over the sink to wash my face and brush my teeth. The problem was, I did those things from a single fixed position without contracting my glutes. Anti-rigidity treated all of these.

Do you ever bend over and reach a point where you know that you will hurt yourself if you continue? This is a corner that is completely missing. Most people have countless postural configurations like this that cannot be loaded at all. Many muscles in the hips and lower back can barely withstand a small fraction of body weight. You want to load these frail muscles very lightly at first, increasing the load over time. To load the muscles with less than body weight, you must lessen the effects of gravity by placing your body into unfamiliar yet supported positions like those illustrated above. The techniques used in Pilates and the poses used in yoga can also be used to this end.

Using Anti-rigidity with Distressed Breathing Is Counterproductive

Performing anti-rigidity will make you want to breathe shallowly. One of the main reasons that dormant muscle stays dormant is because every time you try to use it, it takes your breath away. Pairing distressed breathing with anti-rigidity defeats the purpose. In fact, shallow breathing is enough to turn anti-rigidity work into injurious tension building. When I first started developing the anti-rigidity technique, many friends saw me stretching restlessly and told me, "You know, you look to me like you are just making the tension worse." They felt this way because doing the same exercises would irritate their muscles. Contracting dormant muscle is something that our bodies naturally tend to avoid because, under distressed breathing, the muscle will only become further agitated. Diaphragmatic breathing makes all the difference.

Be mindful that you are breathing diaphragmatically, at no more than six breaths per minute, or else anti-rigidity will lead to more tension. It is imperative that you breathe long, full, smooth breaths, preferably through the nose. Employ a breath metronome when possible. Consider performing anti-rigidity after a diaphragmatic breathing session. You will find that five minutes of breathing along with a breath metronome will make you more limber and make it easier to identify achy muscles. After 20 minutes of paced breathing, anti-rigidity will feel like picking low-hanging fruit.

Anti-rigidity is also accentuated after exercise, massage, or the application of heat. It is far easier to sense and contract dormant muscle after a workout or rubdown. The same goes for a hot shower or bath. This is the rationale behind the practice of "hot" yoga. To experience this, take a shower that is as hot as possible without being uncomfortable. You might want to rub moistened Epsom salt into your neck and shoulders beforehand. Let the heated water hit the back of your neck and stream down your spine. You will notice that your neck cracks more easily, is more flexible, and you can more fully contract the muscles for upwards of 10 minutes.

Rushing Anti-rigidity is Counterproductive

As you get better at performing anti-rigidity, you will become more ambitious and attempt to rejuvenate the stiffest areas in your neck and lower back. By moving slowly and carefully, you can work through these boundaries. However, if you try to force through them, the tissues will become more defensive, not less. Dormant tissues require a gentle approach. Pretend that you are trying to slowly lengthen a piece of a plastic bag without tearing it. At a certain point, you should feel a slight resistance to your movement. Some physical therapists refer to this as a "stretch point." As you hold the position, wait patiently. When the aching sensation fades, your stretch point is releasing.

Bouncing through a stretch can be counterproductive unless it is a very subtle bounce. This is because hard bounces pull quickly on muscle fibers, alerting specialized sensors within the muscle that it has been suddenly overstretched. Nerve signals from these receptors will cause the muscle to shorten further, which is exactly what you don't want. Make your contractions gradual and slow, using only 10-40 percent of your maximum effort. Think of melting into each stretch. If you contract too rapidly or forcefully, you will engage fast-twitch muscle fibers. Contracting slowly will enlist the slow twitch endurance fibers that establish enduring postural tone.

I sought out the most painful and weak cruxes in my body and totally reclaimed them. However, I knew there was a chance that I could herniate a disc or sprain a vital ligament. This is why you must perform anti-rigidity very carefully, especially when starting out. Working through your most frail areas can lead to great injury. However, once restored, they will become highly resistant to injury. Choose consistency over intensity. Avoid movements that prove to aggravate and pursue those that heal. Chip away at your frailty a little each day to make every bit of your body's muscle accessible.

It is necessary to mention that anti-rigidity is not contortionism. You are not attempting to force your body into strange and awkward positions. Also, do not mistake the ache of dormant muscle with the pain of pushing a joint outside its intended range. With time, you will learn to recognize the exact difference between engaging frailty and intruding into the body's natural joint barriers.

You should never hurt, or even be sore, the next day after using anti-rigidity. If you are, you either went too hard or have a serious underlying injury. If you experience a tight pinching or burning sensation, there could be nerve damage. In that case, discontinue immediately. If you have a related disease or disorder, discuss anti-rigidity with a physician before using it. Carefully monitor your pain pattern. If existing pain becomes worse from these activities, discontinue immediately and seek advice from a qualified physician.

Normal cracking is fine, but grating, popping, and crackling sounds indicate a musculoskeletal injury. Do not attempt anti-rigidity if you experience sensations of pins and needles or numbness. Do not attempt if you have been in a recent accident or experience severe headaches. If the pain spreads or radiates to other locations, stop the exercises immediately and consult your doctor. Know your limits and do not overdo it.

Anti-rigidity's Relation to Chiropractic

I have visited five different chiropractors in my life for a total of around 10 appointments. These visits in my late twenties helped inspire me to develop the anti-rigidity method. I recommend visiting a chiropractor yourself so that you can become acquainted with what it feels like to have the body in a configuration where highly dormant muscle is directly engaged and released.

The first time I went to a chiropractor, he commented on how tight my neck was. He was able to crack my spine in several locations. This influenced me to go home and flex into the same spinal configurations he created when performing the adjustments. For instance, I would try to fully extend my neck, looking toward the ceiling, while rotating my head from left to right. It ached deeply, and I wondered if working through this aching could improve my neck. It did.

Only two years later, the same chiropractor told me that he was unable to adjust my spine at all. When he tried to perform spinal manipulations, my joints moved with the manipulation fluidly without cracking. In fact, I can no longer find a chiropractor who can successfully crack my neck or lower back. After feeling the muscles on the back of my neck with their fingers, some told me that my neck is healthy and does not need to be adjusted. This is entirely due to the anti-rigidity method.

Joint cracking is a sign of degenerative activity stemming from passive tension. When the muscles surrounding the spine are held in passive tension, this causes dislocation (subluxation) of vertebrae. These weak, distorted muscle segments are incapable of keeping the vertebrae in ideal alignment. The advantage of the chiropractic adjustment is that it gets straight to the core of dormant muscle, stretching it rapidly and delivering blood. It is common for a patient to report that they can "breathe again" after manipulation. To me this suggests that vertebral misalignment somehow affects the diaphragm's mobility. The cracking also produces endogenous morphine, temporarily relieving pain and bringing patients back for future adjustments. However, chiropractic treatment is only a temporary solution. When a chiropractor performs an alignment, the spine briefly becomes neutral. However, because this does not strengthen the muscles or improve their endurance, the vertebrae fall quickly back out of alignment, sometimes within hours.

Most chiropractors do not insist that their patients exercise the "opened" areas after adjustments. This is why there is limited evidence for the clinical efficacy of chiropractic over physical therapy. However, I have found that anti-rigidity exercises complement both chiropractic and physical therapy. It may take months or years of anti-rigidity training to fully contract a previously dormant muscle, but once you can, it will be fully reintegrated and will no longer require chiropractic or rehabilitative work.

After six months of using anti-rigidity, I could crack dozens of joints throughout my body at will. Because I knew my posture and physique had improved tremendously, I began to tentatively conclude that increasing the ability to crack joints might be the overall goal. However, after another six months of this routine, I found that much of the cracking subsided. As my joints became healthier, they cracked less and less. This made me realize that cracking is a means to an end. In other words, as you employ anti-rigidity, you can expect to go through three phases: 1) an inability to crack, 2) plentiful cracking, and then 3) an abatement of cracking.

I could not crack my joints at first because I did not have the strength in the surrounding muscles to leverage my way into the unhealthy muscle. After six months, my joints were cracking profusely because I finally had some strength in the muscles that would support my efforts to flex into the weakest areas. After another six months of employing the technique, the cracking subsided because even my weakest muscles and joints were no longer degenerative.

The point is that you want to stretch and flex into sore joints throughout your body, using the cracking and aching sensations as diagnostic tools.

Anti-rigidity Is Not the Same as Stretching

Stretching has gotten a bad rap in recent decades because static stretching has been shown to be less effective for athletes than once thought. This is because static stretching on its own is too passive and does not involve muscular contractions. It involves immobilizing a joint and stretching the muscles and connective tissues to their greatest possible length. This increases the resting length of muscles by lessening the sensitivity of tension receptors in the muscle. Studies have shown that excessive static stretching can lead to joint laxity and hypermobility. Stretching muscles too far reduces strength and explosive force. Many stretching programs encourage hyper-flexibility of muscles, which can even result in mechanical instability of the joints. Anti-rigidity doesn't use static stretching, it uses active stretching.

Static stretching increases "passive range of motion." With anti-rigidity, however, we are interested in increasing "active range of motion." Unlike passive, static stretching, you want to perform stretches that accept load throughout the entire range. The stretching aspect of anti-rigidity will increase the joint's mobility and restore proper length to the muscles involved. The contraction aspect will increase the stability of the joint and increase the strength of the muscles. Overall, anti-rigidity should be thought of as a combination of stretching and contracting in which you explore the boundaries of tension while applying low-grade but continuous tensile loads. Yoga, done with active loading, can accomplish anti-rigidity as well.

Employing Anti-rigidity During Yoga

Anti-rigidity methods are implicit in yoga, but there are ways to make them more explicit. When I take a yoga class, I assume the poses as directed and then perform anti-rigidity while inside the pose. For instance, most yoga instructors tell you to keep your neck straight and still while in downward dog because they don't want distressed breathers to hurt their necks. But you and I can safely assume downward dog and use the unique loading properties of the pose to find and strengthen frail joints. From downward dog, it is possible to leverage your way into countless stiff neck positions that are treatable through anti-rigidity. Yoga teachers refer to achy, dormant muscle as "sticky" while practitioners often describe stretches that rouse dormant muscle as "delicious." Use yoga to help you probe for and discover delectable contractions.

In many types of hatha yoga, there is a risk of overstretching certain muscle groups during a pose. Many yoga instructors and practitioners abuse their bodies by pushing too hard in an attempt to achieve an "ideal" form. The best way to improve form is not to force the body into a static stretch but rather to use the pose to gradually rehab the dormant muscle that is keeping you from executing the pose ideally. Ease yourself into the postures and vary your weight while in them so they are not static and isolated. To do this, you want to lean in different directions, play with the articulations, shift your weight, and alter the pose's geometry to achieve various well-rounded contractions. Remembering to use the five tenets of optimal posture from the last chapter during yoga will enhance postural strengthening.

I recommend that anyone interested in yoga start with basic, Iyengar, or restorative yoga to develop proper form and an appropriate emotional relationship with their body. After a few of these lessons, I encourage trying as many types of yoga as possible until you find one that you truly enjoy. You can take classes in a studio or at home using a free internet video. Yoga has shown numerous clinical benefits such as improving emotional regulation and reducing physiological arousal. It has even been shown to assist significantly in the treatment of post-traumatic stress disorder.[1] I believe every person should perform yoga with anti-rigidity on a weekly, if not daily, basis.

The following sketches should help you if you want to practice at home. I strongly recommend moving through the classic yoga poses here as often as possible. Choose at least 10 each night and spend one to two minutes in each while engaging in paced breathing. Another great option is to put something educational on television, then sit a phone or a tablet down next to the TV, using it (on silent) to stream an online yoga class. I do this for twenty minutes every night and learn something while I stretch. An added benefit of performing anti-rigidity and yoga before bed is that it will help you sleep like a baby due to the copious endorphins released.

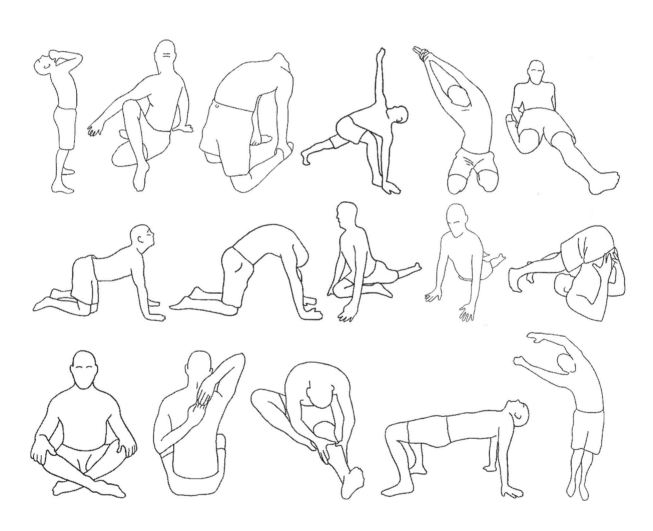

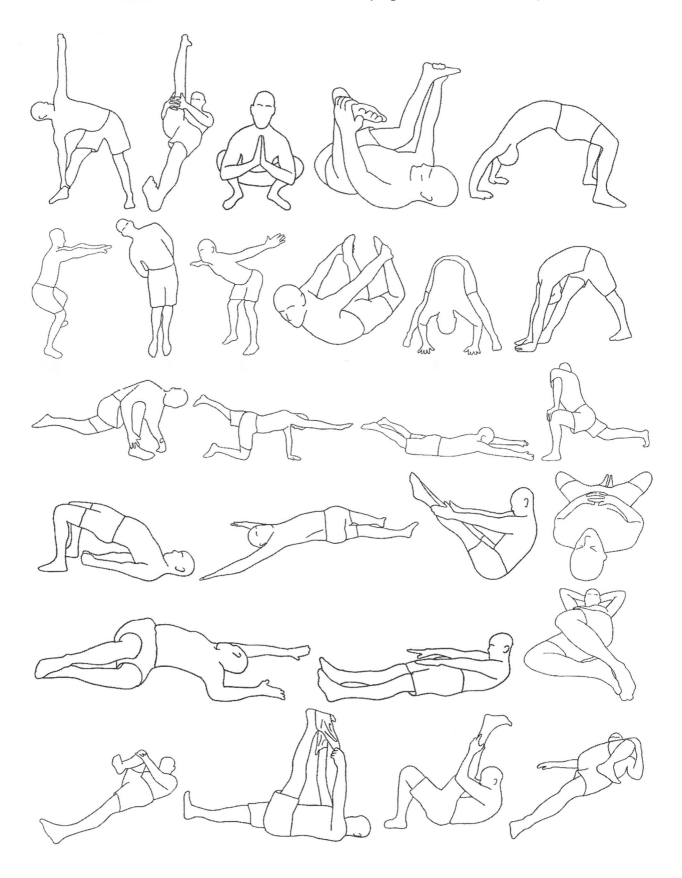

4422

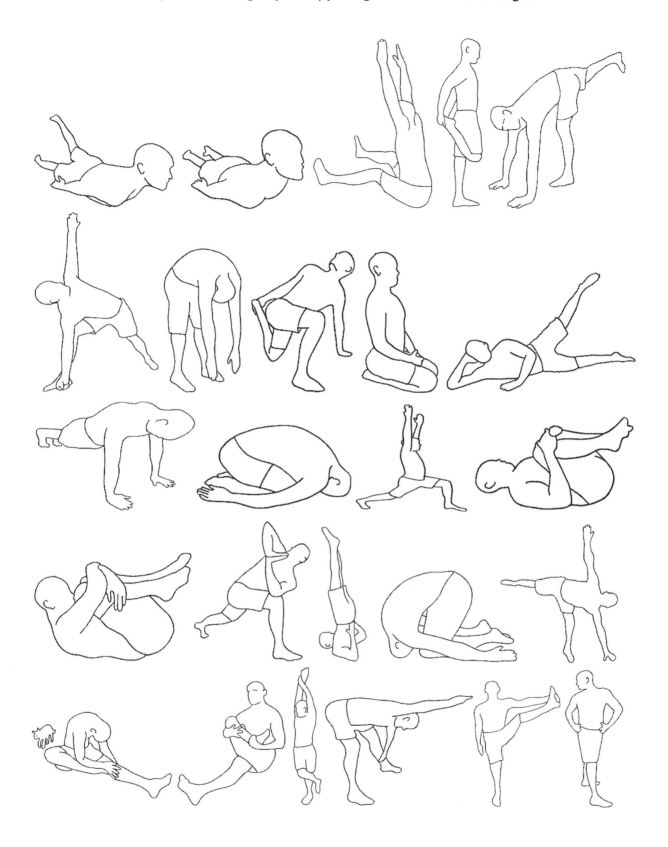

329

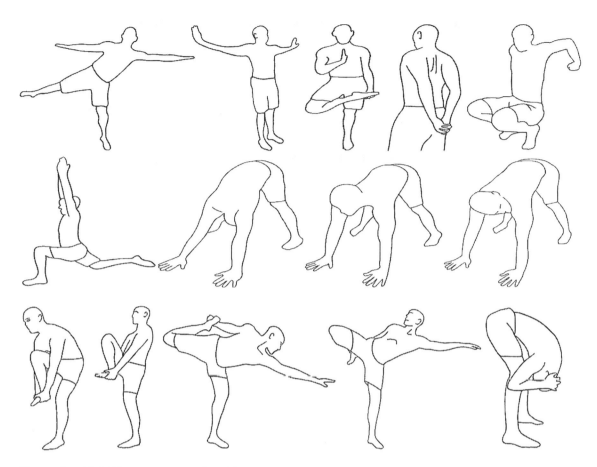

Illustration 14.4: 81 yoga poses and positions.

Health Benefits of Yoga

- Makes muscles, ligaments, and tendons more elastic and resilient
- Stimulates stem cells creating collagen
- Improves fitness, flexibility, and strength
- Reduces pain and improves mobility better than other forms of low impact exercise
- Can reduce blood pressure and risk factors for cardiovascular disease
- Seems to improve symptoms related to depression, PTSD, and anxiety

Conclusion

When I was 25, I went to a nearby court to play basketball. The moves and skills that I developed in my late teens had disintegrated. I felt incredibly clumsy and feeble on the court. I wanted to know why. Because I had not played basketball in years, I assumed that I had lost the memories and neural connections responsible for my skills. I was researching the neuroscience of Alzheimer's at the time, and that influenced me to assume that because I hadn't used those brain pathways, I may have lost them.

However, at age 35, I went out to play basketball again, only to discover that the skills and coordination of my teenage years were back. My poor performance 10 years prior had nothing to do with losing brain circuits and everything to do with frailty. Now, instead of feeling like a dry twig running down the court, I feel like a velociraptor. My body supports me fully in any position I put it in. It is the same with dancing. People don't stop dancing in old age because they forget how. They stop because their joints are immobile and their unnecessarily feeble bodies hurt. Anti-rigidity is like an analgesic but a permanent one. As many yogis insist: "You are only as old as your spine." Another way to put this is: "You are only as old as your spine is frail and painful."

Anti-rigidity Exercise #14.1: *Search Your Body for Rigidity*

Use the illustrations of poses above, along with the Anti-rigidity Protocol, to guide you in a five-minute search for frailty in your body. Once you find the muscular patterns that cause joint cracking and create a feeling of achiness, spend time within them using firm, sustained contractions. Practice paced breathing during this session.

In my 20s, if I got less than four hours of sleep, my back would hurt all day. However, a couple of years of anti-rigidity has made it so that even if I miss an entire night of sleep, I feel no joint discomfort because my spine still supports me. I can stand up straight for long periods while everyone else succumbs to slouching. I can sit cross-legged on the floor for hours while others languish on the couch. The postural reinforcements that anti-rigidity created sometimes make me feel like I am in some kind of supportive harness or mechanical exosuit. Anti-rigidity makes it effortless to hold your body assertively, proudly, and energetically.

The strength gains from anti-rigidity come with muscle mass gains. They don't make you look like a weightlifter, but because they involve postural musculature, they help you look more like an athlete. As the next chapter will detail, anti-rigidity works complementarily with cardio and weight training. You will find that anti-rigidity will not only counteract the tension created by your exercise routine but also that you can employ anti-rigidity during exercise as well.

Chapter 14: **Bullet Points**

- The anti-rigidity technique is performed by searching for dormant muscles whose joints crack or ache, then rehabbing them. To reach these dormant muscles, the body must be placed into unfamiliar positions.

- Rehab is achieved by finding a postural configuration that cracks and then holding it for five to 30 seconds at a time. It feels like a stretch but is a contraction that you want to hold until the muscles involved reach fatigue.

- It is well known in exercise science that firmly contracting a muscle before relaxing it brings it to a deeper level of relaxation.

- Usually, contracting dormant tender muscles makes us breathe shallowly as if we were being submerged in cold water. The key to anti-rigidity is to pair the contraction of dormant muscle with diaphragmatic breathing.

- Anti-rigidity reduces the internal impedance within the contractile tissue, resetting the muscle to its biomechanically optimal orientation. If you want peak performance, you need anti-rigidity.

- Anti-rigidity releases foundational postural muscles from strain. Some of these muscles may have been lying dormant for decades. This results in the reintegration of dormant muscle with active muscle restoring strength, endurance, flexibility, stability, and ideal posture.

- Anti-rigidity will get your muscles firing again, tone and balance your body, reduce fatigue and soreness, and counteract the poor loading profiles of the modern lifestyle.

- For a muscle to be healthy, it needs times during the day when it is pulled to full resting length and other times when it is contracted to its smallest dimension. Use anti-rigidity daily to achieve this.

- Experiment and play with the muscles you have neglected for so long, and with time, you will experience an "incredible lightness of being."

- Muscles are like springs that are bent out of shape. A muscle that has low tone and is not firing properly is like a spring whose coil has become stretched out. Such muscles require anti-laxity.

- A muscle stuck in partial contraction is like a spring that is not at its resting length (relaxed) or its shortest length (contracted) but stuck somewhere in the middle. Such muscles require anti-rigidity.

Chapter 14: **Endnote**

1.   Gallegos, A. M., Crean, H. F., Pigeon, W. R., & Heffner, K. L. (2017). Meditation and yoga for posttraumatic stress disorder: A meta-analytic review of randomized controlled trials. *Clinical Psychology Review*, *58*, 115–124; van der Kolk, B. A., Stone, L., West, J., Rhodes, A., Emerson, D., Suvak, M., & Spinazzola, J. (2014). Yoga as an adjunctive treatment for posttraumatic stress disorder: A randomized controlled trial. *Journal of Clinical Psychiatry*, *75*(6), e599–565.

Chapter 15: **Combine Anti-rigidity with Exercise**

Excessive Exercise Without Anti-rigidity is Detrimental

Unsustainable workout habits played a large role in my stress. Overly ambitious running and heavy lifting were tightening my straitjacket. I was reaping ephemeral, short-term benefits such as muscle gain and fat loss. But the long-term costs of accumulating soft tissue injury were significant. For instance, even though I had developed some strength in my bench press, if I altered the position of my shoulders slightly or turned my elbows or wrists a little, the same bench-pressing motion was painful and incredibly frail. When you put a great deal of tension into an invariant configuration, the other potential arrangements become extraordinarily limited. It is the same with running. Aside from my habitual running pattern, my body was highly immobile.

If you signed a contract to play a superhero in an upcoming blockbuster movie, you would engage in arduous weightlifting and strenuous cardiovascular exercise. A few months of this would tighten existing knots in your muscles but make you look incredibly fit. A few years of activity like this would produce copious dormant muscle, shackling the spine. In kinesiology, this is referred to as "muscular pattern overload." It would make you stronger in the short-term but much weaker in the long-term. This is how I exercised in my twenties: sprinting and grueling weights with no stretching, massage, or recognition of bracing. Combined with chronic panicked breathing, zero postural awareness, and lots of sitting, it wrecked my foundation. The sad truth is that this should sound familiar to many people.

The Cost of Lifting Heavy Weights

Lifting heavy weights was my defense mechanism for dealing with the male status hierarchy. I thought that more muscle would free me from hierarchical worries, but it became my prison, both figuratively and literally. It wrecked my posture by pulling my shoulders forward and my chin away from my chest. I am not alone in this. Postural neglect, excessive bracing, and inattention to hyperfatigued muscle accelerate age-related postural decline in the majority of people who lift weights. Frankly, weightlifters experience significant reductions in all planes of spinal movement.

As a teenager, I read books on lifting weights that proclaimed that 8 to 12 repetitions done to complete muscle failure is the scientifically established way to achieve muscle growth. This is true on the order of months, but without regular anti-rigidity, 8 to 12 repetitions with the heaviest weight you can bear is a recipe for dormant muscle. It took me years to realize that overzealous lifting came with hidden costs. They creep up on you. Lifting heavy weights at low reps causes you to fall into faulty muscle recruitment patterns, leading to strain and cramping all over the body. In my late twenties, I would wake up every morning in agonizing tension. After rising, it would take at least 10 minutes for the circulation in my chest and neck to reestablish and abate the crushing pain.

Most people wouldn't even have described me as muscular, and yet my chest, shoulders, neck, and back were completely locked up from weightlifting. I had trigger points, scar tissue, and chronic inflammation all along my shoulder girdle. The tension of unchecked weightlifting crept up my spine, through my cervical vertebrae, and into the attachments between my neck and skull. At this point, it impinges on one's soul. Like most people that lift weights, I avoided frail muscles altogether. In doing so, we magnify the frailty.

Underused Muscles Need Anti-laxity, and Overused Muscles Need Anti-rigidity

When loading to certain muscles is completely missing, and these muscles sit adjacent to muscles that are unnaturally overloaded you have injury and pain waiting to happen. Underused muscles are usually long and weak. Overused muscles are short and tight. Underused muscles need to be exercised and toned. Overused muscles need to be stretched, massaged, and, most importantly, contracted through the dormant sections of their range of motion.

Bend down and feel your calf. You likely have a lot of soft muscle surrounding a lump of painful, hard muscle. The soft muscle is underused, while the hard muscle is overused. You want the softest lumps to become harder and the hardest lumps to become softer. To do so, increase the tone in the soft portions through exercise and anti-laxity and decrease the tone of the hard lumps using massage and anti-rigidity (It is the same with your spine, face, voice and, as we will see in Chapter 19, the muscles surrounding your genitals). This will develop the calf's ability to contract as one integrated unit through its full range.

It helps to pull the toes up toward the knee (dorsiflexion), which will contract the muscles in the front of the calf. Hold this contraction and breathe deeply. Next, point your toes away from your body (plantar flexion) using the muscles in the back of the calf. Every day, spend one minute flexing the toes back toward the shin and then pointing the toes in the opposite direction. While in both positions, offset the feet to the left and then to the right. Roll your ankles clockwise and counterclockwise. Search for the areas that feel stiff and achy. If you can find this aching, know that contracting into it calmly is accomplishing bona fide anti-rigidity.

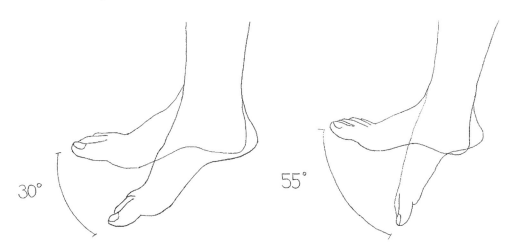

Illustration 15.1: A. The typical range of motion in the ankle is thirty degrees. However, limiting yourself to this range contributes to the development of dormant ankle musculature; B. Exercising the ankle in an extended range will expand the mobility and contribute to healthy ankle joint mechanics.

At first, start these ankle exercises without any weight, even body weight. Just hold the contractions off the ground. Then experiment with partial body weight. Then use full bodyweight calf raises where you try to reach full height during the rise and complete dorsiflexion during the lowering phase. Hold these and breathe. Doing this with the ankles and knees in a variety of positions will allow you to target and tone the underused aspects of your calves. Try new positions like turning the feet out (lateral rotation) or in (medial rotation), and placing weight on the inside of the foot (pronation), or the outside of the foot (supination).

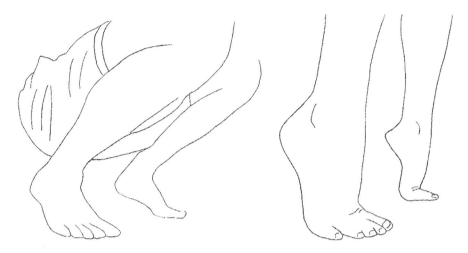

Illustration 15.2: A. Holding the lowered phase of a bodyweight squat to strengthen complete ankle dorsiflexion (ankle bent); B. Holding the full height of a calf raise to strengthen complete plantar flexion (ankle straightened).

Have you heard of "cankles?" It is a pejorative term referring to the combination of "calf" and "ankle" describing an ankle that appears continuous with the calf. They are the unattractive consequence of chronically overused ankle muscles. In other words, a cankle is just an ankle whose muscles are stuck in partial contraction. Cankles are ugly because bulky, hypertrophic muscle in isolated areas leads to swelling, edema, and inflammation. The cankles phenomenon isn't limited to the ankles. Persistent contractions make the whole body look worse for the same reasons. Most people who don't like their physiques are simply unhappy with the appearance of their body's dormant muscles. You want to tone and firm your soft muscles without any underlying musculature being hard and hypertonic. It's a balancing act.

Performing calf raises in the gym with heavy weights turned sections of my calves into very hard muscle segments. This extra muscle was useful for calf raises but otherwise made walking painful. In my late twenties, my ankles, calves, and knees would hurt after just 20 minutes of walking. Percussive massage and anti-rigidity have made it so that I can walk for more than three hours without any discomfort. They also turned my cankles into lean, trim ankles and put a new spring in my step. There are very tangible benefits to replacing our high-intensity, low-variety, repetitious exercises with exercises that use the body more diversely.

Dormant Muscles Expose You to Injury

Tight and shortened muscles dominate movement at the joint disrupting healthy joint mechanics. Some researchers call this "joint compression" (not to be confused with the massage technique). It causes major physical limitations for both athletes and the general population: force leaks, torque loss, and gaps in strength. Shortened and dormant muscle is responsible for why advanced weightlifters fail at entry-level plyometric workout exercises like box jumping.[1] The muscles of many bodybuilders have limited range and tend to fatigue quickly. This is why you don't see them competing in high-level athletics events which demand agility, flexibility, or endurance. Activities that require both speed and strength are often painful for weightlifters. The abrupt forces can even cause cramped, hypertonic muscles to tear or rip.

Dormant muscle and their attachments are highly susceptible to tearing. Sprains (tearing of a ligament) and strains (tearing of a muscle or tendon) are the most common types of soft tissue sports injuries. They are often caused by activities that require muscles to stretch and contract suddenly at the same time. A lack of conditioning, flexibility, and warm-up can contribute, but usually, a strain is a previously existing site of dormancy just waiting to be injured.

When you develop a kink in your neck, lower back, or anywhere else, it is seldom a new development. It is practically always preexisting dormant muscle that has recently been agitated. Usually, kinks are previously locked up muscles that have started to unlock. Unfortunately, immobilizing them until they stop hurting, which most people do, will cause them to relock. Worse yet, trying to move them while breathing shallowly will cause them to close up tighter. But diaphragmatic anti-rigidity will allow you to open and repair these kinks. The next time you pull or strain a muscle, be grateful that a site of frailty has been revealed and is now open to rehab.

I sprained my shoulder wrestling a friend. This was ironic because I lifted heavy weights in hopes of appearing physically powerful. But when it came down to grappling with someone, my uneven tone led to disparities between muscles that could be loaded and those that couldn't. There were muscles along my scapula that couldn't bear even a moderate load and trying to squeeze out of a stranglehold headlock sprained them badly. I learned that it is far preferable to have regular strength throughout the body and little frailty than to have excessive strength in certain areas and extreme frailty in others.

Treating an Injury

Never stretch or use anti-rigidity for the first 72 hours after an injury. You want to give the muscle tears a chance to heal first. This means that any time you strain or even tweak something, just go home and rest. Don't risk aggravating it by continuing to exercise or compete. Soft massage after icing can be beneficial directly following a minor injury. Three days later, it is important to begin proactively compressing and stretching the muscles to stop scar tissue formation. In fact, many medical professionals take untreated scar tissue to be the primary cause of re-injury. I believe that after a week it is safe to start rehabilitating light to moderate strains using anti-rigidity.

Physical therapists often recommend that patients "breathe into" their injuries. If you sprain your wrist, they might advise that you concentrate on deep breathing and the sensations coming from the wrist simultaneously. In yoga and Pilates, instructors recommend breathing deeply when stretching sore, injured, or tight muscles. "Breathing into" tension teaches the brain that it can interact with these muscles without recruiting the fight or flight response. This is why I recommend taking out your breathing metronome whenever you rehab an injury.

I even recommend paced breathing as soon as you sustain an injury to reduce the unnecessary bracing that comes with something like a sprain. Immediately after an injury, people naturally breathe very shallowly, and this causes the surrounding muscles to tense up, potentially exacerbating the extent of the tissue damage. Breathing with the diaphragm and concentrating on progressive relaxation at the injury site can improve the prognosis and decrease recovery time. Just be aware that paced breathing will diminish the body's protective "casting" and immobilizing of the injured area. Accordingly, you must be very careful not to subject this area to any undue loads for the first few days.

I sprained my shoulder in a fall from a skateboard. Of course, it was the locked-up, bench press stabilizing muscles that were injured. Because of the shoulder injury, I had to stop lifting weights completely. My upper body muscle mass atrophied very quickly. I lost almost all my bulk within two months. However, and here is the kicker: the pain, knots, and scar tissue remained as if I had never stopped working out. This proved to me that lifting heavy weights has benefits that are easily lost, while the costs persist. Without incessant weightlifting, you lose the mass but still retain all the cellular scarring. I felt compelled to get this tension from weightlifting out of my body, so I developed an alternate way to lift weights.

Lift Weights with Optimal Posture

Most people lift heavy weights from a compact position. The more you do this, the more ungainly your posture becomes and the more difficult it is to lift from an expansive posture. By exercising with bad postural alignment, you will degrade the structures you are trying to improve. When your vertebrae are out of alignment and you strain under heavy weights, you further reinforce the misalignments. Like trying to erect a massive building on a poor foundation, it will be lopsided and unstable. Thus, when your form breaks down, make that your last rep. With open, expansive, properly aligned posture, any type of exercise you practice will be more effective.

When most people lift weights that are too heavy, they brace and lock up their entire skeleton holding their spine, shoulder girdle, and hips in the same invariant position each time. Merely reducing the weight allows you to lift without bracing. With less weight, you can also alter and vary your posture with each rep and change the distribution of weight loading, stimulating growth in areas that are usually stiff.

Most exercisers perform narrow range repetitions where the muscle lengthens and contracts only a small amount each repetition. This is a surefire way to force muscles into partial contraction. For example, my friend does limited range of motion squats with extremely heavy weight. This means that instead of going from standing to touching his butt to his ankles, he instead only moves a few inches during each squat. Doing this with stacks of weight plates has given him huge knots above his knees. These knots form a buffer for his end range squat, helping him stop the squat halfway down and reverse the motion. But the same knots that help him come back up in that single exercise, limit the general action of his quadriceps in almost all other activities.

I have since helped him get rid of these knots by using full range motion, massage, and anti-rigidity. You can see that this is much like the above example involving my calves. Do you do anything similar to this? If you don't want the knots, lower the weight and increase the range of motion. You may have guessed by now that I can't avoid making a related comparison with animals.

Strength Differences Between Humans and Other Apes

Although chimpanzees are generally lighter than humans (they range between 70 and 140 pounds), they are much stronger on average. The shaved arms of a female chimp look like a professional football player's arms. In captivity, chimps are aware of their strength advantage and are very dangerous because of it. They often physically bulldoze humans. In the wild, they don't know that they are stronger and can be studied safely at closer quarters. Indeed, many scientists think chimps can overpower even the strongest humans. I long wondered how at only 140 pounds, they could be stronger than bodybuilders? I believe their disproportionate strength comes from the way they build their muscles incrementally from all angles.

Apes amass upper body strength gradually from a young age tree climbing and knuckle-walking, which they do with their arms and legs. Using each limb vigorously is an intrinsic part of getting around. They incorporate their entire physique into each smooth, integrated movement rather than wrenching isolated muscles with dumbbells or barbells. Since apes build their muscles naturally rather than lifting heavy weights, trigger points and dormant muscles rarely encumber their movement. If we want to become truly strong, we have to build strength incrementally like a chimpanzee. Now you and I cannot start our childhood over in the trees. But we can start by infusing lightweight exercises with anti-rigidity.

Practice Anti-rigidity During Exercise

Just as you can combine anti-rigidity techniques and yoga, you can also combine anti-rigidity with other workouts, including weight training. By and large, people avoid their trigger points and areas of frailty when exercising. Resist this temptation. You want to work out your short, painful muscles, tailoring exercises to target these sites specifically. To do this, exercise slowly using only light resistance to search for and contract into dormant muscle. Alter your joint configurations until you find a combination that aches or cracks, then hold this pattern and continue to perform repetitions. If you don't let the discomfort disturb your breathing pattern, the muscle will surrender and cooperate.

I want to encourage you to go to your local gym, sit on practically every machine on the floor, use a very low weight setting, and do between 20 and 100 repetitions trying to work through the subtle aching and cracking. Think of each station in the weight room as a tool you can use to employ anti-rigidity from a different angle.

Weightlifting Exercise #15.1: *Anti-laxity and Anti-rigidity with Weights*

Perform standard weightlifting routines with machines or free weights but do so using very light weight. Employ anti-laxity to accustom your body to healthy forces, and employ anti-rigidity to bring blood to and mend dormant muscle. Maintain proper posture and use multidirectional movements with complete range of motion. Add novel curvature to the spine every few repetitions. Vary between kyphosis and lordosis in your neck and upper spine for upper body exercises. Then vary between these in the lower back for lower body exercises. Use spinal flexion, then spinal extension for maximal effect. Bend to each side, twist to each side. Search actively for aching positions to engage.

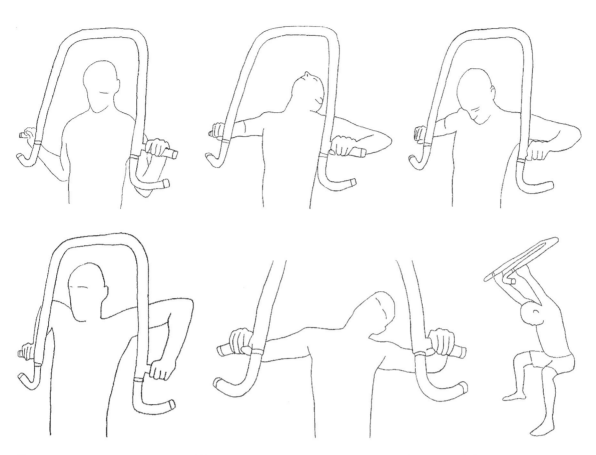

Illustration 15.3: Suggestions for different joint configurations for anti-rigidity during light weight bench press.

Do a few reps with your neck flexed to each side, then with your chin to your chest, with your neck retracted, and then with your neck extended backwards. It should feel like yoga with gym equipment. Any exercise expert would try to persuade you from turning your neck to the extreme left when performing a lateral pull down or from adducting your hip and tilting your pelvis when performing a leg press. They would be right if you were lifting between 50 and 100% of your one-repetition maximum. But if you are lifting less than 30% of your max, you should have plenty of room to play with the joint configurations safely.

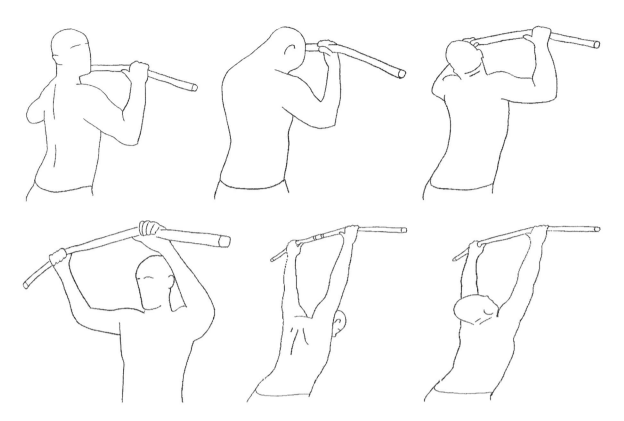

Illustration 15.4: Examples of different joint configurations for spinal anti-rigidity during light weight lateral pulldowns.

One important caveat: I am asking you to vary your spine's position as you work out, but only at low intensity and low resistance. At high intensity, you want to keep your spine straight. This is common knowledge in exercise science. Many athletes refer to any bend in any portion of the spine as a fault or error.[2] Indeed, you commit a fault any time your spine changes shape during any weight-bearing movement. When you lift something heavy off the ground, perform a squat, or a push-up, your spine should stay neutral the entire time. In other words, we should regularly be flexing and extending as many portions of the back as possible, but never when combined with a heavy load or rapid movements.

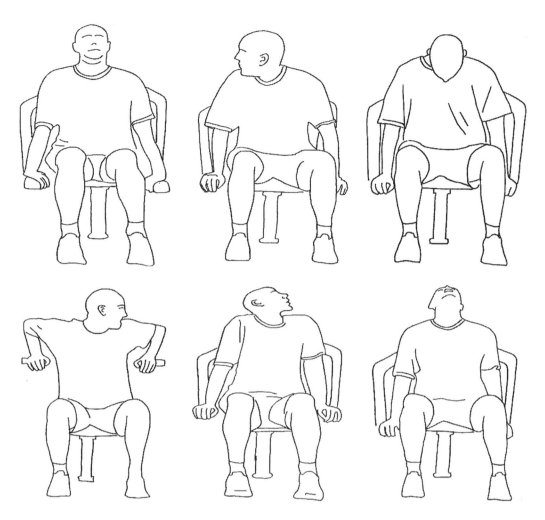

Illustration 15.5: Examples of different joint configurations for anti-rigidity during light weight tricep push downs.

I find using anti-laxity and anti-frailty with weights to be tremendously relaxing. Much like yoga, the blood flow and endorphins make my muscles feel heavy and tranquil. This is a 180 from my previous approach to working out.

Exercise More Often, Not Harder

When mixing anti-rigidity with weightlifting the objective is to gradually increase the load, over the course of months, as your posture improves and your frailty diminishes. Slowly building up to heavier weights and intensities will help you build a broad, stable base to place even more muscle on top of. This is in line with the often-forgotten personal trainer's maxim, "straighten the body before strengthening it."

The common wisdom in personal training, which empirical studies have reinforced, is that muscle typically atrophies at half the rate it took to develop. This means that your gains from six months of squats will completely disappear a year after you stop squatting. To me, the takeaway message is clear. If you gain a lot of muscle from intense training over three months, you cannot expect to keep it for long. So don't plan to work out this way. But if you gain muscle steadily over three years, it will resist atrophy for six years. Instead of stressing the body, plateauing early, and struggling to maintain, envision your workout goal as a slow and steady climb.

This is consistent with a popular weight training routine known as "pyramid training," where you start with very light weights and progress steadily toward heavier weights. You will find that starting lower than bodyweight, then using bodyweight, and then progressing through very light weights will condition your postural muscles with exercise volume as opposed to intensity. For many exercises, even bodyweight is too much. In my opinion, less than 5% of the population is ready for pushups. Ninety-five percent of people will accrue unnecessary damage from pushups, myself included. Instead, they need to spend a few months doing pushups on their knees or simply lowering themselves to the ground from push-up position (working the negative).

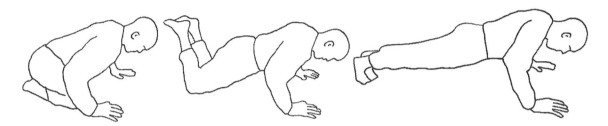

Illustration 15.6: Pushup progression: A. Pushups on the shins and knees; B. Pushups on the knees; C. Lowered pushups, and finally traditional pushups.

Global bodily adaptations to low weights will scaffold a highly balanced system that you can later apply toward heavier weights to achieve surprising results. This takes advantage of the aforementioned SAID principle (specific adaptation to imposed demands). Again, this is how apes, farmers, mechanics, and lumberjacks develop strength. But this doesn't just apply to lifting weights. The same goes for jogging, swimming, aerobics, Program Peace exercises, and anything else. Don't base your exercise duration or intensity on arbitrary factors. Instead, work out from within your frailty until none of your postural muscles are hypertonic, and they all cooperate seamlessly. Then resume traditional full-body workouts.

Starting with low-intensity and focusing on anti-rigidity has another benefit. Recall from Chapter 5 that dormant muscles cannot recover adequately after a workout. They are resistant to growth and strengthening because muscles afflicted with trigger points never rest and can never fully heal.[3] Thus, dormant muscles are equivalent to untapped reservoirs that are full of growth potential. Anti-rigidity allows you to tap into them. Once you convert dormant muscle to supple and tension-free muscle, they will be very responsive to exercise. From there, you will be ripe for a total body transformation.

In my twenties I would visit a nutritional supplement store. The clerks would always tell me, "look man, if you want to gain muscle, you have to take weight gainer." For a long time, I believed they were right and that I needed protein supplementation and hundreds of additional calories every day to put on muscle mass. This isn't true. The real constraint that keeps you from putting on additional muscle is the muscle tension. It is dormant muscle that is responsible for the performance plateaus and diminishing returns. Once you use anti-laxity and anti-rigidity to rebuild this muscle back into your posture, you will find that it will not fluctuate with exercise or diet. Because it moves when you do, and its tone is reinforced by simply standing around, it resists atrophy and does not require overeating.

Practice Anti-rigidity Following Exercise

After almost all forms of conventional exercise, dormant muscle becomes further strained. After a jog, you go home, and your knees hurt a little, or your lower back feels stiff, and this accrues with interest over time. It doesn't have to be this way. Engaging these areas with anti-rigidity exercises directly after a workout is the best way for you to release them. It provides fresh blood to the collateral and stabilizing muscles stiffened by the activity. For every minute of training, you should perform a minute of anti-rigidity.

After you do three sets of bench press, do 3 minutes of anti-rigidity for the neck, shoulders, and upper back. A yoga pose like downward dog is excellent. Whatever you choose, shift your shoulders as you alternate between twisting, flexing, and extending the neck. You'll discover that the increased circulation from a weight lifting or a cardio workout will allow you to contract more deeply into dormant muscle.

You can also use the anti-rigidity and yoga positions pictured in the previous chapter as "counter poses." Counter poses are used in yoga to activate complementary and antagonistic muscles after a pose. For instance, a twist to the left follows a twist to the right and forward bends usually follow backbends. According to yoga practitioners, this "neutralizes" the spine, lengthening it and "calming the nervous system." With practice, you can identify the best counterposes to neutralize the tension created by your exercise routine.

How to Breathe When Lifting Light Weights

Why are some people strong while others are weak? Why are some people muscular while others are not? Most scientists would say that testosterone exposure and genetics determine these characteristics, but I believe these explanations are secondary to a more primary process. This process involves the ability to contract muscles without recruiting the distressed breathing response. Naturally athletic and muscular people had childhoods conducive to combining exercise with unimpeded breathing. In other words, adults with big biceps were kids that learned to sustain hardy bicep contractions without impeding their breathing. But you don't have to be a kid to internalize this. The truth is, we worked on this in Exercises 13.2-13.8 when we combined paced breathing with anti-laxity.

In the same vein, you want to breathe very deeply while pumping iron. Most physical therapists and personal trainers recommend breathing out when major muscles are shortening (the lifting action in a curl) and breathing in during the lengthening (the lowering action of the curl). For a bench press, this would involve breathing out while lifting the bar away from your chest and breathing in while dropping the weight to your chest. This is not bad advice, as it keeps you from holding your breath or breathing at even shorter intervals. However, when using low weight, it is beneficial to breathe at even longer intervals.

Breathing Activity #15.1: *Diaphragmatic Breathing at the Gym*

The next time you lift light weights, start off breathing out for an entire repetition (flexion and extension) and then in for the next repetition. Perform a few sets in this way. Next, inhale for two reps, and then exhale for two reps. This is an advanced technique but will become much easier as you complete the breathing retraining outlined in Chapters 3 and 11. As long as you are breathing deep, complete breaths, you should get plenty of air. Breathing at longer intervals convinces your nervous system that weightlifting is not traumatic, allowing your body to adapt to the challenge rather than resisting it. Deep breathing convinces the body that holding those 15-pound dumbbells in the air is safe, easy, and the new normal.

Lifting heavy weights is stressful on the body and mind, and anything stressful will provoke shallow breathing. The physical exertion involved in lifting heavy weights makes it very difficult to concentrate on breathing diaphragmatically. Lifting definitely contributed to my breathing dysfunction. A high proportion of weightlifters breathe shallowly, and like racehorses, are often high-strung. They are doing the opposite of the Program Peace method, pairing intense muscular contractions with distressed breathing, and further traumatizing them. Also, keep in mind that the anxiety involved in this puts you into a state of catabolism where proteins are broken down rather than built up, ultimately making it harder to put on and keep on muscle.

As you found with your eating routine in Chapter 3, your exercise routines may be tightly intertwined with distressed breathing. You may even find it difficult to exert yourself while breathing diaphragmatically. However, it will be much easier at the lowest levels of exertion, so start there. You can use a breath metronome when exercising or you may just want to tape your mouth.

As you work on your breathing, be aware of your other nonverbals. The stereotypical weightlifter's body language is highly detrimental to their health. Gasping, hyperventilating, jerking, straining, breath-holding, trembling, and bracing the entire body are the exact things you want to avoid. Most people also tighten their vocal tract, raise their eyebrows, make a pained face, sneer, and squint during heavy exercise. For all the reasons described in previous chapters, try to avoid doing these things. The only muscles that should be working are the ones responsible for the load. Rather than being a spaz at the gym, try being poised and laid-back.

Weight Lifting Exercise #15.2: *Breath Metronome at the Gym*

Use headphones and a breathing metronome to perform paced breathing at your gym while lifting light weights and employing anti-rigidity. Set the breathing duration to a low level (e.g. 3-5 second inhalations and 5-7 second exhalations). Don't use a breath metronome while performing heavy resistance or aerobic exercise though. In these cases, let your instincts guide your breath rate, and just try to breathe deeply and nasally (see breathing Exercise 3.8 from Chapter 3).

Using the breath metronome at the gym has another empowering benefit. By the second week of paced breathing, you will be at peace with rather than apprehensive of the muscular and athletic people lifting weights next to you. You will realize that you were previously stifling your breath to appease the other gym members in psychoneurotic ways. In my twenties, I felt like every person in the gym thought they were cooler than me. Paced breathing at the athletic facility changed this completely. By using a breath metronome to calm your thoughts, you will completely escape "gymtimidation." While you're at it, try incorporating other subroutines discussed in this book such as resting face, looking above the eyeline, and the tenets of optimal posture. Paced breathing will help you become the most composed gym-goer at your facility within a matter of weeks.

People also often hold their breath during short but intense athletic performances, like a golf swing, free throw, or cartwheel. Instead, take a deep, slow breath before the feat and breathe out calmly during the feat. As you perform that high jump, penalty kick, sommersault, or basketball dunk, you want to be breathing, and to nurture the execution, it helps to be breathing out. Breathing shallowly or holding the breath tells the body: "hopefully this is the last time we will ever have to do this." Breathing deeply tells the body: "this is something that we are going to be doing regularly now, so you better get good at it."

Anything practiced repeatedly is debraced overtime, especially if you do it while breathing diaphragmatically. A gymnast will have a gorgeous standing backflip if they have done it hundreds of times while breathing calmly. The best backflips come from people that don't have to activate their sympathetic system to pull it off. My cartwheel is still tense, but the more I practice it while exhaling smoothly through the nose, the more I learn which aspects of the motion are overbraced. In movement patterns from layups, to backhands, to football lobs, to jumping jacks, to burpees, don't aim for breathless intensity. Aim for braceless efficiency.

A person new to jumping rope will grab the handles too tightly, brace their spine inordinately, look awkward, and develop an injury if they jump too long. A person who has spent over 10 cumulative hours jumping rope looks and feels like they are skipping on air. Give your exercise activities plenty of time to stabilize under diaphragmatic conditions, and they will become graceful child's play.

Focus on Dissipating the Tension

During an exercise session, tension steadily accumulates in muscles. Some become reset to a harmfully high level, resulting in an elevation in passive contraction. This is why you want to use diaphragmatic breathing to dissipate tension right after you exercise. If you are going to exercise until you feel the burn, then focus on the burn fully subsiding after the set. Lie down if it helps.

Weightlifting Activity #15.2: *Noticing Muscle Tension after a Set*

Simply by paying attention to the mounting tension after you complete a set, you can consciously negate it, thereby enhancing recovery, healing, and muscle gain. When you ignore it, it usually remains contracted. You may feel the muscles twitch or spasm; notice these small intrusions. Because these twitches are uncomfortable, they halt breathing - maintaining the tension in the area. Instead, you want to concentrate on relaxing the tension, and breathing through it until it subsides. Your focus should be on being completely limp between sets.

I used to have disturbing elbow pain from lifting heavy weights. It was tennis elbow, a degenerative condition also known as epicondylitis. Conditions like it have a poor prognosis and no modern medical treatments besides rest, pain relievers, and surgery. Many of these types of surgeries have been shown to be no better than a placebo mock surgery. I used to finish resistance exercises in an extremely agitated state. Then I would spend the rest of the day, and go to bed, in that state. I wondered why my elbows hurt so much in the morning, and I naively attributed it to aging. Most medical doctors refer to such examples of acute tension as disease because they become chronic in so many people. This "disease" is easily remedied.

Now, whether resistance training, swimming, running, or anything else, I stop completely every few minutes. I take a full 30 seconds to bestow the tightness the mental attention it needs to subside. When I get home, I squeeze, compress, and percuss any muscles that hurt. I thought I was going to have tennis elbow for the rest of my life. After less than 10 total minutes of elbow tension awareness and 10 additional minutes of compression and percussion as outlined in Chapter 6, the elbow "disease" has disappeared and never resurfaced. This method has worked for me for dozens of similar issues in the last few years. That is how powerful these simple solutions are.

Rest Once the First Muscle Group Reaches Fatigue

When people lift heavy weights, some of their large muscle groups are prepared to deal with the weight, but other muscles are far too weak. The muscles that are not up to the task are usually those used to stabilize the weight. The stabilizing muscles (such as the scapular muscles during bench press) don't move or rest between repetitions. Some muscles don't even rest in between sets. Between each repetition, you want there to be moments where every muscle is given a microbreak. As we learned in Chapter 5, this break permits the muscles to escape partial contraction, rest, and regenerate so that they can resume proper function.

Because stabilizing muscles stay still at full exertion during the exercise, they learn to do so all the time. This drives the muscle into deep fatigue, freezing it in place. This is highly damaging. It stops the muscle from growing, and it is why some weightlifters appear so encumbered when they move. Stabilizing muscles keep parts of the body steady so that the primary muscles can do their job. But in a different exercise, a stabilizing muscle may need to be used as a primary muscle. If it is rigid, then performing that exercise correctly is impossible. When stabilizers are dormant, your motion comes across as robotic, stilted, and effortful.

Bench pressing 100 pounds may be great for your pectorals and triceps but may be brutal to your rotator cuff. In this case, you should lower the weight until the exercise is optimal for strengthening the rotator cuff. Many exercises are just right for some muscles but way too hard on others, and you owe it to yourself to fall back to the level of the weakest link. Once the first muscle group has fatigued, it is important to stop what you are doing and wait for it to return to its baseline.

Avoid Overexertion

Large increases or changes in exercise activity can cause tendonitis, tendonosis, and delayed onset muscle soreness. You can easily avoid this through more gradual transitions in an exercise regimen. But few people actually do this. Instead, most change their routine abruptly. Or they exercise infrequently but overexert themselves when they do. Soreness and tendonitis are conducive to the creation of dormant muscle so avoid them by increasing your training more gradually. Four days of recovery is recommended for individual muscle groups after heavy training. However, that doesn't mean you should leave the muscles alone entirely.

I recommend you replicate the activity that made it sore to get the blood circulating and to facilitate remodeling. Just do so with less intensity and for only a fraction of the time, so as not to impede the healing process.

The muscles that feel sore the day after a workout are usually the dormant ones and thus the ones most in need of massage and anti-rigidity. Use any hints of soreness after a workout to help you locate your dormant muscle so you can treat it. If you wake up sore, I recommend taking a baseball, knuckle, or knuckle tool and percussing the entire body focusing on the tender areas. If you are going to work so hard that you are sore the next day, you must rehab the sore spots. Working out until you're sore and then letting the muscles stagnate for days until the soreness disappears is irresponsible. This tells us that our modus operandi should be: "exercise, massage, anti-rigidity, repeat."

Don't kill yourself when working out, and don't be a weekend warrior. Training to complete exhaustion is training under duress. If you are forcing yourself, you cannot go into flow and cannot enjoy the process. Training should be addictive, but it can't be if you push yourself into anxiety just to get it done. In the long run, extreme exertion only wears you down, lowers your mood, and leads to injury. It is exacting to generate the mental energy to train strenuously, but you should find it easy to generate the mental energy to train moderately.

Take a rest after laborious exercise. When you come home from the gym, don't go right to cooking dinner and cleaning up. You want to reset the tension you created, so lie down in corpse pose for five to 10 minutes while paced breathing, and practice progressive muscle relaxation (see Unbracing Exercises 1 and 2). Notice pockets of tension while you are lying down and attempt to let them go.

Often the exercise activity is blamed as the cause of the pain, but in many cases the pain is produced by neglecting to stretch, massage, and relax after exercise. The same goes for those days when you didn't exercise but engaged in prolonged sitting, standing, or walking. When you finally get home and collapse feeling stiff and achy, you've pushed your tissues too far without microbreaks or counterposes. Proper use of the techniques in the last two chapters can make the difference between a day that will make you stronger and a day that will make you weaker.

Conclusion

"The world breaks everyone and afterward many are strong at the broken places." — *Ernest Hemingway*

When my posture was at its worst, lifting weights was so uncomfortable that I reached a point where I just couldn't do it anymore. I badly wanted to build muscle, but the pain and frailty made it so that I would just hold the weight in my hand and look at it. Like a broken-down plow horse, I just stood there and couldn't muster the will to take on the burden. I had few acute injuries, but I was covered in chronic injury. I took two years off from intense exercise and instead focused on anti-rigidity, range of motion, flexibility, low resistance, and low impact. The same weightlifting exercises that were drudgery for me, I now find exhilarating.

Here is a list summarizing the primary elements of the Program Peace muscle rehabilitation method:

The Elements of the Muscle Rehabilitation Method

1) Search for and contract into achiness
2) Find configurations that crack and bring them to a gentle fatigue
3) Combine anti-rigidity and anti-laxity with yoga and light weightlifting
4) Rest limply once fatigue is reached
5) Be aware of bracing
6) Use optimal posture
7) Regularly refresh stagnant muscles using full range of motion
8) Reposition intermittently to avoid staleness
9) Use effective counterposes
10) Massage regularly with compression and percussion
11) Breathe properly all the while

I like the saying, "pain is weakness leaving the body." But it is a half-truth. If the pain is derived from straining, it is weakness entering the body. If the pain is derived from the ache of gently transforming dormant muscle into optimal muscle, it truly is weakness leaving the body.

Chapter 15: **Bullet Points**

- Underused muscles need anti-laxity, and overused muscles need anti-rigidity.
- Dormant muscle tears easily leading to injury.
- Perform anti-rigidity while you perform yoga or while you lift light weights so that you can get leverage into dormant muscle.
- Cardio and weightlifting increase circulation, and thereby make subsequent anti-rigidity more productive.
- Employing anti-rigidity with exercise releases muscles from deep strain, reduces fatigue, and restores strength and endurance.
- When exercising, don't put all your intensity into an invariant form. Alter your form, using as many configurations as possible. This creates multidimensional strength.
- Progress from body weight and very low weight toward heavier weights.
- Rest once the first muscle group reaches fatigue.
- Focus on debracing and dissipating tension after a set or workout.
- It is highly beneficial to perform anti-rigidity and massage on any muscles that are sore the day after a workout.
- Always exercise using the tenets of optimal posture.

Chapter 15: **Endnotes**

1.   Starrett, K., & Cordoza, G. (2013). *Becoming a supple leopard: The ultimate guide to resolving pain, preventing injury, and optimizing athletic performance.* Victory Belt Publishing.

2.   Starret & Cordoza, (2013), *Becoming a supple leopard.*

3.   Simons, D. G., Travell, J. G., & Simons, L. S. (1999). *Travell & Simons' myofacial pain and dysfunction: Upper half of body.* Williams and Wilkins.

Chapter 16: **Anti-rigidity for the Neck and Shoulders**

We are all hunchbacks to different degrees. Our upper spines are contorted from the strain involved in carrying the head in front of the body. This "protruding head posture" bends the lower neck forward and the upper neck backward, creating an "S" shape. Over time, this results in "anterior head syndrome," marked by a bulge in the lower neck that is sometimes called a dowager's hump or a buffalo hump. This is also commonly called "nerd neck." Before I knew anything about this, I found my hump very concerning.

During my 20s, I became preoccupied with the deformed structure of my neck. I could tell that my neck was hunched down in pictures, and when I reached back and felt my cervical spine, I could feel the distorted curvature. The muscles in my neck were hard to the touch due to advanced stage trigger points throughout. Moving my neck hurt, its movement was very limited, and it would tire quickly. I had the necessary symptoms for a diagnosis of "cervical neuromuscular syndrome," which includes chronic neck pain, headaches, sympathetic upregulation, depression, and anxiety.[1] That's right: a tense neck contributes to anxiety. Studies show that it may also contribute to general fatigue, muscle strain, arthritis, herniated discs, pinched nerves, and higher overall mortality.[2]

I would ask my girlfriend to stand on my upper back, hoping that the pressure would crack my vertebrae into proper alignment. Of course, this didn't work. At one point, it crossed my mind that the extreme curvature in my neck was due to the cumulative effects of repetitive strain. I quickly dismissed this notion because I realized how difficult it would be to fix if this was the problem. Sadly, it was. I wanted a quick fix, but there wasn't (and isn't) one. Straightening my neck required years of proper breathing, unbracing, massage, postural awareness, exercise, and anti-rigidity.

The lower cervical vertebrae C6 and C7 bulged out prominently while the vertebrae above them were shrunken in. It took a year of anti-rigidity training for C4 and C5 to come into alignment with C6 and C7. Another year passed before C2 and C3 joined them. Gradually, these vertebrae migrated back into place until the bulges and hump went away. Now, my neck has a healthy curvature and all my previous symptoms are gone. This transformation begins with something called neck retraction.

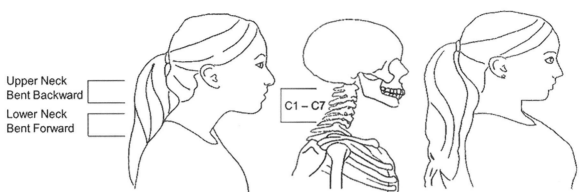

Upper Neck
Bent Backward

Lower Neck
Bent Forward

C1 – C7

Illustration 16.1: A. Neck protracted with the chin poking forward; B. Skeleton with cervical vertebrae visible; C. Neck retracted with the chin tucked.

Neck Retraction Is Tucking the Jaw into the Neck

Crookedness in the neck derives from bringing our head forward, tilting the chin up, and compressing or scrunching the top of the back of the neck. This is called neck protraction. Let's program ourselves to do the opposite: neck retraction. We saw neck retraction in Chapter 13 as the fifth principle of optimal posture. Let's dive deeper.

Neck Exercise #16.1: *Neck Retraction*

The first step is to pull your chin and jaw backward as if you were trying to pull them into your throat. As you keep your chin tucked, lean your head backward relative to your chest until your ears are pulled back behind the chest, in line with the center of your shoulder. Roll your shoulders back and down while looking straight ahead. Adopting this position while doing different activities from different loading positions will help you internalize it. For instance, try nodding yes, shaking no, or bobbing your head to music with the neck retracted.

Another method to achieve this posture is to grab a clump of your hair at the base of the back of your skull and gently pull it up and back. Alternatively, Pilates practitioners imagine a string from the heavens attached to the back of their skull, constantly pulling their heads upward. Think about holding a calm, prolonged contraction in the muscles involved. Spend five minutes holding this posture and performing anti-rigidity within it while breathing diaphragmatically.

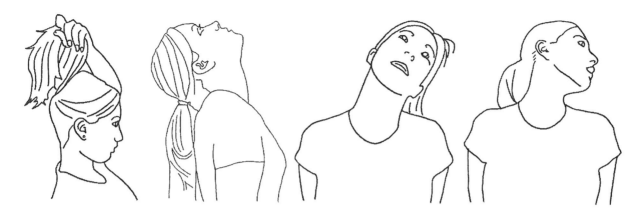

Illustration 16.2: Various neck positions for anti-rigidity.

Most people exercise, socialize, and sit with their necks exclusively protracted. Combined with the stress and strain of daily life, this firmly fixes the neck in a forward slumped posture. Untucking the chin while lifting weights or working at a desk further solidifies this degenerative cervical position. When most people then try to retract their necks, it feels sticky, achy, and scary. Almost everyone butts up against a firm wall of dormant muscle in the back of their neck when they retract it. This wall of dormancy is the hump itself. You will need to use anti-rigidity to chip away at the muscular adhesions responsible for this cramped obstruction.

Stop Untucking Your Chin

The dowager's hump arises from the self-handicapping act of untucking the chin and protracting the neck. This act of jutting the chin out in front of the body declares "I give up" to anyone watching. In my twenties, I would always untuck my chin whenever I passed by anyone. It appears polite and disarming to others but is poisonous to you. This social signal, innate to our biology, is throwing in the towel. Most people untuck their necks whenever they are nervous, and especially during startle. They might as well be placing their head on a chopping block. If anything, you want to retract your neck when startled, as this protects your neck with your jaw.

I held my head as if I were scared that I would bump it against something if I stood up straight. I held it as if I were using my neck to appease angry giants. I held it as if I were trying to tell the world that the pith of my body (the musculature that supports the head) exists in a deeply defective position. The extent of your hunchback is a function of how often you untuck your chin. Everyone is aware of this implicitly, but almost no one speaks of it or does anything about it. Now that you are explicitly aware, use chin retraction to increase your nonverbal dominance. Again, the more often you "fake" it, the more natural you make it.

Making Neck Retraction Habitual

Some people refrain from retracting their neck because it results in a double chin. Paradoxically, not using the muscles responsible for retraction increases the flabbiness in this area. So, retracting your neck often will eventually make that double chin disappear. The chin lock from Exercise 12.4, as well as compression exercises 9.16 and 9.17 for the jawline and jowls, will help greatly in training neck retraction. Combining these exercises will excise the pudginess behind your chin, straighten the back of your neck, increase the extent of ujjayi breathing, and enrich your voice. One of the main causes of weakened voice is postural. When the neck is not retracted, the laryngeal musculature loses proper tone.

Neck retraction will also make your head lighter. The more the head protrudes in front of the body, the more stress is placed on the cervical spine. Straight up and down, the head produces about 10 pounds of pressure on the neck. When the head is tilted toward the floor at 15 degrees, this becomes 30 pounds, and at 45 degrees it is 50 pounds.[3] Thus, neck retraction can lighten the weight of the head by as much as five times. This is enough to turn an overbearing continuous strain into a healthy continuous load.

Neck extension can be a great counterpose to neck retraction. To do this, you bend the head backward.

Neck Exercise #16.2: *Neck Extension to Retraction*

Extend your neck. This means bending it backward, lifting your chin, and tilting your head back as if looking up at the sky. Breathe out for several seconds in this position. For the inhale, flex your neck back into retraction and breathe in for several seconds. Repeat this fifteen times. It can help to use the arms like the model in the pictures below. Repeat the cycle 10 to 15 times.

When your head is extended backward, practice turning/rotating your upper and lower neck to the right and left. Also, practice both neck retraction and protraction from the extended position. Neck retraction from an extended position will reach deeply into the hump in your neck and provide an opportunity for anti-rigidity.

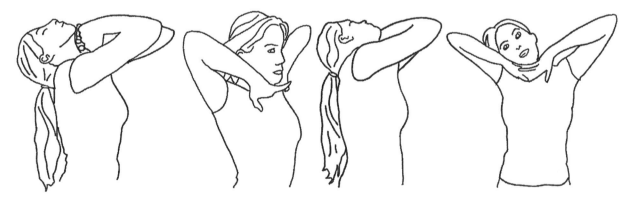

Illustration 16.3: Alternating between neck extension and neck retraction.

An exercise that alternates between neck retraction and extension is often first in a series of hot yoga poses. It is sometimes called "standing deep breathing" because it is traditionally done simultaneously with a form of paced breathing. My initial experiences with this yoga routine strongly influenced the Program Peace method because they made it incredibly clear how effective paced breathing is in the healing process. I firmly recommend these poses as a daily practice. You can easily find videos online. Now for some other exercises that, used daily, will remodel your neck.

Neck Exercise #16.3: *Neck Extension and Rotation*

Lie on your back on the floor. Lift the head an inch off the ground and turn the head from side to side. As you do this, either touch your chin to each shoulder or touch each ear to the ground. Repeat 20-30 times or until you reach fatigue. You can do this with the neck retracted or protracted, flexed, or extended.

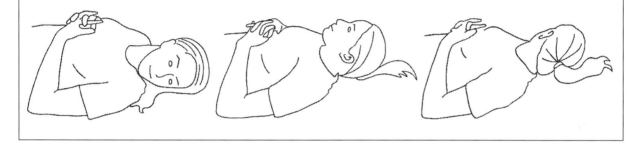

When I socialized in my twenties I must have been bracing and immobilizing practically every muscle in my neck. Looking back on it now, my neck was like an ankle that had been sprained over and over but never iced, massaged, stretched, or exercised. More than anything else, exercises 16.2 and 16.3 have brought it close to optimality. The following lists other helpful routines you can use to limber your neck right up.

Neck Exercises #16.4-13: *Various Neck Anti-rigidity Postures*

Like all the exercises in this chapter, these are intended to be combined with diaphragmatic breathing and the anti-rigidity technique. Use the different positions described here to find and rehab dormant, achy muscle.

4) Lie on your back on the floor with your head on the ground. Lift the chin to the center of your chest (sternum) and then lower it back to the floor. Repeat 20-30 times or until fatigued. To make this harder, each time you lower your head, look to either the right or the left.

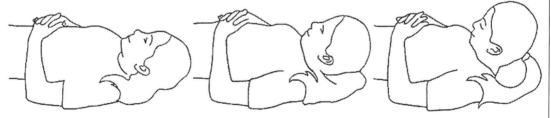

5) Lie on your stomach on the floor. Lift the head off the ground and rotate it from right to left, touching your right ear to the ground, then your left. Repeat 20-30 times.

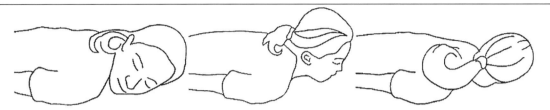

6) Hang your head and neck off the edge of the bed while lying on your back. Tilt your head as far back as it will go and look at the floor. Then, turn your head from side to side 20 to 30 times. Enjoy the stretch as you hang and sway.

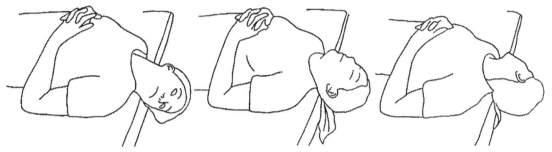

7) While standing, look straight ahead. Retract your neck, then bend you neck to the side so that your right ear approaches your right shoulder. Hold for 1-3 seconds, then bend the left ear toward the left shoulder. Repeat 10-20 times.

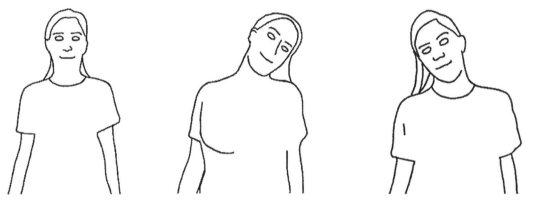

8) While standing, retract your neck and rotate your head to the right as far as it will go. Hold for 1-3 seconds, then rotate to the left. Repeat 10 times. Do this again with the neck protracted.

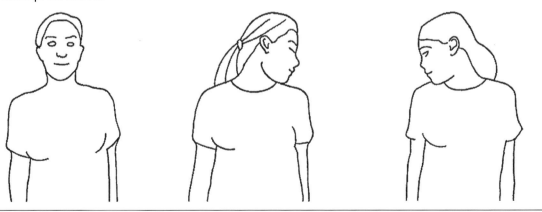

9) Bend your head forward as far as it will go to look at the ground. With the neck in total flexion, gently retract the neck from this position for five seconds, then protract it for five. Rest, focusing on the ache. For additional pressure, interlock your fingers behind your head, allowing the weight to gently pull your neck further downward.

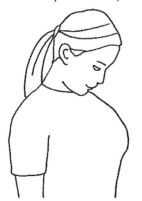 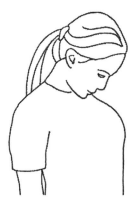 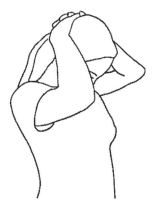

10) Place a towel around your neck like a scarf to provide support. Roll your head in a large circle. Do this 25-50 times. Be sure to alternate directions. Perform this slowly, allowing the neck to hang as much as possible while rotating. This will mobilize the muscles at the bottom of the neck to execute the rotations.

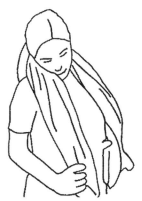 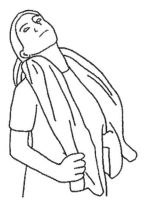 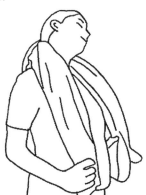

11) Draw a circle in front of your face with your nose. Doing so will utilize the muscles at the top of the neck to execute the rotation. Do this 50-100 times. As you alternate directions of the circle, try varying its size. You might try drawing triangles or squares.

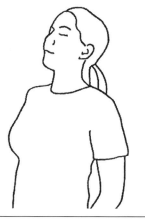 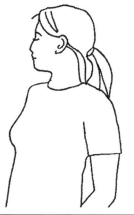 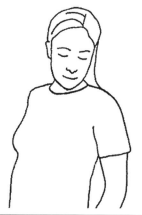

12) Lie on your back on a group of pillows or a large stability ball. The goal is to create a global backward curve in your spine. Let your entire neck relax, extending your head completely back. While remaining on the ball, cradle your head in your hands and pull your chin up to your chest and hold it there. Now retract it actively. Stretch into the aching sensation there between your neck and your shoulder blades.

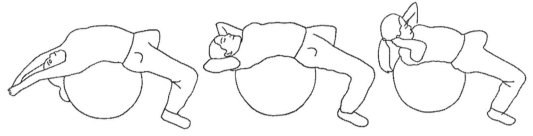

13) Lie on your back and cradle your neck with your hands. Perform tiny sit-ups or crunches that only lift your neck and shoulders off the ground. Focus on kyphosis in your neck—a full forward arch. Use the muscles in your throat to perform these modified sit-ups. The muscles in the back of your neck will stabilize the action, getting a great stretch in the process. Try looking to either side while performing this "neck sit-up."

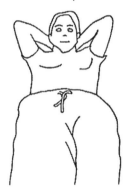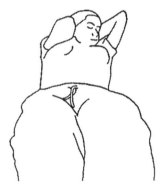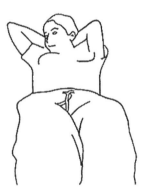

Have you ever wondered why a collared shirt is an essential aspect of proper business attire? I believe it is to obscure the extent of neck protraction so that neck posture does not play a role in corporate politics. The boss or manager may be the best person for a leadership role, but their lack of neck retraction might communicate to their underlings that they do not have a lifetime history of leadership experience. This could undermine their authority. Also, the person with the straightest neck is not necessarily the most knowledgeable and thus should not have undue influence on business matters. You want your company's hierarchy based on diligence and competence. I believe that like suit jackets with padded shoulders, collars level the playing field of physicality.

I believe that people who emerged from childhood with their neck mobility intact have a more dominant physical presence. The way their head is situated absolutely shines and its natural motion is intimidatingly smooth and beautiful. It is also usually easy for these people to build upper body muscle. Your neck may have become stiff and hunched before you reached puberty, but it still has the potential to be remobilized to its optimal extent. These exercises will rehabilitate aspects of your neck that you haven't used in years. After reclaiming your muscles and the coordination to use them, you will find that they contribute subtly to everything you do. A retracted neck with no dormancy or frailty appears striking and even ostentatious, but you won't feel guilty about it because the people struck by it will know you can't help it. Optimal neck carriage is something that cannot be faked.

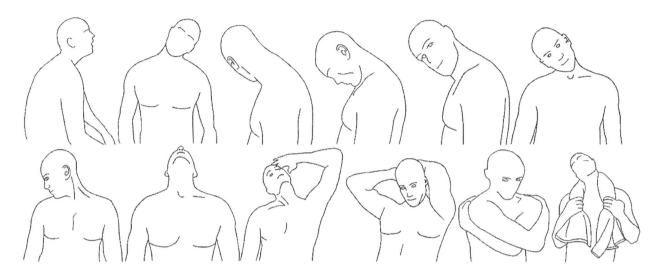

Illustration 16.4: Additional anti-rigidity poses for the neck.

Simulate Vomiting to Stimulate Missing Corners in the Neck

Sometimes when I throw up, I feel a gratifying crack in my neck. An ancient, reflexive motor arc is actuated during vomiting that contracts all the attachments in the neck in series, allowing you to access muscles you normally have no conscious control of. Take advantage of this by performing neck anti-rigidity while you pretend to vomit.

Neck Exercise #16.14: *Simulate Vomiting*
Find your way to your hands and knees and rest comfortably. Simulate the action of throwing up. Dry heaving will induce contractions in muscles from the stomach to the back of the head as part of an innate action pattern. As you use the vomiting pattern to reach into muscles throughout the neck, twist and turn the neck in every direction. You should notice small cracking sensations as well as the achy sensation of activating muscles that rarely get used.

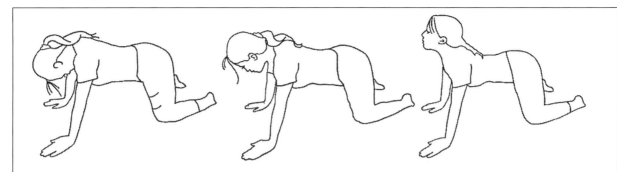

Before Program Peace vomiting was painful for me. This was the case because muscles in my abdomen were braced to the point of stagnancy. At times when retching, my internal organs would feel like they were on fire. As you might have guessed, the diaphragm and stomach produce much of the force used to expel food. This exercise along with those from Chapter 11 and 22 have made it so that vomiting is painless.

Keep Your Shoulders Down and Back

In cartoons, when a character becomes defensive or deferential, they raise their shoulders. Body language experts and animal behaviorists point out that this behavior may represent an effort to protect the neck, specifically the carotid artery and jugular vein. However, prolonged use of this insecure posture causes the muscles along the back of the neck and shoulders (trapezius) to become stuck in partial contraction. This means we walk, sit, and sleep in our beds with raised shoulders.

The simple act of actively pushing the shoulders toward the floor can remodel the upper body. The latissimus dorsi ("lats") that start under the armpits and run along the sides of the torso provide this tug. The more often you use them to pull the shoulders down, the more tone they develop. Pilates practitioners concentrate on keeping the head up and the shoulders down by imagining they are trying to maximize the distance between their ears and the tops of their shoulders. In personal training, this is referred to as "shoulder packing." It involves depressing the shoulders and squeezing the shoulder blades together. Regularly engaging in a practice like this will improve your kinesthetic awareness of what it feels like to appropriately position your neck and shoulder blades.

Neck Exercise #16.15: *Keeping the Shoulders Down and Back*

Bring your neck into a gentle retraction. Next, press your shoulders down toward the floor. The shoulder blades should be lightly squeezed together (adducted), with neck elongated, chin angled down, and chest open. From here, engage your entire shoulder girdle by pressing your shoulders and arms down. You can pretend that you are a gymnast performing a "support hold" on two parallel bars. You could also imagine that you are pressing yourself up out of a sewer hole. Once you have gotten the hang of it, try it pressing down against a hard surface such as a chair, tabletop, or the floor. Again, you want to reinforce this position from as many angles as possible.

Pressing the shoulders down is made easier by carrying (or pretending to carry) a load in the hands. This is the posture of a highly commanding and athletic person. It is also the posture that our body was designed for given that we have been fine-tuned for carrying items while walking. Imagine yourself carrying large hunks of meat or a long spear and a heavy wooden club. The most efficient way to carry these things is with the shoulders fully pressed toward the ground, as our ancestors would have. Whether walking, socializing, carrying things, exercising, or in bed, you want your shoulders back and down.

Neck Exercise #16.16: *Keeping the Shoulders Down with Weights*

Hold a two to 15-pound dumbbell in each hand and allow the weight to pull your shoulders toward the floor. Dynamically shift the position of your shoulder blades and focus on the sensations involved. While letting the weight tug at your shoulders, gently rotate the shoulders outward and inward. Next, try rolling them either forward or backward in circles. As you do so, try to contract all the muscles in your upper torso. You should feel this stretch reaching into previously hidden rigidity all over your upper body.

Puff Up and Open the Chest

Many women hold the breastbone down and inward to withdraw their breasts. Men do it to make their chest less conspicuous. This unnecessary modesty leads to unhealthy posture by depressing the collarbones and lowering the head. Ladies and gentlemen, it is healthiest for you to project your breast forward, so disregard any perceived social consequences.

Neck Exercise #16.17: *Heart Opener*

With your neck retracted, clasp your hands behind your back and pull down. This should draw your shoulders back and down and spread your collarbones wide. Arch the chest upward and forward. Project it out into space. Walk and move in this way with your chest "cracked wide open."

For optimal shoulder stability, you want to strengthen the muscles that externally rotate your shoulders. Do this by turning your wrists outward so that your palms face forward. Allow this to rotate your shoulders toward your back so that they are no longer slumped forward. With this simple change, you should feel your chest and collarbones spread open deep within their joints. Alternately, try lifting your arms to waist height with the palms facing the sky. At the same time, retract your neck, flex your glutes, and puff out your chest. Keep practicing this external rotation of the shoulders until it is habitual. It is especially important during cardio and weight-bearing exercises.

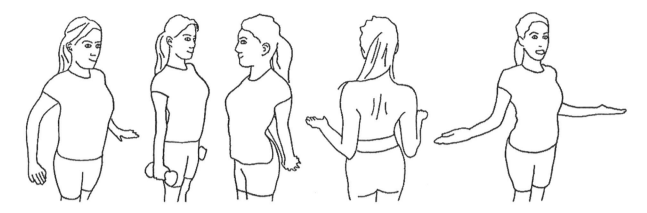

Illustration 16.5: A woman: A. pressing herself out of a sewer hole, B. allowing weights to tug her shoulders down, C. with her shoulders back and down and the hands clasped behind the back, D & E. with her palms facing the sky and her shoulders externally rotated.

Use Shrugging for Anti-rigidity

Apes generally walk on all fours. Their upper body, which we have inherited, was designed for it. To support this form of locomotion, apes assume a multitude of neck and shoulder postural configurations as they press their hands against the ground with each stride. There are many such postures between shoulders completely shrugged and shoulders completely down.
You will find that shoulder shrugging is a great counterpose to shoulders down and that a shrug enhances your ability to find achiness in the neck retracted position.

Postural Exercise #16.18: *Shrugging*
Place your hands on the ground, a table, or a countertop and push away while simultaneously shrugging your shoulders to rehabilitate frailty. Vary this posture in as many ways as possible. Try it with your neck extended and retracted. Try it with the shoulders bowed toward the front of the body and then rotated toward the back.

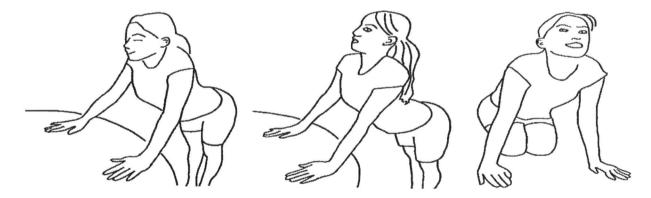

Illustration 16.6: Shrugging positions for anti-rigidity.

Other Methods of Anti-rigidity

Aside from knuckle-walking, apes are also built for climbing trees and swinging between branches. You may know where I am going with this: I recommend using either gymnastics rings or TRX Bands to recreate similar isometric poses to repair your neck and shoulders. You can hang rings or bands from many places, including a tree branch or even a pull-up bar in a doorway. Use these supports to place your body into unfamiliar positions from which to search for areas in need of anti-rigidity.

Neck Exercise #16.19: *Using Gymnastics Rings for Optimal Neck Retraction*

Place each of your hands in a ring with your arms spread out at 90 degrees. Press down lightly on the rings as if you were attempting to perform an "iron cross." Retract the neck, pulling the chin toward the neck. This position should be very frail and unstable and should provide months of productive anti-rigidity training.

You can assume many other gymnastic positions from the rings and receive an excellent isometric workout. The positions include the support hold, Maltese, and various other static strength holds. You can also perform ring push-ups, dips, pull-ups, rows, front levers, muscle-ups, hanging leg raises, and much more. Because you can do these with your feet on the ground, you have complete control of the intensity. As these exercises get easier, put more of your weight into your arms rather than your legs.

Many other tools can be used in anti-rigidity as props to place the body into unfamiliar joint configurations. You can use a trapeze, a pull-up bar, gymnastics supports, a yoga swing, inflatable stability balls, and many others. A long dowel or pole can also be used to help you leverage neglected positions in what are commonly called "stick mobility exercises."

If you have access to a pool or body of water, you should also consider treading water. Treading water is near the top of the list of exercises when it comes to calories burned per minute. Despite this, it is not likely to lead to repetitive strain injuries because it happens in a "weightless" environment where there is very little stress on your joints. Every inch of your body is working while you tread, and unlike other cardio routines, the arms, shoulders, neck, and torso are completely engaged. Also, it presents various opportunities for anti-rigidity, because there are dozens of kick and arm variations you can use. Treading water with your arms while holding your neck in a retracted position may be the fastest way to ingrain retraction. Treading water in a pool never gets boring because you can bring a phone or tablet outside, prop it up on the ground using a towel, and use it to watch videos while you tread.

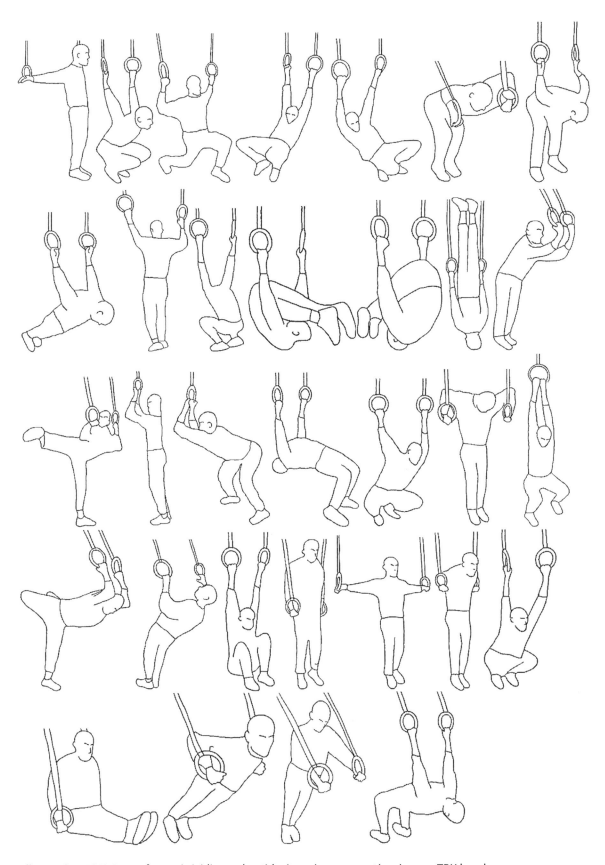

Illustration 16.7: Poses for anti-rigidity and anti-laxity using gymnastics rings or TRX bands.

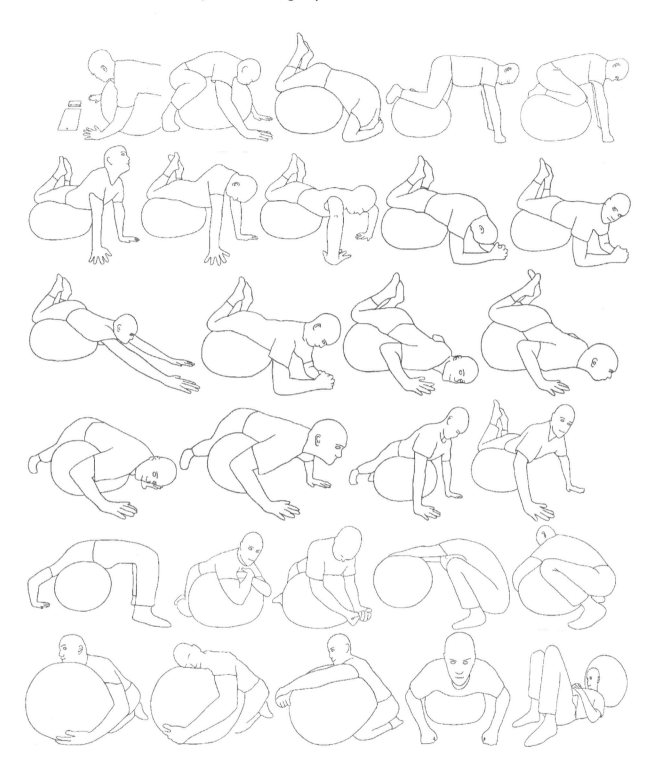

Illustration 16.8: Poses with an inflatable ball for upper body anti-frailty and anti-rigidity. These exercises can easily be performed while watching a program on a tablet and following a breath metronome placed on the floor.

I also recommend contracting into poses of postural strength on a trampoline. For instance, bounce up and down while flexing the glutes, flexing the chin to the chest, and pulling the shoulders back and down. The accelerations and de-accelerations from jumping will expose frailty and allow you to flex deeper into some of your biggest problem areas. Even a mini trampoline can be used to this end.

Compression for the Neck

I strongly advise massaging the neck. You want to use compression, percussion, and vibration on every nook and cranny. Exercises 6.4, 6.5, and 6.6 and Exercise 9.17 provide examples. Consider regularly using percussion with a knuckle tool, baseball, or vibrating massager on the entire neck to reduce excessive tone.

The End Goal for the Upper Body

As you get better at pushing your shoulders toward the ground with a retracted neck, you will find that this integrates your entire upper body into a more cohesive unit. It will allow you to create simultaneous and complementary tone in the muscles that pull the shoulder forward (pectorals), the muscles that pull the shoulders backward (rhomboids), and the muscles that pull the shoulders down (latissimus dorsi). This allows these three sets of muscles to pull against each other synergistically.

Most people tend to contract only one of these at a time, but not all three simultaneously. Generally, only very physically dominant people, with limber necks, feel comfortable having this triumvirate active all at once. You want to walk around with a light contraction in all three of these muscle groups on a daily basis. As you do it, picture yourself as Conan the Barbarian with a giant sword in his hands, as She-Hulk carrying groups of people out of a burning building, or as something in that vicinity.

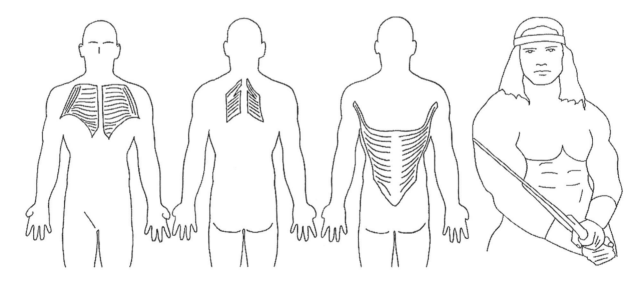

Illustration 16.9: A. Pectorals; B. Rhomboids; C. Latissimus Dorsi; D. All three muscle groups holding a light contraction will result in the conveyance of power.

Conclusion

For two decades, I had a pronounced knot to the right of the C4 vertebra in my neck. It was large enough for people to notice regularly and inquire about. The knot was larger than the size of my entire thumb, and several professionals voiced their concerns. No fewer than four doctors told me it was not muscular and that it was a lipoma or a cyst. However, I knew it was just a knotted muscle. Over the next two years, I used anti-rigidity to leverage my way into this achy, closed-down gnarl. As I gained access to it, by searching for positions capable of making it ache, it shrunk gradually until it disappeared. This general process applied to several other knots in my neck that were less conspicuous. Apply it to yours.

Indian people use a head shake or wobble as a nonverbal signal to indicate goodwill and use it to mean anything from "good" to "I understand." I believe this wobble signifies neck vitality, relaxation, and an easygoing approach. It is a beautiful way to put people at ease, and I think it is no coincidence that this marvelous expression arises from the same culture that brought us yoga and Buddhist philosophy. Incorporate the use of your neck into your nonverbal behavior. Use smooth, playful neck motions to help you build rapport with people and allay their tendency toward neck stiffness.

The simple exercises in this chapter will revise the neural circuitry involved in holding your head up. They will provide abounding coordination, mobility, and strength that will make your neck posture monumental. Raise your head imperiously with poise and majesty and be the master of all that you survey.

Chapter 16: **Bullet Points**

- In most people, the neck is severely underused and holds massive amounts of strain.
- Anterior head syndrome, also called the "dowager's hump" and "nerd neck," is caused by jutting the chin out, bending the top of the neck backward, and pushing the bottom of the neck forward. This is called neck protraction and is a highly submissive posture.
- Counteract this by performing neck retraction, which involves pulling the bottom of the neck backward and pushing the top forward while tucking the chin inward toward the chest and throat. This should include a chin lock.
- You can assume many postures that will help you locate dormant muscle in the neck and shoulders so that it can be rehabilitated with anti-rigidity training. These include neck retraction, protraction, and extension, pressing the shoulders down, shrugging, hugging yourself, shoulder external rotation, opening the chest, clasping the hands behind the back, holding them out to the side, and many others.
- The more you practice bringing dormant neck and shoulder muscles to fatigue, the sooner they will be strong enough to hold an athletic and stable position naturally.
- If you use anti-rigidity to rehab the stiff, rigid muscles in your neck, you will become less tightly wound and you will find the act of exercise to be easier and more rewarding.

Chapter 16: **Endnotes**

1.   Matsui, T., & Fujimoto, T. (2011). Treatment for depression with chronic neck pain completely cured in 94.2% of patients following neck muscle treatment. *Neuroscience & Medicine, 2*(2), 7177.

2.   Kado, D. M., Huang, M. H., Karlamangla, A. S., Barrett-Connor, E., & Greendale, G. A. (2004). Hyperkyphotic posture predicts mortality in older community-dwelling men and women: A prospective study. *Journal of the American Geriatric Society, 52*(10), 1662–1667.

3.   Hansraj, K. K. (2014). Assessment of stresses in the cervical spine caused by posture and position of the head. *Surgical Technology International, 25*, 277–279.

Chapter 17: **Anti-rigidity for the Lower Back**

Lower back pain is more common than neck pain: it is the second leading cause for physician visits in the US. It is so crippling that Americans spend an estimated $50 billion annually on lower back pain alone. This preventable ailment is taxing our wallets and healthcare system. Because our lower backs are foundational to our morale, fortitude, and faith in ourselves, weakness and pain in that area tax our very sense of personal agency.

In most cases, the predominant reason for back pain is muscular imbalance. Vital muscles are left underused and undeveloped while others are overused and strained. We use them at only a fraction of their full range, and usually only while breathing shallowly. This corrupts the muscles with the same ailment we have been discussing all along: dormancy due to partial contraction.

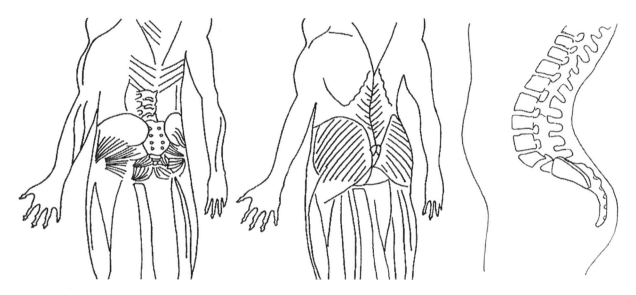

Illustration 17.1: A. Interior anatomy of the lower back with some underlying musculature revealed; B. Exterior musculature of the lower back; C. Excessive backward curve (lordosis) in the lower back.

My lower back was treacherous. The muscles surrounding my lumbar vertebrae were in such bad shape that they hurt every time I coughed or sneezed. I would severely strain my lower back every year due to stress, lack of sleep, or improper exercise, leaving me unable to walk for days at a time. A few times, I was bedridden for a week, forced to crawl back and forth to the bathroom on my hands and knees. Since I began anti-rigidity training, this has never happened. The dormant muscle that used to lock up when I threw my back out was transformed into springy, mobile, load-accepting muscle. I unraveled my entire lumbar region by combining anti-rigidity, spinal decompression, stretching, and therapeutic massage. This chapter will touch on each of these, giving you the information you need to transform your body's most powerful physical asset.

How tense is your lower back? The activity below will guide you through using your fingers to feel the tense, dormant muscles along the back of your hips (iliac crest).

Lower Back Activity #17.1: *Diagnose the Extent of Lower Back Dormancy*

Press your index and middle fingers into your lower back 2-6 inches above each butt cheek. Feel the muscles covering the sacrum (the central bone pictured below) and your pelvis's iliac crests (the bony prominences to each side of the sacrum). As you move your fingers out toward your hips, you will likely feel large, tense cords of muscle fibers right over the sacroiliac joints (labeled below). This is dormancy. This chapter will detail how to bring them to their ideal state, smooth and flat with no perceptible knotting.

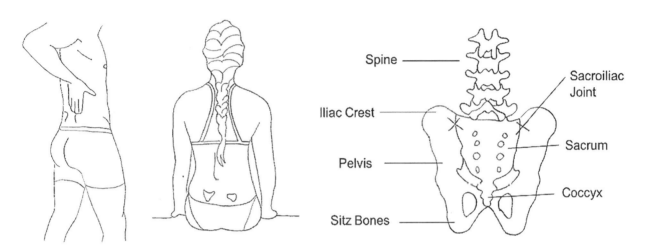

Illustration 17.2: A. Man feeling tense knots at a sacroiliac joint; B. Woman with apparent dimples at the sacroiliac joints; C. Spine and pelvis seen from behind. The sacroiliac joints are marked with an "x."

As you know from Chapter 13, the lower part of our spine, called the lumbar region, naturally curves backward. This backward bend is known as lumbar lordosis. The lower back is bent lordotically to support the legs and absorb impact. In lordosis, the top of the pelvis is tilted forward as if you were pouring a bowl of soup from your waist out in front of you. In most people, this lordotic curve is excessive, making it structurally unsound. When the lordosis is excessive, it is called "anterior pelvic tilt" or "pelvic anteversion." Generally, the more pelvic tilt one has, the less pelvic mobility is available to them.

When my back had excessive lordosis, my belly button was very far from my nipples. Observe your belly button in your default posture. How far is it from your nipples? To correct this, flex your glutes, push your hips forward, and watch your belly button rise. Squeezing your glutes resets your pelvis-lumbar relationship back to where nature intended it to be. That is why it is essential to do this throughout the day.

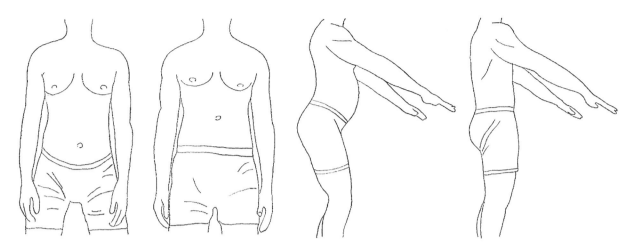

Illustration 17.3: A. Excessive lumbar lordosis is apparent as a considerable distance between the navel and nipples; B. Flexing the glutes and pushing the hips forward results in a neutral lower spine with less distance between the belly button and nipples; C. Excessive lumbar lordosis from the side; D. Neutral spine with glutes flexed.

You can also neutralize excessive lordosis by teaching the lower spine to curve in the extreme opposite direction. To do this, flex the hips inward and up toward the face (lumbar kyphosis). This rotates the imaginary soup bowl backward so that the soup is no longer pouring out in front of you. I like to think of this posture as "shrimping up" because it involves curling the spine's bottom half toward the stomach. Flex your glutes as you do this, and it becomes the equivalent of neck retraction.

Recruiting Your Gluteus Muscles

When the glutes are offline, other muscles, poorly suited for the job, are forced to support the core and stabilize the trunk. It is generally the muscles in the lower back and hips that end up compensating for underuse of the gluteus muscles, taking on heaps of tension in the process. To counteract this and set your pelvis in a neutral position, simply contract your buttocks. Squeezing your butt ensures your pelvic posture and tilt are optimized.

Pilates advocates maintaining a neutral spine by sucking your stomach in, flexing your abdominals, relaxing the lumbar spine, and holding the glutes in a light contraction. During Pilates workouts, practitioners try to maintain this core engagement throughout every exercise. Neutral spine and glute engagement should be generalized to everything you do, not just exercise. Ideally, the glutes should have some form of contractile tone with every movement you make. This will trim your abdomen and increase the strength and size of your butt. Another reason some people don't flex the glutes is they want to increase the conspicuousness of their butt as excessive lumbar lordosis pushes the butt out further. However, lumbar lordosis deactivates the glutes and, with time, their tone will decrease, resulting in a smaller, weaker butt.

Flexing the glutes is a dominant expression that we shouldn't hesitate to make. Most people avoid it, however, because the way their life has programed them, contracting their glutes takes their breath away. Imagine being a naked caveman or woman. The commanding ones had gluteal tone and the unassuming ones had hindquarters that were soft and limp.

So, use anti-laxity to make glute firmness your default by paring firm glute contractions with deep breathing many times per day. While this can make the lower back feel stiff, you can also employ anti-rigidity with the glutes contracted, moving in ways that target unfamiliar, achy configurations.

Perform Anti-rigidity During Cat and Cow Poses

Performing anti-rigidity maneuvers within yoga poses is an excellent way to find dormant lower back muscles that will benefit from being contracted. In particular, cow, cat, and bird-dog poses are the bread and butter of lower back health.

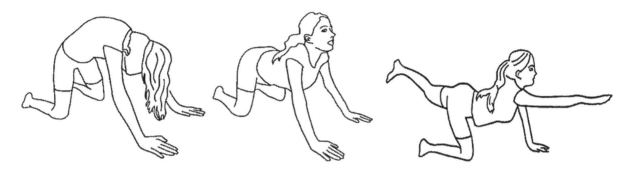

Illustration 17.4: A. Cat or camel pose; B. Cow pose; C. Bird-dog pose.

Backward Bends Straighten Your Spine

A powerful way to counteract lumbar lordosis is to gradually introduce your body to global back extension. You can start by watching TV lying on your stomach. To make this more comfortable, you can prop yourself up on your elbows or place a pillow under your chest. To make it harder, try pressing the pubic bone into the floor until you are balancing on your pelvis and balling your buttocks into firm mounds. When you need something harder still, gently lift your feet and knees off the ground.

Use the back extension exercises in which you rolled over a basketball from Chapter 13 to complement these positions. The simple act of lying on your stomach on the floor will make you feel stiff at first, so remember to perform a forward bend or a few sit-ups afterward as a counterpose. With time, work toward a full upward dog pose. If you can breathe slowly and fully in these positions, you can dismantle your vertebral tension.

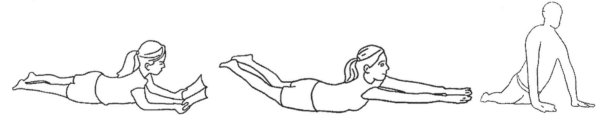

Illustration 17.5: A. Reading on the stomach; B. Pressing the pelvis into the ground; C. Upward dog pose.

Downward Dog Pose

Downward dog is another key yoga pose. After you internalize the mechanics of downward dog, try "walking the dog" by bending one knee at a time. Next, try shifting the butt left and right while holding downward dog. Pivot as much as you can with your hips while doing this. You can access many normally inaccessible muscles all over the spine from this position. This includes muscles in your neck. For example, from downward dog, look to the right, raising and lowering the head 20 times. Repeat this while looking to the left. Spend time walking around in downward dog, doing the "bear crawl."

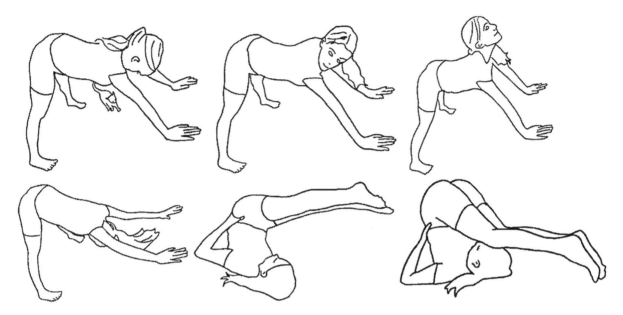

Illustration 17.6: A, B, C, & D. Downward dog pose; E & F. Plow pose.

Strengthen the Hip Flexors: Child's, Happy Baby, and Pigeon Poses

Strengthening the hip flexor muscles on the front side of your waist is imperative for lower back health. To do this, practice the poses below while focusing on bringing the knee closer to the chest in a way that creates a firm contraction in the frontal portion of the hip. If you breathe through the subtle pinch in the hip flexor, you can coax it to contract fully. Doing this regularly will cause your hip flexors to become much stronger and provide integral support for your lower back.

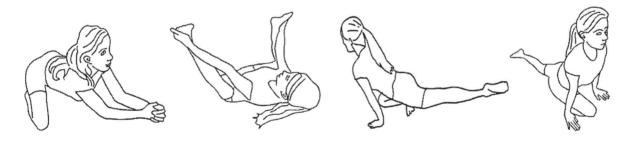

Illustration 17.7: A. Child's pose; B. Happy baby pose; C & D. Pigeon pose.

Trunk Twist

There are many joints in the lower back and hips that articulate very subtly. They amount to a small degree of movement, but their presence or absence affects every lower body motion.

For instance, people with a mobile sacroiliac joint can twist their trunk below the waist. If you sit in a chair and turn to look over your shoulder, you want the turning motion to extend from the neck all the way down to the sitz bones. If the rotation stops at your waist level, you know that your sacroiliac joint is locked up. Regular trunk twists will unlock a multitude of muscles along your spine, allowing your hips to move with your legs during walking and making every lower body movement more graceful, sensual, and stable.

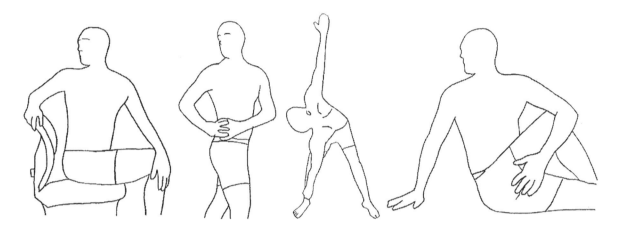

Illustration 17.8: Trunk twist while: A. seated in a chair; B. standing; C. touching the floor; D. seated on the ground.

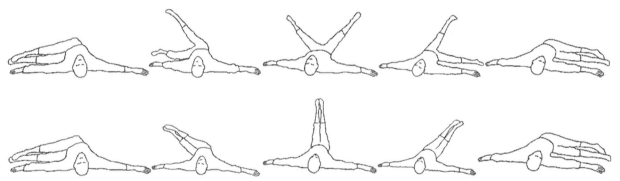

Illustration 17.9: Hip twist progression. The first row shows a version of this exercise where the feet are not touching. The second row shows a much more challenging version where the feet are touching. Performing this 20 times daily will help you progress from the first version to the second over just a few months while building lower back and core strength.

Wagging Your Tail

Next, I will describe a tactic to engage your hips that can lead to better hip mobility. I think of it as wagging the tail. To do this, tilt your pelvis from side to side. This is called pelvic incline or list. One hip goes up while the other goes down, and then, you reverse it. One way to master this movement is to relax on your back, keeping both legs straight. Then, pull one leg in toward you and push the other away. Practice varying the extent, intensity, and speed until you develop coordination. Once you have mastered this hip swivel, you can even do it while seated. The contractions involved will lead you to plenty of achy muscles. Combining tail wagging with anti-rigidity will help restore motor control and fluid motion to the hips and pelvis.

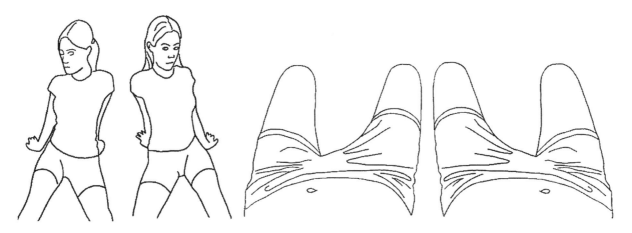

Illustration 17.10: A & B. Sitting pelvic tilt; C & D. Lying pelvic tilt.

Standing, One Leg Up

While standing, place one foot flat on a surface that is between knee and waist height. This will allow you to leverage your way into hip frailty to which you may have previously been oblivious. From here, you can also perform isometric contractions of your side (obliques), abdominals, and one of your glutes. Regularly put one foot up on tables and countertops to achieve these.

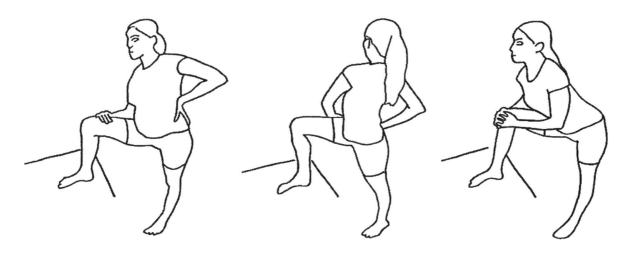

Illustration 17.11: With one leg up perform a: A. side bend; B. twist; or C. forward bend.

Rock and Roll on the Floor

An excellent way to resituate your lumbar vertebrae is to rock up and down your spine from your tailbone to your neck. To avoid injury, do this on a carpet or yoga mat. Lie down on your back and pull your knees into your chest. Roll forward and backward. Attempt to roll smoothly from the first position depicted in the drawings below to the third and back again repeatedly. To do this properly, you want your entire spine curved into a forward C-shape (kyphosis). You should find that as you rock into the third position pictured below, where the man has his weight on his neck, your lumbar region is subject to a pleasurable pulling sensation. Use this for anti-rigidity.

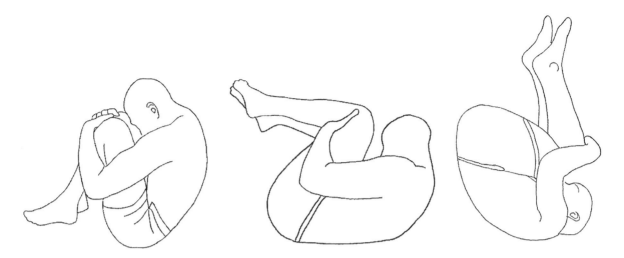

Illustration 17.12: Rolling in a ball to achieve anti-rigidity.

Squats

Squats create formidable strength but also expose us to a high risk of injury. I recommend performing them with absolutely no weight as a way to develop foundational strength. Performing between five and 30 squat repetitions every other day is a great way to improve force and power production in the body. If you aren't using weights, you can play with and vary the forces acting on the disks and vertebrae, distributing them in different ways to intentionally load the weakest segments.

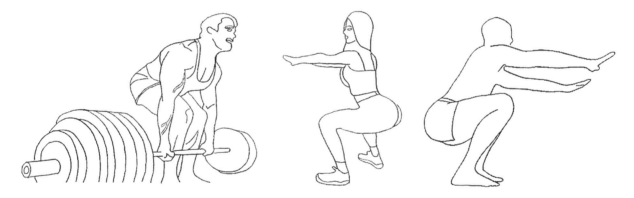

Illustration 17.13: A. Performing squats or deadlifts with heavy weight and invariant posture inevitably leads to injury and pain. As should be clear by now, our bodies were not designed for this kind of strain; B & C. Instead, opt for bodyweight squats with optimal, neutral posture or minor postural variations.

Especially if you perform squats with additional weight, it is imperative to squat using proper form. You want your back flat, feet straight, and your knees slightly outside your feet yet behind your toes. Take a wide stance with your feet just outside the shoulders. As you squat, keep your shins as vertical as possible, not tilted forward. Put your hands at chin height out in front of you. At the bottom of the squat, you want to maintain a neutral curve in your lower back without excessive lordosis or kyphosis. As you stand, flex your butt.

I strongly recommend starting with supported squats. You can achieve this by holding a rail, tabletop, chair leg, pair of doorknobs, TRX bands, or gymnastics rings, and using them to pull yourself up. You can also place your hands on your knees and push against them for support. This will reduce the forces on your hips, knees, and ankles, allowing you to progress into unsupported squats in time. Breathing deeply from a low squat with your knees moderately loaded will recondition them, healing that "crunchy" quality and reducing their tendency to pop and lock up. It will do the same for your ankles and lower back.

Most people cannot perform a full-range, butt-to-ankle squat. While many exercise professionals advise against lowering your butt below the knees when squatting, I recommend lowering your butt to rest on your heels but only if you do so with body weight in a slow, controlled manner. When paired with diaphragmatic breathing, a complete squat will give you a full lower back stretch extending to where your lumbar spine meets your sacrum, excising the tension from this area.

Everyone should do bodyweight squats. Even doing only five a day will inevitably teach your body to do it properly. I recommend trying other advanced weightlifting techniques such as lunges, power cleans, snatches, and deadlifts with either body weight or very light dumbbells. I recommend only adding weight once you have mastered the form and can do 30 repetitions without any discomfort.

Studies have shown that lower back exercises are the most beneficial when practiced daily. More importantly, endurance exercise is recommended over exertive exercise for its protective value. In other words, use low intensity (body weight) and high repetition (10 to 100) to slowly and gently bring these muscles to fatigue. These will establish your unrealized core strength.

Static Squatting

Holding a static squat with your butt at the level of your knees is an age-old yoga technique. In martial arts, this is done with the legs somewhat spread in a pose called "horse stance," which is used to strengthen the lower back and create a feeling of "groundedness." A system called Foundation Training, developed by Eric Goodman, popularized another version of the static squat called the "founder" pose. Check out his version online. A static squat helps isolate and strengthen the epicenter of lower back frailty.

Lower Back Exercise #17.1: *Hold a Static Squat*

With legs shoulder length apart, bend your knees until your butt is just above the level of your knees. Hold a static squat while placing the lower back into different configurations. From squatting position, introduce complete lordosis in your lower back and then total kyphosis. Hold the squat while moving carefully back and forth between the two.

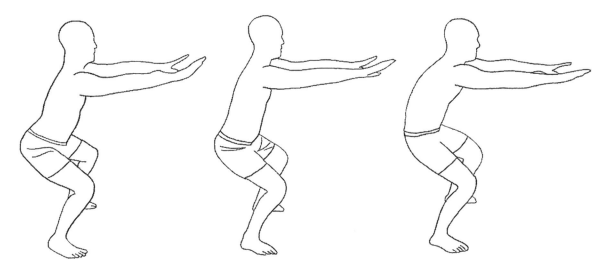

Illustration 17.14: A. Static squat with lumbar lordosis; B. Static squat with lumbar neutrality; C. Static squat with lumbar kyphosis.

Release the Hamstrings

Most of us have hamstring tension that has caused them to adapt to shorter-than-normal resting length. Shortened hamstrings tug insidiously on the sitz bones, placing significant pressure on the lower back. This constant pull forces the pelvis into excessive lordosis. This is why stretching the hamstrings is very important for lower back health. One of the best ways to stretch your hamstrings is to lie on your back with one leg in the air, wrapping a towel or belt around your foot. From here, pull your foot toward your head as pictured below. A ubiquitous lower back disorder called "lower cross" syndrome is marked by short and tight hamstrings and groin muscles, along with weak and underdeveloped buttocks and abdominals. Hamstring and hip flexor stretches will relieve the former while squats and sit-ups will strengthen the latter.

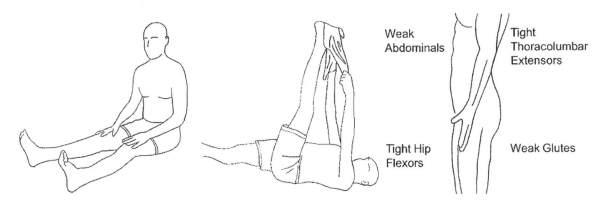

Illustration 17.15: A. Man sitting with legs straight releasing the hamstrings; B. Stretching the hamstring using a towel; C. The features of the lower cross syndrome.

Spinal Decompression and Traction

Age and pressure pull our vertebrae closer together, compressing the spine. This makes the spine like an inchworm that has retracted its telescoping body segments. Decompression (also known as spinal traction) stretches the muscles surrounding the spinal vertebrae, increasing circulation and resting length. Once these muscles are stretched, they can contract more fully and undergo anti-rigidity exercises. Spinal decompression can feel precarious, like you are being pulled apart. Combining it with diaphragmatic breathing, however, will assure your spine that it is safe to expand to full length.

A great way to decompress is to use an inversion table and lie upside down, suspended by your feet, for a few minutes each day. Commonly recommended by physicians, inversion tables have demonstrated significant clinical benefits. A second method to achieve this is to practice "stretchlying,"[1] which I encourage you to read about online. Third, passive motion from shaking can also aid in decompression. Passive motion can come from having someone jostle your spine rhythmically or using a reciprocating "chi machine" that continuously shakes the body. All three of these techniques often cause people's spines to tense up defensively. But, if you give in to it, you can teach your spinal muscles not to resist the passive forces. As you might imagine, paced breathing is immensely helpful to that end.

Massage also has decompressive effects (e.g., Activity 6.1). Consider having a masseuse perform an easy deep tissue massage on your lower back. After a few visits, it should feel comfortable for them to use their elbows to press deeply into every area surrounding your lumbar spine. Having a masseuse stand on your lower back can also be helpful and is common in Thai massage. If your back is very strong, you can ask your masseuse to stand on your pelvis and take gentle steps all the way up your spine. This is a fantastic way to decompress these areas, but it can be dangerous.

Decompressing the spine will help your muscles extend to their intended length. However, because they have yet to be used at this length and have poor tone as a result, they will initially be vulnerable to injury if accidentally contracted too forcefully. This is why, after any form of decompression, you should avoid intense workouts and instead use anti-rigidity carefully and remedially.

Compression and Massage

Compressing the muscles in your lower back by lying on top of baseballs is highly effective. To do this, lie with your back on the ground and bend your knees. Place a baseball on each side of your spine, just above your pelvis, or along the iliac crest. Alternatively, you can use softballs or tennis balls if baseballs are too painful. Once the balls are in place, lift your feet into the air. Use your legs to regulate the pressure placed on the balls, directing that pressure into the sorest spots. You can also use them to compress the muscles around your love handles, as well as the gluteus maximus, gluteus minimus, gluteus medius, piriformis, and others.

You want to rest each portion of your pelvis on the balls for several seconds at a time, ensuring you are breathing deeply and slowly. The tremendous aching sensation results in fresh blood pouring into stale, lifeless muscles. The aching will be vastly reduced after only a dozen five-minute sessions. However, as with the decompression exercises in the last section, it potentially leaves your lower back open to serious injury if you load these newly relaxed muscles too intensely or too soon. Therefore, I recommend performing this after your regular exercises or before bed. Using baseballs in this way will uproot the iliac knots and expel the tension from your lower back.

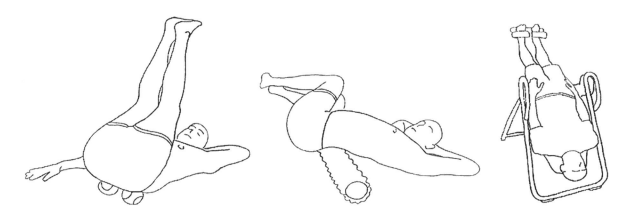

Illustration 17.16: A. Man pressing two baseballs into the sacroiliac joints; B. Man rolling lower back over a foam "rumble" roller; C. Man using an inversion table.

When baseballs are pressing into your back, the pressure will change your back's normal configuration, permitting stretches in planes of motion previously blocked. Take advantage of this and perform anti-rigidity in these planes. You can attain the same effect by placing a football, basketball, or yoga block under your sacrum while lying supine.

I like cankles, love handles form due to dormant muscle. Press a baseball, thumb, knuckle, or tool into the spongey, dormant muscles responsible for your love handles. Focus on pressing firmly into the top ridge of your posterior pelvis. Compressing and percussing these muscles will revive them, introduce new mobility in your hips, and accordingly reduce fat deposition at the site.

To reduce confusion, it is important for me to address the idea of localized fat loss. The majority of scientific studies have debunked the idea of targeted fat loss sometimes called "spot reduction." In other words, working out a particular area of the body may reduce overall body fat, but generally does not reduce fat deposition at that particular site. For instance, doing a lot of bicep curls makes them bigger but does not reduce the fat content of the upper arm. However, it is my conviction that rehabilitating dormant muscle using the anti-rigidity and massage techniques outlined in this book can result in spot reduction. I have seen dramatic instances of it on my own body and on those of my clients. As the crunchy, achy muscle around your midsection is rehabbed, it will become lean and trim.

How to Bend Over

Most people bend over from the waist. This means they hunch their spine forward from the height of their belly button to bend down. This leads to injury. When bending, you want to keep your spine straight by bending a few inches lower, at the hips. This results in a hinge from the hip with a straight back. Hip hinging strengthens the erector spinae muscles and stretches the hamstrings. Fully engage the stomach muscles to help buffer the load on the lumbar spine. Of course, if you are picking up something heavy, you should squat down and lift with the knees. Otherwise, lift small loads by hip hinging.

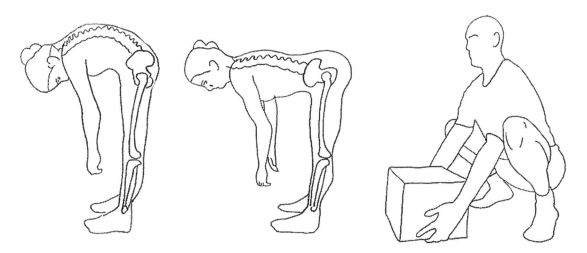

Illustration 17.17: A. Improper bending from the waist; B. Proper hinging from the hips; C. Proper squatting to lift a load.

The more often you can bend over by hip hinging, the better. I shoot for 10 times per day. Put commonly used objects such as your phone charger on the floor so that you must bend to the ground every time you use them.

Perfecting Your Sit-Ups

Sit-ups are the best counterpose for any work with your spine. They will reset your vertebrae from your neck to your tailbone. They place the lower back into neutrality, helping protect individual muscles from the repetitive strain that comes from being out of alignment. For this reason, it is constructive to perform 10-20 sit-ups after performing the other back exercises in this chapter.

A few advanced variations to try when doing sit-ups: 1) Place a small firm pillow (or "sit-up pad") under your lower back so that near the top of the sit-up you have something for your kyphotic lumbar spine to arch against, and press away from. This will help ensure that you are not stuck in lordosis during the sit-up; 2) Straighten your legs and rest the backs of your knees on the ground throughout the motion; 3) Flex your buttocks as you come down from each sit-up; 4) Turn your neck and look to each side.

Doing sit-ups on the floor can irritate muscles that aren't used to the intense forces. This is why I recommend doing sit-ups in bed. It provides outstanding remedial rehab for the entire spine and will accentuate all your other efforts to improve your neck and lower back. Every human should take three minutes to do at least 25 sit-ups in bed every other day.

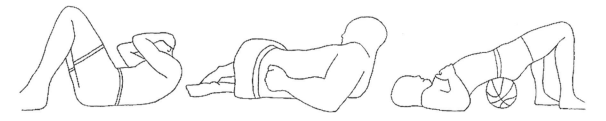

Illustration 17.18: A. Sit-ups; B. Massaging the iliac crests with the knuckles; C. Elevating the sacrum with a basketball into an unfamiliar position for anti-rigidity.

Conclusion

Remember the tense cords of muscle you found with your fingers between your lower spine and hips at the beginning of this chapter? When you compress, stretch, and tone these muscles, you will develop a different diagnostic marker: dimples. Spinal experts claim that people with a dimple just above each buttock on either side of the spine have very healthy lower backs.[2] The dimples demarcate mobility and strength in the sacroiliac joints. I used the methods in this chapter for a whole year, experienced dramatic results, and still lacked these two dimples. I figured the experts were wrong. No, I was wrong. After two additional years of using these methods, I finally developed the dimples.

Over the last five years, I have spent at least five minutes every day reconditioning my lower back. It was chronically painful before, and now there is zero pain. The alignment of my vertebrae has changed significantly. Some vertebrae were far more prominent than others; they even felt crooked to the touch. Yet now they all lie in a straight line. I used to live in fear of the next back injury, but now a back injury seems almost inconceivable. After you use the exercises in this chapter, your body will unconsciously recognize that your lower back will not fail you. If you are like me, once you can trust your spine to support everything you do, immense amounts of unconscious trepidation will be relieved.

Chapter 17: **Bullet Points**

- Portions of the lower back are rarely used, so they remain in a tense state of partial contraction. This leaves them susceptible to injury and causes lower back pain.
- To optimize lumbar mobility, use anti-rigidity exercises in the lumbar region by bending, extending, and flexing it in every direction.
- Doing sit-ups, yoga poses, Pilates, toe touches, trunk twists, hip-hinging, hip-swiveling, deadlifts, squats, and lunges will all help.
- These exercises should be performed with only your bodyweight, at very low intensity, with many repetitions.
- Bend over and touch your toes several times per day. When doing so, bend from the hip, not the waist.
- You can employ traction to decompress the spine by using an inversion table, "stretchlying," or decompressive massage.
- You can unlock the lumbar spinal muscles, glutes, hips, and the entire sacroiliac joint by massaging the area with baseballs, compressing it with your knuckles, or percussing it with tools.
- Put your lower back and hips into as many unfamiliar configurations as possible. Rehab these configurations from all angles using deep breathing, anti-laxity and anti-rigidity.

Chapter 17: **Endnote**

1.   Gokhale, E. (2008). *8 steps to a pain-free back*. Pendo Press.

Chapter 18: Use Optimal Posture and Anti-rigidity While Walking

"Walking is man's best medicine." — Hippocrates (460 BCE – 370 BCE)

"If there is a panacea in medicine, it is walking." — Norman Doidge (b. 1950)

If you place an exercise wheel in a rat's cage, it will use it. They naturally want to move. A rat that uses a wheel is much more mentally and physically healthy than a rat caged without one. It is also more resilient to stress and will live longer. I regularly have to remind myself that I too have a wheel in my cage, and it is the block I live on. Merely walking around your block a few times each day can vastly improve your mental and physical health.

Walking keeps your respiratory and cardiovascular systems strong by providing them with a light challenge. However, for a rat to attain health benefits, its use of a wheel must be voluntary. If the rat feels forced, the exercise becomes stressful, and many of the benefits disappear. So, when I walk I don't hurry, I have no time limit, and no particular destination to reach. For me, the endorphins from a voluntary 15-minute walk make me feel like I am no longer in a cage. Those from a 30-minute walk turn a so-so day into a splendid one.

Modern-day hunter-gatherers average around 19 miles of walking and trotting every day. Like all mammals, we are designed to move. Some doctors urge patients to take 10,000 steps daily, which equates to about five miles and takes about an hour and a half. In my opinion, this is excessive for many people, especially those who do not walk regularly. They quickly develop back, knee, and ankle pain at this rate. Instead, shoot for a healthy fraction of this that is comfortable for you. You might start somewhere between 3,000 and 7,000 steps.

While mortality rates improve progressively with the number of steps taken daily,[1] this positive effect levels off after approximately 6,000 steps (three miles) per day. This demonstrates that you certainly don't need to walk a full 10,000 steps each day to reap the benefits. You might want to use your car or a GPS to measure the distance around your block. Once you have that distance in miles, multiply it by 2,000 (there are around 2,000 steps in a mile) to find out how many steps it takes to circle your block and then how many laps you should shoot for to reach your desired total distance. Wherever you choose to walk, you should find that after a few thousand steps you feel your bracing patterns and emotional tensions begin to wash away.

At the end of Chapter 21, we will discuss the panoply of health benefits from regular exercise in more detail. The remainder of this chapter will discuss how to get the most out of your walks. It will coach you to walk assertively, with impeccable posture, while employing anti-rigidity, and taking appropriate breaks and counterposes. Basically, it details how you can turn your walks into time spent putting Program Peace into practice.

Use Good Posture While Walking in Public

Whenever we encounter someone, the first impulse is to query: "friend or foe?" Unconscious circuits in the brain work to decide: "Are they going to attack me?" "Are they easily provoked?" "Are they analyzing me, waiting for me to submit before they decide whether to be hostile?"

Then we try to determine if they did have ill intentions, would they have the power to enact them? In other words, we size them up to see which one of us would prevail in a physical altercation. Often regardless of whether we think we could win, we let our posture cave in. Don't do any of these things. The inclination to size up others turns our world into a hostile place from the inside out. However, we do want to be aware of how others size us up.

Psychologists, criminologists, and law enforcement personnel agree that walking like a victim increases the likelihood of being mugged or assaulted. They recommend that we "walk with a purpose." Studies have shown that criminals can identify people with histories of victimization by their gait.[2] They walk like an easy target: asynchronously, timidly, with short strides. Depressed people also have a characteristic way of walking. They exhibit reductions in walking speed, stride length, vertical head movement, and arm movement at the shoulder and elbow.[3] When you walk, do the exact opposite.

People who walk like despondent prey are advertising their victimization so others can see that they don't want to compete. They are communicating that they will give in to a bully. But the same self-handicapping that will repel a competitor will attract a predator. There is a fundamental tradeoff to submissive posture, and that is being ripe for predation. This is why the best way to carry yourself is to use the optimal postures described in the preceding chapters, without a hint of either competitiveness or vulnerability.

Your neck should be straight, with your chin tucked in toward your throat. Your shoulders should be pressed down and back. Your eyes should be wide and looking upward. Your face, and your entire body should be relaxed. You should be breathing smooth, slow, long, deep breaths through your nose. This combination of comfort and confidence should help you see the strangers you encounter on your walks as compatriots and allies. A zygomatic smile and a cordial salute can help them see you in the same way.

Walk spryly with nonchalant control and balance. Expand yourself. In becoming more expansive channel a peacock fanning its tail feathers, a cat galloping sideways, or a baboon romping through foliage. Feel the animal strength in your body. Extend your neck and roll your shoulders back so that you can openly display your chest. This gives a signal to others that you are not afraid of being attacked. Hands placed near the hips show readiness for action, hands behind the back signify confidence.[4] Head erect and neck retracted, demonstrate the posture of a military general, an elite athlete, or royalty. Think imperial, dignified...regal. Visualize yourself emanating gravitas and a commanding presence. Good posture leads others to assume that you must have much to be confident about, and they will accept what you project.

Hunter-gatherers have been documented to steal meat from lions by merely walking up to them and taking it. How, you ask? They walk with purpose. They wait until a lion kills a wildebeest. Then as few as three humans will approach a pride of as many as one dozen hungry beasts. They walk directly toward the lions from a distance without a hint of hesitation. One by one, the lions buy into the illusion, grow wary, and flee the site. Walking while projecting assertion, intention, and mettle is incredibly powerful and acts as a self-fulfilling prophecy.

As You Walk, Own the Space Around You

It is common to see a monkey feeding peacefully in one spot but then depart suddenly when approached by another monkey who promptly claims the spot. Behavioral biologists have a word for when one animal makes another animal move. It is called "displacement." It happens when a subordinate animal uses its knowledge of the hierarchy to determine that a confrontation should be avoided. It allows the other animal to evict it from the physical space it was occupying. Preferred spaces can involve food, like a prime spot of grass. They can involve mates, like a spot closer to a fertile female. Sometimes animals are forced to move from unremarkable spaces, where they happen to be. Don't allow anyone to evict you from where you happen to be.

This is not a call to be impolite. Be thoughtful when passing people, share space, open doors, move over to accommodate couples or to make room for children, families, or the elderly. However, don't displace yourself to appease an imposing person any more than you would for someone who wasn't. Hold your ground and expect them to move out of the way as much as you do. When walking, own your immediate space as well as your entire forward trajectory through space. It may feel like you are flouting social customs, but remember that you are not doing anything illegal. You are doing invaluable internal work increasing the boundaries of your comfort zone. When you inevitably bump into someone, be firm but amiable about it.

Many people have told me that my cat is the calmest they have ever seen. This may be because I am calm around him, I treat him like a friend, and I pet him firmly, fluidly, and slowly. But I think the main reason for his composure is that I respect his space. I make an effort not to step over him or walk so close to him that he fears being trampled. I give him authority over his immediate area, which provides him a shield of certainty and control. Take this shield for yourself, wherever you go. Feel complete ownership of the space around you. Wherever you are is your territory because you are in it.

Walk with Exaggerated Posture

When I first went out on long walks exaggerating my posture and standing tall, I could tell that other pedestrians questioned my motives, looking suspicious or even offended. Some people seemed incensed at seeing me standing vertically and looking upwards. My posture looked fake because I was forcing myself to stand straight without the healthy postural tone that should accompany it. Ironically, the best way to develop this musculature is to fake it, standing straighter and taller than our body is accustomed. Once the postural muscles strengthen, standing erect will look genuine, and people will not question it.

Walking Exercise #18.1: *Take A Walk with Exaggerated Posture*
Take a walk in an area where you can avoid worrying about other people judging you. Walk for two minutes with greatly exaggerated posture. Stand tall and straight. Use the five tenets of optimal posture, as well as the anti-laxity method from Chapter 13. The contractions involved should start to fatigue after a few minutes. Once they do, continue to walk but rest your postural muscles completely for at least a minute. Repeat. By letting the muscles go limp, you are giving them the break they need to regenerate.

Pease don't take it overboard. Other pedestrians may be provoked if they can tell that some of your nonverbals are consistent with overcompensation. They may assume that you are putting on a ruse and feel compelled to put you back in your place. You want to avoid this, so be measured and conservative around others as you gradually transform your victim walk into a victor walk. This is also why, at first, I chose to walk and stretch in uncrowded, outdoor places either at dusk or after dark. Find a safe, well-lit park or boulevard where you still have the bit of privacy you need to really swagger. Strut creatively, channeling the gamut of your favorite personality types.

You can work on the timing of your steps by stepping to music. It is as easy as ensuring that your foot strikes the ground on every beat. Try stomping around your block with headphones on. If you let nothing but the drums determine the cadence of your footfall you will learn to walk unhesitatingly. Within two hour of cumulative practice your rhythmic flow will be masterful. You can incorporate a two-step, a spin or turn, and a cross-step (where you are walking sideways and one foot crosses over the other).

Optimal posture only looks natural if it is clear that a person has spent a lot of time there and has interacted with ordinary loads and forces from that position. To get your optimal posture looking authentic, spend time creating these loads and forces using anti-rigidity.

Perform Anti-rigidity Exercises While Walking

The majority of this book's exercises can be performed while walking, but the following exercises are specifically for your walks.

Many people rarely lift their arms above their head because they are afraid it will make others uncomfortable. This complete disuse results in muscle dormancy and neglect of entire sections of the cervical and thoracic spine. The first part of Exercise 18.2 below involves extending the arms directly above the head with the neck retracted. If you do this while employing the anti-rigidity method from Chapter 14 for three cumulative hours, you will find that your cervical spine is completely resituated. You will also invalidate any fears or reservations about lifting your arms in public. The following exercises offer similar postures that you can employ anti-rigidity within. You might take light weights (e.g., one to five pounds) with you to accentuate the forces at play.

Walking Exercise #18.2: *Neck Anti-rigidity While Walking*
Walk for one minute in each of the following configurations while using the anti-rigidity protocol.
1) Raise the hands and arms directly above the head for a few minutes at a time with the neck retracted. You can hold your hands straight up or slightly outward, making a "V" for victory. Search for the achiest configurations and contract your way into them.
2) Hug yourself. Try to grab your shoulder blades with your fingertips as you inch you fingers toward your spine. Do so while varying the retraction of your neck, and the position of your shoulders rooting around for anything that will lead to a crack.
3) Arch the chest inward as far as it will go. Again, this is called thoracic kyphosis in the medical world, and a "hollow" in the gymnastics world. Hugging yourself should give you an idea of how to do this. Next, do the opposite, and arch the chest outward. Then do it laterally to each side.
4) Clasp the hands together in front of you and form the same inward chest arch or kyphotic hollow from #3. Extend the arms as far forward as they will go and press

them together so that you can contract into dormant muscles along the collar bone and shoulder girdle.

5) Place one hand in the air and the other at your waist. Reach as high as you can with the hand in the air, and as low as you can with your hand at your waist. Pivot around in this position hunting for frailty to flex within. Switch arms and repeat.

6) Stand straight with the elbows bent. As you press them toward the ground, make small circles with the elbows as if you were flapping chicken wings. Scour for frailty in the area between your neck and shoulder blades.

7) Walk with your hands out to the side at 90 degrees, making a "t" with your body. Try to bring different aspects of your shoulder blade muscles to fatigue.

8) Walk with your hands clasped behind your back and play with how this changes the forces between your shoulder blades.

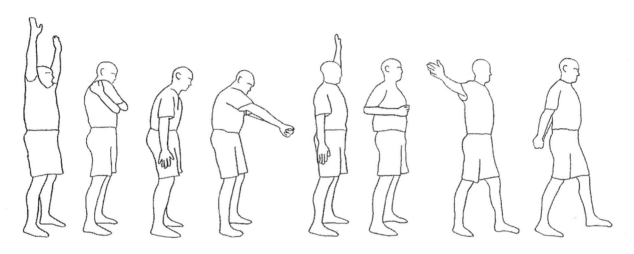

Illustration 18.1: Positions for upper-body anti-rigidity while walking.

Refresh Your Muscles While Walking

Walking requires only a very narrow range of spinal motion. The tension created by walking within this limited range can pull a misaligned spine even further out of alignment. This is why the longer you walk, the more you tend to ache. Simply squatting momentarily, holding a static lunge, or reaching over to touch your toes can completely relieve this by pushing major muscles through their full range. This is why I highly recommend that you do each of these things after every half-mile that you cover.

When you need a break from walking: 1. Stop and crouch down into a low squat. 2. Straighten your back, and flex your ankles, knees, hips, and spine. 3. Then stand and place your fists on your lower back with your elbows at 90 degrees, pointed behind you. You can then bend backwards in this position pressing your fists into your mid and lower back for five to 15 seconds to achieve a full back extension.

Next, use a full back flexion as a counterpose. Slowly bend forward to touch your toes. To make this easier you can support your descent by placing your hands on your upper thighs, and sliding your hands over your knees, down the shins, and toward the feet. Stop for a moment in "forward fold," and then raise up the way that you went in.

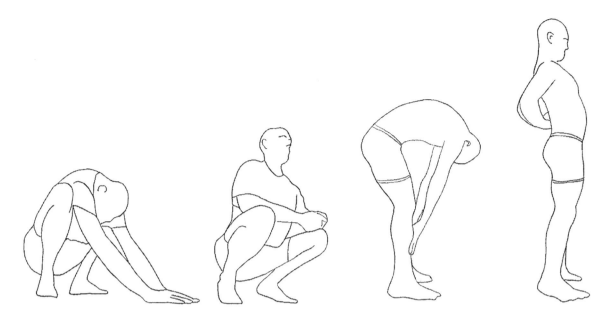

Illustration 18.2: Anti-rigidity poses to use while taking a break from walking.

To make these forward bends harder, you can cradle your head in your hands (as pictured below) and press it toward the ground to engage your neck extensors. This will intensify the active forces in your neck and lower back. For another variation, try this with your legs spread two to three feet apart, or try it with one leg two to three feet in front of the other. I think everyone should be doing 10 of these every day.

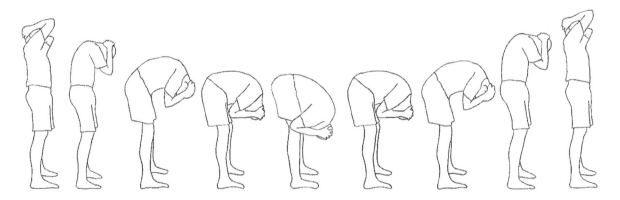

Illustration 18.3: Anti-rigidity routine for the neck and shoulders.

Bent Over Walking Will Tap Into Your Lower Back Pain

There is one particular lumbar position that will reach into the core of your lower back frailty. Maintaining this position while walking will allow you to tap into it so that you can work out the kinks. To assume the position, bend over from the waist (not the hips), and enter lumbar kyphosis (shrimp back), where you curl your hips upwards and inwards toward your face. While you do this, try to keep your glutes contracted. Clasping your hands behind your back can help provide support and balance. Then keep this configuration and start walking, taking small, tempered steps. As long as you ensure that you remain in lumbar kyphosis, you will engage many dormant muscles anchored in the sacrum and ilium.

This will make you feel like a very old person because of the way you are hunched over and because of the intensely brittle feeling in your lower back as you plant each foot. For safety's sake, this bent-over walking should be done very carefully and just a little at a time at first. As you rehab this configuration, you can become more ambitious by bending over further and funneling more power into each stride. It is risky because you can easily pull a muscle. However, if you are careful, it is a vigorous form of rehab that can help you reclaim the lumbar mobility of your early childhood and reinstitute an entire mode of locomotion.

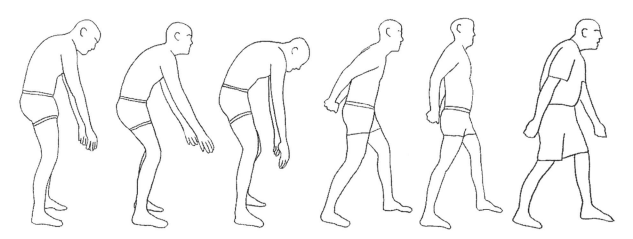

Illustration 18.4: Anti-rigidity routine to engage dormant lower back muscles.

Experiment with walking using both extreme lumbar kyphosis and lordosis. This can also be done on a stair climber, treadmill, or elliptical machine at a low-speed setting. Carefully curl your lumbar spine either backward or forward while on the machine as if you were performing a "cow" or "cat" pose. As your legs move and your weight is redistributed, you will be tugging at various partially contracted muscles. Proceed slowly and carefully, breathing through the pinch you find during each cycle.

Keep Your Feet Straight and Vary the Way You Use Them to Walk

We take every step in almost the same repetitive manner with minimal movement variation at the foot, ankle, or knee. We do this despite the incredible potential for mobility contained within the thirty-two joints, fifty-six ligaments, and thirty-eight muscles of our feet. Unfortunately, many of these are largely immobile in most people. The best way to reengage the dormant muscles in your feet and legs is to spend a few minutes a day walking within various positions, as in the exercise below.

Walking Exercise #18.3: *Vary the Placement of Your Feet*
Strengthening each of the following stepping patterns will help your body find a happy balance and the most efficient walking configuration. Training them will build uncommon mobility, strength, and coordination. To do this, walk for one minute in each of the following ways:

1) Walk with more weight on the outer edge of your feet (supination).
2) Walk with your weight on the inside edge of your feet (pronation).
3) Walk with your feet more than shoulder length apart. Each step should land out to the side. You can even try walking with your feet as many as three feet apart.
4) Walk with your feet less than shoulder length apart. Each step should land close to the center of your body, like walking a tightrope. Consider crossing your feet, such that your left foot lands to the right of center, and vice versa.
5) Walk with your weight on your heels.
6) Walk with your weight on the ball of the foot, digging them into the ground.
7) Walk with your feet turned out toward 45 degrees (lateral rotation).
8) Walk with your feet turned in toward 45 degrees (medial rotation).
9) March like a soldier by raising your knee higher than usual above the ground during each step.
10) Walk backwards.

While walking your feet should face directly forward. My feet used to be dramatically turned out. I was able to fix this completely after only two weeks of walking a couple of minutes a day while concentrating mindfully to ensure that my feet remained straight. I think you may also be surprised by how just paying attention to it fixes this problem. To strengthen both tendencies, you can use 7 and 8 above, walking briefly with the toes turned out and then turning in. As when backbends are followed by forward bends, gently training the extremes will help the body find the ideal midline.

You might also consider getting orthotic insoles prescribed for your shoes. You can get a prescription from a podiatrist or get fitted at your local drug store. Insoles are commonly used to support feet that have been worn out of shape by a walking style that favors one of the above patterns to the exclusion of the others. Wear these arch-supporting inserts less than half the time. Again, you will strengthen and cross-train your feet by exposing them to both conditions.

Practice Glidewalking

Every step we take is supposed to be powered by a forceful gluteal contraction, but most of us have learned to walk without activating the glutes at all. Adding a gluteal contraction at the end of each step is known as glidewalking.[5] To practice this, you want to take long strides with a straight back leg that thrusts you forward due to the extension occurring at the buttock. To ensure that this happens, place your hands inside your pants, just above your back pockets. Cover the top half of each of your glutes with your fingers. Walk so that you feel the top of each glute contract firmly with every step. After a few months of sporadically reminding yourself to train this, you will put your hand on your glute while walking and feel it ball up vigorously. Over time your glutes will become toned and brawny and will add stability and power to your stride.

The same goes for the calves: most people have engineered a firm calf contraction out of their step. Pushing off the ground with the calf muscles of the back leg will challenge and develop them. The heel should make contact with the ground first. Then you should roll forward across the length of the foot to the toes. As this happens, the ankle should pass through much of its full range of motion. The calf should be fully extended as you push the ground away with the ball of your foot. Even the toes should contribute to this push, contracting slightly at the end of each step to help propel you forward. When the toes and calf contract, the glute should contract at the same time.

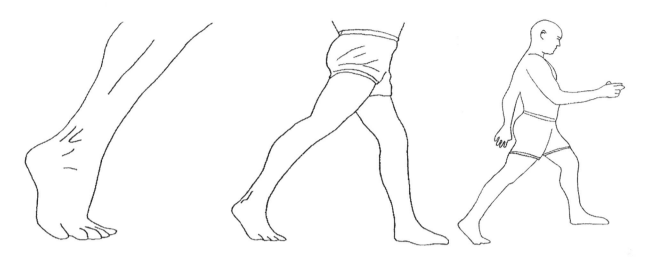

Illustration 18.5: Depiction of glidewalking.

Arm swing is another essential biomechanical component of efficient walking. People reduce arm swing to display subordination, but you should swing your arms blithely whenever you are walking. As you do it, ensure that your shoulders are pressed toward the floor. These elements of proper walking take time to develop, but once they are automatic, they will help you burn calories and build muscle.

Pay special attention to the way you kick your foot forward with each step. Rather than being smooth and graceful, it is likely a violent jerk. This is a major cause of knee pain. You can address it by consciously attending to the jarring motion and making an effort to transform it into a gentle, velvety one. Strolling very slowly helps build the coordination needed. As in tai chi, slow everything down and pay attention to the fluidity of each movement. You are going to look weird walking around your block in slow motion, instituting these exercises. Getting yourself to stop worrying about how others will perceive you will be an accomplishment in itself.

Your routines (e.g., walking) cannot be efficient unless their component subroutines (e.g., extending the ankle, knee, and hip) are optimal themselves. You might feel uncoordinated when you start to slow things down and focus on the individual parts of each action. That's totally normal. You have thousands of steps to take every day, likely for the rest of your life, so you want to re-engineer them to be as efficient as possible. Relearn how to complete the smallest motor movements in ways that don't use anxiety for propulsion. Instead...glide. This goes for writing, speaking, typing, opening a door, handing an object to someone, and everything else imaginable.

Conserve Your Momentum While Walking

Whenever you are walking, you should be taking full advantage of your body's forward energy. Most people walk without conserving their momentum. They break the inertia they have going with each indecisive stride. Poorly timed foot falls eat up their speed, slow them down, and create a bumpy ride. Take some time to analyze how you lose momentum in your default walking pattern.

Each foot plant should not be a collision but rather a brief foothold to push off against. Rolling down your foot from heel to toes will help with this. Also, use the proprioceptive sensors throughout your knees and ankles to help you determine how much momentum from the last step can be reused in the next surefooted step. Placing your foot too far in front of the body, known as over-striding, is one of the most common mistakes people make when walking. It breaks up your glide. Under-striding is also common. So, pay careful attention to the fluidity created by stride length and try to optimize it.

Don't second guess a single step. Conserving your momentum will turn your stride into a buoyant saunter and override any hesitancies deriving from submissive signaling. Done right, you should feel like a freight train. Allay any worries that people will think that you are walking in an aggressive, angry way. It is not angry at all. It is merely efficient.

Don't hobble. Coast. Set sail on your own momentum, and ride like the wind.

Conclusion

"Walk as if you are kissing the earth with your feet." — Thich Nhat Hanh (1926)

It is worth mentioning that there are many ways to multitask while walking. Walking with other people is a great way to bond. You can help each other to develop mutually assertive, out-of-doors, power-walking body language. Instead of taking your phone calls in bed or on the couch, take them as you parade around your neighborhood. A headset with a microphone or a Bluetooth earphone can make this easier. You can also turn your time walking into an opportunity for learning if you decide to listen to audiobooks using headphones. Additionally, you can use the act of walking to create a breathing metronome. For instance, I often inhale for five steps and then exhale for eight. Otherwise, walking can be an opportune time to take in nature, meditate, live in the moment, practice mindfulness, and create a new, improved persona.

Chapter 18: **Bullet Points**

- Walking is highly health promoting.
- Maintain the five tenets of optimal posture while walking.
- Strut and swagger while you walk to build confidence.
- Walk with exaggerated, solider-like posture for two minutes until the muscles involved reach a healthy fatigue. Then allow the muscles at least a minute to rest completely before repeating.
- Perform upper-body anti-rigidity while you walk, by moving your arms, shoulders, and back through different, unfamiliar configurations.
- Walking regularly with your hands in the air and the neck retracted will help put your cervical and thoracic spine into optimal configuration.
- When you walk for prolonged periods take breaks to allow your muscles to regenerate.
- When you break from walking, refresh your muscles by squatting, lunging, and touching your toes. This will bring fresh blood to spinal sections that have become stale.
- Practice glidewalking where the glute, calf, and toes of the back leg are fully deployed with every step.
- Walk with both feet pointing straight ahead.
- Capture the remaining momentum from each stride so that it can be applied to the next.

Chapter 18: **Endnotes**

1.   Lee, I. M., Shiroma, E. J., & Kamada, M. (2019). Association of step volume and intensity with all-cause mortality in older women. *JAMA Internal Medicine, 179*(8), 1105–1112.

2.   Ritchiea, M. B., Blais, J., Forth, A. (2019). "Evil" intentions: Examining the relationship between the Dark Tetrad and victim selection based on nonverbal gait cues. *Personality and Individual Differences, 138*(1), 126–132.

3.   Michalak, J., Troje, N. F., Fischer, J., Vollmar, P., Heidenreich, T., & Schulte, D. (2009). Embodiment of sadness and depression: Gait patterns associated with dysphoric mood. *Psychosomatic Medicine, 71*(5), 580–587.

4.   Van Edwards, V. (2017). *Captivate: The science of succeeding with people.* Penguin Random House.

5.   Gokhale, C. (2008). *8 Steps to a pain-free back.* Pendo Press.

Chapter 19: **Stop Sexually Submissive Behavior**

"The desire for sexual expression is inborn and natural. The desire cannot, and should not be submerged or eliminated. But it should be given an outlet through forms of expression which enrich the body, mind, and spirit." — Napoleon Hill (1883-1970)

Sexual Competition and Submission

Aside from humans, chimpanzees are often considered the most violent and abusive species on the planet, despite competing for just one resource. Ordinarily, they do not compete for food because the fruit and leaves they forage are evenly scattered. They compete for sex, and the competition is often violent. In most primates, dominant males restrict sexual access to females. Nondominant males are thus forced to inhibit their sexuality. They are usually attacked if seen approaching a female for sex and are often forced to either be sneaky or abstain from sex completely. Many primate females are similarly traumatized by sexual competition.

Access to sex is determined by rank in many animals that live in groups. This inevitably leads to stress. Status probably also dictated sexual privileges, to varying degrees, throughout human history. Because our instincts were wired in the past, even in modern humans, this age-old competition leads to unconscious sexual self-handicapping. By employing the same rationale and some of the same tools we have discussed thus far, this chapter will explain how to detraumatize your sexuality and pull your genitals out of this melee.

Sexual Subordination in Animals

The sexual subordination response isn't just found in primates or mammals. There are many examples in the animal kingdom (from vertebrates to invertebrates) of dominant individuals causing the atrophy of reproductive organs in subordinates.[1] For example, the resident queens in honeybees, termites, cockroaches, and many other species suppress the ovaries of their workers. In animals from insects to fish, the less dominant males create fewer sperm that move slower. If given the opportunity to become dominant, many fish can reverse this by increasing the size of their testes and the count and motility of their sperm in as little as a few days.

In mammals, especially primates, alpha individuals from both genders attempt to monopolize breeding through intimidation. This causes a dramatic decrease in sex hormones in their targets. Chronic intimidation can be so stressful that it impairs subordinates' fertility, suppressing the testicular axis in males and halting ovulation in females. This is often called "social suppression of reproduction" or "social contraception."[2] There is an entire body of literature on how conflict in primates creates reproductive disadvantages for the losers.

In many monkey species, the biggest losers are completely celibate. It is common for dominant males to attack or physically displace a subordinate male in the middle of copulation, preventing them from ejaculating. The resulting brain and hormone changes decrease the quantity and quality of the displaced male's sperm. Likewise, repeated conflict with a dominant female can cause subordinate females to lose the ability to conceive. There is every reason to believe that similar coercion and physical repercussions are commonplace in human society.

Indeed, human infertility and sexual dysfunction are both known by medical researchers to be highly exacerbated by the stress hormone cortisol.

Chronically elevated cortisol levels can cause loss of libido and impotence in men mostly by inhibiting the production of testosterone. In women, it can cause severe fertility problems and result in an abnormal menstrual cycle. This antagonism between the cortisol and testosterone hormonal axes is thought to be adaptive because in emergency situations engaging in behaviors that are encouraged by testosterone, such as mating, competition, and dominance is unnecessary and possibly counterproductive.

If you put a mouse in a cage with a more dominant mouse, its testosterone and fertility will decline significantly. Similarly, if you spend time believing that you are inferior or inadequate, your virility will drop. We must avoid sexual bullying and stop ourselves from thinking sexually self-subordinating thoughts. Fortunately, the effects of cortisol on testosterone in both men and women are reversed when the stress goes back down.

You don't want your body to assume you are a pathetic monkey trying to sneak copulations in hiding. So, you need to send it the right messages. You want to develop a mindset of sexual dominance and disinhibition affirming that you can achieve arousal at any time, have sex anywhere, and be in your sexual comfort zone under any social conditions...as long as it is ethical and legal, of course. This starts with slowing everything else down and making your sexual response a priority. Just as subordination causes us to ignore our shallow breathing and protracted neck, it also causes us to ignore both the tension and the pleasure in our genitals. The best way to counteract this is to learn to "listen" to your genitals.

Sexual Exercise #19.1: *Listen to the Sensations Coming from Your Genitals*

Your genitals are continuously sending you sensory signals about their current state of arousal. Most of us ignore this steady influx of cues, leaving us out of tune with our sexuality. Sexual suppression and submission have turned our erogenous zones into blind spots. Feeling good down there is not a sin, not a luxury, and not something you have to earn. It is your basic right as a mammal and an integral part of dealing with stress. If you want to cultivate your sexual response, you must pay attention to any and all pleasurable sensations coming from in between your legs.

Close your eyes, and spend five minutes meditating on this area. Focus on it completely like you are watching a movie. At first, you may not sense much, but with time and patience, you will begin to notice faint instances of erogenous squirming and pulsating. Indulge them. Learn to revel in them. Doing this will help prove to your body that you are a lusty beast unencumbered by sexual trauma. With time, practice, and the use of the other exercises in this chapter, infrequent tingles and quivers will turn into a steady stream of not-so-subtle heaving and throbbing. Monitor your breath while you do this and imagine breathing "straight into your genitals." This will help you develop the laser focus necessary to become reacquainted with the full extent of your aphrodisia.

One of the best ways to improve your awareness of sexual sensations is to stop bracing the muscles involved. This is simply because, if they are constantly strained, they cannot respond actively to sexual stimuli. There is no throbbing in dormant muscle.

Stop Bracing the Muscles Surrounding Your Genitals

Hip or pelvic tension can be a conscious or unconscious attempt to downplay the potency of the genital region and is yet another form of submissive body language. Over time the formation of dormant muscle leads to withered libido, lessened enjoyment of sex, and sexual dysfunction. There are other sources of pelvic bracing. Falling on the bottom, bruising the tailbone, long hours sitting at a desk or a bicycle seat, and all types of physical trauma can lead to tension the area.

Pelvic bracing is linked to medical disorders. Vaginismus is the involuntary contraction of muscles that surround the vagina. The tight muscles make penetration and intercourse painful for women with this disorder. Bracing may also make it harder for some women to orgasm. For a woman to climax, the muscles of her pelvic floor cannot be taut. They must relax during sexual stimulation so that they can contract rhythmically during orgasm. Many researchers believe that various sexual disorders such as male impotence, latency to female orgasm, and vulvodynia (chronic vulvar pain) can be due to excessive bracing of muscles adjacent to the sexual organs.[3] This seems even more likely when you consider that common preceding events for these disorders include sexual assault, rape, domestic abuse, sexual humiliation, chronic pain, and generalized anxiety.

It is well known that the blood vessels surrounding the external genitalia constrict during sympathetic stimulation and dilate upon parasympathetic stimulation. This means that blood flow to the penis, clitoris, and vulva is impeded by stress and accentuated by relaxation. In fact, the pelvic floor is one of the most reactive groups of muscles during startle. When it contracts it results in a retraction of the clitoris for women and the penis for men. Relaxation of the anococcygeal area is thought to be key in improving the sexual arousal response. As a matter of fact, engorgement of the penis, clitoris, and labia results from the relaxation of smooth muscle. In other words, blood doesn't flow until these unconsciously regulated muscles loosen up.

Sexual Activity #19.1: *Brace and Debrace Your Pelvic Muscles*

How do stress and intimidation affect the bracing of the muscles around your genitals? Most people could not answer this because they have little to no awareness of this common reaction. Let's try bracing them to see how it feels. Tighten the muscles in your lower back. Tilt your hips to one side and brace them. Squeeze your legs together. Tighten your urinary sphincter as if you were trying to stop yourself from peeing. Now contract all these muscles, and anything else local you can find, at 90% of their maximum strength. After 10 seconds, let go entirely and register what it feels like to let the bracing here subside. Repeat this contraction and relaxation four more times.

We signal sexual submission by straining sex-related muscles in the abdomen and pelvis. These muscles lose their healthy tone after sexual trauma or feelings of sexual inferiority. Thankfully, like all muscles, you can rehabilitate them. Most people have an untapped reservoir of muscle in the groin that has atrophied. The next two sections will show you how to exercise and strengthen it. I believe proper tone in these muscles allows the genitals increased vascular blood flow (vasocongestion), increases the prominence of arousal, and heightens the accompanying sensations.

Exercise Your Urine Retentive Muscles

You have numerous muscles situated between your sitz bones, pubic bone, and coccyx. These muscles support the pelvic organs, contract during orgasm, aid in childbirth and ejaculation, and provide core stability.

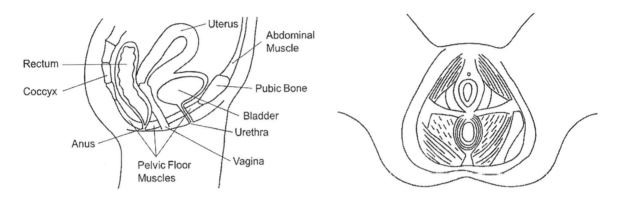

Illustration 19.1: A. Side view of female reproductive anatomy. Note the location of the pelvic floor muscles stretching from the pubic bone to the tail bone (coccyx); B. Frontal view of the pelvic floor musculature which is similar in women and men. Several pelvic muscles are depicted including the ischiocavernosus, bulbospongiosus, coccygeus, pubococcygeus, the urogenital diaphragm and others.

In the 1960s, Dr. Arnold Kegel taught people how to strengthen the perineum (the area between the anus and the genitals). He knew that these muscles are often injured in women during childbirth, and he instructed women how to contract them, reinstating their strength, in an exercise that came to be known as "Kegels." Doctors have prescribed Kegels for many reasons, including treating urinary incontinence,[4] ameliorating erectile dysfunction,[5] and controlling premature ejaculation.[6] Kegels are taught by having the patient repeatedly interrupt their urinary flow. Dr. Kegel recommended urinating a spoonful at a time. Try this in the activity below.

Sexual Activity #19.2: *Contracting the Urinary Sphincter*

The next time you find yourself peeing, stop urinating midstream. Once you can stop the flow completely, you have found the right muscles. Try urinating for only a second at a time until you have voided your bladder. Focus on tightening only the pelvic floor muscles, keeping the abdomen, thighs, anus, and buttocks relaxed. This will allow you to isolate the contraction. Doing this several times will help you identify the muscles and gain conscious control of them. At that point, you should do this exercise without urinating and from any position you want.

Most of us learned to brace the Kegel muscles intensely as young children when "holding it" for long periods to avoid the embarrassing experience of urinating in public. Can you remember an incident in which this muscle was likely traumatized by being braced heavily during the traumatic scenario of trying desperately to find a bathroom as a child? Not only do the muscles surrounding the genitals seize up in these scenarios, but distressed breathing predominates, making the strain worse. Most people have a strong tendency to hold their breath when performing Kegels,[7] and of course, this defeats the purpose. Therefore I recommend pairing Kegels with paced breathing.

Sexual Exercise #19.2: *Diaphragmatic Kegels*

Perform hard Kegel contractions as if you were interrupting the stream of urine. Do this while paced breathing. This will build your capacity to activate the pelvic floor muscles without holding your breath. Hold a forceful contraction during a 10-second passive exhalation and then relax for a few breaths. Do this 10 times in a row. You might also try performing rapid Kegels (i.e., one to three per second) for a minute.

These muscles contract involuntarily during arousal and orgasm. So, loosening them up and developing their responsivity may enliven your sex life. Also, after developing the muscular strength that comes from pelvic floor exercises, men can perform a Kegel at orgasm to withhold ejaculation effectively allowing them to experience multiple orgasms. I also believe that strengthening and unbracing these muscles can facilitate female ejaculation and squirting.

The next section will provide you with an exercise that will dilate these areas rather than constrict them. In a previous chapter, we learned how important it is to perform forward bends after backward bends to neutralize the spine. I believe that performing Kegels without exercising the antagonist muscles leads to similar imbalances. For example, there is evidence that performing Kegels can lead to incomplete emptying of the bladder, and this is a risk factor for urinary tract infection and other maladies. As you might have guessed, the counterpose for a Kegel is complete bladder emptying.

Exercise the Muscles that Expel Urine

Interestingly, the Kegel contraction is braced involuntarily during social competition. Kegels result in a retraction of the clitoris, penis, and testicles, potentially making them less conspicuous to a competitor. I believe that, in this, they are submissive and intended to hide the genitalia. It is like the sea slug withdrawing its gill or the snail withdrawing its eyestalk.

Male monkeys and apes are frequently observed hiding their erections from other males, especially from males above them in the hierarchy. They don't want to be attacked for being aroused. This is why I think genital retraction due to chronic Kegel contraction is an innate defense mechanism protecting subordinates from sexually dominant individuals. It is yet another display equivalent to a collapsed posture. I believe that losing tone and developing partial contraction in the pelvic region is a self-handicapping mechanism that assumes advertising one's level of sexual arousal is dangerous.

If you have balanced tone in your pelvic muscles, your flaccid penis or clitoris will increase and decrease in size with your arousal level. If you have strain or poor tone, the flaccid organ may remain at its smallest possible size until full arousal is reached. Most people are aware that the penis and clitoris shrink in size when exposed to cold. In fact, penile length decreases by up to 50% in the defensive response to low temperature. I believe men with a history of chronic intimidation and sexual subordination are more likely to exhibit this kind of shrinkage when flaccid. This likely corresponds to the "grower" vs. "shower" dichotomy referenced in popular culture. The growers may be men with a more extensive history of being sexually intimidated. This may be reversible by performing the opposite of the Kegel.

It is easy for both women and men to pinpoint the muscles that expel urine. They speed up the stream. These muscles include the lower abdominal muscles and the bladder detrusor muscle. They aid in the expulsion of urine by increasing the pressure applied to the bladder wall. The stream of urine will cease when the bladder has been voided, but the muscles themselves can still be contracted. If you continue to squeeze the expulsive muscles very firmly after you finish urinating, you will realize you can flex these muscles through their full range.

Most people never use this full range, creating a missing corner of dormant muscle. Thus, it is also a reservoir that you can tap into and rehab. Think of the exercise as an "antiKegel." As we have seen in previous chapters, sometimes the only way to free muscles from partial contraction is through hard, full contractions.

Sexual Exercise #19.3: *Contract the Expulsive Muscles*

The next time you urinate, try to expel the urine more forcefully than usual. Steadily increase the force as you empty your bladder. As it nears empty, do not let up. Instead, squeeze the related muscles hard even after the stream stops. Notice the posture that your lower back and lower abdomen have taken on, and remember the feeling of contracting this muscle so that you can do it later. After you have emptied your bladder, continue to squeeze the muscle at 70 to 90% maximum force for an additional 10 seconds. It may ache tenderly, but performing this exercise each time you urinate will make this aching disappear within a matter of days.

Start practicing it away from the toilet as well. You should feel comfortable performing the Kegel and "antiKegel" contractions in the presence of others. There is no reason to brace or self-limit your pelvic range just because other people are around. To really stimulate these erogenous areas and all the tissues and blood vessels involved, you can also try gently performing Kegels and antiKegels while you have an erection, whether clitoral or penile. Together, these exercises will help put an end to neurotic pelvic flinching and straining.

Urine Expulsion as a Posture and Mindset

You want to incorporate proper tone in these urine-expelling muscles into your daily standing, walking, and sitting postures. The muscles involved include the lower abdominals, so imagine being able to take a small punch to the lowest segment of your abs at any time. This means you need to practice walking around with your lower abs engaged as if you were peeing. I want to encourage you to walk, jog, exercise, and socialize as if you are dribbling urine everywhere you go.

"Listen" intently to the sensations involved. It should feel pleasurable. Imagine spurting rainbows and gushing warm velvet from your urethra onto everything in front of you. Experience everything orgasmically. This should be happening as you look at yourself in the mirror, as you walk around the block, and as you squeeze in that last repetition while exercising. Imagine that your genitals are permanently everted rather than inverted. As you strengthen the retentive and expulsive muscles, muscle memory will develop, and they will come to hold balanced tone automatically. I believe this is highly beneficial for psychosexual health.

I suppressed these muscles during my lifetime through acquiescent, self-handicapping behavior. I have always been averse to dirty jokes and overt sex play, which may have led to less sexualized perineal posture growing up. I believe that I unconsciously allowed my Kegel muscles to strain and my expulsive muscles to atrophy because I was sexually repressive, and anal-retentive. Again, the expulsive urinary and anal sphincter muscles work antagonistically with the retentive muscles, meaning that expulsive qualities may be especially weak in "retentive" people. If you think that you may be anal-retentive, you are probably also urinary retentive. While we are talking about poop, please ask yourself whether combining distressed breathing while straining on the toilet seat during defecation may have traumatized your anal muscles. If so, you might consider using paced breathing while defecating, when constipated, and while contracting the anal retentive and expulsive muscles.

Strengthening the muscles involved in expelling urine will make your behavior more assertive. Activity and tone in this area are associated with approach and the seizing of opportunities that are both sexual and non-sexual in nature. It is difficult to maintain a dominant, self-assured demeanor if the tone in the expulsive muscles is low. You have probably noticed that worry or sudden fear makes your retentive muscles tense and the expulsive ones limp. Similarly, encountering something sharp or experiencing fear of heights does this as well. For example, peering over the ledge from the 5th floor of a parking structure can make your whole pelvis seize up. This happens immediately and involuntarily during startle and fright. Your pelvic floor recoils from threat.

When you take an ego blow or get upset or flustered, the muscles that expel urine similarly drop out of flexion. If your machismo is questioned, but you have the gumption to reassert yourself, you might notice the activity waiver and come back. Activity here "shrivels up" when people get their "balls busted." For many depressed and anxious people, these muscles drop out of tonicity during social encounters. For sexually assertive people, the expulsive musculature develops a stronger tone when around others they find attractive. For sexually withdrawn people, the tone may actually decrease in these situations. Losing tone and accumulating strain in these muscles leads to emasculation and/or defeminization.

When I first started to engage the muscles that expel urine, I would become afraid of upsetting the bully introduced in Chapter 2. I realized that I was afraid to engage the muscles even when he was not around. When I tried, thoughts, visuals, and a feeling of being in the bully's presence would intrude into my mind unconsciously. It took me some time to realize that I was bracing these muscles in a restricted range out of fear of "offending" the bully. This bully was muscular, highly charismatic, a felon, and a murderer. On one occasion, I had seen him continue to make fun of and laugh at someone even after that person pulled a gun on him. As many bullies do, he would frequently tell sexually explicit stories describing his sexual prowess in attempts to intimidate other men. This is one of the fundamental forms that sexual toxicity takes.

The man had acquired "pseudopsychopathy," meaning he had developed criminal, antisocial, and hypersexual personality traits after severe brain trauma. He was catastrophically disinhibited after being fully ejected headfirst through the windshields of two cars he stole on separate occasions. I was subverting my sexuality in an attempt to appease this man. Simply becoming explicitly aware of this subversion was enough to end it. After bringing peace to this context, I realized that there were additional contexts that caused me to brace my genital musculature. What contexts of intimidation sting you in the genitals and keep you stuck in a partially contracted Kegel? Don't let anyone keep you in a retentive state in which the genitals are retracted or keep you from contracting your expulsive muscles. Rather than being held taut in a restricted range, these muscles should fluctuate naturally between the two extremes of retention and expulsion as you go about your day.

Once you become comfortable fully contracting the muscles that withhold and expel urine, you should notice them quiver involuntarily more frequently. Toning the muscles and stretching them out of partial contraction will increase the range of motion of your orgasms. You may also notice that you experience increased blood flow and heightened turgidity in your genitals. This suggests to me that formal physical therapy centered around exercising these muscles could treat both diminished sex drive and erectile dysfunction. However, most medical experts on the topic assume that these muscles operate autonomously and needn't be exercised.

This medical opinion is at odds with Ayurvedic medicine and tantric Hinduism, which recognize the base of the spine as a chakra. It is called muladhara, the root chakra, and kundalini yoga emphasizes that it must be used and meditated upon. Additionally, some Japanese Zen meditation practices emphasize the lower abdominal area (dantian or tanden) as a focal point for meditation. I believe the exercises in this chapter can guide you to exert control over and rehabilitate these foci.

At one point, I realized I lacked the coordination to contract my urinary expulsive muscles and gluteus muscles simultaneously. When I tried, I held my breath. Many people have this functional dissociation. When these are dissociated, you are limited to either doing one or the other. However, it is easy to fix. Proper core stability demands that you be able to contract these muscles together actively. Everyone should teach their body to activate both the urinary and fecal expulsive muscles while simultaneously contracting their buttocks.

Sexual Activity #19.4: *Pairing Expulsive Tone with Gluteal Tone*

Stand with optimal posture, as described in Chapter 13. With your feet parallel and the top of your hips rolled backward, contract the gluteus muscles. Now contract either your urinary or fecal expulsive muscles as if you were trying to pee or defecate. Now try all three together. Spend time in this zone varying these contractions to different degrees while engaging in calm, paced breathing.

As with many other examples in the Program Peace system, if holding two dominant displays simultaneously is uncomfortable or difficult, they likely inhibit each other. However, if you can calmly practice them together, you disinhibit them and increase the probability they will arise together on their own.

Walk Confidently as if Your Genitals Were on Display

In Chapter 2, we discussed how submissive animals minimize the appearance of physical assets like horns, claws, and muscles. This includes the genitals. Your everyday posture and mannerisms reveal cues to others as to how comfortable you are naked. Body language evolved during our history as unclothed apes, so even clothed, we often act as if we were naked. Most people conceal their genitals during times of insecurity with their hands, legs, chairs, or tables. When a dominant person makes a power play, it is quite common for other people of the same sex to place their hands in front of their sex organs. The only time you should conceal or protect the genitals is to block a physical blow to the groin.

Most people walk in a way that hides or apologizes for their genitalia. Walking like this involves hunching or crouching of the lower back. Remember the lumbar lordosis and anterior pelvic tilt discussed in previous chapters? We actually use these to withdraw our private parts from view. They obscure the genitals like a dog hiding its tail between its legs. You should do the exact opposite. This means walking around with the back and hips open as if presenting the genitalia. To do this, flex your buttocks. That's right, gluteal contraction puts your genitals on display by pressing your hips forward, and rolling the top of your pelvis back, as discussed in Chapter 17. It is an entirely different style of standing and walking that comes across as much more sexually self-assured.

If you can imagine being comfortably naked in social situations, you will project higher confidence. The more time you spend naked, the more comfortable it will become, which is why I strongly recommend sleeping naked when possible. If you have never slept naked, you may lose some sleep the first night because of how uncomfortable you feel. But you will relax into it within a week. I also recommend spending time alone in your room in the buff as described next.

Sexual Activity #19.5: *Spend an Hour in Your Room Naked*

Make sure no one can see into your room, and you won't be disturbed. Lock the door. Completely disrobe. Place towels underneath you if uncomfortable sitting on the floor naked. Spend a full hour reading, watching TV, meditating, whatever you want, completely naked. It can help to have a mirror in front of you. Use optimal posture. Once you become comfortable, try talking on the phone. How do you hold your body when completely nude? Do you tend to cover up or hide your genitalia? Is your posture retentive or expulsive? Notice these tendencies change as you become comfortable. Experiment with pushing your pelvis out, contracting your glutes, and spreading your legs in different ways. If performed with paced breathing, this activity will transform your relationship with your birthday suit.

Masturbation Trauma

Most of us were petitioned by our parents at a very young age to stop touching our genitals in the company of others. We learned to feel bad for stimulating the area, resulting in a subtle form of trauma. I recommend briefly touching yourself in a sexual/affectionate way at least five times a day. This can be a graze, stroke, or reassuring grope. Some people already do this regularly. To others, it is very foreign. You can do it alone or discretely in public. Even a second of self-comforting can help decrease bracing of the pelvic floor.

I used to worry that frequent masturbation could cause specific forms of cancer until I used pubmed.com to look at the actual medical studies. It does not. There are no diseases linked to masturbation. So, give yourself carte blanche to be completely self-indulgent. However, there are a few important caveats to keep in mind. Masturbating to pornography may desensitize you to real people, potentially leading to sexual dysfunction. Also, masturbating with a lubricant can make it difficult for men to sustain an erection with a condom. Also, consider masturbating while standing up to avoid losing the ability to remain aroused while standing. Definitely consider masturbating while paced breathing. For some people, it takes time and work merely to reach arousal while paced breathing. But the process will steel and gird your sexuality.

Studies have shown that placing tiny vibrators near or on the genitals of mice can increase sexual response, interest, and the production of sex hormones. Studies like these suggest that the external use of vibrators may convince the mammalian body that it resides in some kind of maximally optimal sexual environment and may in turn elicit an optimal sexual response from it (involving changes in gene expression). Keep in mind though that masturbating to orgasm with some sex toys may make it difficult to sustain arousal during regular intercourse.

The fascia and muscles nestled in the pelvis control the responsivity of sexual arousal. Massage and myofascial release are probably beneficial for these muscles; however, there is no existing rubric to help people do this safely and effectively. Moreover, excessive pressure could damage your sexual organs or drastically change the tone of the muscles that regulate blood flow to them. For these reasons, I will not describe a protocol for genital massage here. If you decide to use compressive massage on the areas between your legs, I recommend using only very light pressure. That being said, you should also find that groin stretching and anti-rigidity can be helpful in conditioning these muscles.

Sexual Expressivity

The anti-rigidity exercises for the lumbar spine from Chapter 17 will help free up your hips and lower back, making your sexual expressivity more sensual and enjoyable. Try to incorporate previously dormant muscles into intercourse and use them to explore new movement patterns. Use the next two activities to enhance the coordination of the muscles and joints involved.

Sexual Activity #19.6: *Bump Your Pubis Against the Wall*
Find some privacy and turn on some sexy music. Stand with your feet shoulder-width apart and your toes touching a wall. Press your pubic bone into the wall to the beat of the music. You can bump against it like a bouncing basketball or smear yourself into it with each thrust. Contract your buttocks firmly as you advance. Vary the curvature of your lower back, the distance between your feet, and the placement of each blow against the wall.

After a few sessions, you will develop the coordination to turn it into a dance. You can move each advance from left to right or from top to bottom. Doing this against a door jamb can give you the leg room you need to bend your knees and drop lower. You can also try this exercise by bumping your butt against the wall instead of your pubis. Bang everything from your pubic bone to your hips, your sacrum to your sitz bones into the brick, wood, or plaster. Focus on rhythm, timing, and bravado.

Good sex should provide a massage to the pubic bone, and the muscles that surround it, for both partners. The friction between your pubic hair and your partner's should make rhythmic crackling sounds. Pubic-bone-on-pubic-bone massage increases arousal and is one of the best ways to stimulate the clitoris. Just like the muscles in our lower backs, muscles that surround the pubic bone can take the form of tense cords that form tense cords. Teaching yourself to massage them during the act of sex, along with those of the other person, can be very sexually empowering.

Sexual Activity #19.7: *Hump Your Pillows to Music*

Put on some music or a music video. Stack pillows on your bed to support your pelvis in different sexual positions. You can straddle these pillows, kneel, squat, or lie on top of them. You can also fold a pillow over a couple of times to make a hard, raised surface to nestle your pubic bone up against. As you explore different arrangements, lean your pubic bone into the pillows from different angles.

While propped on the pillows, simulate sexual thrusting, grinding, and gyrating movements to the beat of the music for an entire song. Experiment with reciprocal and circular thrusting in different planes. Think: heaving, stirring, twerking, screwing, wiggling, drilling, pounding, and tapping. Experiment with flair and ostentatious movements that you are normally too inhibited to try. This is your chance to have fun and attempt the different positions and moves you've always wanted to. Practice full lumbar lordosis on the upswing, from there transition gradually into full lumbar kyphosis by the end of the downswing, and back again over and over. You might also look into incorporating a dance move called the "body roll."

See yourself as a sex machine or a sensuous, captivating performance artist. Create a safe environment for you to practice and master dominant, free-flowing, rhythmic, and unhesitating sexual maneuvers. Feel unhurried, with no external pressures and no time constraints. Absorb yourself in the carnality of the experience without any fear of failure. You will quickly become more confident in your ability to deliver your pelvis fluidly.

You may want to consider extending the amount of time you spend near orgasm by deliberately delaying it. This is known as "edging," or orgasm control. Whether practiced alone or with a partner, the idea is to maintain a high degree of sexual arousal for a prolonged period before climaxing. The critical technique consists in building toward orgasm, and then, before it is reached, reducing the level of stimulation to retain arousal, but delay the orgasm. Modulating the pace and pressure in this way can result in remaining near orgasm in a highly aroused state for several minutes at a time. When the decision is made to permit the orgasm to occur, the sensations involved may be amplified.[8] There is good reason to believe that extended periods of heightened sexual arousal could lead to several benefits, such as profound partner bonding and higher concentrations of stress-relieving neurochemicals and sex hormones. Obviously, this technique is the polar opposite of what a submissive monkey sneaking copulation does. Take your sweet time during sex. Survey, probe, and investigate your sensual side because the more you use it, the less you will lose it.

Conclusions

After being stuck in a low-level anxiety attack for years, at age 25, I decided to see an endocrinologist and have a blood panel taken. The doctor said that the most apparent result from the panel was very low testosterone. Usually, this problem worsens with time. But, over a decade later, my blood panels show that my testosterone is back in the normal range. I attribute this recovery to the far-reaching benefits of diaphragmatic breathing and the Program Peace exercises, especially those in this chapter.

Many scientists concur that a satisfying sex life may be as important as diet and exercise in promoting health. However, our culture steals our sexuality from us by making us feel sexually incomplete. Due to our infatuation with status, people willingly expose themselves to things that make them question their social standing. Similarly, our instincts for sexual competition cause us to choose to expose ourselves to experiences and thoughts that question our sexual standing. For this reason, marketers and modern media inundate us with content that makes us feel sexually inferior, and that anything less than human perfection is shameful. This not only makes us feel inadequate, but also makes us feel like our partners are inadequate.

Television advertising, raunchy comedians, photo doctoring on social media, the ubiquity of unrealistic pornography, a lover's thoughtless criticism, and the occasional sexual failure have given all of us sexual inferiority complexes. Most people feel that their sexual endowment or bedroom proficiency doesn't measure up or that their body is not conventionally attractive enough. It is not your responsibility to brood on these things. Get over any inclination you may have to ruminate about how you compare to your partner's previous lovers, the times you have been sexually embarrassed, or what it was like to be cheated on. These thoughts trigger our hardwired sexual self-handicapping response. When we dwell on our shortcomings, we reinforce this response. This eventually robs us of our ability to feel horny and relish erotic experiences. Sexual jealousy and worrying cause us to suppress our sex drive, brace our perineal muscles, and start down an early road to sexual decline. This can be enough to push minor penile or clitoral erectile issues into full-blown sexual dysfunction. Do not let this happen to you.

You have nothing (NOTHING) to feel bad about sexually as long as you treat your partner with affection, have good intentions, and are driven to become a better lover. Sex should be hedonistic, fun, playful, and flirtatious without hang-ups, insecurities, or self-doubts. See yourself exuding sensuality and sex appeal. View you and your partner as sexual Olympians. Follow behind them in the market or the mall, staring at their butt, thinking about how you love them, and lusting after their private parts as you contract those urinary expulsion muscles.

Don't let anything undermine your sexuality. Listen to it. Own it. Magnify it. Celebrate it.

Chapter 19: **Bullet Points**

- Primates are violently sexually competitive, causing all but the most dominant individuals to become sexually submissive.
- Most people have a submissive urogenital posture secondary to suboptimal responses to sexual bullying.
- Sexual submission involves pelvic floor bracing, which is related to sexual dysfunction, and the regression of psychosexual development.
- Pairing diaphragmatic breathing with exercising both the urinary retention and expulsion muscles can rehabilitate your pelvic floor.
- Spend time focusing on the physical sensations emanating from your genitals, and touch them in affectionate and reassuring ways to reduce bracing.
- When alone, spend time naked. When in public, pretend that you are both naked and comfortable.
- Whether you are nude or clothed, flex your buttocks, push your hips forward, roll the top of your pelvis backward, and otherwise use your body language to show that you are proud to have your genitals on display.
- Don't obsess over perceived physical or performance inadequacies.
- Get people and media that are toxic to your sexuality out of your life.

Chapter 19: **Endnotes**

1.   Hermann, H. R. (2017). *Dominance and aggression in humans and other animals: The great game of life*. Academic Press.

2.   Sapolsky, R. M. (2005). The influence of social hierarchy on primate health. *Science*, *308*(5722), 648–652.

3.   Whatmore, G. B., & Kohli, D. R. (1968). Dysponesis: A neurophysiological factor in functional disorders. *Systems Research and Behavioral Science*, *13*(2), 102–124.

4.   Dumoulin, C., & Hay-Smith, J. (2010). Pelvic floor muscle training versus no treatment, or inactive control treatments, for urinary incontinence in women. *The Cochrane Database of Systematic Reviews*, *10*(10), CD005654.

5.   Dorey, G., Speakman, M. J., Feneley, R. C. L., Swinkels, A., Dunn, C. D. R. (2005). Pelvic floor exercises for erectile dysfunction. *BJU International*, *96*(4), 595–597.

6.   La Pera, G., & Nicastro, A. (1996). A new treatment for premature ejaculation: The rehabilitation of the pelvic floor. *Journal of Sex & Marital Therapy*, *22*(1), 22–26.

7.   Vopni, K. (2017). *Your pelvic floor - the inside story: Education & wisdom from pelvic health professionals across the globe*. Pelvienne Wellness.

8.   Bodansky, S., & Bodansky, V. (2000). *Extended massive orgasm: How you can give and receive intense sexual pleasure*. Vermilion.

Chapter 20: Healthy Eating Patterns

"Eat food. Not too much. Mostly plants." — Michael Pollan (1955)

If a pack of wolves kills a deer, the leader gets the choice cuts before the pack shares the rest in an egalitarian way. They eat until the entire deer is gone because they don't know when there will be another. Likewise, for much of our hunter-gatherer past, food was not guaranteed. Thus, when we encountered a glut, we would gorge ourselves. There was no benefit to limiting food intake because an excess of stored calories was necessary to survive periods of famine.[1] The constant hunger drive was a survival mechanism. The same goes for our drive to minimize energy expenditure. The less movement you made, the more calories you conserved. This is why today, some of us have the inclination to be insatiable couch potatoes. In our modern world, these adaptive traits are no longer beneficial. Instead, they have made us susceptible to obesity and related ailments including diabetes, hypertension, and cardiovascular disease.[2]

Rats with a perpetually full food dish that are allowed to self-regulate their own food intake become rotund. They eat as much as they want, engaging in "hedonic hyperphagia." This is food intake motivated by pleasure and independent of hunger. Overfeeding in this way causes them to suffer from metabolic diseases and cancers.[3] These rats die much younger than rats fed appropriate portions. You and I are domestic mammals that are allowed to feed ourselves ad libitum. World obesity statistics demonstrate that humans are not doing so well given these liberties.[4] Unlike rats, we can self-impose limitations on our eating. This can be difficult, but we need to do so if we want to stay healthy. Of course, it is not only how much we eat but also what we eat that makes a difference.

Sometimes an evolved mechanism becomes a liability once certain features of the environment change.[5] For instance, many animals eat brightly colored trash because their visual perception of it excites appetitive circuits in their brains. Animals regularly die from such misplaced instincts, and, due to the modern food industry, so do we. Favoring sweet, salty, fatty foods was necessary for the survival of prehistoric humans. Hence, our taste receptors make us crave sugar, sodium, and fat. Given the glut of hyperpalatable food options today, this adaptation has backfired.[6]

Our bodies produce feel-good chemicals when we consume tasty food and when our stomachs are full. These chemicals reduce bodily pain, stress hormones, and the activation of the fight or flight system. The transient alleviation of stress influences us to adopt unhealthy eating habits. On the other hand, trying to force ourselves to eat less and eat healthy can promote stress. In this chapter, we will discuss some effective solutions for how you can keep weight off without contributing to stress.

Calorie and Nutrient Density

Worthless people live only to eat and drink; people of worth eat and drink only to live. Socrates (470 BCE -399 BCE)

Scientists estimate that 50% of the pets in the U.S. are overweight. Even a little extra weight in our pets reduces their health, lifespan, mobility, and playtime. My cat Niko used to be overweight. Feeding him less wasn't working. He would just cry in desperation until I gave him more food. The solution was feeding him the least caloric cat food on the market. Now, he still eats the same volume of food, so he is just as satisfied. However, because his food has less fat and fewer calories, he is now slim. This solution works just as well for you and me.

Energy density is the number of calories (energy) in a given amount (volume) of food. It is often measured in calories per cup. Most of us eat lots of heavily processed and refined food, which are very energy dense. The problem is, if you fill your stomach with it, you will have far exceeded your healthy calorie limit. Now, if you eat proportionately less of it, you will still be hungry. The solution is to eat decent-sized portions of less calorie-dense food.[7] Foods that are low in calorie density but high in nutrient density include fruit and vegetables, lean meat, fat-free dairy, and whole grains. Consider, for instance, that a large 18-gram strawberry has six calories, but a small 18-gram chocolate chip cookie has 90 calories.

Studies show that people tend to eat about the same overall weight of food everyday regardless of the number of calories it contains. This means that adding low calorie density foods to your meals will allow you to feel perfectly full on fewer calories. Additionally, because they are less addictive than food containing additives like soda, chips, fast food, and candy, you are less likely to overeat.

Most mammals will eat more when palatable food is readily available. Hyperpalatable food is rare in the wild but is commonly eaten by domestic animals. For instance, mice and rats have a strong preference for potato chips over their standard foods. Like us, their pleasure system drives them to make unhealthy choices. And, if they are allowed to live on potato chips, they will consume a larger volume of food. The "tastier" the food you keep in your fridge and pantry, the more you will be tempted to gorge yourself on it.

If you can convince yourself to buy less palatable and more nutrient dense food, you will naturally be less likely to overeat. You may even find that you have no interest in continuing to eat bland food on a full stomach. This will ensure that you eat to reduce hunger rather than maximize pleasure. Start with your morning routine. If you can eat a low-fat, low-sugar, high-fiber cereal, you will be off to a great start. Consider adding some fruit to reward yourself and increase the volume of what you're eating. Fruits and vegetables are the ultimate choices for low-calorie density but high nutrient density.

Keep telling yourself, "If I'm not hungry enough to eat healthily, I must not really be that hungry." Eating bland, healthy food sounds like a chore, but the good news is that you get used to it. My cat didn't like the diet cat food at first, but within a month, he preferred it. You should similarly find yourself developing a preference for healthy food after intentionally exposing yourself to it. The more fruit and vegetables you eat, the more you'll know which ones you like, and in which combinations. After a while the prospect of your favorites will make you salivate. When I eat fruit or vegetables, I often pretend that I just found, dug up, or picked them myself. This makes me savor the taste even more. After eating healthy for a while, many people find going back to junk food to be revolting. I did.

Getting Full on Fruit and Vegetables Will Trick Your Body into Liking Them

In all our heads, there is a spoiled little prince or princess who wants each bite to be as delicious as possible. Their sense of entitlement is the reason we eat so terribly. Banish them. Eating is not about delighting our taste buds. It is about getting essential nutrients while barring unhealthy foods access to the interior of our bodies. However, many people find that they have no appetite for healthy food. This makes it difficult to get started. If this sounds like you, ask yourself whether you have ever gotten full on unprocessed food alone. Having *only* fruit for dinner sounds like a nightmare to many people. But this is only because they have never tried it.

I was pressed for time one day, searching for a lunch I could take on a long drive. The most accessible items in the market were two bananas and a carton of strawberries. I realized that it would take up about as much room in my stomach as a burger and fries, so that was all I ate. I tried to enjoy it, didn't eat anything else after that meal, and didn't give it much thought. That simple experience transformed my perspective on strawberries and bananas because I used them by themselves to get full for the first time.

Your gut's nervous system works in sync with several unconscious areas in your brain, constantly learning about factors related to appetite and feeling satiated. Once you get full on something without getting sick, your body unconsciously learns to trust it. Even your conscious feelings about that food can change. Why do you think chimps salivate at the prospect of a mouthful of insects, leaves, or bark? It is because they have gotten full on them before.

Healthy Weight Exercise #20.1: *Get Full on Fruit or Vegetables*

Plan a meal entirely composed of raw fruit. Eat until you are full and don't eat again until the next meal. Afterward, focus on the feeling of satisfaction. Over the next few days, notice how this experience has changed your orientation toward fruit. Next time, try this with vegetables, then a combination of both.

The exercise above will help you learn to crave nutritious fruit and vegetables. The first few times, you might feel queasy or nauseous, but this will pass. You may notice changes after a single meal, or it may take several sessions, but you will find that simply getting full on healthy food is a fail-safe way to trick your body into trusting and enjoying it. This will set you on a path toward following the USDA's evidence-based recommendation to make half of each meal fruits and vegetables.[8] This is, in my opinion, by far the best recommendation offered by nutritional science today.

Do you know that piercing hunger that drives you to eat things that are unhealthy? Instead of addressing it with fast food, eradicate it with fruit and vegetables. Snack on grapes, nuts, pears, peaches, seeds, dried fruit, and sugar-free trail mix. Dip broccoli, celery, cucumber slices, snow peas, green beans, and carrots in hummus. Cut raw tomatoes, avocados, tangerines or mangos into your meals. Cook legumes, corn, onion, garlic, cherries, mushrooms, or chilies in with your rice or pasta. Place dried cranberries, olives, spinach, sundried tomatoes, figs, and apple slices in your sandwiches. Add blueberries, melons, plums, mangos, guavas, and papayas to your breakfast. Use asparagus, sweet potatoes, beets, cauliflower, and eggplant as sides to your entrees. When you feel like grazing, graze on nature's superfoods, and after a while, you may be surprised to find how they can better gratify your hunger.

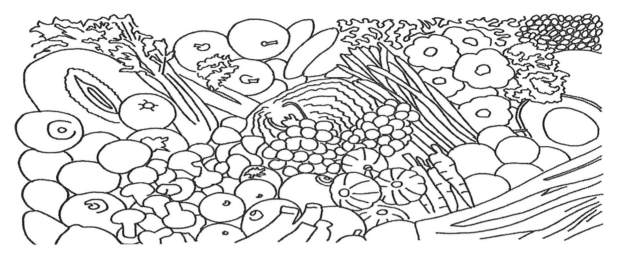

Illustration 20.1: Make half of each meal fruits and vegetables.

Eating plants is more convenient than you might think. If the grocery store near you has a salad bar, skip the lettuce, and fill your bowl with precut fruit, vegetables, lean meats, and low-calorie dressing. Most grocery stores, convenience stores, and big-box retailers carry fresh-cut fruit and vegetables to go. Consider taking advantage of this. If you want to save money and eat inexpensively, you can cut them yourself. Eating several servings of fruit and vegetables daily will help you to get lean fast and get all the vitamins, minerals, antioxidants, and fiber you need.

Make a Smoothie Every Day

Preparing fruit and vegetables yourself can be time-consuming. Cutting them into bite-sized portions, and then chewing them takes time. However, because fruit and vegetables turn to liquid in a blender, you can drink large quantities in seconds. Smoothies, shakes, and liquid meals are much easier for your gut to process and decrease the physical effort of digestion, which some scientists believe may prolong lifespan. Also, the bioavailability of liquid meals is higher, meaning your body absorbs more nutrients. Furthermore, blending fruit and vegetables does not reduce their fiber or vitamin content.

With your fruit smoothies, try adding dates, yogurt, almond milk, cashews, walnuts, vanilla extract, honey, and ripe frozen bananas. With your vegetable smoothies, try tomato juice, cayenne pepper, chili flakes, lemon, lime, onion, or garlic. A daily fruit or vegetable smoothie is an easy, cheap, filling, and extremely healthy meal.

Get Your Essential Vitamins and Nutrients

A diet lacking in certain vitamins can contribute to depression and anxiety. Folic acid, iron, omega-3, vitamin B12, magnesium, vitamin C, vitamin D, selenium, and zinc are all essential.[9] Deficiencies in these can result in fatigue, irritability, apathy, poor concentration, aggressiveness, mood swings, and increased depressive symptoms.[10] This is another reason why it's imperative to eat more of those fruits and vegetables.

Cut out Saturated Fats

Try not to eat any fats that are solid at room temperature. These are saturated fats, and consuming them leads to high cholesterol, clogged arteries, atherosclerosis, and heart disease. Much of the saturated fats we ingest come from just a few culprits. You should seriously consider minimizing pure animal fat, processed meat, poultry skin, whole milk, heavy cream, high-fat cheese, sour cream, lard, butter, margarine, ghee, tropical oils, and mayonnaise in your diet. Avoid full-fat dairy and go for the fat-free variety. Cut the white or clear fat off your meat and stay away from fried food. Altogether avoid hydrogenated or trans fats. Unlike saturated fats, unsaturated fats are essential, so make an effort to eat fish, nuts, seeds, and vegetable oils (e.g., canola, olive, flaxseed, soybean, etc.).

The Paleo Diet Works

The Paleolithic diet promotes the consumption of food that our hunting and gathering ancestors would have eaten. It is rational to eat what our bodies naturally expect and have eaten for millions of years. The paleo diet advises that we eat whole foods, like fruits, vegetables, fish, and grass-fed meats. It also discourages processed foods and added sugar and salt. These recommendations are entirely in line with modern nutritional science, and the paleo diet has been shown to have significant health benefits in controlled trials.[11] However, there are two valid criticisms of the paleo diet. First, the diet restricts some nutrient-dense food such as fat-free dairy and whole grains, which need not be restricted. Second, the high meat intake may lead to health problems if the meat is not lean. Besides these two issues, asking yourself, "Would my ancestors have eaten this?" can be a practical question to help you avoid detrimental foods.

Drink More Water

Many beverages are extraordinarily caloric. Simply cutting soft drinks from your diet can be highly beneficial. Even juice has a lot of calories but no fiber, so despite being calorie dense, it doesn't do much to make you feel full. This is why if you are not drinking smoothies, you should be drinking plain, purified water. Dieticians commonly point out that water is absolutely free of calories and can contribute to feeling full, so let's drink up.

Many people don't get enough water, leaving them with mild symptoms of chronic dehydration. Dehydration is physiologically detrimental and contributes to a lack of energy, discomfort, and the muscular dysfunctions discussed in previous chapters. Try to drink between five and eight 8-ounce glasses (up to 2 liters) of water per day.[12] Never drink less than your thirst dictates.

Detraumatize Your Ability to Chug Water

I used to frequently choke when drinking. This was because my swallowing reflex had become uncoordinated due to hyperventilation. Drinking fast felt perilous, and chugging felt like being waterboarded. Swallowing involves the temporary closure of the epiglottis to keep food and drink out of the lungs. If not synchronized correctly, then the liquid is inhaled into the lungs (pulmonary aspiration). This was happening to me daily. Difficulty swallowing is known as dysphagia; everybody has a little bit of it, and you want to minimize your bit. Use the exercise below so that you drink mightily with no unnecessary encumbrances.

Healthy Weight Exercise #20.2: *Chug Water Mightily*

Pour yourself a large glass of room temperature or warm water. Tell yourself there is no rush. There is nothing better for you to do at this moment than observing your swallowing apparatus at work. Take a deep breath and drink the water slowly and mindfully. Start with small gulps, making each one voluntary. Pay very close attention to the cadence of your gulping. It should be steady. Focus on the following:

1) During each gulp, your muscles should move through their full range of motion decisively and uninterrupted.

2) Much of the swallowing process is an automatic reflex controlled by unconscious neurological mechanisms in the brainstem. Give each swallow sufficient time to progress entirely through its reflex arc before attempting to swallow again. You don't want to interrupt a swallow by swallowing again too soon.

3) It takes practice to know when it is safe to initiate another swallow. It is like two people passing sandbags down a line. The first person must wait until the second person's hands are free before giving them another bag. Passing each gulp of water from the cup to your mouth and then the back of your throat should be efficient and quick but not at all rushed.

4) You can either hold your breath while you chug or try to coordinate nasal breathing with drinking. Either way, don't let involuntary gasps interrupt the chugging process. You can't breathe and swallow at the same time, and you must teach the involuntary aspects of breathing and swallowing to cooperate and wait their turn.

Practicing this exercise twice per day for two weeks should be enough to ensure you have no problem chugging four large glasses of water in 20 seconds. You will be able to put away a bottle of water or a smoothie in a very short time. More importantly, you will never again be afraid of choking on water.

We Overeat to Combat Stress

"It is the nature of the wise to resist pleasures, but the foolish to be a slave to them." — Epictetus (c. 50-135)

We eat unhealthy food for pleasure but also to quell our pain. As discussed earlier, the taste of fat, salt, and sugar and even the activation of our stomach's stretch receptors stimulate the release of endorphins, dopamine, and other feel-good neurotransmitters. Conversely, dieting can increase stress hormones, startling, breathing rate and heart rate. Discomfort from skipping a meal can deplete serotonin, reducing the frontal lobes' ability to regulate the amygdala, resulting in increased anxiety and frustration. In turn, heightened stress makes us hungrier and drives us to keep eating even after we are full.

As you know, eating a meal makes the parasympathetic nervous system kick in. And eating a larger meal emphasizes rest and digest even more. Unconsciously, we know this, and we overeat to subdue the fight or flight mode. Thus, we overeat to turn the volume down on our bodily pain. Many of us eat to the point where we feel tired and slightly nauseous just to reduce our daily stress.

We also eat compulsively because we perceive food binges as mitigating distressed breathing. Hunger indeed makes our breath shallow. Trying to abstain from a piece of cake does the same. That is why it is often preferable to just give in and eat the cake. However, as you will see if you try it, taking deep, slow breaths every time you feel tempted can make you impervious to the siren song.

Combining Fasting with Diaphragmatic Breathing Reduces Your Hunger Drive

Our prehistoric ancestors would not have experienced undue stress the way we do from missing just one meal. Our bodies were designed to go for days without eating. Most people can live longer than a month without food as long as they have access to water. However, we have spoiled our appetitive systems. Every time we are a little late for a meal, our breath becomes shallow and disturbed. Simply, we haven't learned to retain coolheadedness while hungry. I believe that many fasting practices recognize this. However, I think fasting can be much more beneficial if intentionally combined with diaphragmatic breathing.

Try skipping a meal and breathing through the discomfort using paced breathing. Focus on how hunger affects your breathing and internal bracing. However, be prudent about this. Don't skip a meal in the middle of a hectic workday, as this will further traumatize your relationship with hunger. Make it a lunch on a weekend so you can pay attention to how it makes you feel without worrying about distractions. When I fast, I just relax, especially for the three or four hours when I am at my hungriest. When you fast, you will notice recurring pangs of hunger starting a few hours after your regular mealtime. Thoracic breathing fuels these hunger pangs. All your life until now, you have paired hunger with distressed breathing. Dissociate these by using paced breathing to override hunger's ability to highjack your stress system.

Healthy Weight Exercise #20.3: *Diaphragmatic Fasting*

Skip a lunch or dinner and spend time quelling your hunger pangs using paced breathing. Concentrate on the sensations of hunger and how they make your breathing shallow. Breathe along with a breath metronome for several minutes each hour during this fast. Imagine that you are a relaxed caveman or woman who hasn't eaten for two days yet who is confident about finding plenty of food by tomorrow night.

Pairing diaphragmatic breathing with hunger will dramatically soothe your hunger drive. The experience afforded by the exercise above will help you differentiate between a neurotic impulse to eat and the body's valid hunger signal. Resolve to eat only when you feel this honest signal emanating from your gut.

By eating less, you may be prolonging your life. Studies show that modest calorie restriction increases health and longevity in all mammals that have been tested. Temporary calorie deficits cause your cells to break down some of their internal building blocks for energy in a process known as autophagy. Many of these molecular structures were damaged and dysfunctional before they were broken down. The next time you eat, the cells then turn around and rebuild these structures back up correctly, resulting in healthier cells.[13] The fact that our cells regenerate in response to calorie restriction is another justification for why we should learn to tolerate hunger. However, keep in mind that these health benefits do not outweigh the costs associated with anorexia or bulimia.

Shrink Your Appetite by Eating Less

Neuroscientists know that exercising restraint is much like exercising a muscle. Every time you abstain or show moderation when eating, it gets easier to do so in the future.[14] Conversely, every time you binge, you will want to eat more the next few meals. Thus, the next time you flex your willpower by eating smaller portions or healthier food, take some consolation in knowing that your willpower is growing.

It can take up to 20 minutes for the satisfaction signal to reach the brain. This is unfortunate because it means that we are liable to eat 20 minutes' worth of food that we don't need and within just a few short minutes, will not want. Learn to stop eating early and anticipate satisfaction before it arrives. One way to accomplish this is to stop eating once you reach 80% of being full. It can also help to make a concerted effort to eat less while enjoying your food more.

I used to get stressed if a meal was not large enough to make me very full. Now, I find the sensation of being stuffed repulsive because I get tired after eating a heavy meal. Overeating promotes lethargy, making both exercise and concentration more difficult. This phenomenon is called "postprandial somnolence." It can lead to sleepiness and a significant drop in mental acuity around lunchtime.[15] Avoid this in the middle of the day by splitting your lunch in half. Eat one half at noon and the second 30 minutes to an hour later. Eating frequent, smaller meals may help you stay alert and keep your metabolism high.

Dormant Muscle Increases Body Fat

Modern medical experts know that the current worldwide epidemic of obesity and diabetes is attributable to unhealthy eating and insufficient exercise, but they don't appreciate the role of dormant muscle. I believe that the extent of dormant muscle is a major determinant of metabolic rate. It is pretty clear how dormant muscles cause an involuntary loss of lean mass and a progressive increase in fat mass. When parts of your neck, shoulders, spine, and hips are frozen in place, your movement is impeded. When your lower back hurts, your stomach is flaccid, and your range of lumbar motion is compromised, every action is attenuated. For these reasons, I firmly believe that performing the dormancy-reducing anti-rigidity exercises from previous chapters will increase your will-to-move and your metabolism along with it.

Increasing age is associated with decreasing metabolic rate. I believe this relationship is mediated by frailty and that anti-rigidity may allow one to maintain a more active life well into old age. Frailty is the main reason that you have lower energy now as opposed to when you were younger. Thus, anti-rigidity may be the best weight loss tool available. When I was 28, I moved like a grandfather. I also had a "skinny-fat" physique and had to eat small portions to avoid being overweight. Dormant muscle strongly influenced me to be sedentary. Not anymore.

There are two primary reasons for the variability in metabolic rate between individuals. One is the difference in lean body mass. A person with more muscle will have a higher metabolism. The second is voluntary movement not accounted for by exercise, called non-exercise activity thermogenesis (NEAT). NEAT is spontaneous physical activity and is highly variable across individuals, including how you move and hold your body during work, leisure, household tasks, and ambulation. NEAT can vary by as much as 2,000 calories per day between two people. The notion that obesity and overweight may be more related to NEAT than diet and exercise is supported by studies.[16] I strongly believe that reclaiming atrophic and hypertonic musculature using anti-laxity and anti-rigidity is a surefire way to increase lean body mass and NEAT. Getting the dormant kinks out of the back and filling in the missing corners in the abdomen by using the exercises in the next section will shred away one's fatty belly.

Reviving Your Abdominals Through Exercise

Our bellies are fat because our abdominal muscles are flaccid and underactive. In the following exercise, you will learn how to pair isometric abdominal contraction with paced, diaphragmatic breathing using the anti-laxity method from Chapter 13.

Healthy Weight Exercise #20.4: *Standing and Walking with Flexed Abs*

In this exercise, you will breathe to a breath metronome while standing with proper posture and tightening your abdominals. Pull the belly button toward the spine and contract your abs. Notice how tensing your abs makes you want to breathe at very short intervals. Simply contracting the abs stifles the diaphragm automatically, but you can override this. Hold the abdominal contraction and breathe deeply to the pace of the metronome. The longer you pair these two things, the more robust you make your abdominal tone.

Very lightly strike your abs all over with your hand or a rounded object. This will help you keep a solid contraction. When doing this exercise, your chest will tend to cave in, so expand the chest and lengthen the distance between your breastbone and pubic bone. Don't forget to retain proper tone in the muscles that expel urine we discussed in the last chapter.

Allowing the diaphragm to push the stomach out is key to diaphragmatic breathing. The sight of a protruding abdomen, however, is not fashionable in our society. This is why many people habitually suck in their gut, which can keep the diaphragm tense and limit its motion. You should feel comfortable anywhere poking your stomach out as far as it can go. At first, you will look like you have a potbelly, just as retracting your neck gives you a double chin. However, as these muscles gain natural tone, your stomach will slim. Pushing the stomach out is also vital to lower back health, as it cushions the lumbar spine during forward bends. Let's use anti-rigidity (contracting directly into achiness) to fix this.

Healthy Weight Exercise #20.5: *Doubled Over with Protruding Stomach*

Pair paced breathing with the activation of deeply dormant abdominal musculature. To reach the deepest portion of your abs, sit down with your legs in front of you. Bend forward from your hips and rest your hands on your shins. From this position, press your stomach outward as far as it will go. Experiment with pressing your stomach out and tensing the abs to different extents to find the weak areas of your abdomen. You should be able to find several areas that ache very deeply. Be very careful because contracting your abdominal muscles too hard or too much at a time could strain the back or even cause an abdominal hernia. If it hurts, work up to it slowly. Follow the breath metronome while safely contracting into the achy dormant muscle to rehab it.

For maximum results, perform the last two abdominal exercises from several different positions: standing, kneeling, crouching, taking one knee, squatting, lying on the back, etc.

Reviving Your Abdomen Through Massage

Performing myofascial release on the lower back and love handles dramatically diminished my stores of local fat. This got me wondering whether the same technique could decrease abdominal fat deposits. It sounds too good to be true, right? It's not. Much of the rectus abdominis has been traumatized because of the way it instinctually contracts without rest during fear. All this strain leads to a "dead gut" that fails to burn fat. Getting the trauma out will make your abdominals much stronger, make ab exercises easier, and help your core to be more engaged during everything you do. To do this, in the next exercise we will percuss the abdomen while lying on the back.

Healthy Weight Exercise #20.6: *Myofascial Release for Abdominal Muscles*

Use your fingers, knuckles, or a tool to percuss the entire abdomen. Lift your hand three to eight inches above the abdomen before each strike. Strike the abdomen two to three times per second. You want to hit hard enough to break the bracing pattern without creating any real pain or damaging tissue. Each soft strike should elicit an ache. This aching feeling will make you want to brace to protect yourself, initiating the "stretch reflex" and a defensive contraction. You want to inhibit this defensive contraction, instead allowing your abs to remain as limp as possible. Search for areas that feel tight, inflexible, or crunchy. Spend time pressing firmly into the tense cords of muscle overlying the bones of the lower rib cage, hips, and pelvis, all areas that your abdominal muscles anchor into. Each day, the aching will further subside and you will have to strike slightly deeper to access achy tissue. After a session, there should be no bruising or pain whatsoever, so if these occur, you are hitting yourself too hard.

This activity will wake up your core, but as with all forms of massage, overdoing it can diminish muscle mass. For this reason, just do it until you get the intense achiness out.

Conclusion

Restaurant owners know that people don't want to pay for raw, unprocessed food. This is because unprocessed food is cheap and involves very little preparation. Consequently, it is perceived to have very little added value. Restaurants provide a service by processing the food such as frying or baking/cooking in oil. We are all addicted to these unhealthy preparations. Eating bland, chewy, raw, unprocessed food is work, but it is how wild animals and people stay lean and healthy. Employing nonresistance, nonjudgment, healthy breathing, and a bit of old-fashioned stoicism will help.

People who overeat to reduce their stress will find that what their bodies are really hungering for is exercise. The use of cardiovascular exercise in the reduction of stress will be discussed in the next chapter.

Chapter 20: **Bullet Points**

- We don't crave healthy foods because we have not had the experience of getting full on them by themselves. Give yourself that experience by eating full meals that consist of only fruits and vegetables.
- Use a blender to turn fruit and vegetables into smoothies. It is a speedy, healthy, inexpensive, and low-calorie way to get full.
- We overeat unhealthy food to transiently increase our dopamine and endorphins as an attempt to self-medicate against panic and stress.
- We have spent our lives pairing hunger with thoracic breathing. This is why hunger causes distress, which, in turn, causes us to overeat. By fasting for a meal and pairing the fasting experience with paced breathing, you can detraumatize your nervous system's relationship with hunger.
- Stop eating when you feel 80% satiated.
- Only start eating when you feel at least 80% hungry.
- People with copious dormant muscle must diet to a stress-inducing extent to maintain a healthy weight. Reviving dormant muscle using anti-rigidity will increase your metabolism.
- Most people have an extensive reservoir of dormant abdominal muscle. Your stomach will become much leaner if you rehabilitate this muscle with massage and anti-laxity and anti-rigidity exercises.

Chapter 20: **Endnotes**

1.   Reser, J. (2011). Nutrition, behavior, and the developmental origins of the metabolic syndrome. In V. Preedy, R. Watson, & C. Martin (Eds.), *Handbook of behavior, food and nutrition* (pp. 2627–2638). Springer.

2.   Reser, 2011, Nutrition, behavior, and the developmental origins of the metabolic syndrome.

3.   de Gortari, P., Alcántara-Alonso, V., Matamoros-Trejo, G., Amaya, M. I., & Alvarez-Salas, E. (2020). Differential effects of leptin administration on feeding and HPT axis function in early-life overfed adult rats. *Peptides, 127*, 170285.

4.   Haslam, D. W., & James, W. P. (2005). Obesity. *The Lancet, 366*(9492), 1197–1209.

5.   Robertson, B. A., Rehage, J. S., & Sih, A. (2013). Ecological novelty and the emergence of evolutionary traps. *Trends in Ecology & Evolution, 28*(9), 552–560.

6.   Bleich, S., Cutler, D., Murray, C., & Adams, A. (2008). Why is the developed world obese? *Annual Review of Public Health, 29*, 273–95.

7.   Drewnowski, A. (2018). Nutrient density: Addressing the challenge of obesity. *British Journal of Nutrition, 120*(S1), S8–S14.

8.   Haytowitz, D. B., & Pehrsson, P. R. (2018). USDA's national food and nutrient analysis program (NFNAP) produces high-quality data for USDA food composition databases: Two decades of collaboration. *Food Chemistry, 238*, 134–138.

9.   Greenfield, B. (2020). *Boundless: Upgrade your brain, optimize your body & defy aging.* Victory Belt Publishing.

10.   Rao, T. S, Asha, M. R., Ramesh, B. N., Rao, K. S. (2008). Understanding nutrition, depression, and mental illness. *Indian Journal of Psychiatry, 50*(2), 77–82.

11.   Ghaedi, E., Mohammadi, M., & Salehi-Abargouei, A. (2019). Effects of a Paleolithic diet on cardiovascular disease risk factors: A systematic review and meta-analysis of randomized controlled trials. *Advances in Nutrition, 10*(4), 634–646.

12.   Kenefick, R. W. (2018). Drinking strategies: Planned drinking versus drinking to thirst. *Sports Medicine, 48*(Suppl. 1), 31–37.

13. Kobayashi, S. (2015). Choose delicately and reuse adequately: The newly revealed process of autophagy. *Biological & Pharmaceutical Bulletin, 38*(8), 1098–1103.

14. Hofmann, W., Deutsch, R., Lancaster, K., & Banaji, M. R. (2010). Cooling the heat of temptation: Mental self-control and the automatic evaluation of tempting stimuli. *European Journal of Social Psychology, 40*(1), 17–25.

15. Reyner, L. A., Wells, S. J., Mortlock, V., & Horne, J. A. (2012). 'Post-lunch' sleepiness during prolonged, monotonous driving - effects of meal size. *Physiology & Behavior, 105*(4), 1088–1091.

16. Chung, N., Park, M. Y., Kim, J., Park, H. Y., Hwang, H., Lee, C. H., Han, J. S., So, J., Park, J., & Lim, K. (2018). Non-exercise activity thermogenesis (NEAT): A component of total daily living expenditure. *Journal of Exercise Nutrition & Biochemistry, 22*(2), 23–30.

Chapter 21: **The Amygdala, Cortisol, and Chronic Stress**

Trigger warning: this chapter discusses some disturbing, emotionally difficult material.

Traumatic Incidents Affect Your Inner Mammal

I woke up in my bed at 5:15 a.m. to a bright flash of light and an explosion. It was the loudest sound I have ever heard. I could feel the force of the blast resound in my chest. At first, I assumed there was someone in my bedroom with a shotgun. I leaped out of bed for cover and then heard footsteps and yelling just outside my bedroom window. I didn't know what to do. My home had been burglarized before, and I even experienced a robbery a few months prior, so I assumed I was experiencing a home invasion. After a half-hour of walking around maniacally with a baseball bat, I finally got the local watch commander on the phone. He told me police had served a warrant next door and used stun grenades to gain entry.

It had never crossed my mind that law enforcement caused the situation. As soon as I knew the explosions were not criminal, I started to calm down. At least the conscious part of me knew I was no longer in danger. On the other hand, my cat, Niko, couldn't understand this. He engaged in all kinds of nervous behavior that I had never seen from him: looking over his shoulder, pawing at the ground, and shaking. I tried my best to calm him, but I didn't know how to communicate to him that we were safe now. I got dressed and took the bus to work. There were no empty seats that morning, so I stood up, feeling the ice in my blood and the tremors shoot down my spine. Holding the rail, I asked myself: "How am I going to face my colleagues and give my talk this afternoon?" At the time, I knew next to nothing about diaphragmatic breathing, and hadn't developed any Program Peace exercises, so I struggled through it. The audience could tell I was overwhelmed.

That night I couldn't sleep. My conscious self knew I was completely safe. But, my unconscious brain areas—that, like my cat, don't speak English—didn't know this. Like small, scared animals, these brain modules continued to be emotional because they do not have access to the conscious, declarative knowledge that there never was any real threat. Evolution kept these brain modules in the dark because the organism cannot afford to trust the semantic belief that "I'm pretty sure I'm safe now." You may not be able to talk to or reason with these modules, but you can communicate with them using your breath. Deep breathing persuades them to cool off. I didn't have paced breathing back then to help me keep the trauma from sinking in, but I was able to use it years later to dig it out.

My overreaction to that situation was shaped by prior experiences. I have been violently assaulted several times in my life. I have been held up at knifepoint and seen people stabbed, shot at, and beaten. I have never received an official diagnosis, but I believe these experiences caused me to develop a form of PTSD, even if a subclinical one. Panicking didn't help me in any of these situations. The heightened anxiety from one did not serve me in the next. The morning after, I would wake up with my teeth heavily clenched, eyes squinted into slits, lumbar spine contorted, and shoulders up around my ears. Many people suffer heinous traumatic incidents, much worse than these, that go on to desecrate modules throughout their body. I have a few friends that were "jumped" and beaten by groups of individuals. The neurological toll this takes can be ruinous, especially if it happens multiple times.

Car accidents, mugging, battery, rape, gruesome injury, childhood abuse, and anything that involves an incapacity to stop a terrible thing from happening can plant the seeds of trauma. Feelings of entrapment, immobilization, and helplessness make it worse. But it is when we allow these feelings to persist through time that the real damage occurs. Obsessive rumination, bracing, and distressed breathing occurring well after the actual event itself are what prime the body for suboptimality. These three things turn stress into trauma by "proving" to your unconscious that things have not gotten better. Alleviating them starts with the breath because if full, long, smooth, diaphragmatic, belly breathing does not resume, then your muscles won't let it go, and your mind will continue to relive the tribulation. What traumatic episodes are you prolonging?

A Heightened Stress System

As discussed in Chapters 2 and 5, sustained stress changes the body's life strategy. It convinces the body that the environment it was born into is particularly life-threatening. Scientists refer to such environments as high in "extrinsic mortality." This kind of environment communicates to the organism on a cellular level that the probability of it being able to live a long and happy life is low. The genes then reprogram the body to deal with a short and grisly one. This changes your mortal shell from a slow-burning candle into a firecracker. Your body expends all its energy upfront because it doesn't expect to live for long. This happens at the expense of long-term energetic investments such as healing, the immune system, learning, reproductive functioning, affiliation, and investing time and energy in offspring.[1] For example, chronic anxiety inhibits your body's ability to protect itself from oxidation, which is a process that acts on your cells in the same way that rust acts on metal. It also contributes to aging by keeping the body from repairing its telomeres, the protective caps at the end of your chromosomes, reducing the number of times your cells can divide.

As you know, when stress goes on for too long, it results in a chronically heightened fear and startle response. The brain is retuned to enhance performance during life-threatening situations[2] and facilitate cautiousness and hypervigilance, traits that would have been highly adaptive during extended periods of dire stress in prehistoric environments.[3] These changes cause the stress response to become more pronounced and more easily triggered.[4] The brain center that triggers stress, the amygdala, has its own innate response pattern to chronic stress. Let's learn more about this almond-sized nucleus that acts as yet another biological repository of trauma.

The Amygdala Recognizes Threats

As we learned in Chapter 7, threats are recognized by the amygdala. This unconscious, subcortical area becomes active once it perceives a stimulus, or a group of stimuli together, as dangerous. The amygdala responds quickly and automatically to the inputs it receives from the eyes, ears, and other sense organs.[5] If the threat is sufficient, it broadcasts the fear signal to the rest of the brain. It can do this unconsciously (a glimpse of a looming object), or visually (the view of a bus barreling toward you). The recognition of an abstract stressor (knowledge that you missed your bus) involves the prefrontal cortex, which indirectly alerts the amygdala.[6] Either way, once the amygdala is activated, it will signal the hypothalamus which initiates fight or flight.

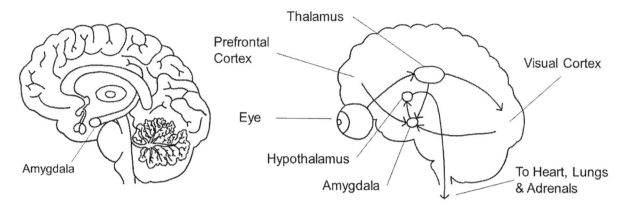

Illustration 21.1: A. Cross section of the brain with amygdala revealed. You actually have two amygdalae, one in each cerebral hemisphere; B. Three fear pathways to the amygdala: 1. The unconscious pathway travels from the eye to the thalamus, to the amygdala. 2. The visual pathway travels from the eye to the thalamus, to the visual cortex, to the amygdala. 3. The thinking pathway travels from the prefrontal cortex to the amygdala.

If the amygdala is strongly and repeatedly activated over the course of several weeks, its default level of activity will increase. Over months of repeated activation, the amygdala develops stronger connections with other brain areas intensifying its influence. It also increases in overall size.[7] This enhanced priority given to the amygdala causes the animal to react to every seemingly threatening stimulus as if it were a full threat.

The amygdala's job is to decide whether a pattern of inputs looks like something that turned out badly in the past. However, it does not use reason or conscious deliberation to do this. Rather, it engages in simple pattern matching in which it adds up seemingly bad inputs to see if they sum to a threshold. If the inputs surpass this threshold, the amygdala triggers the sympathetic nervous system. Thus, our feelings of dread are not prompted by logical thinking. Instead, they are initiated by the amygdala's eccentric way of determining statistics and probability. For example, an offender's voice, clothes, name, or cologne could subliminally reinstate an amygdala highjack.

Allow me to provide an example of how the amygdala's form of logic is susceptible to mistakes. One day when I was in a lousy mood, I picked up the phone and the caller asked to speak to my roommate. The next day when I heard their voice again, it made me angry and I realized my prior bad mood had biased me against the caller for no good reason. Because my brain made this unconscious negative association, hearing the voice later triggered the same negative emotions. It was illogical and unfair to the caller. But my first impulse was to trust it unquestioningly. We accept the amygdala's alarm bells as a type of foreboding intuition. Negative emotions usually feel valid and impelling, but they are often invalid and illusory. This is why we should question them rather than act on them impulsively. Especially after you experience a series of stressors, the amygdala will influence your thinking to be delusionally negative.

When activity in the amygdala surges, the brain is temporarily retuned to perceive everything as troublesome. For instance, it increases the tendency to perceive ambiguous events as bad, such as criticism when none is intended or hostility from a neutral face. This is the opposite of a manic episode, which causes people to perceive everything as a gleeful, lucky coincidence. People with mania often feel like cars on the freeway move to let them through, everyone is their best friend, and everything goes their way. On the other hand, chronic stress makes us more likely to succumb to road rage and the feeling that everyone and everything is against us. Whenever I start to feel disheartened, I try to remember that neurochemicals can paint over reality.

You may have noticed that after one negative interaction, you are much more likely to get stressed out about other, completely unrelated things. With the exception of living in a warzone this displaced negative thinking is irrational in the modern world. Interestingly though, it may not be irrational from an ecological standpoint. It was beneficial for mammals to be prepared for the worst during bad times. Just imagine what life would have been like for early mammals in the Jurassic and Cretaceous periods.

When there are predators on the loose or natural catastrophes strike, they are rarely quickly resolved. For furry varmints from possums to porcupines to panthers, it makes sense to become scared and remain paranoid. From a modern perspective, however, it is preposterous to generalize anxiety to whatever your mind turns to. Don't let one unfortunate scenario lead to a domino effect of suspicion and dismay. Notice when you carry negative emotions from one thought over to another. When you realize it, try to tell yourself that the negativity may feel compelling but that it is probably just residual and misattributed emotion.

Stress and Cortisol: The Mind-Body Connection

"Stand porter at the door of thought. Admitting only such conclusions as you wish realized in bodily results, you will control yourself harmoniously." — Mary Baker Eddy

When the amygdala decides it has perceived a stressful stimulus, it triggers the hypothalamus. The hypothalamus mobilizes the sympathetic nervous system, leading to rapid breathing, tense muscles, reduced sensitivity to pain, suspension of digestion, and a rise in heart rate and blood pressure. It also activates the adrenal glands, prompting the release of adrenaline. The release of adrenaline is a fast-acting hormonal response to an acute stressor. Adrenaline frees up blood sugars to give muscles and other tissues the energy they need to deal with an immediate threat.

After adrenaline, the second principal stress hormone is cortisol. Cortisol a is slow-acting response to a persistent stressor also released by the adrenals. It gives animals extra strength by liberating the energy from fat molecules into the bloodstream. This sounds like it could lead to weight loss, but it doesn't. In the long run, cortisol promotes fat storage and muscle protein breakdown. It also changes the expression of several genes in fat tissue, increasing the likelihood of obesity and type 2 diabetes.[8]

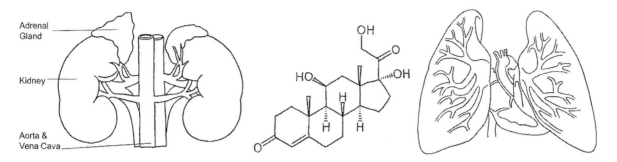

Illustration 21.2: A. The kidneys with the adrenal glands sitting on top; B. The molecular structure of the hormone cortisol; C. The heart and lungs.

Chronic stress upregulates this entire stress hormone system, also known as the HPA (hypothalamic-pituitary-adrenal) axis. The result is that the body is continuously flooded with adrenaline and cortisol. Sustained elevation of cortisol is highly pathogenic and leads to hypertension, elevated heart rate, increased circulating levels of lipids and cholesterol, atherosclerotic plaque formation, decreased high-density lipoprotein (HDL) and increased low-density lipoprotein (LDL) cholesterol.[9] Cortisol makes stress corrosive and is related to disorders like arthritis, asthma, acid reflux, cardiovascular disease, chronic fatigue, decreased metabolism, depression, various cancers, migraines, sleep deprivation, immune system impairment, and ulcers.[10]

Elevated cortisol also causes the immune system to produce inflammatory chemicals (cytokines). This results in inflammation (redness, warmth, and swelling), which increases the immune system's ability to heal wounds from physical attacks. Again, this would have been advantageous in prehistoric times when stress indicated that cuts and lacerations were likely. In modern times however, chronically elevated inflammation can lead to pain, poor digestion, cancer, autoimmune disorders, and other dire disease states.[11] In fact, it has been found to be a player in almost every chronic disease. To escape chronic inflammation, we must stop thinking inflammatory thoughts. But unfortunately, cortisol also acts on the brain.

Cortisol causes mammals to search desperately for a way out. Today, this urge to escape drives us to drink alcohol, smoke, overeat, and displace work-related frustrations on family members. If you are curious to see what highly elevated cortisol feels like, try submerging your entire forearm in an ice bath for two minutes. The pain from the ice causes a rapid spike in cortisol release, and this method is often used in experimental studies. When cortisol is raised like this, it causes subjects to perform mental tasks less flexibly and intelligently. It also increases pessimism, aggression, and the negativity bias.

As you might have guessed, elevated cortisol is common in humans and animals on the bottom of the pecking order. Cortisol is the hormone of status defeat, and it surges in monkeys and apes that are being dominated. Decades of studies on early life exposure to cortisol in monkeys reinforces much of what we have been discussing in this book. Exposure to trauma and cortisol makes a young monkey more psychologically vulnerable to stress and leads to decreased dominance, increased aggression, decreased social competence, reduced ability to find social interactions rewarding, and reduced affiliative drive.[12] When we feel defeated, our serotonin and testosterone drop and our cortisol rises. Intermittent stressors like workplace abuse or even replaying uncivil incidents in one's mind elevate cortisol levels.

Stress expert Robert Sapolsky wrote an excellent book on the neurobiology of stress called *Why Zebras Don't Get Ulcers*. In the book, Sapolsky explains that most animals, other than social primates, do not give themselves ulcers because they don't waste time worrying. Zebras, and most other animals, only get upset when they find themselves in immediate danger, usually involving a predator. If we only got upset when wild carnivores were stalking us, we would all be a whole lot happier! Moreover, zebras probably don't rehearse negative social situations or mull over their place on the social ladder. It is mostly monkeys, apes, and humans that repeatedly model these scenarios in their heads. As a primate, your amygdala is inclined to latch on to social confrontation and cause it to be played out continuously in the imagination. This results in an existential nightmare that Chapter 7 offered you tools (e.g., nonjudgment, nonresistance, and nonattachment) to wake yourself up from. Most of these tools influence the way you assess problems.

The way you appraise a stress-provoking stimulus will program your automatic response the next time you encounter a similar stimulus. In other words, your brain will do its best to remember how you responded so it can expedite that response next time. So, when something alarms, shocks, or unpleasantly surprises you, don't get caught up in it. Instead, try to immediately minimize the negativity.

Whether it is a mosquito whining in your ear, a car honking at you, or a person yelling at you, stop, take a deep breath, and choose to be calmer. Underreacting inoculates the amygdala against stress. Face difficulty with a levelheaded mindset that is as centered, grounded, and poised as possible.

De-Stress Activity #21.1: Maintain Composure Amid Tragedy

Imagine that a terrible crisis is unfolding all around you. You are attempting to stop assailants from battering your friend. You are being lambasted, absolutely torn to shreds by your colleagues. You are experiencing a natural disaster. A large animal is attacking your group. Imagine maintaining complete composure amid this chaos. You are going through hell, but you keep going. You stand straight, put on your game face, breathe deeply, and master the fear in your gut. Other people see your outward appearance and are puzzled by it. You focus on fixing the situation the best way you can, knowing that maintaining your presence of mind will only aid your efforts to help others and right wrongs. If you make these scenarios vivid and extreme, then after you have done this for a while, there should be nothing and no one in real life that can throw you off.

Don't Develop an Unhealthy Fear of Stress

"He who fears he shall suffer already suffers what he fears." — Michel De Montaigne (1533-1592)

After recounting so many of the physical costs of stress in this book, I would be doing you a disservice if I didn't encourage you not to stress out over stress itself. Here is why: Studies have shown that the pathogenesis of physical disease in response to stress is made much worse when someone believes that stress affects their health. Basically, thinking that stress is unhealthy makes it more unhealthy.[13] Also, people who report they actively avoid stress are more likely to suffer from depression. So, what can we do?

When you feel stressed, don't hate it, fear it, or fight it. Appraise it as enthusiasm and allow diaphragmatic breathing and belief in yourself to take away the unhealthy elements. Whenever you believe that you will end up stronger from a stressful incident, you almost always will. This is known as post-traumatic growth. People who see stress as normal and an opportunity for progress fare better. For instance, nervous public speakers who said, "I am excited" were rated as having better speeches than people who said "I am calm."[14] So, decide to see yourself as scrappy, full of grit, and able to bounce back. Believe that stress and arousal will create an advantage for you.

A stressor itself is inherently neutral. It is the way it is appraised that induces either distress or eustress. Eustress is positive stress and comes about when we decide we can cope successfully. Eustress, mounted in response to exciting challenges, drops off quickly rather than lingering like the cortisol response does.

Besides this distinction between distress and eustress, scientists also differentiate between the threat and challenge responses. The threat response is the fight-or-flight response that makes you angry or fearful, priming you for self-defense. The challenge response gives you initiative, helps you focus, and motivates you to confront obstacles. Both responses share several physiological factors, such as an increase in heart rate. However, when you feel challenged, your heart beats stronger, not just faster, giving you more energy.

During the threat response, the body is anticipating physical harm and makes relevant alterations. For example, blood vessels constrict to minimize blood loss due to injury sustained during combat. The body also increases inflammation and mobilizes immune cells to prepare for bruises and cuts. The threat response leads to cortisol and feelings of self-doubt. Studies have shown that, over time, the threat response leads to obesity, brain volume loss, and an increased risk of cardiovascular disease.[15]

The challenge response doesn't do these things. The challenge response leads to tenacity and enthusiasm. Experts say that if you feel you don't have what it takes to meet a situation head on, you experience a threat response. I agree. I also think that the threat response is selected when distressed breathing predominates and that the challenge response is selected when diaphragmatic breathing is retained. Use your deep breathing skills to turn threat responses into challenge responses.

I would also be remiss not to mention that low to moderate stress levels are natural and beneficial. In fact, most excitement is accompanied by a little adrenaline and cortisol, along with an increase in heart and breathing rates. We need some stress, just like we need to contract our muscles regularly. The problem with the stress response is when it is elevated chronically like a braced muscle.

I am asking you to avoid mulling over threats, fights, and abuse. I am not, however, asking you to deny reality or stop thinking about rising to meet challenges. Avoiding what makes you anxious can suspend growth. This is why it is important to expose yourself incrementally to gradations of challenging social situations. Voice that extra comment, joke, or observation to your peers to challenge yourself without pushing yourself into panic. Spark a conversation with a stranger. Chat up the clerk at the cash register. Find progressively larger audiences to share your ideas with and make eye contact for those few extra seconds. Every time you meet a moderate challenge and succeed, you become able to face bigger challenges. Assert yourself in ways you were hesitant to previously and push yourself to gently expand your comfort zone boundaries.

Remember those monkey studies we discussed a few sections back? It turns out that if the young monkey was exposed to elevated levels of cortisol a few times, but only briefly, then they developed increased resilience to stress and lowered cortisol levels. It toughened them up. Your stress system is just like a muscle, you want to push it through its full range regularly, but not for extended periods. Undergoing stress that challenges your cardiovascular and sympathetic system ends up being excellent exercise if you are not defeated by it and if you can relax afterward. Envision your stress system as agile and able to go from 0 to 100 and back to 0 uncomplicatedly. Endure, prevail, and recoup. Be made better and stronger by everything that happens by remaining fundamentally unharmed.

Feelings of Control and Safety

An animal's stress is exacerbated when it cannot figure out how to make things better, feels helpless or powerless.[16] A rat subjected to small electrical shocks will liberate significantly less cortisol if it thinks it has some control over the frequency of the shocks. Tricking the rat into thinking that pushing a lever reduces these shocks helps it remain calm, even if the lever actually does nothing.[17] In a similar experiment, when a beeping noise preceded a shock to a rat's foot, those rats had less severe ulcers than those with no warning. Because the stress had some predictability, the rats could retain a sense of control.

The moral of this story? Don't focus on the elements of disturbing events that are unpredictable or uncontrollable. More importantly, know that your reactions, attitude, and reasoned choice are always under your control. Your breathing is always under your control as well. We all have times we are confused and uncertain. Do not let the nonlinear, chaotic, or unforeseeable distress you. Instead, take the time to identify which aspects of an unpleasant situation are malleable. This can help take the sting away from the unruly and erratic and help you turn threats into challenges.

Challenging yourself and embracing disorder is great, but there are times when you must feel able to completely put down your guard so that you can rest deeply. After the police loudly arrested my neighbor, I felt helpless in my own bed. This is not ok. Do what you must to make sure that you feel in control underneath your sheets, even if it means installing an alarm system or a thicker bedroom door with a deadbolt. The place where you sleep should provide sanctuary and refuge so you can debrace, recharge, and think safe, happy thoughts.
The Buddha sat and slept at the base of the Bodhi Tree because it provided protection and security. He trusted it to have his back. Make sure your resting place makes you feel unconditionally secure.

Preventing Scalp Soreness and Other Forms of Hypoperfusion

Hair loss can be caused by stress. I have a friend who left his ferret alone for two days and came home to find it covered in bald patches. It is common for mammals to lose fur after trauma. The details are unclear, but it may be some kind of social signal. When chronic stress causes hair loss in humans, it is known as telogen effluvium. I started rapidly losing hair at the end of 11th grade. At the time, I had no idea what caused the sudden hair loss. Looking back two decades later, it is clear that it started immediately after having my nose broken. I believe the hair loss was a direct response to some form of high-intensity bracing that I took on after the injury that caused an outpouring of cortisol.

It is cortisol that makes hair follicles thin and fall out (it is also stress hormones that make them turn gray). This is why hair loss is associated with other stress-related illnesses like coronary artery disease, hypertension, dyslipidemia, and increased mortality.[18] Although genetics plays a role in hair loss, abrupt hair loss from an early age is usually caused by extreme stress. By age 30, my hairline had receded to the midline of my scalp, farther than my father or grandfathers' hairlines. Fascinatingly, my hair loss stopped (for eight years at least) immediately after I started paced breathing. Of course, only a little of my hair grew back because the miniaturization of the follicle responsible for balding is irreversible.

Another contributor to hair loss is reduced blood supply to the scalp. Stress and aging can reduce circulation and vasculature in subcutaneous tissues all over the head. This can cause scalp soreness. In the medical literature, sore scalp has been closely associated with hair loss (alopecia and male pattern baldness). I believe that you can reduce your risk of hair loss by increasing circulation in your scalp. Does your scalp feel sore when you firmly press a knuckle into it with five pounds of pressure? It shouldn't. If it does, it may have reduced blood flow and the accompanying reductions in oxygen and nutrients. If the exercise below feels sore or painful, you should do it often to improve circulation. The intervention is simple, quick, and can vastly reduce scalp soreness in less than two weeks. Do the following:

De-Stress Exercise #21.1: Increase Scalp Blood Flow
1) Take the heel of your palm and press firmly down on the top of your head, around your hairline, or on any patch of scalp that feels sore.
2) Move your hand in a circular motion while pressing very firmly. You should feel like you are stretching the skin away from its attachments to the underlying bone.
3) Try to move your hand in wide circles, attempting to stretch the scalp as far as it will go in each direction.
4) Take about one second's time to complete a full circle.
5) Repeat this all over the scalp, focusing on the sorest areas for a total of five minutes. Also use other forms of massage including compression and percussion.

When I started, five pounds of pressure from a single knuckle at the top of my head provoked unbearable discomfort. The sheer amount of pain suggested to me that the scalp is another anchor for trauma. So, I felt compelled to try to get the pain out. Within 10 five-minute sessions of the exercise above it went from puffy and dimpled with inflammation to smooth and sleek. Aside from the scalp there are other areas without underlying muscle that can be affected by poor circulation.

I often use headphones to listen to audiobooks when I take walks. After a few years of this, my ears hurt every time I took off my headphones. They were so painful one day that I figured I would have to stop wearing them. Frustrated with this, I cupped my palms over my ears and bent them forward firmly. This stung, so I spent 60 seconds bending them in different directions. It ached, but it also felt good. When I wore headphones the next day, it was much less painful. Three more sessions like this, and the pain was gone completely.

With age and uneven use, our tissues develop a condition called hypoperfusion. This is also known as diminished blood flow and is the reason my ears hurt. Reduced perfusion of blood can cause pain all around the body. As you know, pain exacerbates stress and drives the production of cortisol so we should be finding these areas and massaging them.

Hypoperfusion develops when tissues and organs receive reduced circulation due to diminishment in the number of small blood vessels. Pinching and bending my ears for less than five minutes overall provided the mechanical deformation of the tissues necessary to stimulate the creation of new small blood vessels (angiogenesis). All our hypoperfused tissues, including dormant muscles, need this kind of tender loving care. If it aches and itches, target it further. I want to encourage you to use compression, percussion, and vibration to address hypoperfusion anywhere you can find it because it will scale down your stress.

Drug Use Leads to Frailty and Chronic Distress

In my early twenties, I had between one and five alcoholic drinks on weekends, a cigarette every Saturday night, and a cup of coffee most weekdays. I wanted to stop, but I couldn't help myself. When I was taking them, the drugs created the illusion of helping manage my stress. Taking them leads to relief because they mitigate distressed breathing for a few minutes, but in the long term, they actually contribute to it. It took me years to realize that even these uncontrolled substances lead to compulsive use, relapse after abstinence, and physical dependence.

Both nicotine and alcohol create a sense of euphoria that lasts a few minutes. However, the accompanying withdrawal from even a single use can lead to minor dysphoria that lasts days. Whether you are aware of it or not, this discomfort affects you emotionally and increases your bracing, shallow breathing, and emotional distress. I never noticed the withdrawal symptoms in my twenties, but after developing sensitivity to my inner states (discussed in depth in the next chapter), they became very apparent. Alcohol withdrawal symptoms include irritability, fatigue, shaking, sweating, nausea, headache, and difficulty concentrating.[19]
But these symptoms don't just affect alcoholics who go cold turkey. They affect everyone who uses alcohol in a dose-dependent manner. The symptoms of smoking cessation can be worse. Withdrawal from any drug robs a user of diaphragmatic mobility, and I believe the resulting shallow breathing is a primary mechanism in addiction.

When you use psychoactive drugs every week, you experience fiendish cravings. I realized that two shots of liquor made me feel fearless for thirty minutes, and a cigarette extinguished my anxiety for an hour, but for the next few days, the subtle pain from withdrawal made me slightly more introverted and submissive. Situations that I would consider to be minor hassles before became calamities that would make me think, "My God, I've got to have a drink." When you feel you "need" a cigarette is precisely when you shouldn't smoke. Instead of masking the pain, work through it by spending some time with your breath metronome.

Intense social interactions that go on too long create loads of tension. Drugs amplify this. This is why after mixing the two, otherwise known as partying, you wake up feeling achy and nauseous, with a headache and stiff breathing. It is also why rock stars and child actors often burn out so fast. You cannot consume caffeine, alcohol, tobacco, or marijuana and hope to keep your latent trigger points from flaring up in social situations. Instead, intoxication makes you intensify your social displays without awareness of the increase in bracing.

When people use drugs recreationally, it makes them feel immune to social stress for a short time. This inevitably leads them to go too hard on their bodies. It proceeds like this: as you work the room, you strain your trigger points and chakras to the limit until you reach the point of needing another drink or cigarette. Using dulls the discomfort and allows you to continue to push your chakras, further deranging and abusing them. Soon, you are in so much discomfort that you're turning to a third drink, a fourth drink, or possibly even harder drugs.

Imagine that you badly strained your neck Friday afternoon. Would you go to a party that night, drink, and do drugs? If you did, do you think it would make your neck better or worse? Would you go to the party if you had a fever? What if you were 95 years old, would you do it then? I offer these hypotheticals to help the reader see that social drug use is characterized by postural neglect, zero muscle refreshing, shallow breathing, and mounting tension. I recently heard a 20-year-old friend who stayed up all night drinking and partying say something the next morning that stuck with me. As she practically limped to her car, she said, "My entire body feels bruised." Episodes like this contribute immensely to frailty and muscle dormancy.

Most recreational drugs, legal and illegal, increase dopamine, making you feel eager and rewarded. Thus, drug use pits two different sections of the brain against each other. One finds the drug stimulating and exhilarating, while the other finds it depleting and impoverishing. As mammals, we are designed to choose whatever increases our dopamine. This is why, for most people, the fleeting reward of drug use outweighs the long-term costs. Drug use tricks the brain's pleasure centers into being delighted at the cost of tightening the vices around our chakras. In the long run, it also saps our dopamine. Within a couple of hours, the dopamine dips below default, and the person feels understimulated and restless, compelling them to want to use the drug again. Moreover, studies show that long-term drug use can permanently lower dopamine and serotonin levels.

I thought I would always crave cigarettes and alcohol, but diaphragmatic retraining abolished my urges. In fact, studies have shown that paced breathing can help addicts maintain sobriety.[20] Cigarettes and alcohol brought so much relief to me before but no longer did once I started breathing diaphragmatically. I believe that this is simply because there is little to relieve now. Instead, cigarettes generally just make my body feel weak, while alcohol makes me feel slow and tired.

There is a growing community of people who believe they can use drugs to achieve spiritual (entheogenic) growth. Sadly, almost all these people are oblivious to their shallow breathing while doing drugs. For this reason, most heavy trips are bad trips, even if the person does not realize it. I believe that if you want to do drugs, you should only do them while paced breathing. Otherwise, they will inevitably increase the extent of bracing going on under your level of awareness. Drugs should be used exclusively under the condition of complete composure. Under any other circumstances, they will unhinge your emotional well-being. However, hypocritically, I do recommend you take a drug for the following exercise.

De-Stress Activity #21.2: *Desensitize to the Sensations of Caffeine*

Commit a whole day to observing your body's reaction to caffeine. Make or buy a caffeinated beverage of your choice, then drink some of it. Caffeine, taurine, and other alkaloids increase adrenaline and cortisol. The caffeine will lead to the amplification of your discomfort, the activation of latent trigger points, and the straining of various chakra-like modules. Lie down and focus on these intense sensations. They may involve buzzing, crackling, heat, or cold and they may come in waves. Do not fight the waves. If you breathe mindfully through the twinges of pain convulsing your innards, you will learn to control and dispel them. Try going to sleep in this state.

If you are a regular caffeine consumer, try to abstain from caffeine and perform this exercise while being exposed to caffeine withdrawal symptoms instead. Having encouraged you to drink caffeine, I want to be clear. Clinical studies show that long-term use of highly caffeinated beverages can result in significant adverse health outcomes, including cardiac and psychiatric conditions.[21] For this reason, I strongly discourage the consumption of energy drinks. My subjective opinion is that caffeine should be kept under 50 mg per day, which is the equivalent of one or two eight-ounce cups of tea.

Several drugs, including hallucinogens, dissociatives, and psychedelics, can induce temporary psychosis. Profoundly disturbing states of nightmarish terror, fear of overdose, or "ultimate entrapment" are commonly reported. A bad trip is not physical and emotional pain caused by a drug. It is preexisting pain from bodily tension and latent trigger points unmasked by the drug. Being exposed to this and being badly and unmindfully distressed by it increases trauma in the body. However, I think that any bad trip can be reversed by 30 minutes of paced breathing. Mental health specialists are searching for a treatment that can be administered to patients shortly after an overdose, panic attack, or horrific trauma. I believe that deep, paced breathing should be used in emergency response and clinical settings because it has the power to terminate these states and, in so doing, help block the formation of traumatic memories.

I have a friend who smokes concentrated THC every day, smokes cigarettes hourly, and drinks between 10 and 15 drinks a night, every night. This sounds like a living hell to most people. But few realize that doing less than this is just a proportionately smaller version of that hell. I have watched this woman's good looks erode over just a few years. Every time I see her, the squinting and sneering are further entrenched. She doesn't even do any hard drugs, but the poor gal is in constant displeasure and dissatisfaction driven by her withdrawal symptoms. She once described her pain to me as claws and teeth, tugging at her internal organs and devouring her from the inside out. I believe this is an insightful description of what it feels like to have your chakra-like modules saturated in inflammation and trapped in partial contraction.

Video Games, Violent Movies, and Loud Music Contribute to Stress

Humans have a tendency to create unhealthy attachments to forms of overstimulation. I was addicted to video games, violent movies, and loud music. Just as with drugs, we become hooked on the dopamine and adrenaline they produce, and the fleeting thrill causes us to ignore the persistent, low-level panic.

Traditional hunter-gatherers had exceptionally low stimulation levels 95% of the time. They were out in nature. Today, we plug into many streams of overstimulation that promote thrill-seeking and hyperarousal. Videos of street fights, "epic fails," people getting injured, combat sports, horror movies and other forms of sensory assault are some of the most popular videos online. As with pornography, these intense but damaging experiences make us dissatisfied with our real lives. I believe that some people's limbic systems respond to intense media stimulation with the challenge response, but I think most respond to them with the threat response.

Social media use, video games, and the violent nature of modern movies and television fragment our attention and foster a gambling mindset that causes us to become addicted to short-lived thrills. News outlets design the daily coverage of current events and politics to incite negative emotions because it grabs attention. Everything from unsolicited emails to our social media feed, to the nightly news report inundates us with shock, confusion, and consternation. Modern media has been documented to decrease the capacity for concentration, discipline, and the kind of work ethic necessary to thrive in the modern professional sector.[22]

Almost any wild mammal placed in a nightclub or movie theater would frantically try to escape. Ironically, these are the places we go to relax even though our innate senses want to retreat from loud sounds, bright lights, and quick movement. They keep our amygdala ringing with fear. Even children's movies today are hysterically paced and feature constant calamity and pandemonium. A large proportion of children are incapable of breathing through their noses under these conditions. As we sit consuming popular media, we hyperventilate, sneer, startle, raise our eyebrows, brace our vocal cords, and protract our necks. As long as you allow media content to impede your breathing pattern, this is inescapable.

De-Stress Activity #21.3: *Disengage from an Action Flick*

The next time you watch a suspenseful movie, television show, or video game, carefully monitor your internal reactions. When the main character is risking their life, and there are big stakes, notice how somewhere deep down inside of you, you hold a conviction that says, "Don't take a full, long breath, or else you will put the protagonist of the movie in jeopardy." Do you see how absurd this situation is? What is happening to a fictional character in a film should not adversely affect your breathing.

The fear of breathing properly is our most limiting belief. At the theater or on your couch, pull out your paced breathing app, dim the screen, and override this tendency as you continue to watch. While you witness the character experience peril, breathe long, slow breaths. You will be amazed by how this allows you to detach from and become desensitized to the nail-biting worriment.

When the diaphragm tenses, it is like a turtle retreating into its shell. It "wants to hide" from loud sounds and fast movement. When it is afraid, it lies still in partial contraction. When it feels safe it ventures out. While we consume entertainment media our tendency is to breathe with the chest and freeze the diaphragm in place. The diaphragm remains buried inside the rib cage like the turtle's head inside its shell. This keeps the belly still. During each inhalation, pay attention to the downstroke of your diaphragm. Imagine it emerging from the bottom of your ribs and pushing on the contents of your belly. As you perform Activity 21.3 above, you should have dozens of breakthrough moments where, little by little, you are able to encourage your diaphragm to come out and play.

As with drug use, intense stimulation from modern media causes us to completely disregard the panic signals our body is sending us. Performing paced breathing while engaging in these activities is an excellent way to learn to retain your composure as you are inundated. If you practice, you will get to the point where you can breathe through your nose at five breaths per minute in a loud theater, digital firefight, or clamoring nightclub for hours at a time. Allow me to point out that it doesn't matter which arena, arcade, or bar you are in; if you breathe at five breaths per minute or less, you are automatically the coolest cat there.

Most video games create suspenseful situations in which players must react quickly to keep their character from being hurt or killed. The simulated danger and time pressure recruits fast-acting areas of the brain, such as the amygdala and basal ganglia, to help perform the hazardous button pressing. These unconscious brain areas don't know they are just being recruited to play a game. They assume the actions are dire, and so involuntarily activate the sympathetic system. This is why playing real-time video games can be affectively detrimental. Each decrement in the character's life bar causes startle and cortisol release.[23] Each startle contributes ever so slightly to one's background hum of anxiety. Moreover, as you hold the controller (as with your phone or keyboard), most of your major postural muscles are completely braced and immobilized. In a very real sense, we are monkeys being terrorized while handcuffed to the keyboard, mouse, or controller.

Videogames have been shown to increase cortisol levels, bolster aggressive affect, and reduce prosocial behavior.[24] Most of my friends who play video games act breathless and panicked afterward, driving them to smoke cigarettes and drink alcohol during gaming breaks. Playing an hour of competitive, online "deathmatches" would strip almost anyone of their composure. Over time, this undermines autonomic balance. In my twenties I didn't realize that loud, violent entertainment was turning me into the stereotype of the high-strung geek.

Many studies have shown that merely reducing television volume can vastly reduce the sympathetic stress response to violent videos and games. In general, the louder the TV, the more frequently and intensely the amygdala is triggered, and the more cortisol is released. Turn your speakers down a few decibels, and you should notice that you feel far less uneasy after a play session or an action movie. We should also seek out activities that put us into a state of flow and stimulate dopamine without stimulating cortisol. What you are doing right now, reading, may be one of the best. Socialization, meditation, massage, sex, singing, and exercise are others.

Some breathtaking things are good for us. But we need to differentiate between the scenic overlook and addictive trauma. Overstimulating media tricks our bodies into thinking we are preparing for tremendous amounts of exercise, even though we usually consume it while sitting on our backsides. Rather than stewing in them, use up your stress hormones by engaging in physical activity.

Conclusion: Exercise Is the Best Antistress Tool

Perhaps the best antidote for stress is regular exercise. There is an extensive body of research documenting the many benefits. Exercise bolsters self-esteem, enhances body image, increases stress resilience, and is an effective treatment for depression and anxiety.[25] Some studies indicate that exercise may even increase life expectancy and the overall quality of life.[26] There are many reasons to exercise.

Health Benefits of Exercise

- Improves circulation efficiency and reduces blood pressure
- Increases pain tolerance
- Increases the number of red blood cells, facilitating oxygen transport
- Lowers total cholesterol while raising good cholesterol
- Prevents bone loss and stimulates bone growth reducing the risk of osteoporosis
- Promotes weight loss
- Reduces risk for heart disease, blood clots, and stroke
- Reduces the risk for diabetes and cardiovascular issues
- Strengthens the heart muscle, improves its efficiency, and reduces resting heart rate
- Strengthens the muscles of respiration

Most people don't engage in daily physical activity because it feels uncomfortable. They assume exercise will add to their distress. It's true: exercise does lead to a slight increase in adrenaline and cortisol. This is why we must appraise the sensation of exercise as positive stress, a challenge, and as under our control. Moreover, mounting a small stress response to exercise repeatedly will diminish your stress response to subsequent exercise. In other words, the more you train, the less uncomfortable it becomes.

Exercise involves the good type of stress that fortifies us against bad types. It does this by teaching the respiratory and cardiovascular systems how to handle heavy loads and recover rapidly. Also, after exercise, stress plummets. For instance, it is known that blood concentration levels of cortisol rebound (fall off) abruptly. On the other hand, cortisol rebound after social stress is sluggish and it won't rebound at all if it leads to rumination. The next time you find yourself overthinking an argument, take a run. You may find it wipes most of your concerns away.

Exercise is a potent antidepressant and anxiolytic that makes us feel significantly less affected by unfavorable events. The reason is that physical exertion, whether aerobic or anaerobic, results in endorphin release. Beta-endorphin is a neurohormone released into the bloodstream from the pituitary gland during exercise.[27] Endorphins attach themselves to specific receptor sites in the brain that affect our perception of well-being and, in large amounts, can even create the feeling of euphoria. Endorphins are the body's way of rewarding us for exerting ourselves. Endorphins not only give you a sense of pleasure; they also suppress appetite, elevate mood, increase memory retention, and improve immune activity.[28]

Aerobic exercise results in the increased creation of new brain cells (neurogenesis) in the same areas that lose cells in people with depression (such as the hippocampus). The concentration of nerve growth factors, like GDNF and BDNF, increases with exercise.

These proteins cause neuron branches to grow and make new connections. They also reduce susceptibility to degeneration. It is no wonder that a sedentary lifestyle is a risk factor for neurodegenerative illnesses in humans. If you don't exercise to improve health, fitness, or appearance, then do it to increase the quality of your level of consciousness. In fact, exercise has many positive biological effects on the brain.

Neurobiological Effects of Exercise

- Boosts energy and reduces stress
- Improves brain structural connections
- Improves cognitive function, cognitive control, and various forms of memory
- Improves mental health, increasing cognitive capacity
- Improves mental wellness by relieving stress, tension, anxiety, and depression
- Improves self-image and confidence
- Improves sleep quality
- Increases gray matter density
- Results in new neuron growth

Exercise enhances the feel-good neuromodulators while having none of the downsides of overeating, drugs, alcohol, or chaotic entertainment. The endorphin release that occurs during exercise is one reason why running around the block once or twice can make you come across as highly relaxed before a meeting, date, or party. The other reason is that it resets the level of tension in your chest.

Unspent, negative energy will inevitably be funneled toward the bracing of your diaphragm. This makes it so that a tense "claw" powers each inhalation and exhalation. Intense cardiovascular exercise that requires heavy breathing forces you to loosen that claw and expand the diaphragm's range simply so that you can get enough air. Additionally, when an exercise thoroughly works out your breathing musculature, it will need rest, preventing it from reverting to its usual pattern of heavy tension. In other words, aerobic exercise stimulates and strengthens the breathing musculature, making it largely incompatible with bracing the diaphragm.

De-Stress Exercise #21.2: *Unbracing Heavy Breathing*

During intense aerobic exercise, you should feel some degree of discomfort in your chest. Some of that discomfort is a normal part of heavy breathing, but a large part comes from breathing muscles that have been chronically braced. The next time you perform aerobic exercise, like running, jumping rope, cycling, or climbing stairs, zero in on this pain. You can retire it if you just stop bracing the muscles responsible. It is an anguished, panicked reaction to exertion that is unnecessary. Part of this is an innate fear of pushing the heart and lungs too far.

While exercising, imagine that you will have to keep up this high level of respiratory output for the rest of the day. To do this, you would need to make your breathing as efficient as possible. Imagine resting in action: accepting heavy cardiovascular demand and relaxing in the face of it. That burning sensation in the center of your chest and around your ribs *will* fade away as you teach yourself to turn it off.

Wolves and wild dogs often travel tens of miles daily while foraging. They are designed for sustained, daily activity. Dog trainers know that daily exercise is the most important aspect of rehabilitating problem dogs. This is because being deprived of activity without an outlet for their natural energy increases neurotic, defiant, and aggressive behaviors. Dismally, many people don't bother to walk their dogs. Professionals dog behaviorists like Cesar Millan argue that walking a dog for less than sixty minutes every day is abusive.[29] Millan walks his dogs in a large pack for at least four hours a day. He doesn't do this for their physical health as much as their mental health. How much exercise is enough for humans? It isn't clear, but many experts and the U.S. Department of Health and Human Services recommend at least 20 minutes of moderate aerobic activity every day. I would say that we should shoot for more like 40.

You need a daily outlet for your natural energy just as much as any other mammal. Every day you skip cardiovascular exercise, you are mismanaging your body and compounding your stress, social defeat, and pain. To stay motivated, make your workouts fun, varied and (as discussed in Chapter 15) not too strenuous. Listen to an audiobook, a podcast, or your favorite music. Become interested in and build skill at as many different forms of exercise as you can. Try out different sports, gymnasiums, and classes in your neighborhood (see table below). Ask your friends if you can join them in their routines. Dance and practice yoga every day. Lift weights using the anti-laxity and anti-rigidity techniques. Get out for a walk using the exercises in Chapter 17. Free yourself from that self-imposed kennel.

Individual Exercises	Cycling, Cross Country, Dancing, Elliptical, Hiking, Jogging, Mountain Climbing, Jumping Rope, Rowing, Running, Skateboarding, Swimming, Stair Climbing, Trampoline, Walking
Group Sports	Badminton, Baseball, Basketball, Boxing, Cheerleading, Cricket, Dodgeball, Football, Handball, Hockey, Lacrosse, Martial Arts, Racquetball, Rugby, Soccer, Softball, Skating, Skiing, Tennis, Volleyball, Wrestling
Group Classes	Aquarobics, Body Works, Bootcamp, Calisthenics, Cardio Kickboxing, Cross Fit, Dance, Jazzercise, Jiu-Jitsu, Karate, Krav Maga, Muay Thai, Pilates, Salsa Dancing, Spinning, Step Aerobics, Tae Kwon Do, TRX, Turbo Kick, Water Aerobics, Yoga, Zumba

Table 21.1: Forms of cardiovascular and aerobic exercises to try.

Chapter 21: **Bullet Points**

- Don't fear stress. Apprehension of stress makes it more physiologically detrimental.
- We can respond to stressors in a healthy way by considering them challenges (challenge response) or in an unhealthy way by considering them threats (threat response).
- Whether your unconscious mind responds to stressors with the threat response or the challenge response may be determined by the quality of your breathing.
- Virtually all drug use leads to withdrawal symptoms that weaken you as a person.
- People who mix socializing with drugs unknowingly brace various muscles and organs for sustained periods.
- Video games, loud music, and violent, suspenseful entertainment lead to low-level panic that can become chronic.
- You are on "no chill" mode. And you need to come off it.
- Consider taking one day a week, perhaps Sundays, to unwind and remove yourself from all worries, work, rushes, and social conflicts. A whole day of rest serves as a "macrobreak." Committing 1/7 of your life to restorative relaxation can make a huge difference over time.
- Regular exercise releases endorphins and enhances our mood, keeping our minds from running our bodies into the ground.
- Anxiety is your body's way of begging you for exercise.

Chapter 21: **Endnotes**

1.   Ellis, B. J., Jackson, J. J., & Boyce, W. T. (2006). The stress response systems: Universality and adaptive individial differences. *Developmental Review, 26*, 175–212.

2.   Wingfield, J. C., Donna L. Maney, Creagh W. Breuner, Jacobs, J. D., Sharon Lynn, Ramenofsky, M., & Ralph D. Richardson. (1998). Ecological bases of hormone-behavior interactions: The "Emergency Life History Stage." *American Zoologist, 38*(1), 191–206.

3   Marks, I., & Nesse, R. (1994). Fear and fitness: An evolutionary analysis of anxiety disorders. *Ethology and Sociobiology, 15*(5), 247–261.

4.   Miller, D. B., & O'Callaghan, J. P. (2002). Neuroendocrine aspects of the response to stress. *Metabolism: Clinical and Experimental, 51*(6 Suppl 1), 5–10; Sapolsky, R. M., Krey, L. C., & McEwen, B. S. (1986). The neuroendocrinology of stress and aging: The glucocorticoid cascade hypothesis. *Endocrine Reviews, 7*(3), 284–301; Lovallo, W. R., & Gerin, W. (2003). Psychophysiological reactivity: Mechanisms and pathways to cardiovascular disease. *Psychosomatic Medicine*, 65(1), 36–45.

5.   LeDoux, J. (1996). *The emotional brain: The mysterious underpinnings of emotional life.* Simon and Schuster.

6.   Bremner J. D. (1999). Does stress damage the brain? *Biological Psychiatry, 45*(7), 797–805; LeDoux, J. (1998). Fear and the brain: Where have we been, and where are we going? *Biological Psychiatry, 44*(12), 1229–1238.

7   LeDoux, J. (2015). *Anxious: Using the brain to understand and treat fear and anxiety.* Penguin Books.

8.   Sapolsky, R. M. (2017). *Behave: The biology of humans at our best and worst.* Penguin Press.

9.   Sapolsky, R. M. (2005). The influence of social hierarchy on primate health. *Science, 308*(5722), 648–652.

10. Sapolsky, 2017, Behave: The biology of humans at our best and worst.

11. Sapolsky, R. M., Romero, L. M., & Munck, A. U. (2000). How do glucocorticoids influence stress responses? Integrating permissive, suppressive, stimulatory, and preparative actions. *Endocrine Reviews, 21*(1), 55–89.

12. Nelson, E. E., & Winslow, J. T. Non-human primates: Model animals for developmental psychopathology. *Neuropsychopharmacology*, *34*(1), 90–105.

13. McGonigal, K. (2015). *The upside of stress: Why stress is good for you and how to get good at it*. Penguin Random House.

14. Brooks, A. (2013). Get excited: Reappraising pre-performance anxiety as excitement. *Journal of Experimental Psychology*, *143*(3), 1144 –1158.

15. McGonigal, 2015, *The upside of stress:Why stress is good for you and how to get good at it.*

16. Glass, D. C., Reim, B., & Singer, J. E. (1971). Behavioral consequences of adaptation to controllable and uncontrollable noise. *Journal of Experimental Social Psychology*, *7*(2), 244–257; Minor, T. R., Jackson, R. L., & Maier, S. F. (1984). Effects of task-irrelevant cues and reinforcement delay on choice-escape learning following inescapable shock: evidence for a deficit in selective attention. *Journal of Experimental Psychology: Animal Behavior Processes*, *10*(4), 543–556.

17. Sapolsky, R. M. (1994). *Why zebras don't get ulcers*. Henry Holt and Company.

18. Gude, D. (2012). Hair loss: A harbinger of morbidities to come! *International Journal of Trichology*, *4*(4), 287–288.

19. Testino, G., Leone, S., & Borro, P. (2014). Treatment of alcohol dependence: Recent progress and reduction of consumption. *Minerva Medica*, *105*(5), 447–466.

20. Elliott, S., & Edmonson, E. (2006). *The new science of breath: Coherent breathing for autonomic nervous system balance, health, and well-being*. Coherence Press.

21. Sanchis-Gomar, F., Pareja-Galeano, H., Cervellin, G., Lippi, G., & Earnest, C. P. (2015). Energy drink overconsumption in adolescents: implications for arrhythmias and other cardiovascular events. *Canadian Journal of Cardiology*, *31*(5), 672–575.

22. Christakis, D. A., Ramirez, J. S. B., Ferguson, S. M., Ravinder, S., & Ramirez, J. (2018). How early media exposure may affect cognitive function: A review of results from observations in humans and experiments in mice. *PNAS*, *115*(40), 9851–9858.

23. Gentile, D. A., Bender, P. K., & Anderson, C. A. (2017). Violent video game effects on salivary cortisol, arousal and aggressive thougthts in children. *Computers in Human Behavior*, *70*, 39–43.

24. Anderson, C. A., & Bushman, B. J. (2001). Effects of violent video games on aggressive behavior, aggressive cognition, aggressive affect, physiological arousal, and prosocial behavior: A meta-analytic review of the scientific literature. *Psychological Science, 12*(5), 353–359.

25. Babyak, M., Blumenthal, J. A., Herman, S., Khatri, P., Doraiswamy, M., Moore, K., & Krishnan, K. R. (2000). Exercise treatment for major depression: Maintenance of therapeutic benefit at 10 months. *Psychosomatic Medicine, 62*(5), 633–638.

26. Gremeaux, V., Gayda, M., Lepers, R., Sosner, P., Juneau, M., & Nigam, A. (2012). Exercise and longevity. *Maturitas, 73*(4), 312–7.

27. Boecker, H., Sprenger, T., Spilker, M. E., Henriksen, G., Koppenhoefer, M., Wagner, K. J., Valet, M., Berthele, A., & Tolle, T. R. (2008). The runner's high: opioidergic mechanisms in the human brain. *Cerebral Cortex, 18*(11), 2523–2531.

28. Anderson, E., & Shivakumar, G. (2013). Effects of exercise and physical activity on anxiety. *Frontiers in Psychiatry, 4*, 27.

29. Millan, C., & Peltier, M. J. (2006). *Cesar's way: The natural, everyday guide to understanding & correcting common dog problems*. Random House.

Chapter 22: **Listen to Your Heart and Gut**

"Go to your bosom; knock there, and ask your heart what it doth know." — William Shakespeare (1564-1616)

"Beauty is not in the face; beauty is a light in the heart." — Kahlil Gibran (1883-1931)

Most of us are unable to localize the sensations of turmoil within our bodies. They compel us to harbor destructive thoughts and take self-destructive actions, though we usually have little awareness of the feelings themselves. This is especially true for the sensations from the thorax and abdomen. I was mostly blind to the constriction in the various organs within my chest and gut, which was unfortunate because recognizing individual sensations and tracing them back to their physical origin is key to disrupting them. And so, whenever you feel particularly stressed, take it as an opportunity to lie down and become immersed in the physical manifestations of your worry. Paying attention to the internal state of your body is called interoception. This chapter will teach you how to create an interoceptive watchtower from which to monitor your autonomic space.

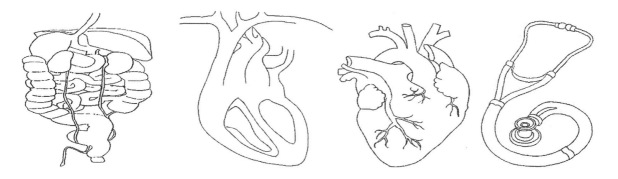

Illustration 22.1: A. Digestive tract; B. Cross-section of the heart; C. Surface of the heart; D. Stethoscope.

How to Find and Quell the Pain in Your Heart and Gut

Your brain receives a continuous feed of sensory information from each muscle and most tissues in the body. In the cortex, this incoming information participates in and contributes to your conscious workspace and train of thought. Sensations of pain coactivate with whatever else is on your mind and influences it to be more negative. In other words, pain twists and distorts your thinking. Most of us don't pay attention to these data streams and, as a result, develop a conscious blind spot (scotoma) for them. When you are blind to them, they control you without your awareness. But if you work on cultivating interoception, and combine this with relaxed diaphragmatic breathing, you gain the ability to send data back to these tissues. This feedback calms them while denying them a hold over you.

The insula and anterior cingulate cortex receive many of the interoceptive signals your body sends to your brain. Neuroscientists think of these areas as pain areas because they light up in a brain scanner when participants experience discomfort. These two areas respond to nausea, stomach pain, fullness, air hunger, food hunger, sexual longing, vibrations, menstrual cramps, butterflies in the stomach, shortness of breath, and much more. They also react to social pain triggered by separation, exclusion, persecution, or disapproval. You should be able to imagine these feelings. You are imagining them within your insula and anterior cingulate. Inhabit these brain areas and "watch" the imagery that unfolds there nonjudgmentally.

Focusing on the minutiae of your physical discomfort is the only way to rein it in. As we have seen, bodily pain involves partially contracted muscles that have reached a state of hyperfatigue. By paying attention to them, you can teach them to relax. Search for constriction, pressure, aching, and tingling. When you find them, remind yourself that they are just physical sensations. They are nothing to fear; they are "fear itself." Remember the corpse pose and "body scan" activities that we performed in Chapter 5 to search for skeletal muscle bracing? Well, the next exercise will feel similar but focuses on bracing awareness for your smooth and cardiac muscle: your internal organs.

Interoception Exercise #22.1: *Listen to Your Heart and Gut*

Find a dark room where you can lay down on the floor and feel totally secure. Bring a breath metronome with you. Bed down and try to relax completely. Notice that partially contracted and quivering muscles in your chest and abdomen keep you from being able to relax. Build as much mental imagery around these sensations as you can. Imagine their location in space. Label where you feel them anatomically in your body. Track their fluctuations in intensity through time. Notice how the separate modules interact and affect each other. Pay close attention to how paced breathing calms them. Work on gaining bidirectional control over these modules in the same way that you can alternate between tensing and relaxing your hand.

Learn to focus completely on the discomfort, feeling it in its totality without panicking, bracing, hyperventilating, repositioning, or giving in to the temptation to stop the exercise. This builds confidence in the face of internal tumult. When you tolerate the discomfort and are even able to feel comfortable, relaxed, and safe within it, you are taking the major step toward vanquishing it. You are invalidating it by proving to your body that it is unnecessary. You want your body to believe that these pains have no informational value because they contribute nothing to the way you should perceive your environment or the way you should act within it.

After several minutes lying in the dark focusing on your heart and gut, you should experience your body as a pulsating sea slug, like the one we discussed in Chapter 2. Ride with the painful retractions, don't fight them. Depersonalize and detach from them. Don't accept them as part of yourself.

The autonomic nervous system is composed of motor neurons that send messages to "involuntary" muscles and glands. It was long described as functioning below the level of consciousness. This is why medical researchers believed there was no way to deliberately calm these organs. Thankfully, recent biofeedback research has shown that we can gain some voluntary control over autonomic governance.[1] It has also shown that merely sensing these pains is key to relaxing them. At first, you will find that many of the sensations I am describing are impenetrable to introspection. This is because they are preverbal and nondeclarative.

You don't yet have words for them and how they affect you. But, just because you cannot articulate how they make you feel, doesn't mean you can't feel them if you concentrate.

Think about the aspect of you that is shocked when you are immersed in frigid water or woken up by an alarm clock set too loud. It should run down the midline of your body from your neck to your lower spine by way of your chest and gut. When you locate the physical borders of this sensation, you will have found your trauma core, the cause of internal agitation that makes you feel panicky, unbalanced, and demoralized. Once you have found it, console it. Usually, you try to rise above the pain, pretending that it is not there. Dive down into it. Incorporate the meditative and mindfulness practices from Chapter 7 into this search.

While alone with your pain, you will experience boredom and impatience. It will make this exercise frustrating until you realize that the boredom is restlessness stemming from the same visceral unease you are trying to dispel. Meditating on your bodily pain can be mundane, or it can be an exciting adventure if you approach it with "shoshin." Shoshin is a concept in Zen Buddhism meaning "beginner's mind." It denotes an openness, curiosity, eagerness, and a lack of preconceptions when exposed to something familiar. Imagine yourself as a psychonaut, a "sailor of the soul," exploring your mind and body. The more you map the territory and understand the "lay of the land," the better you will control your emotions.

Scientists know babies to be experts at self-soothing. They "listen" attentively to their sympathetic nervous system. We forgot how because as we grew up, we realized that paying attention to our internal milieu demands attentive resources. And attention is limited. Babies cannot change their environment, so they are forced to change their response to it. They have no recourse but to calm themselves. Children and adults, on the other hand, learn to change their environment and manipulate people to fix a situation. Unfortunately, by age five, we think that the best way to self-soothe is to bring about an increase in our social standing. You can, however, revert to infancy, bypass the ego and the social machinations, and take a shortcut straight to the center of the problem by confronting the tumultuous activity within your body at its source.

Cats often sit close to a wall and stare at it for minutes at a time. I used to think this was absurd. However, since I expanded my interoceptive senses, I find myself doing this sort of thing frequently—staring blankly at nothing. It is not boring to stare at a wall if you are also gazing into your visceral milieu. The more time you spend surveying and relaxing the activity in your spine, stomach, heart, face, vocal tract, intestines, and genitals, the more you can cleanse them with peace.

Myofascial Release for the Gut

I used to get regular pangs in my stomach during social confrontations. These felt like electrical shocks a few inches behind the belly button. Such pangs are caused by the clenching of the abdominals along with smooth muscle of the gastrointestinal tract. They are responsible for the sinking sensation in the pit of the stomach, resulting in a strong predilection to submit. You lose all will to fight when intense gut pain kicks in.

This visceral pain is due to the activation of latent trigger points, resulting in the stimulation of pain receptors in and around the digestive pathway. These receptors span the thorax, abdomen, and pelvis. They respond to stretching, swelling, and oxygen deprivation. The areas are in chronic pain because they have been braced for so long. Some experts believe that irritable bowel syndrome and a host of other gastrointestinal problems are exacerbated by bracing.[2] In the next exercise, we will use compression to massage these bracing patterns away.

Interoception Exercise #22.2: *Compressing the Internal Organs*

Lay over a large, firm ball and press it gently into your stomach. A soccer ball, volleyball or basketball work well. You can do this lying on the floor or in bed. The easiest way is to stand or kneel by the corner of a bed. Place the basketball on that corner of the mattress and drape the upper half of your body over it. Either way, you want to have good control of how deeply you press the ball into your abdominal cavity. It is important to be stable and comfortable.

The discomfort that this causes in your stomach may be very intense at first. Proceed gently and focus on applying firm pressure to the abdomen from the bottom of the ribs to the pelvis. Pressure applied to the lower ribs will also help stretch and manipulate the diaphragm. You should notice that the tension in your stomach will not give in to the ball unless you are breathing slow, smooth breaths. Relax, pace your breaths, and use abdominal compression to unwind the vice clenching your innards.

This practice pulls stress out of your body by its roots. Once you use a basketball to rid your midsection of the aching, you will vastly reduce your potential for experiencing gut-wrenching pain. The first time I deeply compressed my abdomen, I was immediately reminded of the long-forgotten feeling of being kicked in the stomach in second grade. This indicated that I was finding and releasing points of tension that I had been harboring since early childhood. As I continued, the searing discomfort in my stomach caused me to have flashbacks to other long-forgotten traumatic episodes. My brain was asking, "Hey, are you sure it's okay to relax the abdomen to this extent given these memories?" When your brain asks you this question, reassure it that it is a-okay. This gut compression technique is powerful because, if you can get rid of the pain in your gut, you will become far less susceptible to intimidation.

The gastrointestinal tract, from mouth to anus, is 15 feet long. It is lined by a vast network of neurons, which form a regional administrative center. This amounts to a miniature brain with over 100 million neurons. This is more than the brain of a mouse, which has around 70 million neurons. This miniature brain is needed to perform various digestive behaviors with which your mind cannot be bothered. Chances are your gut's brain has an anxiety disorder, and it braces the muscles it controls endlessly. Compressing away its bracing patterns may be the best way to communicate to this entity that there is no reason for it to be anxious.

Heart Rate

The heart is another entity within your body that you need to convince to loosen up and simmer down. Like the gut, the heart has its own neural network containing over 40,000 neurons. This is less than a fruit fly (100,000) but more than a snail (20,000). This mini-brain allows the heart to perceive and process information, make decisions, and even demonstrate a form of learning and memory.[3] More than likely, your heart's brain (like your gut's brain) has become convinced that your environment is life-threatening. We need to trick our hearts into believing the opposite.

The heart is a hollow muscular organ that uses repetitive rhythmic contractions to keep blood pumping through the body's blood vessels. Even some of the simplest invertebrate animals have hearts. Mollusks like clams, arthropods like insects, and even many types of worms have them. Some animals even have multiple hearts. The human heart beats slightly more than once every second, about 1,000 times per day, as many as 3.5 billion times over one's lifetime. Each beat is powerful enough to send blood spurting up to three meters if the aorta is severed. Every hour, it dispenses around 70 gallons of blood. That's 1,680 gallons per day. It works relentlessly. It works so much and so hard that it is imperative that it works efficiently.

The heart is composed of a special type of muscle called cardiac muscle, which operates involuntarily. Unlike skeletal muscle and the smooth muscle of the gut, the heart muscle is myogenic, which means that it can contract and relax without any input from the brain. It accomplishes this coordination of contraction and relaxation through the sinoatrial and atrioventricular nodes. These pacemakers are controlled by the sympathetic and parasympathetic systems which act as accelerator and decelerator, respectively. A heart that is biased toward acceleration is inefficient. In a sense, your life's trauma is manifested to the extent that your heart beats faster than it should. This is expressed in the following formula:

Your current heart rate - Your optimal heart rate = Accumulated life trauma

The average resting heart rate is 60 to 80 beats per minute. Stress and anxiety cause the heart to receive too much adrenaline, which increases heart rate. Chronically high levels of circulating adrenaline cause "tachycardia," meaning that the heart beats at an unsustainably fast rate. There is a single maximally efficient heart rate for your body size and body composition. Unfortunately, because nearly all humans are inveterate worriers, our hearts beat well above this optimal rate. Clinically, tachycardia is defined as a resting heart rate above 100 beats per minute,[4] but most of us are on a "tachycardia continuum." Even though your heart rate may be well under 100 beats per minute, it is likely above its optimal rate.

Elevated heart rate is perhaps the most detrimental form of sympathetic upregulation. Technically it is a type of stress cardiomyopathy. Aggression, anger, hate, fear, guilt, violence, and drugs all push your heart further from its ideal pace. The faster it beats, the more fatigue it experiences. Fascinatingly, the short rests between beats give your heart the microbreaks it needs to regenerate its strength. But, if your heart is always beating quickly, it misses out on these breaks. When stress is chronic, the microbreaks are vanishingly short, and the heart can never rest. The absence of downtime places excessive pressure on the muscles of the heart and the surrounding blood vessels. This becomes a never-ending marathon, during which the heart's tissues accumulate physical damage. Unremitting elevated rate forces the heart to destroy itself. It slowly tears its own tissues apart. Chances are, right now, you are overworking your heart.

The strain of chronic accelerated heart rate causes morbidity. Morbidity is the condition of being diseased by ailments that reduce longevity. It is the extent to which we have one foot in the grave. Morbidity from elevated heart rate, excessive cortisol, and stress-related bracing is eating your body (and soul) alive. Watching that scary movie, doing that line of cocaine, and throwing a tantrum against your coworker all contribute to terminal decline. When the heart is made to work harder than it should for extended periods, it does not receive adequate oxygen or nutrients, and this can result in pain known as angina. Heart pain[5] and the accompanying heart problems[6] have been strongly associated with hyperventilation. This provides you with yet another good reason to breathe slowly and smoothly through your nose.

Diaphragmatic breathing may be the best way to get your heart to assume that your present reality is safe. When you take deep breaths and override the body's preferred breathing style, you may feel small bursts of panic and a strong impulse to switch back to shallow breathing. An acceleration in heart rate is partially responsible for this panic. Resist the temptation to revert to shallow breathing. As you notice your heart speed up, mentally reassure it, "Hey, there's nothing wrong. I'm just taking deeper breaths."

As you breathe at longer and longer intervals, your heart will try to warn you that what you're doing is dangerous. It assumes that you are ignoring the hostilities of your environment and overriding its defense mechanisms. This is why many patients relive past trauma while performing diaphragmatic breathing in clinical settings. In fact, therapists ask their patients to discuss the psychological associations that come to mind during abdomen expansion, including self-image, emotional release, and vulnerability. As you calmly and assuredly breathe through these, you heal yourself. By teaching your heart that long, deep breaths are safe, you also teach it that a slower heart rate is safe.

Using a Stethoscope to Find Inner Peace

Because your ticker is overworked, it hurts. Nature programmed our hearts to transmit a pain signal when beating at a higher-than-optimal rate. It communicates to the animal that it is functioning at a level of output that cannot be sustained indefinitely without serious functional compromises. The painful sensations emanating from your heart make it a fly drowning in ointment. This is the discomfort that we try to use liquor, smoking, shopping, unhealthy food, risky sex, and overstimulating media to cover up. But because the brain interprets your heart's pain as delocalized and diffuse, you don't even recognize it as coming from the heart.

As with the diaphragm, normally, you cannot hear or feel your heart consciously, so you are blind to your own nervous system's two most fundamental signals. Heart rate controls and modulates behavior in countless ways, but for some reason, nature decided to mask its rate from our awareness. We can only feel it if it is beating in response to intense fear or excitement. Even then, we usually do not pay attention. How can we follow our heart if we are completely habituated to it?

Spend $10 and buy yourself a stethoscope online. Use it as a direct line to your heart. As you listen to your stethoscope, you will come to realize that your heart is like a fearful little animal inside your chest. Cravings for dopamine cause us to excite it, abuse it, poke at it, and sensitize it further to fearful stimuli. However, merely listening to it beat will desensitize you to the negative sensations emanating from it.

Interoception Exercise #22.3: *Listen to a Stethoscope to Desensitize Yourself to Your Heartbeat*

Find a safe place to listen to your heart with a stethoscope. Place the bell in the middle of your chest directly on the skin. What is your first impression of your heartbeat? Does it feel uncomfortable? Does it feel like it is beating too fast? Many people feel that each beat is accompanied by discomfort. You can overcome this by practicing paced breathing while being exposed to your heartbeat.

Imagine that you are breathing in and out through the area surrounding your heart. This will focus awareness on the heartbeat. Notice your tendency to switch to shallow breathing whenever your heart speeds up. Next, notice how a particularly heavy or painful heartbeat makes you switch from exhalation to inhalation. Do not let these small intrusions control your breathing. Your inhalations and exhalations should be influenced by air hunger, not by heart rate.

At first, the pain of listening to my heart made me project my discomfort onto the stethoscope itself. I felt like I hated it. Many people that I have worked with experience this, too. This happens because whatever you think about when you feel pain in your heart can easily become an object of animosity. Your mind will appraise this external object as the problem, transferring the pain onto it. Stop the overreacting. Face the pain. Coexist with it non-resistantly. Eat it with a knife and fork. When I started, each heartbeat felt like a mousetrap snapping shut inside my chest. After several weeks of Exercise 22.3, my heartbeat became the pleasurable and uplifting thump of a drumbeat.

As you listen to your heart, try focusing on your "interbeat interval." This is the length of time between successive heartbeats. With time, you will start to notice when two heartbeats have a longer interval between them than the beats that came prior. This is when you have relaxed. Other times, this interval collapses and becomes shorter. The interval will decrease after a stressful thought. Concentrate on making the interval as long as possible. In doing this, you will be programming yourself for a slower resting heart rate and providing your heart with a longer rest period.

As you listen through the stethoscope, notice that the sound of each heartbeat coincides with a faint feeling in your chest. The stethoscope makes this invisible sensation apparent. This pairing constitutes a form of biofeedback that allows you to understand what your heartbeat feels like so that you can recognize it in the future, even without the auditory cues of the stethoscope. This will help you develop a sense of how fast it is beating. You'll be able to compare the magnitude of the stressors in your environment to the rate of your heart to determine whether the two are commensurate. You should find that your heart is beating in a way that is out of proportion with most experiences. Unless you are having lots of fun or getting lots of exercise, you can allow your heart to beat as slowly as possible.

You can use breath-holds, like those in Exercise 11.5, to accentuate the sensations coming from your heart. Studies show that meditative breath holding makes participants more aware of their heartbeat and helps them calm the sympathetic nervous system's reaction to it by activating the vagus nerve.[7]

The more time you spend listening, the more you will ask yourself, "There is nothing here for me to be afraid of, so why does it hurt and why is it beating so fast?" This is the magic question, and if interrogated enough, you will have an emotional epiphany that only this experience can provide. Repeatedly inhaling smoothly through several heartbeats in a row, then exhaling through several in a row teaches the heart, and your psyche, to let go of trauma. I recommend performing diaphragmatic breathing for at least five minutes every night before bed with your stethoscope on. I find this helps me fall into a deep, restful sleep.

To Overcome Rapid Heartbeat, You Must Overcome Fear of Death

"Think of the life you have lived until now as over and, as a dead man, see what's left as a bonus and live it according to Nature. Love the hand that fate deals you and play it as your own, for what could be more fitting?" – Marcus Aurelius (121-180)

Interoceptive exposure to your own heart can be dreadful. In attending it, you will come face to face with your instinctual fear of death. Fear of dying perpetuates much of your heart's unnecessary exertion. The way to escape this situation is to reach full peace with the idea of dying. Do it now. "Die before you die." Then, you will have already done it and won't have to spend a lifetime in fear of it. The pain in your heart, warning you of impending death, will no longer be informative.

Meditate on your mortality. Take the time now and convince yourself that you have had a good life, that you have done many worthwhile things, and if you were to have a fatal heart attack this instant, you would still feel whole, complete, and satisfied with your time on the planet. In Hinduism, it is common to look forward to death, and the liberation it brings is known as moksha. Death is thought to release us from our mundane, mortal minds and introduce us to our permanent essence. Moksha and the concepts in the next activity helped me come to grips with my own eventual demise.

Interoception Activity #22.1: *Embrace Your Eternal Nature*

I have recently found some consolation in the idea of the eternal moment, and I hope you can too. Modern theoretical physicists as well as philosophers differentiate between presentism and eternalism. The adherents of presentism see the present moment as the only time that is real. They figure that if something happened in the past, it is over, now nonexistent, and generally unrecoverable. Eternalists, on the other hand, believe that all moments in time are equally real. Eternalists believe that there is no objective present, and that our subjective sense that the past is gone and irretrievable is illusory. I prefer eternalism.

Eternalism is sometimes referred to as the "block universe" theory because of its description of space-time as an unchanging four-dimensional block. If you apply this to the human condition, it tells us that all existence in time is equally valid. Therefore, if you existed at all, you will always exist. In other words, time is a dimension that our experience is embedded within, but if you could move outside of time and look down on it, you could see the entire timeline and all of your human existence, any second of which is just as legitimate as any other. So, every one of the moments you ever experienced, every decision, and every

---

thought may be eternal, happening right "now," and recorded somewhere in an immutable temporal continuum. This may all sound pretty abstract, but why not let it give you some comfort, if not let it make you feel immortal.

Allow me some poetic license for the next two paragraphs.

We don't fear or mourn the 13 billion years of nonexistence before our birth. Why should we fear the trillions of years that will come after our death? We shouldn't, especially because "we" will continue on in a different form. As denizens of planet Earth, we are part of the universe. In a very real sense, our conscious minds are manifestations of the universe experiencing itself. After we die, the universe doesn't die. And so, we should recognize our larger identity: that we are not only intertwined with all of reality, but we are all of reality. There will be an end to our human story and our mortal melodrama. However, death is not final. We are recycled back into the biosphere, resubsumed by the cosmos. The matter and energy that was us will be (and already has been) transformed into other things. Things that will inevitably interact with the repercussions of the good deeds we performed while alive.

Every atom that has ever been a part of you, every molecule you have eaten, drank, or inhaled belongs to a larger, more beautiful system. Even the nonmaterial information in your brain, body, and DNA belongs to this system. Your cerebral cortex will decompose. But we don't need the autobiographical memories inscribed in our brain's neural networks to persist meaningfully. You are not merely the character that you have played in your short lifetime. Like a person reading an engrossing novel, don't get so wrapped up in your life's narrative that you forget your larger role, your more permanent selfhood. We are much more than a bag of bones, flesh, and ego. Think of death as an expansion of your sense of being. In playing a part in the macrocosm, we are it. We are other people, we are the birds, bees, and black holes. You won't fear death if you're aware of your larger, eternal identity.

I was dragged around by a large Rottweiler as a four-year-old. The dog grabbed me by the hood of my jacket and pulled me around a backyard forcefully for a few minutes. I believe the dog assaulted me because I didn't act afraid of it. While the dog was dragging me, I realized that I might die or be badly hurt. I felt that if I surrendered, it might let up. Because I was cringing and my heart was racing, my body language caused the dog to sense that I submitted and that it won. It stopped shortly thereafter. It is common for dogs to stop attacking people that fully capitulate. Frightful situations like this one impel an archetype deep in our nervous system: "Full submission can save me from death."

The ultimate source of submissiveness is that we feel the need to display fear of physical attack so that our attacker will decide to be merciful. We are afraid that if our heart stays slow and calm, our persecutor will kill us for our insolence. This is because when our heart speeds up, we involuntarily choke up, tremble, and give numerous other nonverbal signals of submission.

We must renounce the belief that submissive fear will buy us leniency. To do so, imagine being viciously attacked by a stranger or a predator. Neither panic nor submit. Simply imagine yourself swiftly but calmly, taking the steps needed to extract yourself from the danger. Imagine someone or something trying to kill you while you retain total peace. Your tormentor is stabbing you, and you speak to them plainly and honestly while forcefully grabbing the wrist that holds the knife. The beasts are taking bites from your body, and you deftly deliver carefully placed blows to their noses. Your attitude need not be defiant or combative. It must simply be valorous and lionhearted. Right now, commit to dying fearlessly.

Chronic accelerated heart rate is a state of vigilance guarding against impending death. But we generalize this to everyday life by resorting to high resting heart rates with our bosses, friends, and family. We are living as if we are about to die. Using the stethoscope, you are feeling the very essence of your apologetic submissiveness. Know that your racing heart is not helping to keep you alive. Rather, it is keeping you in the land of no tomorrow. Surrendering your cardiac unrest will extract you from a world of death, struggle for survival, and animals ravaging and annihilating each other.

The next time you feel your heart beating out of your chest, focus on it. Accept it, befriend it, love it. It is not there to hurt you. It is literally giving you energy and power. Within a few moments, you can transform that throbbing feeling of impending doom into motivation. People with anxiety tend to be afraid of the sensations involved in stress. Don't let adrenaline scare you. Desensitize yourself to the discomfort by not overreacting to it, as you did in Exercise 5.2. Learn to delight in it and feel comfortable in uncomfortable physiological states. Rather than being afraid of the energy, think about how you are going to channel it.

Vigorous exercise can raise your heart rate to around its maximum. But when you exercise vigorously, you don't feel crushed by panic. Instead, you feel vitalized. It feels normal for your heart to speed up during exercise. But when your heart speeds up in the absence of exercise, you become afraid. When this happens, tell yourself that your body preparing for exercise is nothing to fear. The more you exercise, the more comfortable you become with the sensations involved in rapid heart rate. Keep in mind that athletes have lower resting heart rates, often as low as 30 to 40 beats per minute. Consistently training the heart muscle causes it to push more blood out with each beat meaning that it does not need to beat as often. The more exercise you get, the slower your heart will beat.

Take the warrior approach to panic. Luxuriate in the thumping. Instead of causing you to withdraw in resignation, the beating should make you approach in ascendency. As discussed in the last chapter, appraise it as rising to a challenge rather than descending to a threat. Afterward, if you need to, take a run around the neighborhood to burn up any remaining negative energy.

Vagal Tone is a Measure of Calm

This section and the next will introduce two more medical concepts, vagal tone and HRV. They add detail to the present discussion and highlight the physiological benefits of paced breathing.

Vagal tone is a measure of the activity of your vagus nerve, the nerve responsible for calming you. The vagus nerve transmits a relaxing signal from the brainstem's medulla oblongata to much of your body. This large, diffuse cluster of nerves branches out from the brainstem down to the bladder, affecting several organ systems along the way.[8] It affects the heart, spleen, bronchioles, lungs, stomach, pancreas, liver, gall bladder, intestines, ureters, and more.

The vagus nerve also connects the head's brain with the gut's brain and the heart's brain. It calms them. Its name comes from the Latin word "vagus," meaning "vagrant" or "wanderer," because it is so long and has so many branches. The activity of this nerve, calming multiple organ systems, is called vagal tone. High vagal tone is associated with autonomic balance, emotional stability, lowered inflammation, and better cardiovascular health. Low vagal tone causes the opposite.

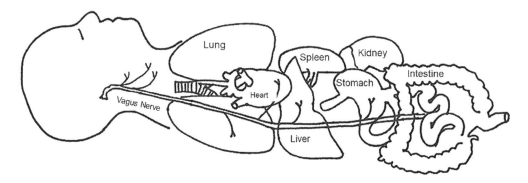

Illustration 22.2: Path of the vagus nerve from brain to intestines.

Interoception Exercise #22.2: *Compressing the Internal Organs*

Lay over a large, firm ball and press it gently into your stomach. A soccer ball, volleyball or basketball work well. You can do this lying on the floor or in bed. The easiest way is to stand or kneel by the corner of a bed. Place the basketball on that corner of the mattress and drape the upper half of your body over it. Either way, you want to have good control of how deeply you press the ball into your abdominal cavity. It is important to be stable and comfortable.

You should also try using your fingers to press into your abdomen. Situate your hands as in the illustration below. Press your fingertips into your belly, especially the area around the belly button. Anywhere that burns lightly should be massaged. Compress, release, repeat. You do not want to do any damage to your internal organs. You can use static compression or active percussion, but either way, press carefully. This is much slower, firmer, and deeper than the abdominal percussion from Exercise 20.6.

Many athletic coaches and trainers recommend a similar "gut smash" technique to mobilize the abdominal muscles. Some massage therapists call it visceral manipulation. People are using it safely. However, this technique, like many of those in this book, has not been tested on large populations in medical studies. A certain proportion of people may seriously injure themselves using it. Again, as with all Program Peace exercises, you should discontinue and seek medical counsel if you have any discomfort after performing the exercise.

The discomfort that this causes in your stomach may be intense at first. Proceed gently and focus on applying firm pressure to the abdomen from the bottom of the ribs to the pelvis. Pressure applied around the lower ribs will also help you manipulate the diaphragm. You should notice that the tension in your stomach will not give in to the massage unless you are breathing slow, smooth breaths. When it does, it should feel warm, pleasurable, and relieving (almost like voiding a full bladder). Relax, pace your breaths, and use abdominal compression to unwind the vice clenching your innards.

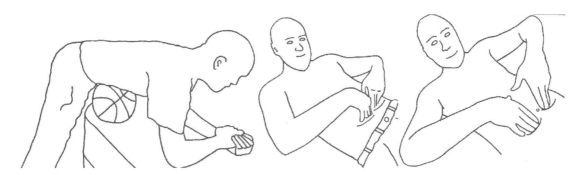

Illustration 22.2: Visceral massage gently reaches into and compresses internal organs.

Mammals have a unique branch of the vagus nerve that supports social engagement. It connects with the larynx to modulate your tone of voice and with the head to make facial expressions emotionally appropriate. When active, your vagus nerve makes your voice and face friendly and approachable.[9] When it is at its most active your voice relaxes and you may notice an improved ability to use melody and prosody. When the vagus nerve is active, we enjoy a physiological state that supports spontaneous social engagement and intimacy. We feel outgoing rather than introverted and vibrant without being overly aroused. As you might have guessed, the vagus nerve is a pivotal component of the parasympathetic system and is largely responsible for lowering heart rate, breathing rate, and blood pressure. Vagal tone decreases heart rate by inhibiting the firing rate of the sinoatrial node (the heart's pacemaker). Vagal tone also acts through the phrenic nerve to slow and smoothen the strokes of the diaphragm. When it is active you stop bracing, stop feeling the need to send submissive displays, and regain your composure.

Low vagal tone makes you feel irritated and restless. Vagal tone is reduced when the amygdala sounds its alarms. Many people who live lonely lives also have shorter lives. This may be because loneliness is associated with chronic low vagal tone. High vagal tone is the calm, pleasurable feeling you get when petting an animal, taking care of small children, or looking after a loved one. High vagal tone is correlated with purpose, love, friendliness, compassion, affection, and tenderness. If you have felt these things before, then you know exactly what vagal tone feels like. Imagine that you can feel this branching structure inside you, descending from your emotional brain down to your heart, gut, and diaphragm. You want it to feel warm and fuzzy as often as possible. Allow this feeling to help you debrace.

Vagal tone decreases with distressed breathing and increases with diaphragmatic breathing. Slow, deep breathing is one of the best ways to stimulate the vagus.[10] A range of biometric responses indicates this. For instance, diaphragmatic breathing elevates hand temperature, reduces electro-dermal response, reduces high-frequency beta brainwaves, and increases calming alpha brainwaves.[11] It also increases heart rate variability, which is our next topic.

Heart Rate Variability (HRV)

Want to know your level of vagal tone? Unfortunately, directly measuring vagal tone requires inserting electrodes into the nerve to test its level of activity. Since that requires invasive surgery, scientists indirectly, but accurately, measure vagal tone using the body's ability to synchronize heart rate and breathing. This is known as heart rate variability, or HRV.

The concept of HRV, along with its relationship to health and relaxation, is strongly scientifically supported[12] and it has become prevalent in stress reduction and self-improvement circles. The idea is that during negative emotions, the heart's rhythm is erratic and disordered, resulting in low HRV. During positive emotion, the heart's rate increases slightly during inhalation and decreases during exhalation. This equates to high HRV. Many psychophysiologists call this ordered pattern "coherence."

Heart rate variability is used as an index to measure autonomic imbalance due to trauma.[13] When high, it is considered a marker of stress resilience.[14] Vagal and HRV dysregulation are among the main clinical features of complex traumatic syndromes following early-life relationship trauma.[15] Calm infants have high vagal tone and high HRV. They tend to be less irritable than other infants and have a secure attachment to their mothers. Children with high vagal tone and high HRV have less social inhibition, improved mental health, and better emotional regulation.

Having a higher HRV is associated with a healthier cardiovascular system, improved executive brain function, decreased stress, increased immune function, improved mood, and overall greater health and longevity.[16] HRV declines with age and predicts future health problems.[17] People with relatively low HRV are less likely to recover after a heart attack.[18] Low HRV amplitude correlates with a highly elevated risk of sudden cardiac death, coronary heart disease, and mortality from a range of causes.

There are accepted ways to raise your vagal tone and HRV. First, stop obsessing and ruminating about negative things. Studies have found that daily worry is strongly associated with low HRV.[19] Science also recognizes that you can increase HRV by focusing on happy thoughts, deliberately curtailing anger, and exercising regularly. But there is another way.

You can increase your HRV through biofeedback. To do this, you can purchase a pulse sensor and the accompanying software for your computer or mobile device. The application shows your heart rate variability and positively reinforces you for bringing it into coherence. This HRV biofeedback has been shown to decrease depression, anxiety, and stress.[20] Take a guess at how these electronic devices coach you to raise your HRV. They do it by providing you with a breath metronome. Breathing deeply at long intervals is effective at increasing HRV. I want to encourage you to look into them, but you probably don't need to buy an HRV biofeedback device. I believe that the paced breathing regimen set out in this book can dramatically improve your HRV.

Many scientists believe that heart rate variability is maximized at around five breaths per minute (i.e., five-second inhalations and seven-second exhalations).[21] Breathing deeply at this rate allows your heart rate to drop 10 to 20 beats per minute at the end of every exhalation. This drop in heart rate during exhalation gives your heart the microbreak it needs to regenerate properly and beat sustainably. Breathing shallowly at something like 15 breaths per minute decreases HRV by keeping your heart rate from dropping with every exhalation, sacrificing the critical rest period.

Bracing the diaphragm during the exhalation may also cause us to miss that rest period. Breathing Exercise 5.1 asks you to allow your diaphragm to go limp throughout each exhalation. After you do the work of inflating your lungs, the air pressure itself should do the work of deflating them. I believe that allowing your lungs to deflate passively during exhalation may not only give your breathing muscles a short respite, but may also allow your heart to slow down during the exhale, increasing HRV.

The relaxing effects of paced breathing on the heart are also seen in blood pressure. Several experimental studies have published results showing blood pressure to be reduced when participants breathe at a rate of six breaths per minute, with the exhalations longer than the inhalations. In one study, paced breathing for merely 15 minutes resulted in elevated mood, higher HRV, and lower blood pressure.[22] Another study had patients perform paced breathing twice a day for three months. They experienced significant drops in blood pressure that would be expected in an individual taking one or two blood pressure medications.[23]

Don't drive your heart like it's a car that you stole. Stop redlining, downshift, and put less wear and tear on the vehicle.

Conclusion

The commotion of distressed breathing causes so many sensations within your chest that it completely obscures your heartbeat. If you can't feel the pain in your heart, you can't correct its overreactions, and they will continue to mount. When you are ignoring the pounding in your chest, your body is going to assume that this is because your current situation is so desperate. Like running on a broken leg, this should only happen during life-or-death situations, never on a daily basis.

Paced diaphragmatic breathing is so smooth and quiet that it allows you to feel your heart beating in your chest. In other words, long, deep breaths make your heart rate apparent to you so that you can tell whether it is beating too fast and make the necessary corrections. Of course, paced breathing with a stethoscope magnifies this even more. Find the pleasure in slow breathing, find the bliss in a slow heartbeat, and find the combination of the two as nourishment.

Chapter 22: **Bullet Points**

- Interoception is the ability to perceive the sensations going on within your body. Developing interoception will allow you to learn how to unbrace your internal organs.
- Preexisting tension in your abdomen combined with stress causes that sinking feeling in the pit of your stomach.
- Compressing your abdomen with a basketball will relieve this tension and make you immune to gut-wrenching episodes.
- Your heart chronically beats too fast, causing cumulative damage to it.
- If you listen to your heart with a stethoscope, you should be able to sense that it is beating too fast and out of proportion with environmental demands.
- Listening to your heart with a stethoscope while paced breathing provides a form of relief that you cannot get anywhere else.
- As you do this, imagine breathing into and out of your heart.
- Paced diaphragmatic breathing causes your heart to slow, your vagal tone and HRV to increase, and your blood pressure to decrease.
- Tell yourself that you are the kind of person whose heart beats slowly.
- Your thought process is playing a game of table tennis with your diaphragm. Your heart is the ping pong ball. Each time the ball strikes a paddle, you have a heartbeat. Right now, they are playing at a furious pace and none of the players are enjoying themselves. You want to slow them down. You want them to be lobbing the ball to each other, keeping an easy volley going, and having a fun, non-competitive game.

Chapter 22: **Endnotes**

1.   Schwartz, M. S., & Andrasik, F. (Eds.). (2003). *Biofeedback: A practitioner's guide* (3rd ed.). Guilford Press.

2.   Whatmore, G. B., & Kohli, D. R. (1968). Dysponesis: A neurophysiological factor in functional disorders. *Systems Research and Behavioral Science*, *13*(2), 102–124.

3.   Longo, D., Fauci, A., Kasper, D., Hauser, S., Jameson, J., & Loscalzo, J. (2011). *Harrison's principles of internal medicine* (18th ed.). McGraw-Hill Professional.

4.   Ostchega, Y., Porter, K. S., Hughes, J., Dillon, C. F., & Nwankwo, T. (2011). Resting pulse rate reference data for children, adolescents and adults, United States 1999–2008. *National Health Statistics Reports*, *41*, 1–16.

5.   Miller, M. A. (2011). Association of inflammatory markers with cardiovascular risk and sleepiness. *Journal of Clinical Sleep Medicine*, *7*(5 Suppl.), S31–33.

6.   Clark, A. L. (1997). The increased ventilator response to exercise in chronic heart failure: Relation to pulmonary pathology. *Heart*, *77*(2), 138–146; Fanfulla, F., Mortara, A., Maestri, R., Pinna, G. D., Bruschi, C., Cobelli, F., & Rampulla, C. (1998). The development of hyperventilation in patients with chronic heart failure and Cheyne-Strokes respiration: A possible role of chronic hypoxia. *Chest*, *114*(4), 1083–1090.

7.   McKeown, P. (2015). *The oxygen advantage: The simple, scientifically proven breathing technique that will revolutionize your health and fitness*. Harper Collins.

8.   Porges, S. W., Doussard-Roosevelt, J. A., & Maiti, A. K. (2008). Vagal tone and the physiological regulation of emotion. *Monographs of the Society for Research in Child Development*, *59*(2-3), 167–186.

9.   Porges, S. W. (2001). The polyvagal theory: Phylogenetic substrates of a social nervous system. *International Journal of Psychophysiology*, *42*(2), 123–146.

10. Lichstein, K. L. (1988). *Clinical relaxation strategies*. Wiley-Interscience.

11. Elliott, S., & Edmonson, E. (2006). *The new science of breath: Coherent breathing for autonomic nervous system balance, health, and well-being*. Coherence Press.

12. Jonsson, P. (2007). Respiratory sinus arrhythmia as a function of state anxiety in healthy individuals. *International Journal of Psychophysiology*, *63*(1), 48–54.

13. Thayer, J. F., & Brosschot, J. F. (2005). Psychosomatics and psychopathology: Looking up and down from the brain. *Psychoneuroendocrinology, 30*(10), 1050–1058.

14. Appelhans, B. M., & Luecken, L. J. (2006). Heart rate variability as an index of regulated emotional responding. *Review of General Psychology, 10,* 229–240.

15. van der Kolk, B. A., Pelcovitz, D., Roth, S., Mandel, R. S., McFarlane, A., & Herman, J. L. (1996). Dissociation, somatization and affect dysregulation: The complexity of adaptation of trauma. *American Journal of Psychiatry, 153*(7 Suppl.), 83–93.

16. Luskin, F., Reitz, M., Newell, K., Quinn, T. G., & Haskell, W. (2002). A controlled piolet study of stress management training of elderly patients with congestive heart failure. *Preventive Cardiology, 5*(4), 168–174; McCraty, R., Atkinson, M., & Thomasino, D. (2003). Impact of a workplace stress reduction program on blood pressure and emotional health in hypertensive employees. *Journal of Alternative and Complementary Medicine, 9*(3), 355–369.

17. Zulfiqar, U. I., Jurivich, D. A., Gao, W., & Singer, D. H. (2010). Relation of high heart rate variability to health and longevity. *American Journal of Cardiology, 105*(8), 1181–1185.

18. Kristal-Boneh, E., Raifel, M., Froom, P., & Ribak, J. (1995). Heart rate variability in health and disease. *Scandinavian Journal of Work, Environment, and Health, 21*(2), 85–95.

19. Brosschot, J. F., Van Dijk, E., & Thayer, J. F. (2007). Daily worry is related to low heart rate variability during waking and the subsequent nocturnal sleep period. *International Journal of Psychophysiology, 63*(1), 39–47.

20. Sutarto, A. P., Wahab, M. N. & Zin, N. M. (2012). Resonant breathing biofeedback training for stress reduction among manufacturing operators. *International Journal of Occupational Safety and Ergononics, 18*(4), 549–61.

21. Elliott, S., & Edmonson, E. (2006). *The new science of breath: Coherent breathing for autonomic nervous system balance, health, and well-being.* Coherence Press.

22. Steffen, P. R., Austin, T., DeBarros, A., & Brown, T. (2017). The impact of resonance frequency breathing on measures of heart rate variability, blood pressure, and mood. *Frontiers in Public Health, 5,* 222.

23. Adhana, R., Gupta, R., Dvivedii, J., & Ahmad, S. (2013). The influence of 2:1 yogic breathing technique on essential hypertension. *Indian Journal of Physiology and Pharmacology, 57*(1), 38–44.

Chapter 23: **Serotonin, Optimism, and Cooperation**

"There is something at once sobering and absurd in the extent to which we are lifted by the attentions of others and sunk by their disregard." — Alain de Botton (1969)

Competition, Defeat, and Brain Chemicals

For the last 60 million years, the dominance hierarchy has been the primary regulator of primate life. This requires monkeys and apes to spend a great deal of their mental energy making estimates about how they stack up relative to each member of their group. But how do animals reliably make these sorting predictions? As this chapter will explain, it has much to do with fluctuations in brain chemicals, especially serotonin. Animals that win fights or spats increase their serotonin levels while losing animals lower those levels.

In all of us, serotonin contributes to feelings of wellbeing, happiness, relaxation, and self-confidence. It increases the expectation of social dominance and causes animals to stand up for themselves. When humans or primates take supplements that increase serotonin, they have reduced stress responses to external threats such as pictures of fearful and angry faces. There is reduced serotonin production in panic disorder, generalized anxiety disorder, and depression. In simple terms, low serotonin causes the trivialities of life to terrorize us.

In adult primates, serotonin levels are more causally related to dominance than body size or testosterone levels.[1] In fact, dominant male monkeys have up to twice as much serotonin in their blood as non-dominant ones. Similarly, humans in leadership positions have higher serotonin levels than their subordinates.[2] One study found that fraternity officers average 25% higher serotonin levels than other frat members. The same pattern is seen in the military, where higher-ranking officers have more serotonin, and in corporate America, where higher-ranking employees have more and executives and CEOs have the most.

When a dominant primate is overthrown, usually after a fight, its serotonin levels plunge while the replacement's surges. During most exchanges between people, there are few overt hostilities. Covert factors such as level of relaxation and verbal fluency determine each person's relative status. If you come across as tenser than the other person, chances are you both perceive this. After the encounter, your serotonin may lower while theirs rises. Being snubbed or getting negative feedback causes serotonin to drop as does becoming aggressive or angry. On the other hand, successful social assertion results in the release of serotonin.

Every primate in a troop knows its status relative to every other animal, just as high school students give remarkably consistent rankings for the popularity of their classmates.[3] In other words, our brain's limbic system paints the world as one big popularity contest. Whether you think others perceive you as having high status is the decisive factor influencing your serotonin level. In other words, if you believe others hold you in low regard, your serotonin may stay low. Because our brains are wired to derive self-worth from others' evaluations, we need to push back against our biology.

Many social insect species are born into a caste, either the aristocracy or the working class. However, a mammal is constantly negotiating its status. Do you want to be renegotiating your rank every day for the rest of your life? If not, you will have to change your mindset. You need to develop a healthy sense of self-esteem that others cannot push around, but also that doesn't involve putting others down or even putting yourself above them. What would it take for you to have optimal self-esteem? Let's explore that in the next activity.

Serotonin Activity #23.1: *Imagine Extreme Superiority*

What would be needed for you to feel triumphant? How would you feel if you heroically saved the lives of every person on the planet and are now taking interviews on international television? Imagine that you have been the most charismatic person on earth your entire life and everyone already expects effortless magnetism from you. Imagine being the world's most famous superstar or the emperor of the galaxy. Imagine being the undisputed boss gorilla in a jungle full of tiny monkey friends. Imagine being thousands of years old, the oldest soul, and the wisest, most centered person on the planet.

Now, imagine not being corrupted by this absolute power and being a calm, measured, beneficent leader and protector. How would all this influence you to hold your body and face? How would your bracing and posture be affected? How would you breathe? How would it make you feel deep down in your gut and heart? Inner peace at last? Can you live your life feeling this way without needing these outlandish scenarios? You can.

Serotonin and the Ego

"For all those who exalt themselves will be humbled, all those who humble themselves will be exalted."
— Jesus (c. 6 BCE – 30)

The human ego is a specialized neurological system found in all primate brains that causes us to analyze whether we should be more or less insecure and, consequently, whether our serotonin should be lower or higher. The monkey that thinks more about their place in the hierarchy has more objective notions about their station and the social appropriateness of their actions. Consequently, a monkey that is highly concerned with its ego may do well relative to the other members of its troop. Hence, the ego is sometimes referred to as the "monkey mind."

In primates, serotonin level is also a fertility indicator. The most dominant males have the most offspring. Individuals that excel in status-seeking contribute more to the gene pool. Thus, we are self-conscious and ego-obsessed today because it was good for our ancestors' reproductive success. But as modern-day human beings, we are not looking to maximize our number of offspring or even our sexual partners. What we really want is to be happy without being controlled by our egos. So again, we are at odds with our biology.

The egotistical thoughts that you experience are not you, and you have little control over them. Realize that the negative, conceited thinking going on in your head likely has nothing to do with your aspirational self, your true self. These thoughts that you think are "yours" are generated by your brain's instincts to be endlessly competitive. The social concerns you find yourself ruminating about come from this monkey mind and the way it has been programmed by the other monkey minds you have interacted with up until today. The real you is not concerned with reputation and comparison. The real you, who is now gradually taking over your thinking process, is not even interested.

Because this instinct is so strong, status is most people's ultimate goal. This means that they have no overarching ambition in life other than to increase their sense of status relative to the people around them. Once you see this clearly, you can become motivated to choose goals other than the one that natural history selected for us. To disconnect from your ego, you must stop feeding it. Make your goal to starve it in the following exercise.

Serotonin Activity #23.2: Imagine Extreme Inferiority

Imagine being the weakest, most poorly composed person on the planet. Imagine that you have been utterly rejected by your parents, every friend, and each romantic partner. Imagine that people have been turning away from you in disgust as soon as they see you for years. Imagine that you have been jumped and beaten by a gang of people more than a dozen times. Imagine that you were completely embarrassed in the most humiliating way possible on a popular reality show and that it is now all over the Internet. Imagine having a job in which the patrons or clients treat you in a haughty and cavalier way. Imagine constantly being treated like you are less than a person.

At the same time, imagine being at complete peace with all of this. Picture being a servant without a chip on your shoulder, a whipping boy with optimal posture, or a mistreated but ever-cheerful golden retriever. Put yourself through the fire by imagining the most denigrating scenarios you can and, in so doing, inure your psyche against even the harshest flames. Retain complete cool in these situations without letting them ignite your pain.

In Activity 23.1, I asked you to pretend to be superior to everyone, and then in activity 23.2 I asked you to be inferior. Surely, we are neither. But we can intentionally take the best aspects but none of the negative aspects out of these two extreme scenarios (see Table 23.1 below). Unfortunately, many people take the worst from both scenarios and develop a personality as pernicious to themselves as others. They can neither take criticism nor compliments well. They are boastful but also engage in abusive self-talk. They love to argue with and gossip about others but can't stand up for themselves when it counts. They apologize when they shouldn't and often don't apologize when they should. Rising above this kind of behavior is as easy as accepting your shortcomings and being comfortable and calm when confronted with them.

	Best Attributes	Worst Attributes
Dominant	Self-satisfied, confident, assured, assertive, effective, powerful, honored, content, spirited, stately, self-respecting, valiant, calm, courageous	Self-absorbed, pompous, vain, egotistical, bossy, domineering, despotic, privileged, scornful, imperious, contemptuous, arrogant, snooty, pretentious
Inferior	Humble, easy-going, respectful, nonresistant, meek, accommodating, amenable, ingratiating, patient, modest, uncomplaining, unselfish	Wimpy, resigned, acquiescent, deferential, obedient, passive, compliant, pliable, servile, cowardly, doubtful, unsure, shy, timid, pessimistic, rootless, fearful

Table 23.1: Take only the best attributes of dominance and submission.

Our Brains Ration Serotonin

If animals are self-interested survival machines, then why don't their brains maximize serotonin production? It would undoubtedly be a simple adaptation. Animals have not evolved to do this because it would be dangerous to be a non-dominant animal with a dominant mindset. If you are an animal losing a fight, it is actually beneficial to lower your serotonin because it makes you act submissive, shielding you from further harm and retaliation. When researchers artificially raise serotonin in a non-dominant ape, it will act dominant. Merely acting dominant convinces the other monkeys that it is dominant, but only for a few days. Before long, it will be tested, exposed as a pretender, and likely injured in the process.

Your mammalian brain does not release serotonin and other mood-boosting chemicals (dopamine, oxytocin, and endorphins) whenever you want. It uses them to reward you for accomplishing specific survival criteria. It releases them in spurts when unconscious brain circuits perceive an improvement in survival and reproductive prospects. Most people are frustrated by their inability to fulfill the stringent requirements used by their neurochemical guidance system. Frustratingly, the criteria for attaining happiness chemicals are usually held just beyond our reach, making it nearly impossible to win and thus impossible to be happy. This is why using our cortex to try to pry serotonin from our subcortex (limbic system) often leads to self-destructive status-seeking.

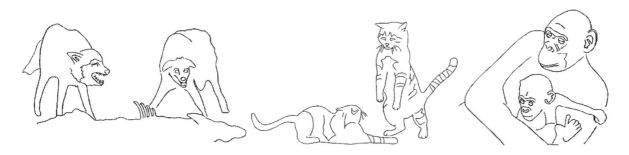

Illustration 23.1: A. One wolf (left) asserting dominance over another (right) with a threat display. Note that the teeth are bared, the ears are flattened forward, and the hackles are raised. The submissive wolf lowers its head, presses its ears backward, splays its legs, and turns away to appease the dominant individual; B. Similar body language is seen in cats; C. A mother chimp protects her baby.

A signal that is constantly on has no informational value. Consequently, our serotonin levels have evolved to fluctuate dramatically and subside quickly. Humans spend their entire day trying to boost their mood from a brain trying to ration the relevant chemicals for the proper circumstances. To transcend this, we need to choose to feel satisfied with precisely the amount of social power we already have. By being fully content with whatever level of dominance you currently have, you give your unconscious the same level of security that comes with being an alpha. When other people see this healthy, non-dominating self-satisfaction, they will instantly respect you.

Changing your outlook on your wins and losses is essential. Otherwise, no number of victories will satisfy your serotonin system for long. Take pleasure in past accomplishments, no matter how old. Think about all the hard work you have put in over your life and feel good about it. Focus your attention on the small triumphs you have every day. Once you learn to celebrate each win for a bit longer, you will not find yourself hurried into the next risky scheme for serotonin. Rather than focusing on the most shameful or embarrassing moments, concentrate on the laurels that stick out in your mind. We need to take responsibility for coaxing our brain's happiness chemicals to change rather than waiting on the world to change.

Serotonin, Abundance, and Gratitude

"...all things work together for good..." — Romans 8:28

Low serotonin promotes fear, fleeing, and submission in many animals, from reptiles to insects. Even crustaceans such as lobsters utilize serotonin to establish hierarchy. We share a common ancestor with lobsters over 500 million years ago. This shows how ancient our status system is. In fact, it goes back to worms.

In the microscopic roundworm, C. *elegans*, serotonin acts as a signal that follows the discovery of a new grazing area. When the worm finds food, serotonin acts to slow down its incessant burrowing and activates the muscles used for feeding. Depletion of serotonin in these little guys makes them act as if they were in a low-food environment and causes them to travel faster in their search for food. It also suppresses mating and egg-laying. Across species, depletion of serotonin convinces animals that they are experiencing food scarcity. This action of serotonin caused scientists to reframe its purpose more broadly. It is now conceptualized as an indicator of the availability of natural resources.

We have discussed how serotonin indicates social rank in primates, but rank is just a special case of serotonin's broader significance: resources. High-ranking primates have high serotonin levels because they have priority over mating and food. Just as with the worm, serotonin convinces them that it is okay to relax and take advantage of the opportunities available to them. In a sense, primates are just hairy, four-legged worms whose social lives have grown more complex. Self-subordination is just the strategy of a worm that has become convinced that resource availability is low in the current environment.

This knowledge enables us to easily sidestep status as a means for attaining serotonin. Instead, we can go to the primordial root of serotonin release: feeling like the resources in our life are abundant. The magic button for increasing your serotonin and happiness does not lie in putting other people down. It is found in cultivating gratitude by focusing on the resources available to you.

Scientists have found that gratitude stimulates the brain's pathways involved in reward, social bonding, and positive appraisal.[4] It facilitates the recording and retrieval of positive memories.[5] Gratitude stimulates serotonin release, the parasympathetic response, and the actions of the vagus nerve. Feeling thankful counteracts tendencies toward social comparison, narcissism, cynicism, and materialism. Let's accomplish all of this by expressing gratefulness daily.

Serotonin Activity #23.3: *Practice Feeling Grateful*

What can you feel glad about right now? What about the last year, yesterday, or the present moment can you savor? Fill any sense of scarcity or deficit by changing your mindset from one of deprivation and neediness to one of abundance, fulfillment, and plenty. Reminisce about past achievements and cherish moments of joy and connectedness. Treasure your friends and family. Feel appreciative of everyone in your life. Imagine that you are a content microscopic worm with all its needs met and not a worry in the world.

Common gratitude-building exercises include thinking of one thing to be grateful for every day, writing a letter every week thanking someone who helped you, or simply using the word "grateful" during conversation once a day. Exercises like these are some of the most effective happiness enhancers known to psychology.[6] When you do this, permit yourself to feel enthusiastic, starry-eyed, and naively idealistic.

Keeping a gratitude journal has shown significant clinical benefits.[7] Simply writing down a few things that you are grateful for one to three times per week can raise serotonin, increase life satisfaction, and reduce depressive symptoms. Gratitude journaling has been well researched and validated far beyond anecdotal self-help.[8] Numerous studies have shown that journaling for just a few weeks can create dramatic positive changes in brain activity that remain for months. The clinical results have been shown to rival those of antidepressants. The scientific justification for focusing on gratitude is so strong that it encouraged the

Program Peace Gratitude Journal, which is available on the website. But you certainly don't need that to get started.

Serotonin Exercise #23.1: *Make Entries in a Gratitude Journal*

Locate a journal, find a pad of paper, or create a new file on your computer. Start making entries where you write about what you have to be grateful for. Here are some questions to get you started:

1) What can you feel thankful for right now? This could be an experience, a conversation, a meal, or the weather.
2) Has someone done something nice for you recently? List people you are grateful for and explain why.
3) What places are special to you?
4) What have you learned recently that you value?
5) What activities make your life better?
6) What fills you with wonder?
7) What do you have to be optimistic about?
8) What have you accomplished recently that makes you proud?
9) Has someone done something nice for you recently? Have you had the opportunity to help someone else?
10) What are commonplace things you can appreciate right now?

As you write, allow the gratitude to permeate your body. Make an effort to remember what that feels like and how it affects the bodily systems we have been discussing in this book thus far. Remember this feeling, take a mental snapshot of it, so you can recall it whenever you want.

As a few examples, you may find yourself grateful for the earth, the moon, the stars, the sun, the ocean, rain, animals, pets, friends, your talents, skills, and unique qualities, setbacks that have made you stronger, your senses, fond memories, your favorite songs, movies or shows, foods, the marvel of electricity, the world's food supply, and all the kind souls out there. I feel especially grateful for the generations of people who made sacrifices for the rights and freedoms we enjoy today, as well as those who made the innovations that resulted in our modern technology and our extensive knowledge base.

Raise Your Serotonin through Cooperation and Creating Value

In primates, domination of others is not the only way up. Brute physical strength and fighting prowess are only partial factors in determining status relationships. Social bonds, friendships, past feats, and examples of helping others count as well. Most primates will support or even fight for those that helped them in the past. This is why an open conflict between two primates is usually decided by who has the most allies.

It is also important to note that dominance does not equal influence. The dominant ape is often not the most liked or even the most influential politically. Dominant primates have fighting prowess, boldness, and a characteristic that ecologists call "resource holding potential." But this does not necessarily make them trusted or revered. In fact, the oldest group members, not the alpha, are usually the most influential. Apes will approach influential members to moderate spats, make decisions, or seek comfort.

Dominant individuals are fit to be revered to the extent that they serve the interests of those that revere them. If you want to be justified in being calm and nonsubmissive, you must promote positivity in the lives of those that allow you to remain so. Thus, the next time you notice an urge to belittle someone, remember that bonding with them instead will provide a larger, more sustainable neurochemical boost to happiness and esteem.

Because our biological past also rewards camaraderie, teamwork, and solidarity with a boost of serotonin, there are many healthy ways to get an ego boost from others without bringing them down. It's our job to think creatively about positive ways to interact with others rather than being destructive.

It is usually the youngest and most immature of adult primates that are preoccupied with establishing dominance. Senior group members are less nervous greeting each other and are more concerned with confirming partnership and cooperation than securing dominance. We love people who cooperate, reinforce our confidence, and raise our status. Consequently, if you want to be loved and held in high regard, then work on raising other people's status in their own eyes as well as in the eyes of others. Offer valid and specific compliments, help them argue their point, align your goals with theirs, stand up for them, laugh at their jokes, and beam zygomatic smiles at them.

The higher a chimp's rank, the more likely it is to support inferior parties during disputes. High levels of serotonin cause us to have compassion for and side with the underdog. Dominant apes routinely break up fights, usually intervening on the side of the weaker party. They especially defend the young, the wounded, and the old. In many primates, the alpha male and female play a control role, where they mediate equitably, restoring peace and security. Interestingly, it has been found that the most dominant schoolchildren tend to intervene in playground fights, protect losers, and share more with classmates. It appears to be some form of natural noblesse oblige that we lose sight of as adults.

Monkeys choose to share with one another frequently, both in the wild and in captivity. However, they do not share out of fear of reprisal. We know this because the most dominant monkeys are the most generous, which is part of what earns them their increased status. The best way for low-status individuals to improve their status is to prove their value to the group. Similarly, humans gain status by developing a skill that benefits the community. This is why we should be useful rather than pretentious and entitled. Don't be the person working on their wardrobe, biceps, or tan. Instead, be the person people go to for help with their problems. Don't focus on status threats. Focus instead on expanding your influence and significance to your community. Gain status not from physicality, offensives, and violations, but collaboration, contribution, and earned esteem.

Serotonin Inhibits Fear and Aggression

Serotonin makes many animals from a range of different taxonomic groups less fearful in response to perceived threats. Much of this is due to its actions at the amygdala (the brain's fear center discussed in previous chapters). By default, the cells of the amygdala are quieted by the inhibitory neurotransmitter GABA. This makes it so that the brain's panic button must be pressed firmly for it to actuate. This inhibition has been called the "GABA guard." It is why something surprising must happen for you to become scared.

Serotonin further excites GABA-producing cells in the amygdala, increasing this tonic inhibition and increasing your threshold for getting scared. This is why antidepressants like Prozac, a drug that increases serotonin levels at the synapse, decreases amygdala activity. This is also one of the reasons dominant animals are not unnecessarily aggressive. Their amygdala and sympathetic system are difficult to highjack. The stress hormone, cortisol, acts in a way that is opposite serotonin. It inhibits GABA cells in the amygdala, disabling serotonin's ability to calm the amygdala.[9]

Keep in mind that not only is the amygdala the brain's fear center, but it is also the area most implicated in the initiation of aggressive acts. Thus, high-stress animals are more aggressive while animals with high serotonin levels are less aggressive. This is why, as discussed in Chapter 2, alpha individuals are not combative but friendly. The alpha chimp grooms others more, shares more of its food, and patrols the perimeter to keep its friends safe. As you might expect, artificially elevating the serotonin in a monkey's brain makes it groom and share more. It is more capable of prosocial behavior because its amygdala has been bound and gagged. To me, this strongly suggests that being stuck in fight or flight keeps us from acting altruistically and civil-mindedly.

When serotonin levels are low, animals show signs of being irritated.[10] The threshold for taking offense drops, and fatigue and crankiness rise. Low serotonin chimps pick fights and take unnecessary risks. For instance, monkeys with low serotonin are more likely to jump between distant tree branches and lash out in anger. Similarly, studies have shown that low-status men are much more likely to aggress by yelling, insulting, or using violence. While these behaviors are meant to increase dominance, they often lower status because they result in estrangement. When you find yourself being aggressive, acknowledge that you probably wouldn't be as threatened if your serotonin levels were higher.

Now you understand the neurological mechanism for why serotonin-depleted animals are more belligerent: their amygdala overreacts to anxiety-provoking stimuli, increasing their heart rate and breathing, making them feel cornered. Low serotonin is one of the best predictors of impulsive hostility in mammals.[11] Antisocial behavior in humans also increases with decreasing serotonin. This is why feeling rejected leads to aggression. I think the take-home message is clear. We should avoid destructive rank games. We should comport ourselves with the composure of an alpha monkey with nothing to prove, in the company of equals. Adopting this as a lifestyle may be the most successful strategy to achieve sustainable happiness.

The Healthy Dominance Mindset

"Never depend on the admiration of others. There is no strength in it. Personal merit cannot be derived from an external source." — Epictetus (50-135)

When a baboon ignores the status hierarchy, the members of its troop will kill it. Similarly, if you flout the status hierarchy, you could alienate yourself from others. Therefore, I don't recommend that you completely ignore or go against it. I do, however, recommend reinventing yourself as a cool-headed alpha. It all starts with a little imagination.

It can be helpful to internalize the mindset of being everyone's parent. Parents usually feel like they don't owe their kids submissive displays. Given that a healthy parents' dominance of their offspring is not based on competition, but on a desire to teach and guide, imagine yourself to be the Mom or Dad to every person in the world. I'm not asking you to patronize people. Just be as relaxed as you would be if everyone was your child and you were the only adult present.

You want to be a good parent, even to a bad child. In Japan, mothering has been described as "patiently molding the intractable." Children and infants can be inherently stubborn, but this is best countered by persistence and patience. Even mother chimps reprimand misbehavior without bearing any grudge. They offer reassurance and comfort after disciplining their young. They do this naturally. Use this philosophy with adults. Adults can be as tricky and immature as children, but rather than aggress against them, patiently mold them. Be a father or mother figure. Like a good parent, act permissive yet authoritative.

Just as a good parent doesn't owe their children submissive displays, neither does a warrior owe their fellows submissive displays. They are too busy either risking their life or resting. Take on the rugged exterior of a special forces commando, a mythical god, or a legendary hero. You have corrupt governments to topple and dragons to slay. You have no interest in minor squabbles and infractions. When you are with friends, envision yourself as a champion who has just bested a mythical monster, like the Minotaur, Jabberwock, Medusa, or Cerberus. Now that you, the gladiator, are resting between feats, you do not have the time or energy to raise your eyebrows, hyperventilate, or smile nervously. Feel free to rest between your heroic efforts. Given the chance, you would do the selfless, intrepid thing, so take the hero's poise and grace for yourself right now.

My Experience with Serotonin Supplements

"What man actually needs is not a tensionless state but rather the striving and struggling for some goal worthy of him." – Viktor Frankl (1905-1997)

I used to be clinically depressed. As a preteen, I cut myself with knives. As a young adult, I put a gun in my mouth on a few occasions. I sat on a 20-story rooftop ledge intending to jump a few times. I never followed through with suicide though. I would tell myself that I wanted to tie up a few more loose ends in my life before I fully committed. I know what serotonin depletion feels like and that a person is willing to do almost anything to escape it.

I have never been to a psychiatrist and thus have never been prescribed an antidepressant, but I have taken an over-the-counter nutritional supplement called SAM-e. It is similar to other mood enhancing supplements like 5-HTP, L-theanine, and Saint John's wort and is available at most drug stores. I took SAM-e for two months in my late 20s because I wanted to find out what high serotonin levels felt like. I wanted to experience happiness for a few weeks to understand it and attempt to recreate it later after going off the drug. Without question, it made me a joyous, more composed person...while it lasted.

Like an antidepressant (e.g., Prozac, Zoloft, Celexa, etc.), SAM-e increases serotonin availability at the synapse. In doing so, it also fortifies the GABA guard mentioned earlier, inhibiting the amygdala. It takes two weeks for SAM-e to elevate mood appreciably, but I felt that I noticed changes with the first few doses. I felt lighter on my feet, happy-go-lucky, and less stymied by social concerns. I completely stopped worrying that other people might think that I looked too calm.

After 14 days of taking it, I woke up in the middle of the night feeling euphoric. I had been slightly scared of the dark since childhood, but suddenly I felt completely safe in the dark. I walked through my home without turning on any lights. I found myself sitting on the carpet in the darkest places and reveling in my fearlessness. I stayed awake for three hours, just walking around outside in the shadows, feeling intensely happy. Interestingly, even a single course of antidepressants can end phobias, lifelong bad habits, negative quirks, and antisocial behaviors. Since that night, I have not been afraid of the dark.

That Wednesday night from 2 to 5 am was a vertiginous and ecstatic experience. Nothing remarkable happened, and I was all by myself, but it was the happiest night of my life. All my social status concerns disappeared, replaced by pure excitement for the things going on in my life at the time. I didn't realize it that night, but I was filled with pure gratitude.

I continued to take the drug for six weeks. On it, I was less abusive but more insistent and decisive. I was demanding of people but direct rather than passive-aggressive, so people complied. I would say exactly what was on my mind without sugarcoating it. People liked me more, respected me more, and treated me like I was charismatic. I was more personable, more outspoken, and I craved interaction instead of shrinking away from it.

While on SAM-e, I started making natural eye contact with people for the first time in my life. I even sought out eye contact. It came easily, and my eyes didn't dart away. I was more extroverted and started assuming leadership positions in group projects. People also started laughing at my attempts at humor, despite my jokes not changing. Confident delivery made all the difference.

When I was on SAM-e, I didn't talk or think negatively. Bad experiences were very short lived, and I didn't keep them active in my mind. I didn't trash talk others, even in my head. Most of my previous insecurities felt like faint memories. I felt like such a different person on SAM-e that at one point, I asked myself, "Why were you so afraid of your friends and coworkers before?"

I would take one pill in the morning and then come home in the evening needing another. Sometimes I would take one and then lie down on the couch and wait for it to kick in. As the stiffness in my brow, jaw, and sneer melted away I could feel the tension in my mind slowly evaporate. This was my first clear indication that facial tension, negative emotion, and serotonin all hold hands. But the relief was not just in my face. My whole body felt light and easy, as if all my trigger points had been excised. I wondered whether having increased serotonin levels had healed them.

Interestingly, serotonin increases the threshold of activation for latent trigger points. In so doing, it eases the chakra-like modules in the body, soothing you. Its role in muscular relaxation is why low serotonin is thought to be a major player in fatigue, headaches, gut tension, heart problems, muscle pain, joint pain, and diffuse discomfort. Now that I couldn't feel the tension,

I was less neurotic. For example, increased serotonin levels are also known to curb nightmares, panic attacks, and unhealthy eating, and I noticed these as additional side effects.

A couple of months passed by, and a fledgling business venture initiated with some acquaintances turned sour. So sour that I felt gutted. Within a month, my hairline receded by at least an inch. I realized that my underlying biological trauma had resurfaced from beneath the artificially elevated serotonin. I felt manic anxiety for hours on end and had significant trouble sleeping. I knew that mania was one of the listed side effects of SAM-e, and combined with my preexisting anxiety, it was unbearable. I went off the drug. As the mania went away, the depression crept back in, along with all the previous muscular tension. The experience showed me that serotonin does not fix or heal the brain. It just alters it temporarily. Similarly, it does not fix trigger points or heal chakras. It merely subdues them, allowing our behavior to be less affected. When I went off SAM-e, I noticed my body trembled. It was substantial, and I realized I had to do something about it.

Don't Let Yourself Tremble

In the last chapter, I mentioned a friend of mine who was a drug addict. She had a small kitten that she played roughly with. She would squeeze it, and tease it, and swing it around. Some aspects of this play were pleasant to watch at times, but other elements bordered on abuse. At one point, she asked whether I thought she played too roughly with it. The kitten's interminable trembling answered her question for me. With beautiful, pained eyes, this little furball was constantly glancing around skittishly. It shuddered even when standing still, startled at every sound, and grew into the most nervous cat I have ever seen. The truth is, the owner herself trembled and probably wanted her small friend to share her weakness.

Muscle trembling is a sign that an animal is under duress. It is related to the startle response discussed in Chapter 2 and similarly signals submission. It results in a shaking, quaking, and shuddering that makes us feel weak in the knees. Chronic distress and social defeat cause trembling to become more pronounced. It is quite common for the runt of the litter to tremble because it rarely wins in competitive play and often has the lowest serotonin of the group. Trembling destroys fluid, measured movement as well as timing and rhythm. It occurs all over the body, not just in the voice and hands. Dormant or partially contracted muscles frequently tremble because those muscles can neither relax nor fully contract, making them susceptible to shaking involuntarily between these extremes.

When a poorly-socialized Chihuahua is placed among bigger dogs, it tends to tremble more than usual. We are all shaky Chihuahuas, whether it is perceptible or not. Also, we tremble for the same reason: to keep others from being threatened by us. Trembling goes on in the background and usually becomes apparent under duress, by old age, or after a heavy workout. You may think you don't tremble but may notice it when performing small, fluid movements like knitting. This is why I urge you to spend time focusing your awareness on trembling in an attempt to "get ahold of yourself." Working out with light weights (Chapter 15) and performing anti-laxity while slow breathing will firm your grip.

The slower you move, the easier it is to iron out trembling, flinching, and startling. Moshé Feldenkrais, the founder of the Feldenkrais exercise method, propounded the idea that practicing slow movement is essential to grace and psychological wellbeing. This general philosophy dates back hundreds of years to Taoist and Buddhist monasteries and the art of tai chi. Tai chi is a superb practice that will smooth your movements and help you tremble less. Some forms encourage you to move mindfully, as a "needle in cotton," and develop the ability to leverage joints using coordination and relaxation rather than tension. I strongly encourage you to take a tai chi class, even if you do it from home using free internet tutorials.

Serotonin Exercise #23.2: Take a Class in Tai Chi

Sign up for a tai chi class, or simply follow a beginner's instructional tutorial video on the internet. Practice the movements and motions while trying to move as smoothly and gracefully as possible. Your motions should feel relaxed, fluid, frictionless, and occur at a constant rate. It can help to act as if there is a slight resistance to every movement as if you were in a pool of water. When you stop bracing, notice how you can move more steadily. Sense your body and be present within it.

You should be able to concentrate so deeply on even, tension-free movement that your stream of thought evaporates. To do this, you must activate very primitive brain structures. Every second of mindful "nontrembling" movement teaches them that slow, steady movement is safe and won't be misconstrued by others as an attempt at intimidation.

Remember that prey rush. Predators do not rush because they do not feel threatened or pressured. Move at an unrushed pace that is self-determined and centered on unshakable inner confidence. While you practice, use the tenets of diaphragmatic breathing, optimal posture, and anti-rigidity.

As you become better at diaphragmatic breathing, you will become more aware of your pre-existing tendency to tremble. Focus selectively on each tremor you notice and try to soothe it. Certainly, don't incorporate trembling into purposive movement. Don't allow your fingers to fumble as you use your phone, button down your shirt, or zip your purse. Slow down every movement and engineer it for precision. Hurried, hasty movements require bracing, ruining composure and finesse. It takes patience to eliminate trembling and establish flowing dexterity. Imagine moving like a sloth: slowly, deliberately, and mistake-free. Just like paced breathing irons the apneic disturbances out of your diaphragm's tidal range, slow, purposive movement will iron the discontinuities out of your actions.

Use Dominant Gestures

Dominant people with high serotonin naturally use commanding gestures. Dominance is conveyed preemptively by actions indicating strength, comfort, and fearlessness. Simply practicing and automating these gestures will increase your nonverbal dominance, thereby increasing your serotonin. Let's get into the specifics. Dominant people have towering posture, whereas submissive ones try to hide their height. Dominant people lean toward others and approach others directly rather than haltingly and uncertainly. Dominant people initiate increased proximity, more handshaking, and a higher frequency of touching.[17] So, put your arm around people, touch their hands, slap their knees, rest your arm on their shoulders, and strike their backs when you embrace them.

As far as general posture, we have already discussed retracting the neck, flexing the glutes, pressing the hips forward, and looking upward, among many others. When standing, place your feet at least shoulder length apart and don't fidget. Refrain from folding your hands in front of you, placing them in pockets, or using them to cover your genitals. Because submission is conveyed by the lack of hand movements and hidden hands, gradually work more hand gesticulation into your speech.

Bring your hands into full view, don't brace them in contorted ways, and never worry that the position of your elbows, wrists, or fingers will be taken as offensive. Finding a comfortable place for your hands can be difficult. The key is not thinking about it, or whether people will perceive it as uppity or proud. They are your hands. If other people don't like how you are holding them, that's their problem.

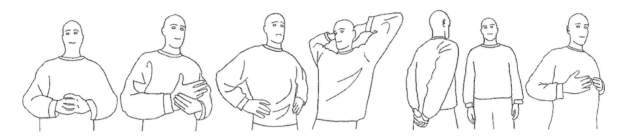

Illustration 23.2: Positions for the hands while standing. A. Holding the fist; B. Holding the hand; C. Hands on the hips; D. Hands supporting neck retraction; E. Hands behind the back; F. Hands simply dangling at the sides; G. Kelly Starrett's position to train pulling the shoulder blades together (scapular retraction/shoulder packing).

Another technique to increase your nonverbal dominance is reducing reassurances such as excessive nodding. Don't stop nodding altogether but reduce how quickly and how often you do it. Definitely smile at people and laugh at their jokes, just don't do it too much. Excessive smiling and laughter directed at another's efforts at humor are submissive. And use the optimal smile and laugh discussed in previous chapters. Nonverbal tics, rapid blinking, prolonged tilting of the head, touching the back of your neck, wringing the hands, coughing artificially, and scratching imaginary itches are all nervous behaviors meant to fill space when you don't know what to do with your body.[13] Omit all of that.

Televised athletes that suffer anything from a crushing defeat to a narrow loss immediately take on stereotypically submissive body language.[14] Their eyes are downcast, their head lowers, they untuck their chin, and their entire back curves forward into the characteristic "C" shape. Most of us take on these postures after somebody else makes a good point in a conversation. No one and nothing should be able to crush your posture. Instead, think of your favorite Olympic sport and imagine what stance you would take on if you just won a gold medal in that event in front of a cheering crowd. Use that hourly.

As we have seen, many submissive displays keep our muscles tense and prevent them from refreshing, hurting us in the long run. However, some displays communicate modesty without doing this. These include feeling comfortable turning your back to another individual, sitting lower than another, or placing yourself in any such position where someone else would have an advantage if they decided to attack you. If you walk into a room and sit in the lowest chair, you make a strong statement, showing that being physically lower doesn't make you feel lower.

I frequently sit, kneel, or lie down next to people that are standing. It gets people to lower their guard. When I do it, it is usually to stretch or allow my muscles to refresh. If you do this, other people will get the point and see that you have no fear that others will attack you.

In chimpanzees, submissive individuals greet dominant ones. This involves a sequence of short, shallow pant grunts that probably represent a form of handicapped breathing. The subordinate will assume a position whereby he looks up at the individual he is greeting. He makes a series of deep bows known as bobbing. In the words of primatologist Frans de Waal, he practically "grovels in the dust." The dominant individual will stand up higher and may step over the individual greeting him. When this happens, the submissive chimp ducks and puts his arms up to protect his head. Thus, even greetings can confirm the dominance relationship, explaining why the alpha is greeted by everyone in the group but greets no one. Adults never greet youngsters, and dominants never greet subordinates. Ceasing to greet is a direct challenge. What should we take from this? I think it is gracious to be the one who initiates a greeting, but be aware of your posture and composure when you do so, and keep in mind that you never have to be the one who initiates a hello.

Conclusion

I used to often feel like prey. Walks in metropolitan areas would trigger concerns of being followed by assailants. Being in nature would trigger fears of being stalked by wild animals. Swimming in an ocean, lake, or even a pool would trigger visions of sharks and prehistoric marine predators. I would have frequent nightmares, causing me to wake up yelling. Every other night in bed, I would give myself chills by imagining a home invasion scenario. This is all a distant memory to me now. I believe that I am utterly free of these fears today because my confidence and serotonin levels are constitutionally higher, thanks to Program Peace.

Besides massage, exercise, gratefulness, cooperation, and assertiveness, how else can we raise our serotonin? Every exercise in this book aims to increase serotonin levels. After you have thoroughly practiced walking while breathing deeply, with wide eyes above the eye line, shoulders down, and a retracted neck, it will be legitimate. And here is the key: Other people's inevitable recognition of this legitimacy will cause them to respect you. Strangers will see your posture and address you as "boss," "chief," "sir," or "ma'am." Even a subtle increase in the tokens of respect you receive from your social environment, relative to what your serotonergic system was previously accustomed to, will be enough to boost your serotonin.

Researcher Michael McGuire and colleagues performed an illuminating experiment. They took a monkey troop's alpha member and placed him in a separate room where he could watch the other monkeys. They placed a one-way mirror between the alpha and his subordinate troopmates so that he could see them, but they could not see him. Because the alpha could see his mates, he made his ordinary dominance gestures. However, because they were oblivious to him, they did not make their submissive gestures in response. Even though the alpha had far higher serotonin levels than the other monkeys, his serotonin levels fell each day of the experiment. He needed visual signals of their submission to stroke his ego. When the experimenters replaced this one-way mirror with a piece of glass, his friends submitted and his serotonin levels rose again.

The trouble with our brain circuitry is that we necessitate submissive displays from others just to feel normal. Many find it impossible to retain a sense of self-worth if others withhold

483

signs of deference. But you shouldn't. Accept a confidence boost when others exalt you but retain your confidence when others ignore you. There is a deeper lesson to take from this: Your social interactions are not fights but sparring sessions. They are not wrestling matches but wrestling practice. Don't see interactions as a competition; see them as cooperation. You are working together to help each other become more and more ascendant. When people fail to show you the esteem you feel you deserve, think of it as part of the game, and let it make you tougher, not weaker.

Before I started this reprogramming journey, my eye-related body language (see Chapter 4) was worse than most of the human population. If I had to ascribe numerical values, I would say that I was in the bottom 10% for having open eyes, the bottom 5% for looking upward, and the bottom 2% for capability for eye contact. I would guess that just around 10 hours in total of using the exercises from Chapter 4 placed me at least 60% higher in each of these categories. Can you imagine how much less frequently social interactions leave me feeling like a weirdo and a loser? Now, I come out of them with more serotonin rather than less.

Take a moment to consider how other exercises in this book will make additional contributions to your confidence. Once you get the excessive tension out of your face, neck, and diaphragm this will be apparent. But remember this is not a zero-sum game. As long as you are not combining your confidence with aggression, your improved body language should not detract from the body language of others. In fact, if you use your optimal demeanor equitably, and show others the respect they deserve (and perhaps more than they deserve), you will become a role model helping and training others to be more like you.

We have seen that there are many ways to increase your serotonin without drugs. However, I think the most powerful way to increase your confidence is to have faith in your skills to mitigate conflict. The next chapter will tackle this topic.

Chapter 23: **Bullet Points**

- Dominant or alpha primates have higher serotonin levels in the blood and brain than the other members of their group. If they are deposed, their serotonin plunges, and the new alpha's serotonin will soar.
- Being an alpha with high serotonin that can never be deposed is a state of mind you can create with time.
- Increased serotonin makes you feel less stressed in response to threats and less concerned with other people's expectations regarding your subordination displays.
- We act in ways to increase our serotonin, but this often brings us into conflict with others and can lead to self-destructive behavior.
- Any wins garnered through aggression or hostility are temporary and unsustainable.
- Increase your confidence not through pitting yourself against or comparing yourself to others but through appreciating the abundance you already have.
- You don't have to be a high-energy extrovert to be assertive and high in status.
- You have reached ego dissolution once your breathing is no longer controlled by pride or prestige.
- The same boost you used to get from pulling others down, you can double it by being successful at building rapport or making a new friend.
- Your nervous system supports a mode of operation in which all movements are fluid and unwavering, as in tai chi.
- Social submission interferes with fluid movement. Your gesticulations at a party should be as smooth and effortless as your motions in tai chi.
- Camaraderie, gratefulness, and a mindset that is not attached to status and not dependent on the regard of others will help us transcend serotonin blows.
- It shouldn't feel socially awkward to have dominant body language.
- Get your confidence boosts by competing with yourself and aiming to beat your personal bests.
- Master the belief that no matter what, you will be just fine.

Chapter 23: **Endnotes**

1.   Raleigh, M. J., Brammer, G. L., Yuwiler, A., Flannery, J. W., McGuire, M. T. & Geller, E. (1980). Serotonergic influences on the social behavior of vervet monkeys. Experimental Neurology, 68(2), 322–334.

2.   van Vugt, M. & Tybur, J. M. (2015). The evolutionary foundations of status hierarchy. In D. M. Buss (Ed.), *The handbook of evolutionary psychology* (2nd ed.). John Wiley & Sons.

3.   Cheng, J. T., Tracy, J. L., & Henrich, J. (2010). Pride, personality, and the evolutionary foundations of human social status. *Evolution and Human Behavior*, *31*(5), 334–347.

4.   Hill, P., Allemand, M., & Roberts, B. (2013). Examining the pathways between gratitude and self-rated physical health across adulthood. *Personality and Individual Differences*, *54*(1), 92–96.

5.   Lambert, N., Fincham, F., & Stillman, T. (2012). Gratitude and depressive symptoms: The role of positive reframing and positive emotion. *Cognition & Emotion*, *26*(4), 615–633.

6.   Emmons, R. A. (2009). Gratitude. In S. J. Lopez & A. Beauchamp (Eds.), *Encyclopedia of positive psychology* (pp. 442–447). Oxford University Press.

7.   Emmons, R. A., & McCullough, M. E. (2003). Counting blessings versus burdens: An experimental investigation of gratitude and subjective well-being in daily life. *Journal of Personality and Social Psychology, 84*(2), 377–389.

8.   Hanson, R. (2013). *Hardwiring happiness: The new brain science of contentment, calm, and confidence*. Random House.

9.   LeDoux J. (2003). The emotional brain, fear, and the amygdala. *Cellular and Molecular Neurobiology*, *23*(4-5), 727–738.

10. Gothard, K. M., & Hoffman, K. L. (2010). Circuits of emotion in the primate brain. In M. L. Platt & A. A. Ghazanfar (Eds.), *Primate neuroethology* (pp. 292–315). Oxford University Press.

11. Hermann, H. R. (2017). *Dominance and aggression in humans and other animals: The great game of life*. Academic Press.

12. Carney, D. R., Hall, J. A. A., & LeBeau, L. S. (2005). Beliefs about the nonverbal expression of social power. *Journal of Nonverbal Behavior*, *29*, 105–123.

13. Shariff, A. F., & Tracy, J. L. (2009). Knowing who's boss: Implicit perceptions of status from the nonverbal expression of pride. *Emotion*, *9*(5), 631–639.

14. Tracy, J. L., & Matsumoto, D. (2008). The spontaneous expression of pride and shame: Evidence for biologically innate nonverbal displays. *Proceedings of the National Academy of Sciences, 105*(33) 11655–11660.

Chapter 24: **Rise Above Status Conflict**

"You do not need to defend against the intrusions of others, there is no pressure on you to defend yourself. Recognize that they intrude upon themselves." — Eckhart Tolle (1948)

We Act in Uncivil Ways to Increase Our Serotonin

Humans, like other primates, are constantly testing one another in an often-unconscious attempt to either raise their serotonin levels or reduce someone else's. We are driven to do it because putting others down can give us a little neurochemical boost. The tendency is instinctual but it can become addictive and sadistic. It is not psychologically healthy to belittle our friends, family members, and coworkers for little hits of pleasure. Neither is it healthy to fail to recognize when others do this to us. I think of this as the "struggle for serotonin" and it is going on in schools, homes, and workplaces everywhere.

Workplace disharmony has been documented by recent research to be a substantial economic cost for American business that is largely preventable but rarely addressed.[1] One in five people claim to be the targets of occupational abuse at least once a week, and ten percent said they witness it every day. Mistreatment does not rouse workers into better focus; it actually impedes their performance. People that have been treated cruelly or thoughtlessly show decreased ability to perform simple tasks, distracted attention, impaired working memory, diminished creativity, and reduced helping behaviors.[2] Inhumane behavior is virulent and negatively affects all involved: the targets, the offenders, the firm, and its customers. After reading about what incivility does in a workplace, imagine what it does to a circle of friends or a family. Let's talk about how to stop it.

We Provoke Each Other Constantly

"As a solid rock is not shaken by the wind, even so the wise are not ruffled by praise or blame." — Buddha (563 BCE - 483 BCE

When I was young, my mother taught me the expression "out to get your goat." This helped me understand from a young age that it is common for people to say or do things just to "get a rise" out of you or try to make you lose your cool. It is ubiquitous. People try to activate the other person's amygdala, sympathetic system, and inferiority instincts to control them, however temporarily. A large proportion of our social interactions revolve around testing each other's composure with jokes, slights, and provocations. When my mom told me, "Don't let him get your goat," she was underscoring my responsibility to safeguard my temper and ignore people's attempts to fluster me.

Etymologists believe that the expression comes from the once-common practice of keeping goats with racehorses. Racehorses are high-strung animals due, in part, to the unnatural levels of strain placed on their muscles. Goats were often used as companion animals to help keep racehorses calm. They were also commonly placed with dairy cows for the same reason. Goats naturally have an exceptionally low outward expression of stress. They are not the most beautiful animals, neither are they the smartest, nor largest, but they are great at keeping their cool. I think this should be a lesson for us; we don't have to be the biggest or best to be the

PROGRAM PEACE *Self- Care Exercises to Reprogram Your Mind and Body*

calmest. We may be far from being the dominant individual in a group, but we can still be so well composed that it inspires everyone else.

There are many physical traits in animals that exist to convey social dominance. These include plumage coloration in Harris sparrows, horn size in mountain sheep, graying in the mountain gorilla, and square jaws in humans. It is common to assume that flashy traits, imposition, musculature, and physical strength make a person dominant. But it is really emotional strength that makes people dominant. Emotional stability keeps people from "getting your goat." It is the only status symbol that is universally, albeit unconsciously, recognized as more important than physical size, looks, reputation, or money. Often, people with great physical strength are accorded respect. This, in turn, helps them build confidence and emotional strength. However, the physically weakest person can certainly have the most control over their emotions. I think of emotional strength as the ability to exhibit sturdiness in the face of negativity.

Emotional weakness starts when someone feels violated by someone else and then tries to fight that feeling like any subjugated monkey. The problem is, if others can tell that you have been stung, they are going to want to sting you again. Children high in rejection sensitivity are more likely to be bullied. Those kids who do not readily feel rejected are much less likely to be victimized. Envisioning yourself as the underdog or the victim is counterproductive because it sensitizes you, lowers your serotonin, and invites further abuse. Dominant animals have thick skin, are the last to feel rejected, and so are the last to *be* rejected. What would it feel like to have zero rejection sensitivity? Can you imagine yourself as inviolable?

Treat everyone like you have known them forever and like they can't easily hurt you. See them as playful monkeys that are bluff-charging, sham-sneering, pretend-scratching, and feign-biting. Only the primates with low serotonin are hurt emotionally by fraternization. All the things that people used to do that made you feel enraged, reframe them as rough-and-tumble monkey play.

We Contradict Each Other Compulsively

If you carefully analyze the way people speak, it is almost shocking how much we contradict one another. Most people are obnoxiously argumentative, disputatious contrarians. For many listeners, the first thing that pops into their mind is a way to poke holes in your line of reasoning. They look for any suitable exception to what you are saying. They often are not even emotionally invested in the contradictions that they place against you. They are merely playing devil's advocate, and throwing out red herrings, to stifle and trip you up. When people do this to you, they are testing your limits and trying to push you down into the lower echelons. They are expecting to feel good and get away with it after they discredit you. But if we recognize the ploy and respond skillfully to it, we can help them reduce this dysfunctional behavior that is certainly hurting them more than it is helping. We can do this by responding without any hint of pain.

When others attempt to shoot you down, try to see what is right about what they are saying while pointing out how it doesn't invalidate what you were saying. Do this with peace in your heart. Remember that you need not get defensive when someone hastily comes up with an irrelevant exception to a statement you made. Take their objections as requests for elaboration, and be happy to give them more details. Reframing people's intrusions and giving them the benefit of the doubt is what the emotionally healthy person does.

We should be looking for what is right in what others are saying to provide support. This is much more constructive for them and us. In the words of Nick Bostrom, this involves resisting "the temptation to instantaneously misunderstand each new idea by assimilating it with the most similar-sounding cliché available in (your) cultural larder." Give people's ideas a chance to marinate in your mind, then help make those ideas better. If you strongly disagree or have something to teach them, prove that you are comfortable in disagreeing by being polite yet assertive. Explain where you agree prior to disagreeing, but don't disagree just to disagree.

Never Fail a Confidence Test

People's jokes, contradictions, and snide comments are "confidence tests" to assess how cool you are under pressure. This is like a dog's first bark. It is a probe used to assess your level of composure. These tests exclaim, "I'm pretty sure that I can break you down, so I'm going to say something rude and see how you respond." If you don't do anything about it, you will fail the test, your rank will drop, and others in the group will try to test you in the same way. If you laugh nervously or go along with it, others will also see this as failing the test. Crying, complaining, or trying to gain sympathy are other ways to fail. Flinging out an insult or becoming furious will create more hostility or get yourself excluded from the group. This is because responding with anger just shows that you are volatile, threatened, and emotionally immature. But if you can respond using the challenge response rather than the threat response, you pass the confidence test with flying colors.

To quote Schopenhauer: "Every reproach can hurt only to the extent that it hits the mark." Thus, when you lose your cool, and distressed breathing kicks in, it becomes clear that the person's comment resonated with you. The only surefire way to win is to react assertively and refrain from showing any hint of discomfort in response to your confidence being tested. Don't search other people's words for things to be offended by. Don't scrutinize voicemails, text messages, or tone of voice for threats or put-downs. There is no reason to investigate.

Confidence testing is primal behavior. Friends, lovers, coworkers, strangers, men, and women alike do it. Sometimes it takes the form of creating drama out of a tiny issue just so that they can scope your ability to withstand stress. They are trying to see what they can get away with. This may take the form of impatience, discourtesy, or asking for endless small favors. Most people fail these tests because they cannot recognize them for what they are. Once you realize that you're dealing with a confidence test, however, it is very easy to pass.

The best way to handle confidence tests is to see them for what they are: monkey business that is not worthy of your stress response. Treat them as jokes and make humorous comments in return. You can turn a confidence test back around playfully or you can even make a self-deprecating joke to show how unflustered you are. The absolute best way to deal with confidence tests is to accept them as invitations to play, as discussed in the next chapter. The second-best way is simply to retain your composure.

Recompose Yourself When You Feel Disrespected

"The mental arrow shot from another's bow is practically harmless unless our own thought barbs it."
— *Mary Baker Eddy (1821-1910)*

People provoke each other because they want to compare bodily pain. When you feel disrespected by someone, your heart rate, blood pressure, and general level of discomfort all go up. Your vagal tone and HRV come down. When someone contradicts you with a trifling point, they are looking to see how your face, voice, and breathing will change in response to this new stressor. They are expecting to take your breath away from you. When they make a haughty innuendo or an untoward comment, they want to see how you will tolerate it physiologically. Recomposing yourself is the best way to stop reinforcing their transgressive behavior. When someone says something that crosses your boundaries, ensure that you:

1) Are breathing slowly and deeply through your nose
2) Are not squinting and your eyebrows are not raised
3) Are not sneering at all and your face is limp
4) Relax your spine, gut, and vocal tract
5) Retract your neck and lower your shoulders

Responding in this way removes all positive reinforcers, dissuading the offending party from provoking you again. If they disrespect you and your eyes remain wide while you respond calmly in a deep and steady voice, they are going to feel stupid. When you react to someone in a way that is otherwise non-optimal, you relinquish your power. When our chi-like or prana-like bioenergy is wasted on negative emotions, we have none left to improve our lives or give to others. Conserve yours, especially in the face of provocation.

We get mad at other people for "making" us lose our composure. However, we should be angry over our own unconscious rules for what makes us tighten certain body parts. Once we change those rules, other people can't upset us. When I get mad at something that someone did, I remind myself that I am only mad because my own rules caused my breath to shorten, my nasopharynx to tighten, and my face to wince. No one else "made" me do these things. *I* did. Breathing with the diaphragm will automatically create the right mindset for dealing with power politics. It will allow the conflict to pass right through you without impacting you. Even taking a single 10 second inhalation will give you more control over your behavior, quell your anger, and allow you to de-escalate potentially explosive situations. Misunderstandings that would have been large-scale crises will now be subtle victories.

I used to look nice and act tough. Like most people, I was doing it backward. Instead, we want to look tough and act nice. Playing submissive nonverbally and dominant verbally makes you a servant to the hierarchical game and turns you into a jerk. Instead, you want to be tightfisted with your nonverbals but easygoing with your words. This gives the impression that you are a well-composed team player rather than an anxious and alienated loner.

If you tense anything, let it be the procerus, pulling your eyebrows down. In other words, when someone is mean or rude to you, try frowning. You practiced this highly dominant expression in Chapters 4 and 8. You can also flare your nostrils. Then, without saying anything angry, ask them to clarify their statement: "Okay, explain that one to me."

The primary way I show others they did something that I didn't like is by making my face calmer. They always get the point. When a problem dog is ignored, it usually calms down in seconds. When abusive people see that you are unagitated and uninterested, it will take them down a peg. Shrug it off—literally. When they see you shrug, they will realize that they are powerless to upset you.

Many of the men I was friends with in my twenties wanted to hurt me and see me in pain. At least a part of them did. They were just doing what their instincts and environment programmed them to do. People often encourage those who subordinate themselves to do so even further. This is not necessarily spiteful because they usually don't even realize what they are doing. Regrettably, I have noticed myself unconsciously helping people play a subordinate role. I try to catch myself. We should treat and speak to everyone, including people such as the homeless and developmentally disabled, as equals, friends, and trusted confidantes.

The best way to cultivate inner freedom is to learn to relax around petty and aggressive people. You will find that the need to defend yourself will diminish until there is nothing they can do to aggravate you. Make them realize that they don't have the power to bite, scratch, or sully you with their words. Chimpanzees fling feces to denigrate one another. Every time someone says something degrading, they are just flinging feces. Lucky for us, words can't stain our clothes.

No matter what, if you have more composure, you will win the argument because you look like you don't care too much. Once they realize they have no access to your physical pain, they will let up. You want people to be able to sense that you are not interested in their antics. They will recognize that they cannot blame you for not being pulled in by shenanigans. You want to communicate: "We're not playing that game of scrutinizing the things we say to each other for slights. Trust me, I'm simply not going to intentionally offend you."

Underreact to Their Offenses

"God gives nothing to those who keep their arms crossed." — West African Proverb

Aside from the struggle for serotonin, your average person acts like a jackass because they are in pain. They offend in a poor functioning attempt to hide the outward manifestation of their trauma. It is like they are trying to show us: "I wouldn't be acting like this if I were scared, would I?" In trying to look strong, they become offensive. Because they see being nice as a form of self-handicapping, they think that they must be mean so as not to handicap. This is a fundamental socio-cognitive error. You can be the strongest, most ambitious version of yourself with zero negativity. However, remember that it is an entirely normal response for other people to resist your efforts to become more assertive. So, roll with any resistance.

When someone is rude to you and you are not rude back, you pull the rug out from under them. By not allowing them to incite your pain, you expose theirs. They may then use a strategy to pretend as if your response to them was rude or sarcastic. They do this in another attempt to make it seem that you are the one who is quick to anger. The best response is to continue to keep your cool. Don't get bullied into becoming angry. Take their harassment in stride. Or simply sidestep it; you don't even need to acknowledge their misdeed. Feel free to ignore it.

It is our right as humans to completely ignore other people's abusive behaviors if we don't do it in anger and if we are willing to engage the person in an alternate topic or activity.

Ignore rudeness without brooding or becoming sullen. The moment you do this, the other person will realize that you are choosing not to respond because they put you in a position where you didn't have the option to respond in a nice way. After ignoring them, give them another chance to engage whenever they want. You can alternatively ignore the rude part of what they said and continue addressing only the positive or intellectual side of their position. Do this magnanimously and they will realize that you gave them a pass. They will also respect you for it. Even if they don't mention it, they can't help but realize, "Wow, he could've taken that opportunity to strike back or discredit me but chose not to." Don't let them pull you down to their level. That's the first step in winning them over.

Let the other person bluster and be brash and make no attempt to do the same. Because you don't counter their display, they will think that they have beaten you. Then, when you act cheerful, not attempting to win or lose but being oblivious to the dominance game in general, they will go through a series of emotions. First, they will feel like they have lost, then they will try to win again to make up for it. They may get stuck in that cycle for a while, and that's fine. Eventually, they will recognize that you intend to act as equals. When this happens organically, it is usually the starting point for an alliance or a friendship. Why not accelerate the process?

Can you imagine negotiating with an angry person without using either appeasement or aggression? What would that look like? Many spiritual teachers say that a sign of someone enlightened is that they cannot be provoked or argued with. They are open to discussion and debate, of course, but not argument. The next activity asks you to explore how you can stand up for what you believe without losing your composure.

Conflict Activity #24.1: *A Relaxed Argument*

The next time someone is critical or accusatory, prepare yourself for a fully relaxed argument. This involves asserting yourself using calm, cool logic without getting offended and without escalating the conversation in any way. Try to achieve the following:

1) Do not raise your voice.
2) Do not whine or speak in a high voice.
3) Do not fake smile, smirk, or laugh.
4) Do not say anything sarcastic.
5) Monitor your breathing rate, heart rate, and level of gastric distress.
6) Breathe calmly through your nose for the duration. Let your exhalations be passive.
7) Present your side of the argument in a straightforward, matter-of-fact way.
8) Show empathy for their feelings and try to coax them to do the same for you.
9) If the other person escalates the conflict, act in ways that deescalate it.
10) Create awareness of your (and the other person's) impulses to become angry or make it personal. Notice how these originate from sensations of pain within the body.
11) Make your intended outcome not to win but to convince the other person that any transgression you may have committed was unintentional.

12) Do not attack them or try to shift blame toward them. Just focus on getting them to see your perspective and why you did what you did.
13) Explain how you will continue to act in the same way in the future, or how you are willing to try to change for them.
14) Feel free to offer an apology for whatever part you played in the disagreement.

Meditate on the term "unassailable," which means unable to be attacked or defeated. You are unassailable because you are a good person and do wrong only by accident. You are also unassailable because you respond to criticism dispassionately but with accountability. You underreact, but you take responsibility for what you may have done wrong. By being happy to completely own up to any mistakes or any trouble you may have inadvertently caused others, you are made invincible. If someone refuses to say, "I'm sorry," "Thank you," and "You were right" to you, it doesn't mean that you should stop saying such things to them. Make yourself honor-bound to say these things whenever they are applicable.

Be at ease with everyone, from the discourteous to the genteel, and treat everyone as if you have known them your whole life. This means when they say something with a pinprick embedded in it to get a rise out of you, act like you have heard the same line a thousand times. You are unfazed and remain sociable with full parasympathetic and vagal tone. At the outset, you will need to override any impulses to respond in kind. Soon, it will become automatic, and you will experience how and why being unfazed is much more powerful than lashing out.

Set Your Expectations of Others to Zero

Competition and aggression are relatively inescapable. It is essential to come to terms with the fact that, at any moment, anyone could say something that will rile you up or make you feel demeaned, disregarded, or disrespected. Everyone, even (if not especially) your closest friends harbor instincts and impulses to dominate you. Ask yourself: "Am I open to being exasperated by anyone at any time?" The answer (without being jaded or cynical) should be: "No, I govern my own emotional reactions. I'm prepared for the worst, even though I treat others as though I only expect the best from them."

Conflict Activity #24.2: *Imagine Your Friends Abusing You*

Imagine that everyone in your social world is trying to abuse you verbally. They are resorting to personal character attacks in foul and underhanded ways. People are screaming and yelling expletives at you, denouncing everything you have ever done. Imagine yourself staying calm and untroubled amid this derision. Imagine yourself not taking it personally, not taking it to heart, and continuing to be productive and accomplish your personal goals. Imagine yourself unperturbed by the abuse. Allow this imaginary activity to take the emotional shock away from personal attacks when they happen and help you appreciate how good your social life really is.

We've got to remember not to take offenses personally. When someone says something snide, you might find yourself immediately starting to wonder if the offender doesn't like your face, your personality, or the way you talk. If a person is rude to you, they are probably rude to everyone. It reflects on them, not you. You need to resist the tendency to ask, "Why me?" One of the best approaches to regaining peace in your life is to avoid taking any personal offense.

Conflict Activity #24.3: *See People As Animate Matter*
Spend a few minutes thinking of everyone on Earth as being made of atoms and molecules that are completely controlled by physical laws. Imagine them with no free will of their own. Everything they do comes from their current physical structure: the existing circuits in their brain and the prior experiences that made them that way. Allow this to help you feel unoffended by their actions. See everyone as automatons, aggregations of cells that move and act in predetermined ways. Like a tumbleweed that has run into you, you cannot rationally be offended by anything they do. Sometimes it can help to see people as deterministic robots in this way. What you put in is what you get out. This holds you responsible for any errors. You should find that when you stop blaming others and hold yourself responsible, you have well-functioning encounters more frequently.

Aggression is Inherently Weak

Aggressive acts are almost always mutually destructive in the sense that they hurt all parties involved. Any positive outcomes won by aggression are usually "pyrrhic," meaning they are achieved at a high cost, often to the point of negating or outweighing any benefits. Tell yourself that there are no "acceptable losses" with aggression and that because it damages everyone, aggression is self-defeating.

Aggression is violent in tone and contains elements of despair, defensiveness, self-pity, fear, and desperation. It invokes and is invoked by the threat response. It is ironic that people often act aggressively to gain respect but only rarely do others respect aggressive people. This is because aggression is inherently weak. Aggression turns the world into a zoo and a "struggle for serotonin."

As discussed in Chapter 1, there is a big difference between acting dominant and trying to dominate others. Cultivating dominant nonverbal behavior is good for your health—it helps you avoid stress. But trying to dominate others is just another source of conflict and, as such, a source of stress. Studies with monkeys and apes have shown that stress, as measured by elevations in the stress hormone cortisol, is often more pronounced in individuals attempting to dominate than in their targets.[3] In trying to subject others, these primates damage their health. People that are constantly trying to assert their rank by being aggressive are similarly exposing themselves to cortisol, inflammation, tachycardia, hyperventilation, bracing, and so much more. The clear implication is that the best way to free ourselves from our egos is to cultivate a non-submissive personality while abstaining from attempts to dominate.

Heal Your Composure with the Most Dominant People in Your Life

Your relationship with your parents is primordial. Everyone picks up aggressive, nonoptimal, nonpeaceful tendencies from their folks. These are usually the hardest to break. Also, the body language and mannerisms you feel comfortable using around Mom and Dad set a foundation for how you act with everyone else. Because so much of our formative time was spent with them, we hold our posture and countenance as if in their presence. It is important that you feel comfortable using dominant, non-submissive body language around your mother, father, and siblings. As soon as you stop bracing your body in a way that is subservient to your family members, you will gain new freedom. The next time you find yourself on a car ride with your parents, family members, or anyone you are uncomfortable around, discretely pull out your breath metronome and teach your body to inhale and exhale freely in their presence.

Primates respect gradation in rank, meaning that a baboon will act much more subservient around a group member five stations above him than it will around a member one station above him. The way you hold yourself around the most dominant people in your life similarly affects you. Think of the largest, strongest, most charismatic, and most successful people in your life. You should act like there is no pressure on you to send them tribute. Take special note of which aspects of your body language are non-optimal when you are with them and work on these. Even when they are not around you may find yourself trying to convince them of things, monitoring their moodiness, and rehashing old disagreements. If this is the case, your thoughts about them are likely influencing you to hold submissive postures. Let all of this go.

Don't Feel Compelled to Sacrifice to Dominant Individuals

"Care about people's approval and you will be their prisoner." — Lao Tzu (571 BCE - Unknown)

Subordinate apes often seek reassurance by putting a finger in the dominant animal's mouth. They are risking their intact finger to pay their respects. This is like a sacrificial offering. Monkeys do this, too. Among stump-tailed macaques, formal rank is reinforced by a mock bite on the subordinate's wrist. The subordinate approaches and places their arm under the dominant individual's nose to invite this ritualized bite. It communicates: "If you don't trust me, you can chew my hand off." Similarly, it is very common for humans to sacrifice disproportionate amounts of time and energy to curry a dominant person's favor. Don't do this. They will not respect you for it.

Nondominant primates are obsessed with the dominant ones. Apes and monkeys spend a lot of time watching or making frequent, furtive glances at dominant members of their troop.[4] In experimental settings, male monkeys are willing to give up precious juice to view pictures of two things: 1) female hindquarters (not surprisingly), and 2) dominant males. In the wild, monkeys constantly inspect the dominants, watching their every move and often giving them their full attention. Scientists suppose that this behavior plays a role in the "acquisition of important social cues."

People do this as well. Have you noticed your tendency to search out high-status members of the same sex and observe them jealously? Do you seek out pictures of female hindquarters and buff dudes on social media? Don't secretly worship the bodybuilders, the CEOs, the fitness models, or the celebrities. Giving them undue attention keeps you locked in a hierarchical mindset, so don't pay them any more attention than you would anyone else.

Have Compassion for Your Transgressors

"If we could read the secret history of our enemies, we should find in each (person's) life sorrow and suffering enough to disarm any hostility." — Henry Wadsworth Longfellow (1807-1882)

In your mind, think of discourteous people as unsophisticated people. Remember that the most offensive ones are likely to have had extreme life challenges such as early trauma or abuse. Further, inappropriate aggression can be a symptom of brain damage, PTSD, or a range of neurological or psychological disorders. When someone is inconsiderate, remind yourself that they may have serious maladjustments and that, more often than not, they could use your help. Everyone is a jerk in their own eccentric way due to their unique pattern of deficits in social intelligence. Don't be surprised or upset by their idiosyncratic manner of being discourteous just because you haven't gotten used to it yet. Most people realize that they are rough around the edges. Many even want to change but find it difficult or do not understand how. Unfortunately, their uncouth behavior causes people to be rude back to them, perpetuating their problem. We don't want to perpetuate people's issues. We want to help resolve them.

Aggression derives from weakness, pain, unfortunate experiences, and mental shortcomings, so we should respond to it with empathy. Those who want to humiliate others have low self-esteem themselves. It is sad that their priorities, judgments, and word choices are impoverished. Had you experienced everything they did, perhaps you would have turned out just like them. Think of quarrelsome people as flamboyant actors who are suffering offstage. Most everyone is a sob story, and we are all walking wounded. Don't let wounds beget more wounds. Everyone you dislike just needs a little recognition, validation, and friendliness. When you give them a chance, odds are they will end up making you revise your opinion of them.

Another thing we should keep in mind is that what we take to be premeditated, personal affronts tend to be defense mechanisms or, even more innocuously, coping mechanisms. Most difficult people do things out of desperation because their sympathetic nervous system is set too high. People who are short of breath, shaken, and choked up lash out. That is what they do. Almost everything that you don't like about people is just them trying ineffectively to maintain their dignity. Work around them if you have to but help them if you can. Let your natural assertiveness and your compassion for them work together.

Anger and Rage

"He that is slow to anger is better than the mighty." — Proverbs 16:32

The brain's rage system starts at the medial areas of the amygdala that perceive anger-inducing stimuli. From there they proceed to the areas that act on anger (including the stria terminalis, the medial hypothalamus, and the periaqueductal gray). Certain stimuli from the environment naturally increase electrical activity in these areas: physical restriction, pain, hunger, and thwarted desires. You can see how these incendiary stimuli are similar to those that evoke fear in the amygdala (e.g., loud sounds and fast movement). As with fear, adrenaline, cortisol, and pain heighten anger, whereas endorphins, oxytocin, and serotonin halt it.[5]

In all mammals that have been tested, rage can be evoked by electrically stimulating these brain areas. We know they find it aversive because lab animals will go to lengths to avoid electrical stimulation of the rage system. When the electrodes in their rage circuit are fed a current, the animal will spring toward whatever object is in front of it and bite. The attack becomes more intense as the current is increased. Humans report that the stimulation of rage via electrodes placed in the brain is a terrible experience. They tend to clench their jaw and sneering muscles and report feelings of intense hatred.

Electrical stimulation of rage causes small-brained mammals like mice to attack inanimate objects. More intelligent mammals like cats and dogs won't attack an object because they understand that this is meaningless, but they will attack the nearest living animal. Primates show a further level of abstraction. Stimulating the rage system in apes and monkeys will cause them to vent their rage toward animals below them in the hierarchy but not above.

A monkey whose rage system is persistently stimulated will ascend in rank. An animal whose rage system is physically damaged in the lab (septal lesioning) will become tame and descend in rank. This suggests that we don't want to completely suppress anger. However, many of us were expected to suppress all outward manifestations of anger by our parents and teachers. I believe that many people fall down the well of anxiety simply because they are reluctant to demonstrate anger. Convince yourself that it is fine to use anger in the form of righteous indignation to stand up for yourself or what you believe in. In Exercise 8.2 we discovered how briefly feigning anger can clear fear from your face. Used in the next exercise it will clear it from your chest.

Conflict Activity #24.4: *Briefly Feign Anger to Overcome Fear*

The next time you anticipate anxiety or experience intimidation from social conflict use anger to overcome it. Imagine, even if just for 10 seconds, that you are very angry at the other person. You might be enraged at everyone in the boardroom. Without letting your blood pressure rise or wanting to attack them, flip the tables by allowing the anger to drain every ounce of fear from you. Then reengage without either anger or fear.

Anger erases social anxiety because when you are angry, you stop caring about what other people think and about the intricate hierarchical games of judgment, evaluation, and apprehension. For those few seconds you are ready to throw it all out of the window. Even a brief flash of anger lasting seconds will harden you, making you callous, unsympathetic and allowing you to start over with renewed composure. Sometimes just reminding yourself that you are capable of feeling angry and expressing anger in front of others can give you the confidence you need to be assertive.

Don't expect people to read your mind or recognize when things are not in your favor. If something bothers you, speak up. Don't be afraid to ask for what you want. Say what you want to say. You should be at a point in your life where you don't feel like you have to act like anybody but yourself. Make sure that you establish non-negotiable boundaries. Don't tolerate intrusions upon your health, family, morals, or psychological well-being. Keep in mind though that you must take responsibility if your assertive words or actions ruffle other people's feathers.

Extreme anger in animals is often called a "red-zone" case. You cannot reason with an animal whose rage circuit is fully active. It is so focused that injuring it will only intensify its ferocity. Its objective to kill overpowers any pain you might inflict. It would rather die than cease its attack. When the rage circuit is activated in a human, you cannot argue or reason with them. Their bodily pain launches a sustained, uninhibited verbal offensive. Don't ever feel like you have to pit yours against theirs. Rather, when someone gets angry at you, think of it as an opportunity to explain your true intentions and give them the information they need to feel less threatened. There is a good chance that their accusation is totally valid given that they don't have the information they need to see it from your point of view. Also, a person cannot stay mad at you if you don't get defensive. Like a truly dominant mammal, tackle the situation with assertion, not infuriation.

In Chapter 1, we learned that the neurological systems for predation and aggression are distinct. When a predatory mammal attacks prey, its rage circuit is entirely inactive. However, when a mammal attacks a member of its species out of anger, the rage circuit lights up. Be a person that doesn't attack members of its species. Rather, attack the misunderstanding at hand. Imagine being a cat stalking in the grass without an ounce of anger or aggression aroused, calmly approaching your prey completely naïve of negative intent. Wouldn't it be more effective to use this manner in a hostile social situation than outrage or defensiveness?

You might ask whether avoiding anger will cause suppressed emotion. It is commonly supposed that if people suppress anger toward others, they will end up "bottling it all inside." But this act of bottling is equivalent to nothing more than muscle tension, something you have now been trained to recognize and release. As long as you do not start bracing and continue to breathe diaphragmatically, you are not suppressing anger. You are deflecting it. And this is healthy. As any endocrinologist will tell you, getting angry is like taking a small dose of slow acting poison. It raises blood pressure, strains the heart, damages arteries, and causes cholesterol-filled fat cells to empty into the bloodstream.

As with fear, every time you become adversarial, the emotion fortifies related brain pathways, making you a more petulant person. Every time you "indulge" in negativity, you encourage tiny incremental alterations in your neural architecture that make it harder to be positive.[6] Conversely, every time you transcend anger, your capability to rise above it is increased. So, the next time you find yourself using your imagination to plan a tirade or spew venom, just stop and move on to something else.

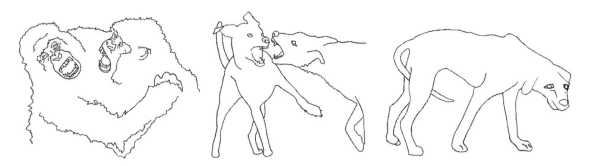

Illustration 24.1: A. Gorillas fighting; B. Dogs fighting; C. Dog with tail between the legs.

Use Proximity, Touch, and Eye Contact for Reconciliation

Physical conflicts are frequent in both monkeys and apes. Heart rates skyrocket, suppressed anger is unleashed, and the fur can fly. What happens afterward is what is important. Most conflicts, even violent ones, don't create distance because the animals tend to be intimate soon after the aggressive incident. They want to make up. As with our hunter-gatherer ancestors, chimps in a troop are usually stuck with each other, so reconciliation is necessary.

After a fight, chimps first seek out eye contact. The former opponents may sit opposite each other for 15 minutes or more, trying to catch the other's eye. One makes the first conciliatory move, holds out a hand, pants in a friendly way, then approaches for mutual grooming. Sometimes within a minute of a fight, apes will rush toward each other, kiss, embrace fervently, and then proceed to groom each other and even lick each other's wounds. This close physical contact is what makes reconciliation possible.

As they groom and make up, their heart rates and breathing rates return to ordinary levels. If the two primates don't spend time in close proximity, giving their hearts a chance to calm down in each other's presence, they may never salvage their relationship. Think of some people that you have trouble getting along with. How do you make up with them after a spat? Failure to reconcile may stem from the fact that you have not made time to decrease your cardiorespiratory output in their immediate presence. If you have relationships that you want to heal, all it may take is a one-on-one "chill-out" session involving togetherness, eye contact, physical touch, and mutual diaphragmatic breathing.

Making Your Calm-Assertive Energy Composed and Nonconfrontational

Animal trainer Cesar Millan uses the term "calm-assertive energy" to describe the aura of a pack leader. In his book, *Cesar's Way*, he underscores that when an owner leverages this aura with their pets, it convinces them to trust and value the owner's authority.[7] He explains how even a small child can gain command over a 150-pound Pitbull if they exude calm-assertive energy. To wield it, you must appear austere, like you have strong expectations that others will respect your boundaries.

Millan explains that your pet dog does not want to be your equal. It either wants to be dominant or inferior. He describes how most problem dogs that he treats try to assert their dominance over their doting owners. Dominance displays used by pet dogs include jumping at people, insisting on being fed, being the first out the door, pulling the owner by the leash during walks, excessive barking, being unresponsive to commands, and many others. They tend to develop these behaviors when their owner is neither calm nor assertive.

Most dogs will gladly accept their owner's dominance unless they believe that the owner's energy is too weak. Dogs know that when a leader has wimpy energy, the "pack" is compromised. For its safety and your protection, it will try to pick up the slack by asserting its dominance. The same goes for children. Many well-intentioned parents are unwittingly submissive to their offspring and end up with aggressive, frustrated kids. The same goes for everyone in your life. If you are not using calm-assertive energy, they will want to keep you down so that you don't compromise the chain of command that is so important to survival. Thus, your coworkers, friends, and family have instincts that tell them they don't want to be your equal. Because they want the tribe to have the most strong-minded leader, they prefer to either lead or follow someone stronger.

Near the end of his book, *The Ape in the Corner Office*, Richard Conniff concludes: "Status competition and hierarchy are inescapable facts of primate life. Though we disparage them, they are also essential tools for encouraging high performance and domestic tranquility." He is right. When the pecking order is stable in groups of chickens, the hens fight less and lay more eggs. Fighting is vastly reduced in chimps where the dominance hierarchy is established. This is also true in humans. For example, when dominance roles are well defined in a business merger, it usually goes smoothly, but if roles are left undefined, there is much more friction.[8] Conniff believes that prosocial dominance is what we should strive for. To him, it is about making friends, employing compromise and persuasion, and getting people to work with you toward common goals and the better good.

I mostly agree with Conniff. But I have this to add: Let us make our posture and body language as stable and secure as possible, our speech as rational and friendly as possible. Beyond this, let us not try to force our eminence on anyone. Instead, we should let others make inferences about relative dominance without attempting to persuade them or twist their arm.

Thus, I recommend using calm-assertive energy combined with a non-dominating/non-submissive demeanor to convince others (against their instincts) that the best strategy is to be equals. I think that these comparisons with animal behavior suggest a golden rule of social hierarchy: Treat others as if they are neither above you nor below you in the status hierarchy and as if they have never done anything wrong. We will build on this in the next section.

Forgiving Transgression

"The best way to destroy an enemy is to make him a friend." — *Abraham Lincoln (1809-1865)*

Although I think we should be quick to forgive, we must let wrongdoers know what they did was unacceptable. If someone wrongs you, address it assertively and immediately. Tell them which of your boundaries they crossed and by how much. Even tell them exactly how you expect them to proceed. However, if they are not doing anything wrong in the next moment, treat them as if they have never done anything wrong in their life. This proves to them that you trust them to improve. This involves not saying things like: "You never listen to me," "You're always doing that," "You don't care about anyone else," and "You'll never change." Keeping score or holding grudges only leads to bitterness on both sides.

Conflict Activity #24.5: *Treat Others as if They Have Never Done Wrong*

Imagine what it would be like to treat everyone in your life as if they had never done anything bad, hurtful, or thoughtless. Imagine relating to each person as an equal and a trusted soulmate that has never harmed or insulted you in any way. Imagine your parents this way, followed by your siblings, extended family, friends, children, coworkers—everyone. Start over with a clean slate. Even better, throw the slate away and stop keeping tallies. This will free you from the encumbrance of having to keep score, withhold affection, and mete out extended punishments. Doing so can play a massive role in making relationships more peaceable and equitable.

Don't Punish Because People Don't Sympathize with Your Aggression

No one is going to perceive your anger as valid if it is directed toward them. Even if you feel like you are justified in getting angry, as long as it is directed toward them, they will perform whatever mental gymnastics necessary to frame you as the victimizer. You may see your actions as retaliation, but they see it as arbitrary abuse. That is why I don't chastise even when I have a clear opportunity. Resorting to belligerent tactics is the best way to provide an antagonist with more ammunition. Also, keep in mind that every time you get upset, a negative part of the other person wins. Every time you keep your cool, that same part is diminished. Punishment is not a sustainable way to get what we want out of people. Rewarding them with stern attention, compassion, and love is.

When someone acts rude, treat them as an animal that you are training that has not performed a trick properly. Anyone that has trained a pet knows that you withhold the food, you wait, you keep talking to it, and you just give it another chance. You don't take punitive action against the animal unless it has physically harmed you or someone else. It is not our place to punish anyone unless they have physically harmed us. Cultivate the same kind of patience with people that you might use with an abused pet. Be a lenient but firm master.

Recognize Psychopathy in Yourself and Others

In computer science, there is a concept known as "device hardening" by which a computer's vulnerabilities are reduced by various means. These constrain the available methods of attack by hackers and viruses. Such methods include changing default passwords, disabling unnecessary services, applying patches, closing network ports, and setting up firewalls and intrusion prevention systems. Reading this book has put you through a process of hardening. The exercises provide stress tests and stress proofing. You have been fortified, and the vulnerabilities in your head, thorax, and abdomen will continue to be reduced as long as you take part in the exercises. This hardening process has strengthened you but also made you susceptible to psychopathic behavior. This is why I want to address the nature of psychopathy so that some readers do not let their newfound composure corrupt them.

In this section, I will try to convince you that we have something to learn from the psychopath. They have a form of strength that we want for ourselves but also a tendency to hurt others, which we don't. Let's start by describing what we don't want. Psychopathy is a personality disorder characterized by bold, disinhibited behavior, as well as impaired empathy and remorse. Many psychopaths are serial bullies. They often parasitize the people around them, constantly committing offenses, many of which are non-arrestable. They exhibit Machiavellian self-interest and are often not concerned with the psychological damage they inflict on their targets. They are frequently negativistic, impatient, intemperate, embittered, oppositional, over-competitive, petulant, and mean-spirited. They can be easily slighted, quickly disillusioned, and have a penchant for wanting to punish others. They use pain as an instrument of power and leave people worse off than they found them. We don't want to follow suit.

The people that I know personally on the psychopathy spectrum set people up to cross their lines of decency so that they can retaliate. They love their "mean" personality. They think that it is smart, witty, and cool. But no one that I know who is proud of being mean is respectable. And I know several. They are all socially disabled hypocrites. They all cross their close friends and family more than anyone else, and their behavior inevitably results in tragedy.

Psychopaths make up only around 1% of the population. However, each of us can become psychopathic in certain contexts. People are more likely to callously abuse others in situations when they become angry or when they believe they are dominant. When someone is calmly rude to you, they are attempting to be a cat toying with a mouse. In other words, they are trying to build the experience of being a predator with a total disregard for how it might be affecting you. Never let yourself be that mouse. If someone is psychopathic with you, I think it is fair to be psychopathic back. In the next few paragraphs, I will explain what I mean: that it is fair to be without empathy, although not sadistic.

The research literature on the psychology and neuroscience of psychopathy is extensive. To boil it down, psychopaths exhibit alterations in emotional brain areas that cause them to be callous and fearless. Interestingly, their amygdala can be utterly unresponsive to many types of social stressors. Psychopaths have reduced sympathetic responsiveness while looking at distressing pictures. The same is true when they look at pictures of other people in distress. This has caused researchers to conclude that they have a lack of empathy. They are poor at naming fearful emotional expressions.[9] They also exhibit a diminished response to conditioned punishment, less fear, and reduced startle reflex to myriad startling stimuli.[10] Social conflict doesn't increase their heart rate or breathing rate, and does not cause them to brace. They are often reported to be charismatic and exhibit superficial charm. They are capable of these things because they do not feel pressured to self-handicap.

But none of these neurological predispositions toward insensitivity necessarily make them bad. A biological predisposition to being unafraid, in and of itself, doesn't make the psychopath evil. Unfortunately, it often causes them to make social mistakes and flout norms. The people that they unintentionally hurt punish them for these mistakes. I believe the resulting constant conflict turns them into bad people over time. But the "bad" doesn't derive from their innate fearlessness; the bad comes in if the repercussions of that fearlessness cause them to start taking delight in others' pain.

Some people find pleasure in hurting others. These people show activity in the brain's reward circuit (the ventral striatum) when shown videos depicting deliberate infliction of pain.[11] When they watch someone maliciously prick another with a needle, they feel amusement and gratification. Some psychopaths exhibit this, but many do not. Psychopaths don't necessarily want to hurt people, but they are willing to hurt them if they can get what they want.

Psychopaths don't feel another's pain, sadists enjoy it. Reveling in another's pain is known as sadism and schadenfreude.

Schadenfreude is defined as the feeling of enjoyment that comes from seeing or hearing about other people's troubles. In German, it means "harm-joy." Sadism is enjoyment in being cruel. Sadists don't choose to feel satisfaction from someone else's misfortune. It is neurological and usually derives from a combination of early experiences and genetics. However, you can confront any tendencies you may have toward sadism, and you and I are obligated to do so. Harm-joy is evil. Draw a hard line in the sand.

Activity #24.6: *Analyze Your Tendencies Toward Sadism*

How do you imagine your brain's reward centers respond to other people's pain or misfortune? Can you think of a time when something grim happened to someone, and you became excited or experienced pleasure? How could you become more aware of this tendency as it happens? How could you interrupt or undermine it if you recognized it? Ask yourself, "How can I take the strength and fearlessness from psychopathy without any hint of sadism?"

You want to be psychopathic when it comes to the dominance hierarchy. You want to be stone-cold when people attack you. To be assertive, sometimes you need to throw excessive empathy out of the window. I am advocating a type of ruthlessness that is not destructive, where you don't worry about what other people think of you, and your heart bleeds for no one. You are not doing anything wrong though because, outside of self-defense, you are too confident and compassionate to feel the desire to hurt others in revenge.

Lessons from Breaking My Nose

In Chapter 8, I recounted how my nose was broken at a McDonald's at age 17. I didn't tell the whole embarrassing story. I walked up to the McDonalds restaurant with an exaggerated posture. I was trying to be a little cooler than I really was. Another 17-year-old in the parking lot didn't like it. He said several unkind things to me, and I asked him to leave me alone. He followed me inside and continued to menace me. While I was standing in line to order food, he made a final, unprovoked, disparaging comment. I didn't consider him a threat, so I reached out and gently pulled the brim of his baseball cap down below his eyes. I expected that it would take a couple of seconds for him to fix his hat. Without even pushing the brim back up, he immediately tilted his head upward so that he could see me and threw a swift right cross to my nose.

There are four things we can learn from this. First, I shouldn't have pushed his hat down. It was the wrong thing to do. It leaped over the line from assertion to aggression. When we touch someone else without being welcomed to do so, it is a violation of something sacred. We shouldn't ever touch people in anger unless it is in self-defense.

The second lesson I found in this is that any fight can do a lot of damage. The blow broke my skull in multiple places. Parts of the nasal bone, maxilla, and septum were fragmented. The surgeon said he had to pick out many bits of shattered bone from my face. The emergency room doctors told me the injury was consistent with being hit with a bat or a club. But I wasn't hit with a club. I remember distinctly being hit with a fist. I was only hit once by a 17-year-old boy that must have weighed less than 150 pounds. I think this should be a lesson for all of us. Any act of physical violence can have severe costs, and just one strike from anyone has the potential to do grave damage. We don't want our faces broken, and we don't want to break anyone else's face, either. Tell yourself that fighting is not worth the costs. Prepare yourself to skillfully and gracefully decline physical violence when it confronts you. This will give you the peace of mind to rise above it.

Third, if you are going to walk around with optimal posture, you must be well-prepared to deal with people trying to call your bluff. I was assaulted because I had my chest puffed up. But I have since proved to myself that it is all in the way you do it. I walk around expressionless with my chest inflated and neck completely retracted all the time now. But I am not putting on airs, it is not a form of submissive threat, and I do it with no remorse but also with no animosity. No one seems to question it or get angry about it. To be honest, I'm not sure that I could pull it off in a penitentiary. But I can pull it off safely in any neighborhood in the world. I promise you that. And I promise that you can do it too. The key is just to do it without an ounce of anger in your heart.

Number four. As recounted in Chapter 8, having my nose broken changed my facial posture and increased the amount of repetitive strain in my facial muscles, but it did something else much more insidious. It stopped me from breathing nasally. A few months after the incident, I started having difficulty breathing through my nose. I resigned to being an obligate mouth breather. Contrary to what I assumed, however, my nasal passage hadn't been narrowed by the damage. Rather, the disuse narrowed it.

After the nose break, it was packed with gauze for two weeks, so I learned not to breathe nasally. Because I learned by habit to breathe through my mouth, my diaphragm atrophied, and my tidal range shrunk. Nasal breathing became difficult—not because my nasal passage was any smaller but because my diaphragm had grown weak. I was no longer able to breathe slowly, smoothly, and at long enough intervals to make nose breathing tenable.

After the cascade of physical and social repercussions of being a mouth breather, I went from being moderately popular in high school to very unpopular in college. As recounted in Chapter 11, I recently forced myself to start breathing through my nose again, and it was difficult at first. Taping my mouth helped. Now it is second nature, and it helped me reclaim the calmness and composure of my youth.

Four interesting lessons from one traumatic incident. Funnily enough, it took me more than 20 years to learn them. How many of our instances of trauma hold important lessons for us?

Prepare Yourself to Avoid Physical Confrontation

In this book, I ask you to walk around like you are a superhero. This can be dangerous as it can arouse insecurity in others and could cause them to assault you. You need a few good conciliatory displays in your arsenal. There are many things you can do at the last second to forestall an attack. Just knowing that you have these is empowering and will help you keep unphased when provoked.

Practicing a head nod greeting can prepare you to extract yourself from tense situations. The head nod consists of two movements: a quick motion either up or down and then a slightly slower motion resetting the head to its original setting. Nodding up is more assertive and can be perceived as a challenge if it is not accompanied by a smile or an eyebrow raise. Nodding down is more modest.

Nodding down can be a helpful way to acknowledge someone and diffuse tension created by eye contact between strangers. The fact that you stayed composed while you acknowledged the other person civilly with a nod before they acknowledged you shows that you do not feel threatened and are not trying to threaten. Practicing a several head nods in front of a mirror will train you to nod reassuringly after a tense or unexpected encounter with a stranger.

Conflict Activity #24.7: *Head Nod Greeting*

Practice a friendly head nod. It may help at first to do this in front of a mirror, making eye contact with yourself. Start by nodding down quickly and then back up. Practice both upward and downward nods. Repeat a few dozen times until you get the hang of it. Nodding once is a positive display that will usually invite the other person to nod back and relax.

Use the mentalis muscle at the bottom of the chin to raise the chin toward the mouth. You might combine this with a risorious smile by drawing the corners of the lips outwards without smiling up into the cheeks. Then combine this with the nod. Using the mentalis muscles to raise the chin while flashing a risorious smile sends a stern but friendly signal that diffuses suspicion.

Prepare yourself with dispassionate lines that will alleviate anger. These include: "Excuse me, friend," "I'm not looking for any trouble," or, simply, "Hello, may I help you?" Say something peaceful while breathing deeply. This will advertise that you are neither afraid nor angry. If the person looks upset and confronts you physically, you might want to diffuse tension by calmly introducing yourself. You could advance a single fist for them to "bump" their fist against or advance an open hand to initiate a handshake.

What is the best way to shake hands? It is pretty easy. Open the web between your thumb and index finger wide and make an effort to stick it firmly into their web. Keep your palm flat rather than cupped so that you can increase the surface area of contact between your palms. Wrap your hand around theirs and squeeze firmly. Don't allow anyone to twist your wrist during the shake. Shake athletically from the elbow and linger for a moment. A firm handshake that moves fluidly up and down shows that you are not trembling. Much of the same goes for hugs. Hugs should be nourishing; long, firm, and without startling or any sudden involuntary movements.

Negative Physical Encounters

"If someone succeeds in provoking you, realize that your mind is complicit in the provocation."
— *Epictetus (c. 50-135)*

Come to grips with the fact that you may have to fight to protect yourself or others. Animal behaviorists almost always recommend that you fight back fiercely if attacked by an animal. Criminologists recommend that you do the same if assaulted by a human. Don't attack until after they have launched the first offensive, but once they do, you have carte blanche.

Fight fair, but fight with zest, gumption, and a determination to end the altercation quickly and with as little destructiveness as necessary. Keep in mind that you can be legally and financially liable for any injuries you cause and that if you gravely hurt the person or kill them, you could end up in jail for decades or even for the rest of your life.

In most escalating situations, if the person can tell that you are not afraid of fighting them but are also not intentionally provoking them, they will leave you alone. The best way to avoid a fight is to show with your face that you are not scared at all and that you are not interested. No one is going to want to fight you if you look like you are disinterested in fighting. You want your attitude to say, "Oh, we can certainly fight, but only as a last resort." I have found that it can help to tell yourself that you do not fight civilians, just monsters, supervillains, evil robots, invading aliens, and extreme threats to good.

It can also help to stop thinking of physical combat as traumatic. Don't fear it or give it more power than it deserves. People that fight frequently think little of it. Think of it as a right of passage or as a game that you are willing to play if necessary. It is an undertaking that serves as a final deciding factor in a dispute. Even if you lose, remain relaxed: "Hey, I lost, you got me." or "Well, the fella whupped me pretty good, so I suppose he can have his way this time." There should be no shame in declining to fight or in losing a fight.

Many people find themselves pulled into fights due to an immature sign of petulance on their faces. They are displaying an air of submissive threat. Primates generally make two kinds of threats: confident and subordinate. Subordinate threats are reckless. They come from a place of fear and pain and have startle embedded within them. Most threats in humans and primates are subordinate.

Monkeys will stare, jerk their head, lunge forward, or fake-charge to try to get another group member to submit. These are usually bluffs. Many wild animals will stop altogether if the other merely holds its ground. Even 14,000 pound charging elephants are known to turn away at the last second from a human standing calmly with planted feet. People relying on physical intimidation are looking for easy targets. It is the same when people try to criticize you. Those who crumble get picked on forever. Don't be intimidated. Plant your feet. If you act afraid of a carnivorous mammal, this "forces" it to become more aggressive. If you act afraid of other people, it similarly "forces" them, instinctively, to persecute you further.

How would you act if you encountered a wolf or mountain lion on a hike? Ideally, you would want to act dominant and indifferent (but always letting the animal know you're aware of its every movement). If you do this properly, it will keep a safe distance most of the time, as you're telling it you feel secure enough to claim and remain in your territory. You are communicating that you pose a greater threat to it than it does to you. This is the mindset to use in public places. You want to implicitly communicate that you pose a bigger threat to others than they pose to you but that you have no desire or intent to harm.

If we can resolve to refrain from physical violence until it is the very last option, we can greatly reduce our level of stress because the expectation of physical conflict is one of the main things that causes us to brace our chakra-like modules. Actively refraining from violence is an age-old practice. The Hindu and Buddhist practice of "ahimsa" (from the Sanskrit word for "noninjury") is a doctrine of renouncing any form of violence toward any living being. It is a beautiful way to live life.

Conclusion

"A great man shows his greatness by the way he treats little men." — Thomas Carlyle (1795-1881)

Because our brains expect that we will be actively competing for food and sex, they expect us to have enemies. Genetically prepared instincts influence us to take the closest thing they can find to an enemy and villainize them. This is also why, if you put two unfamiliar adult cats into a room, they will probably not get along. You might desperately want them to get along—they might be happier if they did—but, often, they cannot get past their reflexive defense mechanisms. This confused, displaced hostility is also present in the modern workplace, and home where conflict seems to be the norm. It is all too easy for values and prehistoric programming to clash. Anger often erupts out of an interaction between two people who both feel they are completely reasonable. As with the cats, this is largely neurological.

A large proportion of animals will attack their reflection when they see a mirror for the first time. Apes will commonly take offense from their own body posturing. They send and receive threatening displays to their reflection until they provoke themselves into assaulting the mirror. If you saw a mirror image of yourself and didn't recognize it, would you be offended by your own social displays? Could you get along with yourself?

Some animals see their reflections in the mirror and want to play. Isn't that beautiful? Let us be that way. Why not carry ourselves in a way that influences others to be playful? We will delve into this in the next chapter.

Chapter 24: **Bullet Points**

- Hostility is associated with heart disease, high blood pressure, insulin resistance, and inflammation.
- There is no need to be right or make anyone else wrong.
- Don't embed barbs in your comments.
- Never let anything anyone says cause you to beat yourself up from the inside.
- Use skillful assertion to bring out the best in people.
- Do as much as you can to see others as tribe members, collaborators, and players on the same team rather than rivals.
- You should never feel forced to choose between being a nice guy no one respects and being a jerk who gets everything he wants.
- When dealing with a difficult person, you want to sidestep their negativity and take the shortcut to the outcome that you want while remaining fair and equitable.
- Resist the emotional urge to take offense and pursue vengeance.
- Respond to provocation with calm non-contention.
- Handle conflict charismatically.
- Never respond as if you are reacting to bullying. Never be a victim.
- Trying to be better than other people and outdo them is exhausting and ends up taxing your health.
- Cultivate self-awareness for your tendency to take out frustrations and transfer blame.
- Don't let anyone grab you by the breath.
- Acknowledge that your actions and opinions are fallible.
- Feel comfortable apologizing and offering clarification for your behaviors.
- Avoid implicitly condoning acts of incivility that you witness.
- Lower your constant guard against perceived diminishment and loss of ego.
- Reframe the offenses of others as shortcomings in priorities, judgment, social maturity, and word choice.
- Demonstrate more interest in finding a solution than in defending a position.
- Retain your peace regardless of the other person's disposition.
- Listen to and make an effort to understand others' perspectives without interrupting.
- Instead of contradicting the contribution of another, think about how you can build on top of it.
- Be a psychopath with a heart of gold.
- Be absolutely unflappable. Pretend you are a god if need be. That calm exterior starts as a bluff but becomes a way of life.
- Assume the best or neutral motives in others. Maintain an objective stance when conflict arises.
- Instead of taking in the worst from everyone and reacting against it, selectively take the best and channel it into everything you do.

Chapter 24: **Endnotes**

1.   Andersson, L., & Pearson, C. (1999). Tit for tat? The spiraling effect of incivility in the workplace. *The Academy of Management Review*, *24*, 452-471.

2.   Porath, C. L., & Erez, A. (2007). Does rudeness really matter? The effects of rudeness on task performance and helpfulness. *Academy of Management Journal, 50*(5), 1181–1197.

3.   Sapolsky, R. M. (2005). The influence of social hierarchy on primate health. *Science*, *308*(5722), 648–652.

4.   Shepherd, S. V., & Platt, M. L. (2010). Neuroethology of attention in primates. In M. L. Platt & A. A. Ghazanfar (Eds.), *Primate neuroethology* (pp. 525–549). Oxford University Press.

5.   Panksepp J. (2010). Affective neuroscience of the emotional BrainMind: evolutionary perspectives and implications for understanding depression. *Dialogues in Clinical Neuroscience*, *12*(4), 533–545.

6.   Maletic, V. M., Robinson, M., Oakes, T., Iyengar, S., Ball, S. G., & Russell, J. (2007). Neurobiology of depression: An integrated view of key findings. *International Journal of Clinical Practice*, *61*(12), 2030–2040.

7.   Millan, C., & Peltier, M. J. (2006). *Cesar's way: The natural, everyday guide to understanding & correcting common dog problems*. Random House.

8.   Conniff, R. (2015). *The ape in the corner office*. Random House.

9.   Blair, R., & Coles, M. (2000). Expression recognition and behavioral problems in early adolescence. *Cognitive Development*, *15*(4). pp.421–434; Stevens, D., Charman, T., & Blair, R. J. R. (2001). Recognition of emotion in facial expressions and vocal tones in children with psychopathic tendencies. *The Journal of Genetic Psychology*, *162*(2), 201–211.

10.   Blair, R. J. R. (1999). Responsiveness to distress cues in the child with psycholopathic tendencies. *Personality and Individual Differences*, *27*, 135–145; Levenston, G., Patrick, C., Bradley, M., & Lang, P. (2000). The psychopath as observer: Emotion and attention in picture processing. *Journal of Abnormal Psychology*, *109*, 373–385.

11.   Buckholtz, J. W., Treadway, M. T., Cowan, R. L., Woodward, N. D., Benning, S. D., Li, R., Ansari, M. S., Baldwin, R. M., Schwartzman, A. N., Shelby, E. S., Smith, C. E., Cole, D., Kessler, R. M., & Zald, D. H. (2010). Mesolimbic dopamine reward system hypersensitivity in individuals with psychopathic traits. *Nature neuroscience*, *13*(4), 419–421.

Chapter 25: **Finding Happiness Through Playfulness & Composed Kindness**

"No one can live happily who has regard to himself alone and transforms everything into a question of his own utility; you must live for your neighbor, if you would live for yourself." — Seneca (c. 4 BCE - 65)

"Trust men, and they will be true to you; treat them greatly, and they will show themselves great." — Ralph Waldo Emerson (1803-1882)

People are often hesitant to be "nice." It is stigmatized. When we see polite people, they often cause us to wonder: "Are they so friendly because they are weak?" This is a common contention because being kind often involves slowing down, letting others have their way, and handicapping oneself. But equating niceness with weakness is fallacious because being nice doesn't necessarily mean that you allow others to take advantage. This is because it is entirely possible to be self-composed when kind. Composed kindness has very few costs. Employing it will improve your interpersonal functioning and restore your good faith in others. In Chapter 1, I said that people were taking my anxious kindness for weakness, making me into a bitter person. You will find that people take your composed kindness for strength, making you into a people person.

Every encounter you have with another person is an opportunity for you to practice composed kindness. Keep spreading goodwill whether others reciprocate or not. Starting with unilateral kindness can help you surmount the other person's defense mechanisms. Be prepared to be the cheerful, helpful chap in a world full of miserable Scrooges. Presume good faith and positive intentions. This eventually brings the best out in everyone. You cannot lose so long as you maintain your sense of enlightened benevolence, guided by your personal code, and centered by unbothered breathing.

Being Cool Is Disarming

One of the best ways to bring composure to your kindness is by being cool. Done right, it can disarm pettiness. What does "acting cool" mean to you? To answer this, think of the top five coolest people you know. Who would be on your list of the coolest celebrities? Who were the people you looked up to in your youth? When have you been cool in the past? Channel this energy. Think urbane, suave, garrulous, jocular, and levelheaded. You want sangfroid, verve, cachet, and moxie. Think firmness of character, force of determination, steadiness of nerves, unruffled tact, and being powerfully good-natured. Keep the word "savoir-faire" and its definition in mind: the ability to speak or behave appropriately and at ease in social situations.

Being cool means not being afraid of being too calm. This can make you come off as numb or detached, and that is okay. Don't be afraid to zone out on your friends. They may take it as aloofness and try to push you away. But if you don't push back and you leave the door open, allowing them to linger, many people will choose to hang out and hang loose with you. Try to get them to detach as much as you have, proving that forced extraversion isn't necessary. Take breaks from talking and just take in your surroundings. Never feel pressured to keep interacting. Lounge in comfortable silences. Don't use adrenaline to help you complete your sentence or help you find that term on the tip of your tongue. Don't allow cortisol to dictate your personality at the event. Instead, use serotonin, endorphins, and oxytocin to help you build rapport.

Being cool is about having sustainable body language in social situations. You want to operate in a way that would not fatigue even if you had to socialize for 48 hours straight. How would you behave if you knew that you would be awake, surrounded by people and face-to-face interactions for two full days? You would have to pace yourself. This would require you to allow plenty of micro-breaks to each of various modules. Your face, voice, breath, and posture would have to be indefatigable (invulnerable to fatigue). And if you were to maintain your assertiveness for the duration, you would have to be very "cool." Almost every one of the exercises in this book will enhance your cool. Facial massage, gut compression, vocal rehab, and increasing diaphragm range will all contribute significantly.

For your coolness to be tenable in the long term, you must act like everyone else is cool. When you treat someone else as though they were cool, you validate them. Thus, the best way to make yourself seem normal and well-functioning is to treat everyone else as normal and well-functioning. So, act as if you expect the other person to be confident and at ease in everything they say and do.

Act as if Nothing Is Awkward

Most people's attempts at social dominance center around making others feel as if they are less socially skilled. The people around you try to gaslight you into thinking that you are socially incompetent. Over time, this caused me to act as if everything I did, and most things that others did, was awkward. I felt that I had social shortcomings and owed it to others to use my body language to recognize this, or else I was shameless. I would also subtly patronize others for their uncouth blunders, thinking it would be dishonest to ignore these. This led me into a downward spiral of awkwardness.

One day I tried the opposite; I acted like nothing anyone did was amateur. I pretended to be comfortable with every aspect of the interactions I had. I quickly found that this tactic works wonders and that it is at the heart of being cool, as well as being simultaneously nondominating and nonsubmissive. The more we treat others as if they are adroit socially, the better they feel about themselves and the more they like us. Do this and be shameless about it. Act as if you and whoever you're with are the coolest people on the planet. Once you put this into effect, you will find that your gallant speech and actions send chills up your spine. Your own behavior will become your primary source of endorphins, and you will get hooked on being assertive in a debonair way.

Treating people who are awkward or socially defeated as if they are normal will liberate them. We should strive to make everyone feel socially facile even if talking to them is uncomfortable at first. Ignore the unrefined aspects of their presentation and express enthusiasm for what they are trying to communicate. Move on quickly from their embarrassments and bloopers. Ignore any tension leakage they may exhibit. Most people focus on all that is ugly and inept in others. When you don't even perceive these things, you give them a chance to blossom.

Being Humble Rescues You from Status Competition

Because our genes have been subjected to the primate status hierarchy for tens of millions of years, our brains have a propensity to interpret every occurrence as either a promotion or a demotion. It is instinctual. Boasting, for example, becomes common in children as young as three. The ego wants to turn relationships into self-aggrandizement. Left unchecked, it will turn everyone, even friends and family, into a means to an end. This instinct to constantly defend ourselves drains us of the same composure that it intends to conserve.

Indeed, confidence is necessary, but egotism is incredibly tiresome. Paradoxically, taking yourself too seriously is a submissive trait. Developing a side of yourself that is humble and modest is necessary for being happy. Counterintuitively, it is also empowering because it allows you not to be affected by constant demotions. We need humility and unobtrusiveness. They afford us a type of confidence that is unconditional and not based on external circumstances.

Happiness Activity #25.1: *Renouncing the Ego*

Consider the Buddhist concept of "non-self." The Buddha recommended that we imagine having no social identity to protect and obsess over. He asked us to recognize the unreality of the self-concept and the need to be better than others. Buddhists use the word "sunyata" to describe both the emptiness and the spaciousness that is achieved when the ego disappears. Can you get yourself to feel it?

Imagine voluntarily relinquishing your identity, pride, and ego. Imagine having no name, no body, and no physical attributes. Imagine having no possessions, education, resume, accomplishments, and no reputation in the world. There would be nothing to gloat about, but also nothing for others to criticize. There would be no striving for prestige and no social comparison. It would mean being formless and self-transcendent. What would it be like to have no ego for the rest of your life?

Another aspect of being cool is not being focused on yourself. Don't think about how you are perceived when you are actively socializing. Pretend to have as little self-awareness of your appearance as possible. Over time, this will manifest. Impression management and self-monitoring can be critical, but at times try to stop thinking about others' social evaluations of you. Tell yourself that you have already had enough approval, compliments, and praise from others to last a lifetime and that you don't need any more. This will help you stop identifying with the evaluations of others. An old cliché tells us that confidence isn't thinking you're better than others; it's not even bothering to make the comparison. This logic holds. As the charitable, big-hearted, alpha-minded individual you are, work toward being oblivious to your conceits.

Healthy humility will make it so that you don't have to look for evidence of your worth anymore. Bring an end to the need to measure yourself against other people. You want to be a strong presence that doesn't glorify or advertise itself. Being humble also precludes you from having to continually prove yourself so that you are not embarrassed when you inevitably make mistakes. We should be willing and happy to play a game with a friend, even when we know she is much better than us. The only person you should be working toward being better than is the human being you were yesterday.

This next activity is sometimes regarded in Buddhism and Hinduism as the single most potent metaphysical practice. It will tear your false pride to shreds and reveal emotional maturity underneath it. It involves resisting the temptation to defend yourself in front of others. Spiritual author Eckhart Tolle has an insight about this practice: "When you are seemingly diminished in some way and remain in absolute non-reaction, not just externally but also internally, you realize that nothing real has been diminished, that through becoming 'less,' you become more."

Happiness Activity #25.2: *Allowing Diminishment of the Ego*

Allow another person to say something to diminish your standing without making any attempt to restore it. Allow other people to strike blows to your pride, whether by being brusque, criticizing you, blaming you, or saying something explicitly wrong about you. Notice how it makes you feel inside. Become comfortable with the discomfort that it creates. Notice what your normal response would be and inhibit it. Remember that you are never required to retaliate or defend yourself. If the other person is waiting for your response, perhaps agree with the part of what they said that is reasonable.

The best way to cultivate inner freedom is to learn to relax around petty, rude, and aggressive people. The need to defend yourself will diminish until it becomes clear to everyone that there is nothing they can do to aggravate you. Every time you stop yourself from overreacting, it gets easier. Likewise, every time you stop yourself from status maneuvering, social chess, jockeying for power, and pretending to be someone you are not, it gets easier.

Endearing But Still Composed

This book has argued that we should not act submissive because of the way it increases tension in the body over time. However, body and voice movements that take effort or briefly compromise composure endear people. There are many ways to do this that come across as warm but that are not inferiority displays and won't lead to repetitive strain. For example, some endearing forms of body language include keeping your palms up, moving closer to people, pointing your feet toward them, and rubbing your hands together.

We should even use self-handicapping displays at times. Do this judiciously, a little bit at a time, without letting it cripple you. If you don't brace them and give them the micro-breaks they need, the modules involved will recharge and can be used again right away with no cost. It is endearing to squint, raise the eyebrows, raise the shoulders, crinkle the nose, speak in a high voice, and stoop over for brief periods. As long as it only persists for a few seconds and trigger points are not made active, it won't drain you.

Embracing Composed Submissiveness

Up until now, this book has denigrated submissiveness. We have discussed various ways that it damages both composure and health. But it is entirely possible to be composed *and* submissive. There are times when composed submissiveness is not just appropriate but also beneficial. These are the times when we let or encourage others to lead.

It can be freeing to be mellow and passive and to support the leadership of others. Allow other people to take over and yourself to relax when they do. Relish the relief from being in charge. Do so while exuding balanced, non-confrontational energy. Perpetual assertion takes its toll. It involves intense face time, eye contact, talking, decision making, and an overtaxing of existing bracing patterns. It leads to social fatigue and is why high-pressure executives and CEOs can age so rapidly. We should be handing over the pack leader role constantly, passing it around from person to person, sharing the stage, the crown, and the accompanying burdens.

Often, in real life, we are forced to play an inferior role. At our workplace, we must submit to higher-ups to keep our jobs and advance our careers. There are many reasons you should treat your boss as the dominant individual. What's more, it may be best for you, your boss, and the business to allow them to act superior in some ways. That said, don't hurt yourself just to let the boss be the boss. Acquiesce appropriately to your employer, law enforcement, judges, and other authority figures without diminishing your posture, shortening your breath, or surrendering your pride. This will allow you to maintain a healthy serotonin level regardless of your place on the corporate ladder.

Just because you don't try to stop someone from acting dominant doesn't mean they are dominating you. They are only dominating you if you are inhibiting yourself or avoiding confrontation with them out of fear. They can never dominate you as long as you stay composed. Take sovereignty from needless one-upmanship.

Keep in mind that everyone has essential observations and keen insights to impart. All humans are our fellows and our equals. As Ralph Waldo Emerson said, "Every man I meet is in some way my superior." So, let every man and woman be your superior at times, especially when they have something to teach you. When you see someone do better than you at something you value, don't feel envious or threatened. Instead, feel eager to learn. This is ego stability and emotional strength.

When threatened by an intruder, a dominant gorilla will let out a tremendous roar, charge, and knock down the newcomer with an immense hand swipe. However, outside of defending themselves and their group members, dominant gorillas do not generally overtly assert their rank.[1] Even though gorillas are immense powerhouses, animal behaviorists often describe them as shy because, most of the time, they don't feel like they have anything to prove. It is not that they are shy; it is that we are arrogant, pompous, and flagrantly adversarial.

The only way to transcend the dominance hierarchy is to be content when you temporarily find yourself in a subordinate position; to be comfortable when others perceive you as subordinate without trying to change their mind. You don't want to be a doormat, but neither do you want to be consumed by resisting looking like a doormat. Only doormats worry about being doormats.

Our unconscious mind values prestige over happiness. The two are often at odds. You can change this by intentionally pursuing happiness over prestige.

Optimism, Excitement, and Feeling Good

It pays to be happy. Optimists live longer, have stronger immune systems, recover from injury more quickly, and have increased mental and physical health. Happiness and positive emotions are linked to higher earnings, better appraisal at work, relationships of higher quality, and increased likability.[2] Happy people are perceived as more intelligent, competent, and physically attractive. Optimists cope more effectively with stress, are generally healthier, and are less likely to become depressed.[3] When optimists have coronary bypass surgery, they heal more quickly than pessimists.[4] Positive thinking results in a cardiovascular system that is less reactive to stress.[5] But how do we become happy in the first place?

Optimists attribute the cause of adverse events to external, specific, and transient factors. In other words, they see a tragedy as a one-off fluke. Pessimists, on the other hand, attribute failures to their own internal, global, and permanent shortcomings. They see themselves as useless and assume the world is out to get them. If this is you, stop it. Regain your optimism by recognizing that you have the potential to fix anything and everything that has ever been wrong with your life. Recognize that the "future you" will be skilled and competent enough to solve any problems that arise.

We are constantly making expressions to ourselves as we go about our days alone. Whatever these expressions are, they constitute our true selves. For most people, it's wincing. If that's you, make the gestures and facial expressions of happiness when you are by yourself. The smiling and the postural alterations from previous chapters will help with this. If solitary happiness is not practiced regularly, attempts at appearing happy among others will be fake. Remember how excited you could become as a child? You had no reservations about expressing exuberance and enthusiasm. Nothing is stopping you from feeling zestfully happy right now aside from the force of habit.

I have spent much of this book describing how we use our bodily energy to traumatize our tissues. This might make you assume that our life force is destructive. It is not. You must redirect that same life force away from anxiety and tension toward happiness and joy. The more you do this, the less energy there is to sustain stress. Doing so actively reprograms how your body routes energy, setting you up for hardwired happiness. Accordingly, all the exercises in this book should be done with joy and optimistic expectations. This will make them much more powerful.

Be a lifeless corpse when it comes to tension, ego, and pessimism. When it comes to playfulness, however, that's when you want to be alive and spend your chi-like energy on positive social displays. Let's start with laughter.

Laughter in Other Animals

Many mammals laugh. For example, most rodents emit long ultrasonic vocalizations during rough and tumble play. The sounds rats and mice make have been described as chirping and occur in the 50-kHz range (inaudible to humans). When chirping, they actively seek being tickled and played with. They chirp when wrestling, chasing, or searching for one another. They chirp during courting and before copulation. Researchers have interpreted rat chirping as an expectation of something rewarding and it appears to elicit friendly social approach in other members of their species.[6] It also nullifies anxiety. If you tickle a rat after a fearful situation, it will neutralize the negative emotions and vastly decrease any fear-related learning going on in its brain.

Dogs can pant using heavy, forced exhalations in a way that suggests a form of modified laughter. They use it during play. Dogs exposed to a recorded "dog-laugh" exhibit significantly reduced stress behaviors, increased tail wagging, the display of the canine "play-face," as well as prosocial behavior such as approaching and licking another dog's lips.[7]

Chimps, gorillas, and orangutans all exhibit laughter-like vocalizations in response to physical play, including friendly contact like chasing, wrestling, and tickling.[8] It is a shallow pant, conveying nonaggression that is highly reminiscent of suppressed laughter in humans. Their laughter shows the same sonographic pattern as that of human babies. They also use similar facial expressions while laughing and are ticklish in the same areas that humans are. Ape laughter consists of a series of exhalations and inhalations (like panting). On the other hand, human laughter consists of a series of exhalations with no intervening inhalations.[9]

Mice, dogs, apes, and humans make their breath shallow to create rapport. Insistence on breathing at long intervals caused me to stop doing this. I was so focused on diaphragmatic breathing that I refused to breathe shallowly even when joking with friends. This is like refusing to make anything other than an expressionless face. Think of shallow breathing during fun, jovial play as a form of healthy panting that serves as a temporary micro-break or counterpose to diaphragmatic breathing. Refusing to pant is refusing to play.

Rehabilitating Your Laughter Will Make It Much More Pleasurable

Gelotology is the study of laughter and the positive effects it can have on the body. Proponents advocate the induction of laughter on therapeutic grounds.[10] Laughter yoga (hasya yoga) and laughter meditation also use voluntary laughter for therapeutic purposes. Studies have shown that it alleviates both stress and pain.[11] These practices assume that voluntary or forced laughter provides some of the same benefits as spontaneous laughter. Voluntary laughter is often done in groups and may turn into real laughter. Participants are instructed to facilitate laughing by using "childlike playfulness" and eye contact. These practices are great, but I think they do not get down to the issue's crux. From what I have seen, people who engage in this practice are mostly laughing superficially. To reap the benefits, we must isolate and strengthen the core laughing reflex.

The muscles involved in laughing have been traumatized by life stress. As an infant, your laugh was primordial and bona fide. Years of anxious laughter and worrying that your laugh is too aggressive have damaged your instinctual laughing pattern. As you might expect, people who are depressed or anxious have the least convincing laughs. Extremely dominant people laugh loudly, without hesitating, at whatever they like. Most people, however, stifle their laughter in the same way they stifle their posture and breathing. This explains why most adults' laughter is eccentric and deviated from the innate laughter pattern.

A baby's laughter is vivacious and natural. To relearn to laugh genuinely, it is helpful to watch infants and toddlers laughing. Take the time to search for videos of "babies laughing" on the internet and mimic them. You will see that infants don't stifle their laughter. They don't worry about their laugh being too forceful or about offending someone. Neither should we. Your laugh should shake you to your core and be intensely pleasurable.

A hearty and progressive emptying of the lungs applies a significant load to the diaphragm and the muscles of the chest wall, triggering the endorphin system.[12] This is why social laughter is correlated with an elevated pain threshold.[13] However, most adult laughs hardly activate the pleasure system at all. After years of stifling laughter, we have forgotten how to laugh in a way that produces this response. For many people, the diaphragm's role in laughter has been weakened so much that laughter no longer recruits endorphins and is draining rather than energizing.

Fake or nervous laughter comes from the throat and often results in increased tension there. During natural laughter, the diaphragm does most of the work. By training yourself to laugh through deep contractions of the diaphragm and abdominals, you can rebuild an authentic laugh. These muscles should reach exhaustion and start to fail during a good laugh. If your diaphragm and abdominals begin to burn like they did when you were a child, you know that you are doing it right. The next exercise will show you exactly how to retrain your diaphragm to fully participate in the act of laughing.

Happiness Exercise #25.1: *Diaphragmatic Laughing*

Practice laughing while exhaling completely. This involves an uninterrupted emptying of the lungs. Inhale completely only after you laugh/exhale completely. Your exhale should consist of a long series of laughing sounds punctuated by vocal (glottal) closure ("haha" equals two glottal closures). The brief closing of the vocal tract (glottis) against the exhalation allows pressure to build and makes the laugh sound like a series of rapid-fire punches. They should roll out somewhat like the Rs when you roll your tongue. Practice this as an exercise and attempt to make the laughter last for at least five seconds, but shoot for 10 to 20 seconds. Laugh all the way to the bottom of your range of exhalation. Use the principles of anti-rigidity. Try the following variations:

1) Focus on and coordinate the laughs (glottal closures) so that they proceed at a smooth and steady rate.
2) Notice inadvertent irregularities in timing, as well as the tendency to gulp, choke, or falter, and iron these out. It's okay if it sounds mechanical and robotic at first while you are relearning the basics.
3) Cause the punctuated exhalations to roll out as fast as possible while maintaining a fixed rhythm. After you gain coordination in speeding them up, try slowing them down.
4) Do this using your voice at various pitches but focus most on using a deep voice to create a deep laugh.
5) Explore your preferred ways of laughing, varying resonance, inflection, and timing. Modulate each in as many ways as possible.
6) Employ different melodies and model other people's laughs. Spend time listening to and imitating actor Mark Hamill's maniacal Joker laugh.
7) Try laughing while exhaling completely until it turns into a wheeze and you feel you don't have a cubic centimeter of air left in your lungs. Ensure that the laughing pattern remains coordinated even at the bottom of your exhalation. This will greatly strengthen the muscles involved.
8) Don't raise your shoulders when you laugh and focus on keeping them pushed toward the floor. Maintain the tenets of optimal posture. Don't allow your spine to curve into a forward "C" shape. You might try lying on your stomach while you laugh to ensure that your spine is straight.
9) Do this with a thoroughly relaxed face or while you massage your face so that you can laugh heartily without intense facial constriction. Induce paroxysms of

laughter without raising the eyebrows, squinting, sneering, or tensing any other muscles.

10) The pressure to keep exhaling should be forceful and have a life of its own. It should feel like a boa constrictor is wrapped around your chest, squeezing you hard and only giving you a short period to inhale every few seconds.

11) Laugh authoritatively, compellingly, boldly, forcefully, mightily. Work on making it contagious.

Because the muscles are strained, stagnant, and uncoordinated, your laugh may sound like that of an insane villain at first. But, with practice, it will become friendly and ebullient. It is important to do this exercise loudly, gleefully, and unhesitatingly, so make sure that you are not worried about others hearing you. Do it in a closet or, better yet, in the car.

It will be uncomfortable at first. The muscles you engage may be so weak that they feel susceptible to damage. Mine certainly were. If so, take it easy the first few days and build up to doing it vigorously. Use laughter to work out the cramp in your diaphragm. This exercise is a powerful complement to diaphragmatic breathing exercises and will help you reach muscles that you otherwise could not. To this end, try it while lying on your stomach, from a forward fold, or from happy baby pose with your belly pushed out.

At first, the laughing exercise should make you feel weary. After only one week, you will be able to push harder and be more adept at coordinating the pulses of laughter. After a few weeks, you will be good at it and find yourself laughing more often. This exercise transformed my laugh from a flimsy, perfunctory, courtesy laugh into something enjoyable. Now I laugh spontaneously, heartily, resolutely, and much more frequently. I find laughing tremendously gratifying, and things that were barely amusing to me before are now hilarious.

I believe that laughing evolved to help humans let off steam. It may have allowed instances of camaraderie and social bonding to influence an individual's life strategy to place less value on the adaptive aspects of trauma. In other words, the more conducive your environment is to laughing, the more your body assumes that your environment is a good one and that it is safe to be optimistic. A real laugh was probably designed by evolution to help us attain a full-range, hard contraction of the diaphragm. As with pant-hooting (Exercise 11.6), this contraction relieves the diaphragm of the partial contraction caused by stress and shallow breathing.

The more you rehabilitate your laugh, the more you increase your diaphragm's potential for providing you with endorphins. Remember that endorphins are most reliably produced by grooming, singing, laughing, and play.[14] These are addressed in Chapter 6, Chapter 12, this section, and the next section, respectively.

Some people with relatively calm nasopharynxes can clear their nasopharynx in the same way others clear their throats. It is like snorting, except it involves breathing out rather than breathing in. Some people call it a nose laugh. I see it as a dominance signal conveying that the person's nasopharynx is not tense. When my nasopharynx was tense, I was incapable of doing it. Once you have compressed your nasopharynx using the exercises in Chapter 11, you can build the coordination to perform this empowering laugh.

Some people use this signal to laugh at something they find inferior, like rolling the eyes. Please don't use it derisively or to ridicule people. Instead, use it as a heartfelt laugh to communicate that you are enjoying absurdity. People usually find it exciting, and it makes them want to laugh along with you.

Happiness Exercise #25.2: *Laugh through the Nasopharynx*

Use a brief (0.5 to 3 seconds) but powerful exhalation to force air out through your nasopharynx with the mouth closed. This snort is similar to a scoff or chortle. It sometimes arises when you try to withhold laughter. First practice doing it in small, short bursts to develop the proper coordination so that you can build up to doing it in a prolonged way. With practice, you will be able to hold convincing, three-second nose laughs. It is a convivial way to express amusement that improves quickly with practice.

Be Playful

"We don't stop playing because we grow old; we grow old because we stop playing" — *George Bernard Shaw (1856-1950)*

Play, like laughter, is a form of medicine, but certain conditions must be met for it to be genuine. All stressors (anger, fear, pain, hunger, and separation) reduce play. Animals must be well fed, comfortable, and healthy for play to take place. When these conditions are met, rats and mice chase and pounce, wrestle, pin, nip, poke, and knock each other over. This is the kind of play that generates high-frequency laughter-like chirps at 50 kHz. Physical rough-and-tumble play is the most fun of all. At one point, I thought all aggressive acts were unpleasant, but judging from play in other mammals, feigned aggression can be joyous.

It is important to note that when mammals play, rapid role reversal is a defining element. In other words, they know it is friendly when everyone gets a chance to be on top. Knowledge of this should influence us to pass being dominant back and forth with our friends. The rat that ends up on top more often during pins becomes dominant. The continuation of play necessitates a willingness on the part of the winner to self-handicap. Dominant rats that go easy on others always have playmates, but those that bully are ignored when they try to solicit play. Play helps animals determine who to avoid and with whom they can develop cooperative relationships. They learn to dominate but also accept defeat without being "defeated."

Dominant animals would rather play, but aggressive animals would rather fight. Rats involved in a fight bite each other and box. This can lead to injury. They stand on their hind legs and strike each other with their front paws. When they do this, the 50-kHz "laughter" turns into 22-kHz "complaints." This is similar to chimpanzees among whom play is accompanied by wrestling, panting, and a play face, whereas fighting involves boxing, tearing, scratching, biting, and barking.

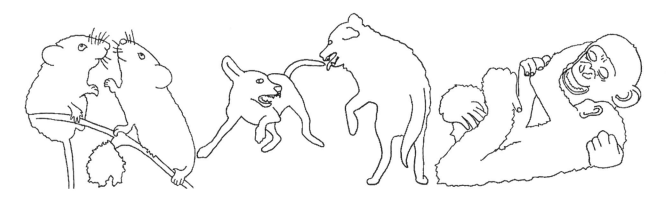

Illustration 25.1: Animals playing.

Rather than being based around wrestling, human play focuses on verbal interchange and banter. Repartee involves provocation, rejoinders, biting commentary, and, if friendly, laughter. As in other mammals, this form of verbal jousting can engender friendship, respect, and cooperation. It can be made more fun with the use of bombastic quarreling, absurd braggadocio, frivolous histrionics, grandiose pretentiousness, and ostentatious balderdash. When you do it, be spunky, employ exuberance, and enjoy it. You don't have to act excitable to be sparkling and bubbly; you just need to be playful. Usually, if you manage to entertain yourself, others will be entertained as well.

Remember to be like the mice during play and allow others their opportunity to be on top, lest you risk losing playmates. This includes giving others equal chance to talk and refraining from dominating conversations. A dog initiates play by crouching. A monkey initiates it by exposing its rear end. Both of these actions involve self-diminishment and vulnerability. Showing others that you don't take yourself too seriously or exposing a vulnerability can make them want to play with you. After experimenting with this for years now, I have concluded that you can be as vulnerable and nice as you can, and as long as you are playful, it won't be mistaken for weakness.

Play ranks among the most beneficial neuroplastic interventions. Placing rodents into enriched environments where they can socialize, wrestle, and play with others results in heavier brains and higher levels of dopamine, endorphins, and serotonin. Studies have found that rats deprived of play are more fearful and aggressive toward other rats. Encouraging playfulness in animals is one of the few behavioral interventions known to reverse anxiety and depressive symptoms.[15] This is probably because it allows them to shift from the threat response to the challenge response.

Social play involves creativity and requires that we learn to approach others in diverting and lively ways. Imagination and fantasy can also facilitate play. My favorite way to play with people is to make up imaginary scenarios: "What would you do if...?" I am animated, shameless, and immature when doing this. My scenarios include helicopters, ninjas, dinosaurs, and hats with pinwheels on top of them. When other people do this, recognize it as play, participate, and egg them on by laughing with them. Whenever someone uses an analogy or poetic license to describe a situation, help them flesh it out until you have created a whimsical, comical cartoon world. Feel at home with wordplay, punning, nonsense, and silliness.

Ask outrageous questions, set up outlandish hypotheticals, and feel comfortable acting like a kid. If you have genuine, heartfelt fun, they will, too, so entertain yourself and your sense of humor first.

Reawaken Your Play Face

A simple open-mouthed expression in primates called the "play-face" communicates that play is either underway or about to begin. It often accompanies primate laughter. The jaw is wide open, and sometimes, the corners of the mouth are slightly drawn back. Unlike the primate sneer or grin, the expression is relaxed, and the teeth are usually covered completely. All apes, as well as macaques, patas, vervets, and rhesus monkeys, use the play-face. Common during play sessions in juveniles, it is also an adult expression. It is used to enlist others to play and is accompanied by a jaunty, sprightly air. The display is usually reciprocated immediately. It is often interspersed with tumbling, tickling, chasing, wrestling, play-gnawing, and lip-smacking sounds.

We know the primate play-face as gaping in childlike wonderment. Our ability to gape has been reduced by our uptight attitudes and by excessive tension in the jaw. However, we can refurbish it. Recover yours because, in some ways, the play-face is better than the smile.

Happiness Exercise #25.3: *Gaping in Childlike Awe Is the Play-Face*

Bring back your childhood ability to express astonishment and delight. Relax your eyebrows, widen your eyes, and allow your jaw to gape widely. Gape without baring the teeth. Gape as if you have no inhibitions about how your wide-open mouth will appear to other people. Imagine that your wide mouth influences others to share your sense of playfulness and excitement. Pretend you are seven and just discovered something wonderful that you can share with your buddies. Alternate this expression with your smile. When you use it, think: "That's incredible!" or "Wanna play?!?" It also makes a great greeting or a reaction to a surprise.

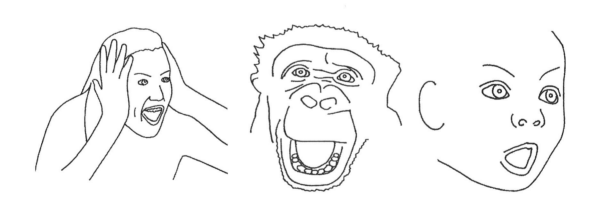

Illustration 25.1: A. Woman in awe; B. Chimpanzee play face; C. Baby excited.

Happy babies open their mouths wide when laughing. Socially defeated adults open their mouths the least. In my twenties, I wasn't able to open my jaw fully, and trying to was painful. Any gaping would make my jaw creak and crack. Dropping my jaw in any social situation seemed like dropping my guard. Pairing gaping with diaphragmatic breathing for less than 30 minutes gave my jaw an oil change. It has never creaked or cracked since. Now that gaping feels natural, I feel less serious and more encouraged to have fun. Master your play face.

Become a Great Conversationalist

One of the best ways to play with and love others is through conversation. Unfortunately, most of us have learned to converse competitively. The conversational narcissist wants to keep the attention on themselves and control the conversation as much as possible. We are all narcissistic in this way, and we all see conversations as competitions to some extent. We pretend to listen but are really just thinking about what we want to say once we have found an opening or way to interrupt. This is like the mouse that always wants to be on top. Nobody wants to play with him.

Lavish your attention on the other speaker. Support their topics of choice. Question how you can get this person to open up further. What is their underlying interest? Keep asking "why" until you get to what they want to say but aren't saying. "Why" helps you discover their motivations for speaking. It also helps to ask what, where, when, and who. Keep your interrogatives open-ended. They should act like bridges, not dead ends. Ask open-ended questions that cannot be answered with a simple yes or no. Ask, "And what did you say next?" and "Then what happened?" Focus on positive topics and use the word "you" more than "I." Turn "Yeah, but" into "Yes, and." Separate asking for clarification from disagreement and separate debate from criticism.

Without empathic listening and anticipating the motivations of others, talking becomes socialized egoism. So, urge them to elaborate. Active listening involves engagement, empathy, and validation. Refer back to what they said earlier. Reiterate their point but put a spin on it. Use your knowledge to help them flesh out and provide evidence for their ideas and opinions. The more interested you are in them, the more interesting you will be to them. Make people feel like they matter. The more you treat them as mature, intelligent, and well-functioning, the more they will see those qualities in you.

Have you ever had a night out with a friend during which an absorbing conversation left you feeling deeply satisfied? Try to attain this kind of satisfaction for you and the other person during every conversation. Pursue a deep feeling of connection that makes the rest of the world feel less important. Good conversation is the primary form of social engagement for us humans, and the emotional connection it provides is one of the best ways to bond, play, and laugh. It is also a surefire way to activate the vagus nerve and the parasympathetic nervous system. Even simple things like brief face time, short chats, small talk, and meals with others are vital to our health. Maximize your time spent with people who make you feel good after being with them and try to be that person for others.

Practice Dancing as a Form of Play

Dancing is one of the best forms of play. It has been squelched for most of us due to social apprehension, self-inhibition, and contamination from distressed breathing. The following exercise will address this by teaching you to rest while dancing.

Happiness Exercise #25.4: *Uninterrupted, Free-form Dancing*

Put on your favorite type of music to dance to. Don't worry about using a breath metronome, but you might want to place some tape over your lips to ensure nasal breathing. If you don't have natural rhythm, start by sitting down and making a fist. Strike your fist softly on a stable surface to the beat of the music. Try to synchronize as best you can with the rhythm. Next, bob your head in the same way.

Take this synchronization with you as you stand up and start to pound your feet on the floor to the music. Step forward and back, left and right, so that your foot makes contact with the ground at the exact time the beat hits. Bend, sway, whirl, and move your arms in time with your feet. If you don't know what to do with your feet, then look up the "two-step."

Here's the key: Don't stop no matter how awkward it feels. Continue dancing completely uninterrupted for at least one entire song. Then, try to dance through several songs while imagining you are a professional performer or go-go dancer on a stage. Since you are being paid to dance, you cannot stop. By not stopping, you force yourself to close the gaps in your performance. These gaps are where you usually stop dancing because you start to feel self-conscious and you look around at your friends with a sheepish smile while breathing shallowly. Push right through them. Also use startle awareness to ensure that you are not startling while moving.

You brace certain body parts while dancing. These tend to fatigue very quickly. However, if you force yourself to keep moving, you will learn to stop bracing them out of necessity. As you continue to fatigue, you will have no choice but to learn to rest while dancing. You may have to dance continuously for at least 10 minutes to reach this point. In doing this, your dance moves will become less neurotically charged, more fluent, jubilant, and playful.

Let loose. If it helps at all, dance in the dark. Dance as if no one is watching, with no fear of being seen as a quirky goofball. The only reason you might look goofy is that letting loose is unpracticed.

Savor Goosebumps to Strengthen the Response

The full-body tingling that you feel when you get goosebumps comes from a surge in endorphins. It is also known as the aesthetic chill response or frisson. This happens when you feel victorious, encounter something beautiful, hear a moving melody, or even when you find yourself strutting in the face of danger. The goosebumps on your skin come from the bristling of tiny hairs in a reaction called piloerection. It makes furry animals look bigger by forcing their hair to stand on end. This is responsible for the "raised hackles" on a surprised wolf, the plump tail of a cat before a fight, and for the bristling fur on a chimp that is marching around, putting on a dominance display.

There are ways to elicit the response deliberately. You can try listening to your favorite music, singing loudly and unabashedly, pant-hooting, partaking in "ASMR" via online videos, or by using the massage and caressing techniques discussed in Chapter 6. Another way to send a shiver up your spine is to combine the postural exercises from various chapters to walk around in public as if you have an "S" on your chest. Regardless, the best way to strengthen the bristling response is to savor it when it happens to you. Savoring a sensation in this way is often called "sensate focus." Focus on extending the feeling and pass your hand over the gooseflesh to heighten the sensation. Like all positive feelings and emotions, every time you get goosebumps, relish the feeling and prepare yourself to welcome its return.

Concluding Activity #25.3: *Awaken to the Pleasure in Your Body*

Scientists recognize multiple painkilling substances that are produced naturally within the body: endorphins, enkephalins, endocannabinoids, endogenous morphine and others. Each are being released, more or less, all the time. They have powerful analgesic effects blocking the communication of pain signals. If you pay careful attention, you can feel their effects. Too often we look for the pain. Instead, look for the pleasure.

There is bliss to be found in everything you do. Every breath, every heartbeat, every quiver of every muscle holds a small amount of gratification. You can magnify these pleasures just by paying attention to them. Most people know to look for the pleasure after they use alcohol. They ask themselves: "Wait, I just had a drink, I am supposed to feel euphoric, where is that feeling in my body? Oh, there it is." That same feeling is constantly being generated within us all the time, just at a smaller scale. All we need to do is sensitize ourselves to it. I'm still not good at it yet, but I believe we can all build this skill. As often as you can, remain open to, and delight in, the sensations involved in your body's natural production of pleasure.

I wish I had a more reliable method of activating and strengthening the pleasure response because I believe it is very positive. But I can report that the frisson response is much more frequent in my life since I have been using the Program Peace exercises. I believe that the improvements that anti-rigidity has made to my posture played a large role. As your confidence increases, your charisma will start to give you goosebumps.

You Have Everything It Takes to Be Charismatic

I want you to develop charisma in the same way that you developed your dancing abilities in the section above. In other words, practice it under relaxed conditions, hitting all the beats without stopping. Assert your opinions in front of others with conviction and panache, and keep them rolling at a sustainable pace. This will unshackle you from all the bracing patterns that typically bar you from doing it fluidly.

To master charisma, you need to indulge in a little showmanship. You can never be the life of the party until you start trying. Hazard risks with a take-charge demeanor. Be fully present when speaking to people. Give them your full attention, and expect theirs. Don't try too hard to impress people. Instead, focus on impressing yourself. Let your style and positivity make them want to impress you. Think of your social abilities as inexhaustible. Imagine that they replenish infinitely.

When you deliver a line or story and you feel like it fell flat, don't let that get you down. Often, listeners just don't know what to say in response. Don't let their silence take away your momentum. If you keep hitting them with smooth deliveries, they will eventually show some appreciation.

To exhibit charisma, you need to act in a way that makes people think that it would be a good thing if you were in charge. You must show the competence of a leader. You want to come across as strong, decisive, and a person others can rely on for guidance. To do this, create a sense of constructive forward motion. As a leader, boss, or manager, express high performance expectations of the people around you, combined with confidence in their ability to meet those expectations. By having faith in others, you build their confidence in themselves, and in you. You want to send out indicators of alliance so people unconsciously assume that you like them, that you respect their opinion, that you will include them, and that you will back them up when it counts.

Did you know that psychologists generally consider optimism to be the key to charisma?[16] Charisma is a set of nonverbal behaviors giving the impression that you have not only strength but also a positive attitude. It is a special mix of power and warmth that makes charismatic people influential, memorable, persuasive, and inspiring.

Caring for Others Will Make You Happier

Moral integrity is key to happiness. People who have ethical social habits are happier than people who do not. The first reason for this is that people are more likely to value you if they see you as a good person. Psychological research has found that the most important traits to increase your likability are trustworthiness, forthrightness, warmth, and kindness. So, choose your words politely, honor boundaries, compromise, show consideration, admit when you are wrong, honor your word, and show respect.

Get over your issues. Don't be petty or vain. Don't seek attention. Don't be racist or sexist. Never hate anyone. Be a good sport and a good loser. Don't say bad things behind people's backs. Acknowledge other people's contributions, helpful advice, and good decisions. State explicitly what they did to help you and how it helped. Acknowledge people's success, no matter how small, and pay a compliment every time you notice something good. Don't judge people. Be courteous. Ask whether you can lend a hand. Make an effort to be a friend. Remember that you must be a friend to have a friend.

The second reason why moral integrity will make you happier is it stimulates an old part of the brain responsible for tending and befriending. All mammalian brains have a care and nurturance system. This system initiates instinctual behaviors meant to take care of the young. In female rats, stimulation of this area promotes nest building, licking, grooming, arched-back nursing, hovering over pups, and gathering those that stray from the nest. Caring for young is as vital to reproductive success as obtaining food and sex. This is why it has similarly strong connections to the brain's pleasure systems. In other words, instead of using food and sex to make yourself feel better, use nurturance.

When you care for others, you activate this brain system along with the related reward pathways. This is why nurturing others naturally produces endorphins. Helping others has been shown to protect against the harmful effects of life trauma. Volunteering after a natural disaster, protecting others during an attack, caretaking, community service, and becoming a peer counselor have all been shown to reduce stress. It quiets the amygdala and decreases inflammation. It is sometimes called the "helper's high." People who volunteer in any capacity have lower rates of heart disease and stroke, lower mortality risk, less depression, and an increased sense of purpose. Activating the brain's nurturance system also subdues the defeat response because they are inherently incompatible. Be a good, kind person; the best person you can be. Dig up all the good that you want in your life from within your own heart.

Practice Being Pure of Heart

Being pure of heart has a reciprocal relationship with being free of nasty thoughts. Seeing yourself as wholesome and virtuous is the quickest route to becoming free from negative rumination. Repeatedly ask yourself whether your actions are noble and pure. Holding yourself to high standards sounds like an adult burden but will make you a kid at heart.

Goku from the original *Dragon Ball* comic and TV show is a small, naïve child who doesn't have a bad bone in his body. He has a trusty cloud (Flying Nimbus) that he rides like a magic carpet. Only people who are pure of heart can ride the cloud. Billy Batson is another small boy, this time from the world of DC comics, whose purity allows him to take on the mantle of the superhero Shazam. Thor from the Marvel universe has worthiness that enables him to lift Mjolnir, his enchanted hammer. I have asked myself on many occasions, "Would I be able to ride that cloud, don that cape, or lift that hammer?" Would you?

Let us practice indiscriminate and promiscuous kindness. Let us do this not to be rewarded but because it is the right thing. I like the saying that tells us, "Love the one that you are with." I take this injunction further to mean that you should love whoever you find yourself with at any moment. Love thy neighbor. Love thine enemy. Use "agape," which is the Greco-Christian term for selfless, unbiased, non-possessive, universal love. Or, experiment with using the "unconditional positive regard" that many psychotherapists use with their clients.[17] When your primary aim is to broadcast goodwill, you act much less defensive and your composure quotient will soar. Thus, a pure, lighthearted mentality not only gives you access to the moral high ground but will also affect many minutiae of your body language and microexpressions, improving your overall aura. This is the bravery of the innocent.

The key to being popular is to like more people. Research has shown that likable people like others. On average, the most-liked people like larger numbers of people and they like those people more.[18] So, forgive those you feel have wronged you. Forgive your parents, siblings, all your family and friends. Then, forgive everyone else from your past and present, and even your future. Forgive people from every walk of life. Forgive the rich, the poor, all sides of the political spectrum. Forgive humanity, then fate, and then the entire universe. Have no fear of rejection from others, have no need to be accepted. Be able to say "I love you" with no regret. Cherish yourself and your body the way it is and know that you, along with everyone else, are absolutely worthy of being loved.

Human kindness is the surest step toward deep healing from any kind of trauma. Expect only good from others and project this expectation in the form of positive overtures. People won't be able to help but respond to you in positive ways, and their responses will reinforce your view of the world as a pleasant place, further entrenching your expectations. If you work hard at becoming pure of heart, you will earn your way to peace. Combined with altruistic acts, you'll find pleasure. And, combined with assertiveness and composure, you will find power.

I used to have a stinging pain in my chest that would surface during stress. It was healed after I made a deliberate effort to be pure of heart. The notion that I had pure intentions reassured some last bastion of muscles in my thorax that they could stop their defensive bracing. I could feel these muscles release. And, because they could finally relax, I was able to bring them to a full contraction using exercises such as the coughing, laughing, pant-hoot, and diaphragmatic stretching exercises. Being pure of heart is the most foolproof way to ensure that you are breathing easily, and I consider it the eighth and final tenet of optimal breathing.

Conclusion

Most people have a secret fear of being bad or having done things for which they can never atone. But it is never too late to start being pure of heart. You can do it at any point in time. Start now. As you take on the Program Peace system, I recommend that you imagine yourself turning over a new leaf. Decide to let go of the regret, shame, and guilt you have carried with you from past misdeeds and mistakes. Turn any ounce of self-hatred that you may harbor into self-forgiveness. Guilt keeps us from becoming good people, so use your participation here as an excuse to get rid of it. Purify your heart by allowing yourself to make it a clean slate.

Trauma has made it difficult to be cool, playful, humorous, and pure of heart. By removing the trauma, you will make these things much easier. See yourself as going from afflicted to blessed. See yourself as principled, incorruptible, and salt of the earth. When you think "pure of heart" think dominant but non-dominating. Think non-subordinate but non-aggressive. Think assertive but lighthearted. Having faith in your goodness is the key to making optimism and relaxation possible. Know that what you're doing comes from a good place with other people's best interests in mind. As long as you know that you mean right by others, you don't have to worry about offending them with your composure. Expect yourself to be pure of heart in everything you do and conceive of your life from here on to be a hero's journey.

Chapter 25: **Bullet Points**

- Treat everyone as if they are the least awkward person you have ever met.
- There are so many ways to be endearing. There's no need to forfeit your composure or health to do so.
- Creating a "pure of heart" mindset will make many of your troubles disappear.
- When mammals are playful, they are truly wonderful creatures.
- You can directly reduce stress by stimulating the play and nurturance areas of your brain. To do this, you must be playful with and nurture others.
- The "feel good" neurochemicals like endorphins, serotonin, oxytocin, and vasopressin derive from kind behavior. Nature endorses morality.
- Remember that real virtue does not complement itself and is not even aware of itself as a virtue.
- Laughing exercises will give you a bold laugh and fortify your innards.
- Every laugh should almost sound antagonistic, as if you were laughing at someone, but only because it is assertive and unaffected by submissive tendencies.
- A night full of fake laughing and smiling will increase the tension you feel the next morning. And yet, one minute of genuine, unadulterated laughing can relieve all that strain.
- Self-stimulating happiness is key to perpetuating your upward developmental spiral.
- Self-amusement is very healthy and a trait of dominant people.
- Feel free to be silly.
- Act like every day is your birthday and every night is Saturday night.
- When you are mistreated, think of it as an opportunity for personal growth. Consciously deciding to under-react to negativity is regarded by many to be the most powerful way to achieve spiritual growth.

Chapter 25: **Endnotes**

1.   Hermann, H. R. (2017). *Dominance and aggression in humans and other animals: The great game of life*. Academic Press.

2.   Snyder, C. R. & Lopez, S. J. (2009). *Oxford handbook of positive psychology* (2nd ed.). Oxford University Press.

3.   Taylor, S. E, & Armor, D. A. (1996). Positive illusions and coping with adversity. *Journal of Personality, 64*(4), 873–898; Carver, C. S., Scheier, M. E., & Segerstrom, S. C. (2010). *Optimism. Clinical Psychology Review, 30*(7), 879–889.

4.   Scheier, M. E., Weintraub, J. K., & Carver, C. S. (1986). Coping with stress: Divergent strategies of optimism and pessimists. *Journal of Personality and Social Psychology, 51*(6), 1257–1264.

5.   Frederickson, B. L., & Levenson, R. (1998). Positive emotions speed recovery from the cardiovascular sequelae of negative emotions. *Cognition & Emotion, 12*(2), 191–220.

6.   Wohr, M., & Schwarting, R. K. W. (2007). Ultrasonic communication in rats: Can playback of 50-kHz calls induce approach behavior? *PLoS ONE, 2*(12), e1365.

7.   Simonet, P., Versteeg, D. & Storie, D. (2005, July 31-August 5). *Dog-laughter: Recorded playback reduces stress related behavior in shelter dogs* [Paper presentation]. Proceedings of the 7th International Conference on Environmental Enrichment.

8.   Panksepp, J. (December 2000). The riddle of laughter neural and psychoevolutionary underpinnings of joy. *Current Directions in Psychological Science, 9*(6), 183–186.

9.   Provine, R. R. (2000). *Laughter: A scientific exploration*. Viking.

10. Folkman, S., & Nathan, P. E. (2010), *The Oxford handbook of stress, health, and coping*. Oxford University Press.

11. Godfrey, J. R. (2004). Toward optimal health: The experts discuss therapeutic humor. *Journal of Women's Health, 13*(5), 474–479.

12. Dunbar, R. I. M. (2017). Group size, vocal grooming and the origins of language. *Psychonomic Bulletin & Review, 24*, 209–212.

13. Dunbar, R. I. M., Baron, R., Frangou, A., Eiluned, P., van Leeuwen, E. J. C., Stow, J., Partridge, G., MacDonald, I., Barra, V., & van Vugt, M. (2012). Social laughter is correlated with an elevated pain threshold. *Proceedings of the Royal Society B. Biological Sciences, 279*(1731), 1161–1167.

14. Dunbar, R. I. M. (2017). Group size, vocal grooming and the origins of language.

15. Wohr, M., Kehl, M., Borta, A., Schanzer, A., Schwarting, R. K., & Hoglinger, G. U. (2009). New insights into the relationship of neurogenesis and affect: Tickling induces hippocampal cell proliferation in rats emitting appetitive 50-kHz ultrasonic vocalizations. *Neuroscience, 163*(4), 1024–1030.

16. Van Edwards, V. (2017). *Captivate: The science of succeeding with people.* Penguin Random House.

17. Rogers, C. (1980). *A way of being.* Houghton Mifflin.

18. Sanders, T. (2005). *The likability factor.* Crown.

Chapter 26: **Conclusions**

"Most men pursue pleasure with such breathless haste that they hurry past it." — Soren Kierkegaard (1813-1855)

"Spite and ill-nature are among the most expensive luxuries in life." — Dr. Samuel Johnson (1709-1784)

The Exercises and Activities

The results you will gain from this program come in many forms and interact synergistically. They don't merely complement one another in an additive way but in a multiplicative one. For example, the benefits derived from paced breathing, diaphragmatic jogging, passive exhalation, and stretching the diaphragm supplement each other. As you get better at one, you get better at the others. Because these skills are all interrelated, they promote and reinforce each other. This leads to recursive improvement in which the skills form structural platforms, elevating you into an upward spiral.

I hope you now feel that you have a tool kit of actionable exercises and access to deep wells of strength that had previously laid untapped. You may not be sold on all the exercises here. Choose the ones you like the most and practice those for now. As you monitor your progress, you may realize you have largely rehabilitated certain body parts. This may motivate you to go back to other exercises that didn't seem as appealing at first. In this book, I wrote about what I found helpful to pair with paced breathing. What benefitted me is not necessarily what will best benefit you, so I encourage you to experiment with your own forms of diaphragmatic generalization. If you come up with a new technique, please share it on the web with our online community.

Do keep in mind that a few days of changed perspective might feel like enough to gain the full benefits of Program Peace. However, it may not be sufficient to override your ingrained routines permanently. This system is all about rehearsal. Sustained weekly practice is key. Be persistent, and your efforts will pay off. Some of these activities may feel onerous at first, but they will quickly become comfortable after you have completed them a few times. Most of the exercises in this book are at least partially routinized after the first five sessions. This means they can be done with minimal concentration from that point on (i.e., while on the phone or in front of the TV).

It was incredibly heartening to know that these exercises were slowly making me a stronger, happier person. I knew that I was making daily progress and that something of value was germinating within me. Anticipate positive results with pleasure and excitement. When this happens, the exercises become intrinsically rewarding. As you watch yourself change, you will realize that all these attributes you assumed were genetic and fixed at birth are trainable.

By the end of this book, the first table from Chapter 1 should take on an entirely new meaning. Employ as many of the dominant displays from that table as you can in the exercise below.

Concluding Exercise #26.1: *Diaphragmatic Phone Conversation*

Perform paced breathing with a breath metronome while on the phone with a friend. Breathe nasally guided by a metronome when the other person is speaking. When you are talking, take complete inhales without gasping and then speak over a complete exhalation. Try it in front of a mirror and look yourself in the eye calmly as if you were looking at your caller. Next, use a hands-free attachment for your phone and walk around your house, back yard, or neighborhood while using as many of the elements of optimal body language described in this book as you can.

Stress and Overexertion

As this book has contended, operating without composure can gravely deplete our health. When we live in distress, we are borrowing health from our future. It is the toll exacted on a methamphetamine addict or a president during an eight-year term. We are talking about a constant state of overexertion in which the body takes a lot of abuse at the expense of your charisma, physique, intelligence, mental health, and spiritual growth.

Distress is an appropriate strategy for an animal with strong evidence that it may die in a few seconds. It is a terrible strategy for you and me. We have discussed how your fight or flight response is seldom directed toward actual fighting or taking flight. Instead, it is directed to bracing, strain, paradoxical breathing, hyperventilation, apneic disturbances, rapid heartbeat, pain, egoism, and submission. To prove to your body that you are not at risk of premature death, you have to divert your focus away from the bad toward gratitude, playfulness, purity, and optimism.

The retraction of the gill by the sea slugs discussed in Chapter 2 shows that they don't have faith in their world. The slugs exhibiting this defensive reflex in response to being uncontrollably prodded and shocked in the lab are "on high alert." Their defensive and escape responses are exaggerated, and their responses to positive events are blunted. The slugs that have not been subjected to this don't show the same defensiveness and are referred to by scientists as "naïve."

Just because you are not on high alert doesn't mean you are naïve. Be the sea slug that has seen it all and yet, still knows that the best way to live is never to brace its gills. Don't treat every threat as novel. Generalize your desensitization to negativity toward every conceivable peril. Do it now. Drop your façade, let your gills hang, keep drawing long, deep inhalations, and learn to expect the best from the world.

Your Transformation

Before Program Peace, I was uncomfortable with my own presence. I exuded tentativeness and a lack of any conviction. I would wring my hands constantly. My dreams were always desperate situations. Once a week, I would wake from sleep yelling in terror. Between the ages of 25 and 30, I would find myself whispering the words "Oh my god" over and over, every day. "That was a nightmare" was my mantra. I had unbearable tension welling up inside of me, gushing out in the form of tortured body language. I hated my home, everything in my room, everything on my desk, all things, and all people because I experienced them through the throes of distressed breathing.

When I turned 20, I discovered that everything hurt a little bit. It hurt to stand up, it hurt to run, it hurt to sit for too long, it hurt to turn my neck, it hurt to use the restroom, it hurt to swallow, and every social interaction hurt. I concluded that this was an irreversible effect of aging. But now I am twice that age, and none of those things hurt. After two years of Program Peace, you should find that you feel much younger than when you started. You will experience a personal metamorphosis internally and externally. You will have acquaintances ask what kind of antianxiety or antidepressant drugs you have been prescribed. Others will ask which cosmetic procedures you have undergone.

Now that I breathe diaphragmatically and send very few subordination displays, the core of my personhood has changed. I used to take dangerous risks that bordered on having a death wish. I never do that today. I am less impulsive, less compulsive, and less codependent. The "imp of the perverse" no longer haunts me, and I no longer play the part of a scapegoat, jester, martyr, or victim. I am no longer consumed with melancholy and self-pity. I am no longer a defeatist or misanthrope. These were recurring themes in my life since childhood. Now, they are distant memories.

All my favorite fictional works involve going on an epic adventure, encountering bad guys, converting them into allies, and then recruiting them to the team. The antagonists in this story are really good guys waiting to be reformed. The thoracic breathing muscles, the sneering muscles, the muscles involved in headaches, and those that make us sick to our stomach are all potential allies. Once converted, your chakra-like modules will become trusted comrades. You will find yourself using them to transform other people into comrades as well.

Breath Mastery

Breathing slowly and deeply with the diaphragm is difficult at first because your respiratory musculature and the nerves that control it have developed their own default pace. You must overcome this default. It is a bit like standing chest-deep in the ocean, trying to keep your balance amid turbulent, unpredictable waves. As you reprogram your breathing, accept the occasional unexpected breaker. Embrace the uneven gushes, the chaotic swells, and the startling surges knowing that, with time, you will control the tides. Permanently. This final exercise will engage your diaphragm using anti-laxity to help accomplish just that.

Concluding Exercise #26.2: Slow Inhale from a Deep Squat

Rest in a deep squat where your butt is nearly touching your ankles. Lean your torso forward and downward so that your chest is touching your knees. You might place your knees in your armpits. This position will push your diaphragm up against the internal organs of your abdomen making it much more difficult to inhale fully. Take 5 prolonged inhalations that each last between 10 and 30 seconds. Feel free to rest and catch your breath between these inhalations. You might use a stopwatch or your paced breathing app to ensure that these breaths are long. This can be made more challenging if done after a meal.

As you are inhaling and your diaphragm descends, it will be exposed to a much heavier load than usual. It may feel shaky or tremble. Use the anti-laxity protocol from Chapter 13 to engage the diaphragm firmly as it expands. Doing this slowly and smoothly using the "belly breath" technique from Chapter 3 will build strength and stability in the diaphragm and enhance your control of it.

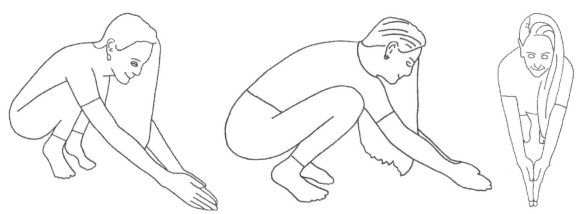

Illustration 26.1: Inhaling slowly from a deep squat can challenge and strengthen the diaphragm.

Whether squatting, lying, sitting, or standing, taking a deep diaphragmatic inhalation for more than 10 seconds is a long trek across a barren desert. After the first five seconds, you realize that you're not going to make it to the other side unless you let go of excess baggage. The baggage consists of those burdensome bracing patterns you are incapable of setting down until you are engrossed in respiration. Try it now. Take a 10-second inhalation. Halfway through, you will feel strain throughout your body begin to drop away. When breathing at long intervals, you don't have the craze and furor to haul this luggage around with you. Every time you cross this desert by taking a prolonged inhalation, you further program your chakra-like modules to let go of their unnecessary burdens.

Allow me a final analogy. You may be familiar with the Greek mythological figure of Sisyphus, a man condemned to rolling a boulder up a hill. As soon as he gets the boulder to the top, it rolls back down, and he must start over—for all eternity. It is a sad story and is considered a tragedy. Now, imagine that Sisyphus didn't let the boulder roll down the hill. Imagine that he unnecessarily lowered it down using his hands, step by step, at great effort. If this were the case, then the poor guy would *never* have a chance to rest. Right?

"One must imagine Sisyphus happy." — Albert Camus (1913-1960)

Relating this back to the body, merely being an animal is hard work. We must labor every day just to provide our bodies with what they require. When stress causes our muscles to remain tense, even when they should be resting, this work becomes Sisyphean. The same goes for breathing. The inhale takes work. Your exhale is your diaphragm's only chance to relax, so if you keep it braced during those few seconds of outflow, you are completely depriving it of rest. In Exercise 5.1, you practiced allowing your diaphragm to go completely limp during the exhalation, thus giving it the brief respite it needs to stop contracting so that it can regenerate properly. Whenever you notice that your muscles are not passive during rest, imagine letting go of Sisyphus' boulder and letting it roll down the hill on its own.

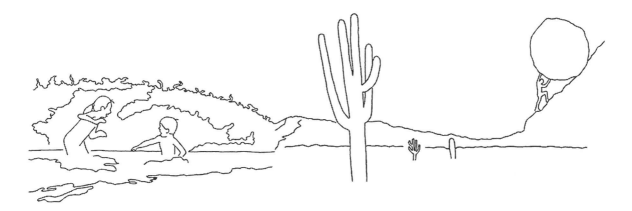

Illustration 26.2: Concluding analogies.

This book has laid out eight tenets of peaceful breathing. I think of them as an eightfold path to optimal respiration. Here they are:

The Eight Tenets of Peaceful Breathing:

1) Breathe deeply (high volume): Breathe more fully, breathing most of the way in and out in a way that pushes the belly forward during each inhalation.
2) Breathe longer (low frequency): Breathe at longer intervals in which each inhalation and exhalation lasts for more time.

3) Breathe smoothly (continuous flow): Breathe at a steady, slow, constant rate.
4) Breathe assertively (confident): Do not let social concerns or stressors conflict with the other rules.
5) Exhale passively: Allow your breathing muscles to go limp during each exhalation.
6) Breathe nasally: Breathe through the nose with nostrils flared.
7) Ocean's Breath: Relax the back of your throat and breathe as if you are fogging up a glass.
8) Breathe with purity of heart: Knowing that you have only the best intentions, and that you exemplify the combination of nonsubmissive and nondominating, will infuse your breathing with peace.

I used to imagine how mind-bogglingly complex it would be to use brain surgery to reduce someone's propensity for negative thinking. For instance, you cannot just cut out the amygdala because this produces all kinds of unwanted side effects. Instead, it would involve complex submicroscopic manipulations of billions of neurons and trillions of synapses. Where would you start? Diaphragmatic breathing retraining does precisely this but requires no neuroscientific knowledge, no futuristic technology, and no invasive techniques. By placing you in a state of calm from which you can reconceptualize your life, paced breathing will make precise, peace-producing alterations to your cerebral cortex, amygdala, hypothalamus, brainstem, heart, diaphragm, gut, adrenal glands, and other organ systems all over the body. The figure below depicts the curative effects as a virtuous cycle to be contrasted with Figure 5.2.

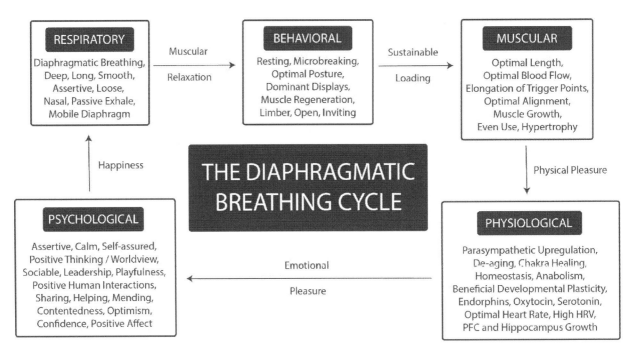

Figure 26.1: Diaphragmatic breathing creates a virtuous cycle.

A Gene's Eye View

The scientific evidence suggests that we are here on Earth because a complex molecule got stuck in a rut of self-replication. Our situation as survival machines for DNA can be given a negative or positive valence. Our pain and the pain we inflict on each other can make this situation a curse. It is too often a frenzied free-for-all where, as Tennyson said, nature is "red in tooth and claw." But if we are actively engaged in improving the quality of our life and other sentient beings' lives, then we transform the condition from a curse to a blessing. I believe making this transformation gives life meaning. Your every action, display, and word may have reverberating repercussions on reality that will continue to echo in the physical universe forever. Instead of contributing to pain through abusive communication, contribute to peace and love.

The nerves that course trauma through our bodies are the reigns by which our selfish genes control us. From our genes' perspective, happiness and confidence are risky and might get us killed. They are only to be expressed in utopian environments. Our cells operate on the assumption that aggression and submission keep us on the straight and narrow; that living without them is problematic, applicable only when our environment is sending us reliable cues that it is unrealistically hospitable. We must overcome the genetically hardwired negativity bias and fear of relaxation. To do this, we can use diaphragmatic breathing to trick our organs and cells into thinking that our world is an unparalleled paradise. This will give you the elbow room you need to coddle your inner pet, encourage your inner child, and admire your inner caveperson. If we can do this, we all, no matter our age or the extent of our trauma, have the developmental plasticity to become genuinely happy.

Turn Off the Behavioral Inhibition System

Jeffrey Alan Gray proposed the "biopsychological theory of personality" in 1970, and it remains a widely accepted model. The theory hypothesized two systems: a) the behavioral inhibition system, which stops us from doing things out of fear, and b) the behavioral activation system, which causes us to do things out of positive motivation for reward. He proposed that these two systems are constantly interacting and that people vary in the extent to which these systems influence their behavior.

People who have an overactive behavioral inhibition system spend their life repressing their impulses and restraining their desires. They are sensitive to punishment and perceive it as highly aversive.[1] A predisposition toward behavioral inhibition starts in infancy. Toddlers who are behaviorally inhibited have higher heart rates, higher stress hormone levels, tighter vocal cords, and highly reactive amygdalae.[2] I would assume that they are also predisposed to distressed breathing.

The behavioral inhibition system has been proposed to be the causal basis of anxiety and depression. It is what keeps us from dancing, laughing, and improvising and pulls us to retreat into our shells.[3] The behavioral activation system is the opposite. It promotes approach behavior: cheerfulness, spontaneity, and sociability. As you might have guessed, the exercises in this book aim to activate the behavioral activation system. The following table offers further detail.

	Behavioral Inhibition System	Behavioral Activation System
Emotion	Fear of pain	Excitement for pleasure
Motivation	Avoid punishments	Approach rewards
Arousal	Sympathetic	Neutral / Parasympathetic
Personality	Introverted / Reserved	Extraverted / Outgoing
Personality Disorder	Anxious / Depressed	Impulsive / Exploitative
Hierarchical Station	Submissive	Dominant
Affect	Negative	Positive
Outlook	Cynical	Hopeful

Table 26.1: Comparing the Behavioral Inhibition and Activation Systems

You will find that the consequences of these two systems reach into every facet of your life. For instance, as I shot a basketball in my twenties, I would retract from the ball in a cringing motion. This was the behavioral inhibition system in action. Today, my hand follows through and remains briefly in the air at full arm extension. Disinhibiting your follow-through is integral to your ability to score. Be an exhibitionist and treat everything like a game you are playing to win.

We need to be accepting of the fact that we will continue to suffer social failures. We will displease some and not be liked by others. But, if we let our fear of these things lead to inhibition, social defeat will be inevitable. Never choose to withdraw when confronted by a stressor. Always approach. When you find yourself upset, don't pull away. Push back playfully. You deserve to be loved and respected while being your true, unfiltered self.

See the roadmap for your life as a long series of green lights and ease off the breaks. At every fork in the road, ask yourself: "How would an undamaged, badass version of me deal with this situation?" Start visualizing this person when you think about yourself. When you imagine doing something, picture this person doing it. In time, you will become that person.

Within a pack of mammals, status roles are often initially determined by an animal's intrinsic energy level. The boisterous youngsters become the pack leaders. These are usually animals that have very low activation of the behavioral inhibition system. The animals that expend more energy in play, foraging, and socializing rise to leadership positions. How can you get your energy levels up? This book has detailed how: how to remove knots, how to reverse frailty, and how not to leak energy.

Dominant people proactively pursue their interests without being hindered by unproductive social fears. They have faith in their ability to succeed and trust that others can't stop them. They are not embarrassed easily. Neither do they second-guess themselves or worry about what others will think. Don't stifle the pleasure principle and hide your desires just to get along with others. Like a rambunctious wolf cub, learn to be okay with the social conflict that arises when you try to gratify your wants.

Don't be a zoo animal released into a wildlife park that still crouches within the invisible confines of its old cage. Having put yourself on a short leash, you are the only one who can take it off. To beat the behavioral inhibition system, you must be spontaneous and do the first thing that comes to mind more often. Don't be afraid to let your inner animal free. Be resolute in your opinions. Charm people with pizzazz. Make bold and audacious announcements about positive things. Show some backbone, sing with your heart, and live with guts and gusto.

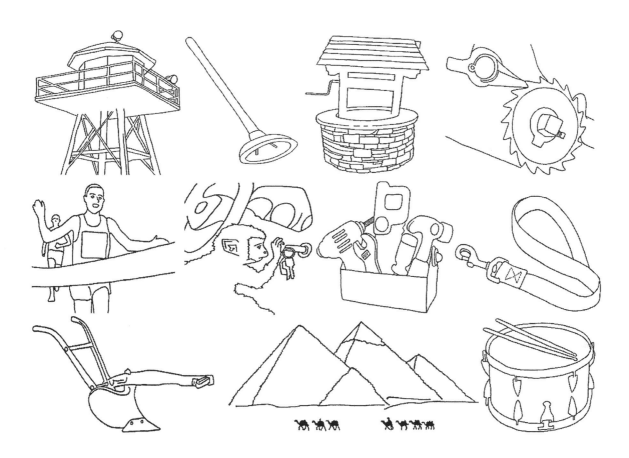

Illustration 26.3: Analogies used in this text.

Being Pure of Heart Will Free You from Retaliation Apprehension

Let me leave you with a description of one final concept from psychology: retaliation apprehension. This is when we feel worried that someone will take what we are saying or doing in the wrong way and get offended. Retaliation apprehension shows in your face, breathing, and body language. It is difficult to describe verbally, but people recognize it immediately when they see it.

My brother has extraordinarily little retaliation apprehension. This is why he can make a personal joke about someone, and they never get mad. Often, it seems that he can say whatever he wants to anyone at any time and get away with it. If I were to say the same thing in the same tone, people would be miffed. My brother can do this because he shows zero concern about the other person retaliating. This allows him to poke fun at people and things in a playful way without offending.

Retaliation apprehension is not just an admission of remorse for known wrongdoing. It is a state of mind we have even when we have done nothing wrong. A tendency toward retaliation apprehension can start very early in life. Many adults have "anxious attachment" issues that stem from their early relationship with their parents. The child with anxious attachment is preoccupied with what pleases and displeases their caretaker. They see their relationship with their mother and father as fragile and they feel at risk for rejection and abandonment. This leads to fear of, and obsession with, the emotions of others.

Refrain from scanning others for a hint of displeasure with you. It is submissive. The best way to do this is to not think about it. Drop any worries about defending yourself. Expecting the other person to like you and not being offended should be presumptive and implicit in your demeanor. Regularly dropping your defenses in this way should lower your cortisol, blood pressure, and heart rate while raising your feel-good neurotransmitters and HRV. It should also make it easier to breathe with the diaphragm.

Acting with zero retaliation apprehension is one of the most dominant things you can do. Still, it must be authentic. To do it properly, you must have good intentions. This is where being pure of heart (discussed in the last chapter) comes in. When you feel completely secure in the fact that your actions are well intentioned and that you are a force for good, fear of retaliation won't even cross your mind. It will make social harmony a default that you don't have to work or strive for. When using the "pure of heart" mindset your retaliation apprehension can be nil even when your behavioral activation system is running at full force.

Conclusion: How to Play the Dominance Game

Humans have a strong instinctual predilection for submissive behavior. When submissive body language goes on for too long, it makes us vulnerable to various forms of muscular tension, which in turn make us vulnerable to disease. This biological propensity should be studied through both basic and applied research and fully addressed by medical science. There should also be explicit social contracts that limit the extent of submissiveness we "require" from one another in both personal and professional sectors. The more awareness you and I can create, the sooner this will happen.

Hopefully, this book has made it clear that the abysmal repercussions of submission and aggression hamper human potential. If we can minimize our tendencies toward destructive status striving and the social tensions that eat us up inside, we can increase our productiveness. If we can help others do this, we can increase humankind's productivity and problem-solving potential.

If someone has better posture than we do, we should still stand tall. If someone has a more powerful voice, we should continue to speak powerfully. If someone has a bigger smile, we should keep smiling wholeheartedly. Comparing ourselves to others, like arming ourselves against others, is for animals in "submissive mode." Put your sword (anger) and shield (rejection sensitivity) down. Let your burdensome armor (retaliation apprehension) drop to the floor. Recognize that the combination of being non-aggressive and non-submissive has made you not only invulnerable but incomparable.

If you are going to play the dominance game, play it with a competitive spirit, play it fairly, play it without malice and without exposing yourself to trauma. Play it breathing diaphragmatically all the while. Don't flaunt your position or be embarrassed by it. Don't puff up when things go your way, and don't shrivel up when they don't. Think of yourself as dominant without having to dominate. Keep in mind that no one really wins in the end, so there is no reason to keep score. Instead, see competition as "iron sharpening iron." See it as productive play that makes every participant stronger. Turn contests into friendly cooperative games in which everyone is a teammate whether they know it or not. This will not only earn you friends, but it will also make you imperturbable, indomitable, and self-possessed.

Chapter 26: **Endnotes**

1.   Braem, S., Duthoo, W., & Notebaert, W. (2013). Punishment sensitivity predicts the impact of punishment on cognitive control. *PLoS ONE*, *8*(9), e74106.

2.   Moehler, E., Kagan, J., Oelkers-Ax, R., Brunner, R., Poustka, L., Haffner, J., & Resch, F. (2008). Infant predictors of behavioral inhibition. *British Journal of Development Psychology*, *26*(1), 145–150.

3.   Gray, J. A. (1970). The psychophysiological basis of introversion-extraversion. *Behavioral Research and Therapy*, *8*(3), 249–266.

Program Peace: *Paced Breathing App for iPhone and Android*

Download the free Program Peace app as a companion to this book. Using the app will train you to breathe deeper and longer. It also provides an easy-to-use interface without bloat, clutter, ads, sign-ins, in-app purchases, or full version upgrades.

Place the app next to a book, computer monitor, tablet, or TV so that you can pace your breathing while you attend to other things. Listen to music or audiobooks while using the app. Place it in your pocket and select vibrate if you want to use it in silence, hands-free. Select how long you want your inhales and exhales to be. Peruse the preset breathing rates to learn about various breathing methods. Practice the Program Peace exercises to build confidence, a positive mindset, and rehabilitate systems throughout your body.

Scientific studies have shown that paced breathing lowers blood pressure, heart rate, muscle tension and calms the mind. Research has also shown that breathing at longer intervals can improve mood, focus, and flexibility, increase athletic performance, reduce recovery time, mitigate fatigue, and help people get to sleep at night. This app is designed to help you take full advantage of those benefits.

For more information, you can visit www.programpeace.com.

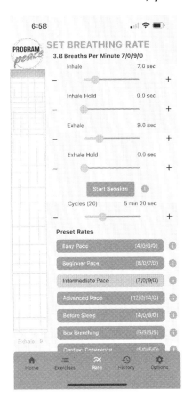
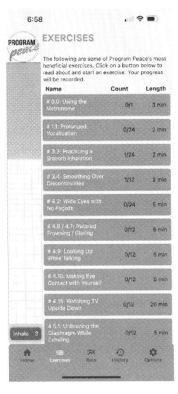

FEATURES:

* Customizable breathing bar
* Choose your breathing intervals
* Over a dozen preset rates
* Optional breath holds
* Current and longest streaks
* Track your history and progress
* Multiple sound effects
* Rank system
* Multiple color themes
* Custom reminders
* Recommended exercises
* Vibrate function
* Multiple audible cues
* Dark mode
* Color palette options
* Original informative content

Program Peace: *Fitness Manual & Journal*

Download this free journal to keep track of your Program Peace exercise sessions and progress. It also includes a 90-day program that teaches you the fundamentals of exercise, nutrition, and fitness according to current scientific research. Whether your goal is weight loss, muscle gain, flexibility, cardiovascular health, or just logging your exercises, this fitness planner can help.

Track numerous fitness metrics and establish monthly goals. Make records about your exercise, diet, sleep, stretching, meditation, strength training goals, daily steps, heart rate variability, and other important data. By completing the worksheets and following the recommendations, in just 90 days, you can build new, long-lasting habits. Buy the paperback on Amazon or download the free PDF at www.programpeace.com.

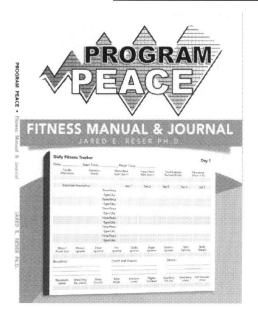

FEATURES:

* Customizable, undated worksheets to log your favorite exercises, sets, and reps.
* Keep notes about duration, intensity, and impressions to keep track of your progress.
* Space to record nutritional intake, body weight, self-massage, blood pressure, flexibility, balance, cardio, heart rate, skin fold measures, body circumference, BMI, TDEE, RMR, and workout goals.
* Record hours of nightly sleep, breathing exercises, flights climbed, hours standing, and much more.
* Read detailed fitness and diet recommendations to help you understand your body and achieve results that last.

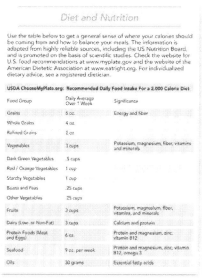

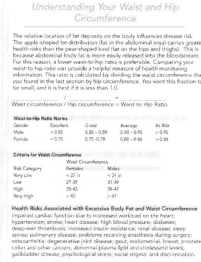

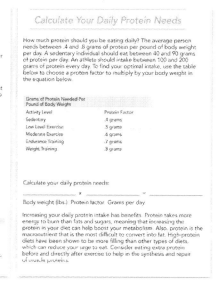

Anti-Rigidity: *How to Release Muscle from Partial Contraction*

Anti-rigidity is a rehabilitative method for releasing muscles from excessive tension and partial contraction. Because it was used throughout the book it is outlined here.

Optional Preparation	Anti-Rigidity	Afterwards
Increase blood flow using: • Stretching • Cardio • Weightlifting • Heat • Massage	Assume stiff, rarely used positions and postures Firmly contract the muscles involved until they fatigue Explore configurations that crack Use diaphragmatic breathing Search for and contract into aching or soreness until it fades	Help the muscles rest using: • Repeated contraction • Full relaxation • Heat or cold • Massage • Vibration

Muscle in Partial Contraction	Muscle in Full Contraction	Muscle at Resting Length
Before Anti-Rigidity	During Anti-Rigidity	After Anti-Rigidity

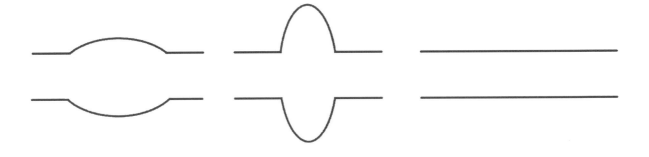

Program Peace: *Tools and Ways of Being*

Personal Care	Paced Breathing, Prioritize Composure, Exercise, Hydrate, Sleep Eight Hours, Walk, Take Time for Yourself, Live in the Present, Awareness of Startling / Flinching / Trembling, Fasting, Interoception, Using a Stethoscope, Optimism
Social	Optimal Body Language, Nonsubmissive, Nondominating, Nondefensive, Grooming / Caressing / Massaging Others, No Unnecessary Competition, Camaraderie, Steady Eye Contact, Annunciating Clearly, Playfulness, Laughing, Smiling, Connectedness / Bonding, Nurturance, Healthy Sex, Free and Open Body Language, Taking Up Space, Humble, Indomitable, Forgiving, Affectionate, Breaking Up Fights, Sharing, Helping, Mending, Loving
Breathing	Paced Breathing, Long / Deep / Smooth / Assertive Breaths, Passive Exhale, Belly Breathing, Rehab the Diaphragmatic Speedbump / Dormancy / Apneic Disturbances, Nasal Breathing, Taping the Mouth, Diaphragmatic Vocalization, Reading Out Loud, Throat Limp, Voice Deep and Relaxed, Pant-Hoot, Ocean's Breath, Diaphragm Stretch, Breath Holding Exercises
Muscles	Anti-rigidity, Anti-laxity, Microbreaks, Postural Awareness, Massage / Compression / Percussion / Vibration, Delocalized Pressure, Bidirectional Control, Progressive Relaxation, Body Scan, Stretching, Yoga, Firm Contractions, Full Range of Motion, Decompression, Stretchlying, Glidewalking, Counterposes, Postural Variety
Mindset	Egalitarian Worldview, Nonjudgmental / Nonresistant / Nonattached, Empathy and Compassion, Desensitization, Control, Rising to Meet Adversity, Eustress & the Challenge Response, Coolness, Pureness of Heart, Watching the Thinker, Mindfulness, Gratitude, Fearlessness, Fun-loving, Composed Kindness, Emotional Maturity, Dominance, Imperturbable, Self-possessed
Avoid	Retaliation Apprehension, Rejection Sensitivity, Timidity, Domineering, Gasping, Breath Holding, Lack of Rest, Lack of Sleep, Overeating, Overly Sweet / Salty / Fatty Foods, Lying / Gossiping, Vanity, Taking Offense, Addictive Behaviors, Violent Media, Horror, Unnecessarily Loud Music, Drugs & Alcohol, Inhibition / Withdrawal / Avoidance
Postural	Neck Retracted, Shoulders Back and Down, Abs Contracted / Chest Spread, Glutes Contracted, Feet Parallel, Urine Retention and Expulsion, Eyes Wide, Eyes Fixated, Eyes Up, Head Pointing Up, Ability to Glare and Frown, Eyes Unblinking, Relaxed Eyebrows, Expressionless, Mewing, Sneer Awareness, Smiling

Made in United States
Orlando, FL
04 October 2024

52356406R00300